Colitis and Crohn's: Understanding and Managing Inflammatory Bowel Disease

Colitis and Crohn's: Understanding and Managing Inflammatory Bowel Disease

Edited by Ella Young

hayle
medical

New York

Hayle Medical,
750 Third Avenue, 9th Floor,
New York, NY 10017, USA

Visit us on the World Wide Web at:
www.haylemedical.com

ISBN: 978-1-63241-911-8

Cataloging-in-Publication Data

Colitis and crohn's : understanding and managing inflammatory bowel disease / edited by Ella Young.
    p. cm.
Includes bibliographical references and index.
ISBN 978-1-63241-911-8
1. Colitis. 2. Crohn's disease. 3. Inflammatory bowel diseases. 4. Inflammatory bowel diseases--Diagnosis.
5. Inflammatory bowel diseases--Treatment. I. Young, Ella.
RC862.C6 C65 2020
616.344 7--dc23

Table of Contents

Permissions

List of Contributors

Index

Preface

Every book is a source of knowledge and this one is no exception. The idea that led to the conceptualization of this book was the fact that the world is advancing rapidly; which makes it crucial to document the progress in every field. I am aware that a lot of data is already available, yet, there is a lot more to learn. Hence, I accepted the responsibility of editing this book and contributing my knowledge to the community.

Inflammatory bowel disease (IBD) is a set of inflammatory condition affecting colon and small intestine. There are two kinds of inflammatory bowel diseases - colitis and Crohn's disease. Crohn's disease can affect any part of the gastrointestinal tract from mouth to anus wherein colitis affects the colon and rectum. Common symptoms of Crohn's disease are abdominal pain, diarrhea, fever and weight loss. Common symptoms of colitis disease are abdominal pain, tenderness, loss of appetite, fatigue etc. These diseases are caused by a combination of genetic and environmental factors leading to inflammation and immunological responses to intestine. It can happen in any age group but it majorly occurs in teenagers and youngsters. The treatment of these diseases however depends on how severe they are. Although they are not completely curable, Crohn's disease is treated with the help of antibiotics, aminosalicycate and corticosteroids, colitis disease is treated with the help of antibiotics and surgeries. This book unravels the recent studies in the field of Colitis and Crohn's disease. The book presents researches and studies performed by experts across the globe. The extensive content of this book provides the readers with a thorough understanding of the subject.

While editing this book, I had multiple visions for it. Then I finally narrowed down to make every chapter a sole standing text explaining a particular topic, so that they can be used independently. However, the umbrella subject sinews them into a common theme. This makes the book a unique platform of knowledge.

I would like to give the major credit of this book to the experts from every corner of the world, who took the time to share their expertise with us. Also, I owe the completion of this book to the never-ending support of my family, who supported me throughout the project.

Editor

Deficient Production of Reactive Oxygen Species Leads to Severe Chronic DSS-Induced Colitis in Ncf1/p47^{phox}-Mutant Mice

Tiago Rodrigues-Sousa[1], Ana Filipa Ladeirinha[2], Ana Raquel Santiago[3], Helena Carvalheiro[1], Bruno Raposo[4], Ana Alarcão[2], António Cabrita[5], Rikard Holmdahl[4], Lina Carvalho[2], M. Margarida Souto-Carneiro[1]*

1 ImmunoMetabolic Pharmacology Group, CNC- Centro de Neurociências e Biologia Celular, Universidade de Coimbra, Coimbra, Portugal, 2 Departamento de Anatomia Patológica, Faculdade de Medicina, Universidade de Coimbra, Coimbra, Portugal, 3 Instituto Biomédico de Investigação da Luz e Imagem, Faculdade de Medicina, Universidade de Coimbra, Coimbra, Portugal, 4 Medical Inflammation Research, Karolinska Institute, Stockholm, Sweden, 5 Departamento de Patologia Experimental, Faculdade de Medicina, Universidade de Coimbra, Coimbra, Portugal

Abstract

Background: Colitis is a common clinical complication in chronic granulomatous disease (CGD), a primary immunodeficiency caused by impaired oxidative burst. Existing experimental data from NADPH-oxidase knockout mice propose contradictory roles for the involvement of reactive oxygen species in colitis chronicity and severity. Since genetically controlled mice with a point-mutation in the *Ncf1* gene are susceptible to chronic inflammation and autoimmunity, we tested whether they presented increased predisposition to develop chronic colitis.

Methods: Colitis was induced in Ncf1-mutant and wild-type mice by a 1st 7-days cycle of dextran sulfate sodium (DSS), intercalated by a 7-days resting period followed by a 2nd 7-days DSS-cycle. Cytokines were quantified locally in the colon inflammatory infiltrates and in the serum. Leukocyte infiltration and morphological alterations of the colon mucosa were assessed by immunohistochemistry.

Results: Clinical scores demonstrated a more severe colitis in Ncf1-mutant mice than controls, with no recovery during the resting period and a severe chronic colitis after the 2nd cycle, confirmed by histopathology and presence of infiltrating neutrophils, macrophages, plasmocytes and lymphocytes in the colon. Severe colitis was mediated by increased local expression of cytokines (IL-6, IL-10, TNF-α, IFN-γ and IL-17A) and phosphorylation of Leucine-rich repeat kinase 2 (LRRK2). Serological cytokine titers of those inflammatory cytokines were more elevated in Ncf1-mutant than control mice, and were accompanied by systemic changes in functional subsets of monocytes, CD4$^+$T and B cells.

Conclusion: This suggests that an ineffective oxidative burst leads to severe chronic colitis through local accumulation of peroxynitrites, pro-inflammatory cytokines and lymphocytes and systemic immune deregulation similar to CGD.

Editor: Katrin Schröder, Goethe Universität Frankfurt, Germany

Funding: H. Carvalheiro was funded by Fundação para a Ciência e Tecnologia grant SFRH/BD/60467/2009. This work was funded by the Marie Curie grant PERG-GA-2008-239422 to M.M. Souto-Carneiro, by the Swedish Research Council and the EU FP7 project Neurinox to R. Holmdahl and by the FEDER/COMPETE/ Fundação para a Ciência e Tecnologia project Pest/C-SAU/LA0001/2013-2014. The funders had no role in study design, data collection and analysis, decision to publish, or preparation of the manuscript.

Competing Interests: The authors have declared that no competing interests exist.

* E-mail: margarida.carneiro@cnc.uc.pt

Introduction

Mutations in the components of the NADPH oxidase 2 (NOX2) complex compromise the normal oxidative burst by phagocytes and B cells and are related to hyper-inflammation phenomena and recurrent opportunistic infections in patients with chronic granulomatous disease (CGD) and several animal models of inflammatory diseases [1–5]. Since the majority of CGD patients present mutations in the gp91^{phox}/Cybb subunit (about 70%) or in the p47^{phox}/Ncf1 subunit (about 20%) of NOX2, several studies have focused on understanding the immune response in corresponding animal models [6–9]. In particular, a point mutation in the *Ncf1* gene of B10.Q mice impairs the production of reactive oxygen species (ROS) leading to increased susceptibility to infections with *Staphylococcus xylosus*, *Staphylococcus aureus* and *Burkholderia cepacia* [10], and to the development of severe chronic autoimmune disorders such as collagen-induced arthritis and experimental autoimmune encephalopathy [11–13]. These hyper-inflammatory responses are directly related to the incapacity of producing ROS, since the administration of oxidants or reestablishing the burst capacity of macrophages with a functional *Ncf1* lead to permanent recovery in treated animals [8,11–14]. In knockout mice for either *Cybb* or *Ncf1*, an increased susceptibility to infections and to chronic inflammation was observed [6–9]. Since bowel inflammation, resembling Crohn's disease (CD), is a common complication of CGD, with patients presenting elevated titers of Crohn's associated antibodies even in the absence of active colitis [15], $gp91^{phox-/-}$, $Ncf1^{-/-}$ and –more recently- $p40^{phox-/-}$ mice have been used to understand how the lack of ROS-production associates with colitis [19–21]. However, the results in $Ncf1^{-/-}$ and $gp91^{phox-/-}$ mice were not consistent with those observed in CGD patients, since dextran sulfate sodium (DSS)-induced colitis was indistinguishable between $Ncf1^{-/-}$ mice and their wild type (WT) counterparts, whereas in $gp91^{phox-/-}$ mice DSS-induced colitis was milder than in the WT groups [16]. Furthermore, these studies focused on a single-round of colitis induction, without addressing the possibility of differences in repeatedly challenged mice. Contrasting to the studies on $Ncf1^{-/-}$ and $gp91^{phox-/-}$ mice, when DSS-colitis was induced in $p40^{phox-/-}$ mice the colon tissue was more injured in the mice deficient of ROS production than in the control group. This was associated with a more severe disease and poor recovery [17]. However, since Ncf4 interacts directly with Ncf2, knocking out $p40^{phox}$ might induce a broader phenomenon, making it difficult to assess which is the unique contribution of $p40^{phox}$ to colitis severity. By inducing two cycles of colitis with DSS intercalated by a resting period in BQ.$Ncf1^{m1J}$ mice with a point mutation in the $Ncf1$ gene, similar to that in CGD patients, we propose a new colitis model to study how the lack of oxidative burst can lead to the development of chronic inflammatory bowel disease (IBD).

Materials and Methods

Animals

6–8 weeks old male homozygous Ncf1-mutant BQ.$Ncf1^{m1J/m1J}$ (Ncf1*, n = 15) and wild-type (WT, n = 15) BQ mice (C57BL/10 expressing H-2^q) were obtained from breeding heterozygous mice, as previously described [14]. Animals were bred and maintained under standard conditions, with food and water *ad libitum* in a specific pathogen–free environment. All procedures were done under anesthesia in order to reduce discomfort and stress during sample collection. All animal studies were approved by the internal CNC Ethics Committee, and were in accordance with EU legislation for experimental animal welfare.

Induction of colitis

Colitis was induced by oral administration of 3% (w/v) DSS (average 40,000 g/mol, AppliChem, Darmstadt, Germany) *ad libitum* in drinking water for 2 cycles. The induction protocol consisted of 7 days of treatment with DSS, followed by 7 days of resting on normal water, and a second 7 days cycle with DSS (Fig. 1D). Five Ncf1* and WT mice were sacrificed at the end of each time point: day 7; day 14; and day 21, for histopathologic assessment of colitis and blood collection.

Clinical Evaluation

The clinical scores of colitis: weight change, diarrhea, colorectal bleeding and survival were monitored every other day. Blood scoring: 0- no blood; 1- visible blood; 2- rectal bleeding. Consistency scoring: 0- Normal; 1- Soft but formed; 3- very soft; 4- diarrhea. For all clinical scores the number of mice evaluated at each cycle was for both groups: Days 0 to 7 n = 15, Days 8 to 14 n = 10; Days 15 to 21 n = 5.

Histopathological evaluation of colitis

Separate swiss-rolls of distal, transverse and proximal colon were fixed in 4% neutral buffered formalin and stained with hematoxylin/eosin (HE) according to standard protocols. Additionally, immunohistochemistry was performed on proximal colon sections. In brief, endogenous peroxidase activity was quenched by 15 minutes incubation with 3% diluted hydrogen peroxide. Nonspecific binding was blocked with Ultra V Block (Ultra Vision Kit; TP-125-UB; Lab Vision Corporation; Fremont CA; USA). Incubation with primary antibodies against B220 (Instituto Gulbenkian de Ciência, Oeiras, Portugal), CD11b (clone Mac1, Instituto Gulbenkian de Ciência, Oeiras, Portugal) and CD3 (polyclonal, DakoCytomation, Glostrup, Denmark) to detect B cells, macrophages and T cells, respectively, or against FoxP3, IL-6, IL-10, IL-17A, IFN-γ, TNF-α (all from Biolegend) and Dundee-MJFF LRRK2 PhosphoSer935 (phosphorylated Leucine-rich repeat kinase 2; clone UDD2 10(12), RabMab/Abcam) was followed by incubation with biotin-labeled secondary antibody (Ultra Vision Kit; TP-125-BN; Lab Vision Corporation; Fremont CA; USA). Primary antibody binding was localized in tissues using peroxidase-conjugated streptavidin (Ultra Vision Kit; TP-125-HR; Lab Vision Corporation; Fremont CA; USA) and 3,3-diamino-benzidine tetrahydrochloride (RE7190-K; Novocastra Laboratories Ltd, Newcastle, United Kingdom) was used as chromogen, according to manufacturer's instructions. Hematoxylin was used to counterstain the slides. Morphological alterations and infiltration by inflammatory cells were screened by two pathologists in a blinded fashion.

Inflammation was scored for each colon section according to the number of inflammatory foci present: 0- no inflammatory focus; 1- one inflammatory focus; 2- two inflammatory foci; 3- three or more inflammatory foci. Dysplasia was scored for each colon section using a semi-quantitative scale: 0- no dysplasia; 1- nuclear pluristratification and hypercromatic independent glands; 2- nuclear pluristratification and hypercromatic independent glands and complex glands; 3- nuclear pluristratification and hypercromatic complex glands with scattered mitosis. The infiltration of lymphocytes, neutrophils and plasmocytes was scored based on cell morphology, and corresponded to the percentage of each subset within the total inflammatory cells. Infiltration of B220$^+$, CD3$^+$ or Mac-1$^+$ cells was scored based on the immunohisto-chemistry cell-specific staining as 0 (absence of cell type); + (<50% positive cells); ++ (50–75% positive cells) and +++ (>75% positive cells), considering the total inflammatory infiltrate in each case using the web-based ImmunoMembrane image-analysis software (http://153.1.200.58:8080/immunomembrane/).

Relative quantification of cytokines and pLRRK2 was performed using the web-based ImmunoRatio image-analysis software (http://153.1.200.58:8080/immunoratio/).

Superoxide anion detection

Formalin-fixed, paraffin-embedded sections (4 μm thick) were mounted on polysine-coated glass slides. Sections were deparaffinized in xylene and rehydrated in PBS. The sections were incubated for 90 min at 37°C with the fluorescent probe dihydroethidium (DHE, 5 μmol/l; Molecular Probes, Life Technologies, USA). In the presence of superoxide anions, DHE is oxidized to ethidium, which intercalates with DNA, and yields bright red fluorescence. After washing with PBS, sections were incubated with 4′,6-diamidino-2-phenylindole (DAPI) for 20 min. Sections were rinsed in PBS and mounted on glass slides using Glycergel mounting medium (Dako, Denmark). From each section, four random sections were acquired in a laser scanning confocal microscope (Zeiss LSM 710, Germany). The specificity of the staining was evaluated by the omission of the dye (negative control). Densitometric analysis of DHE fluorescence intensity was performed using ImageJ Software 1.46r (NIH, USA).

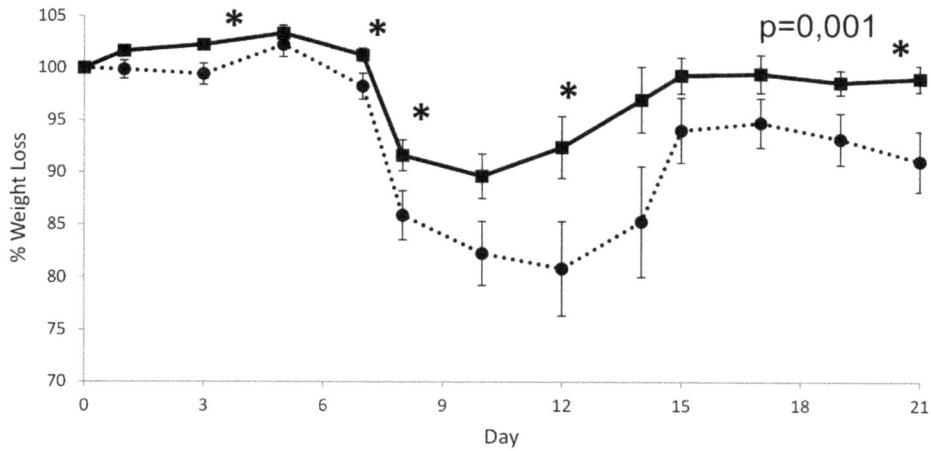

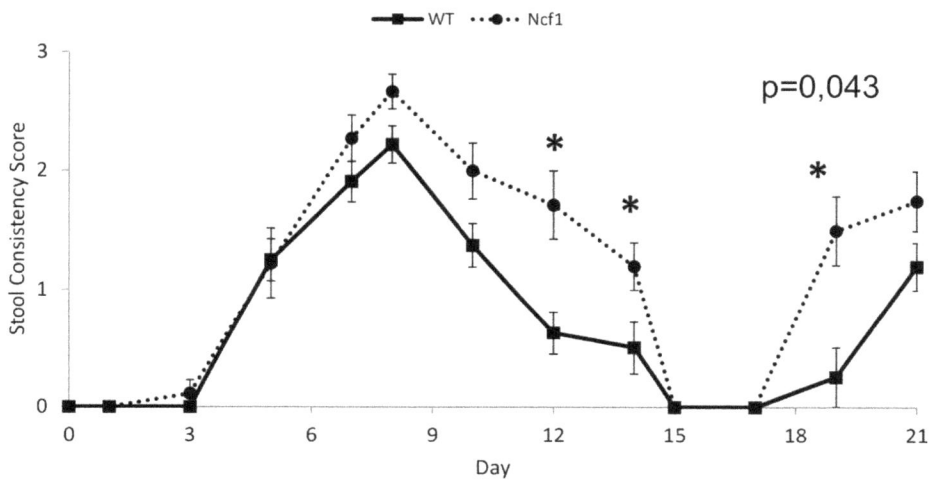

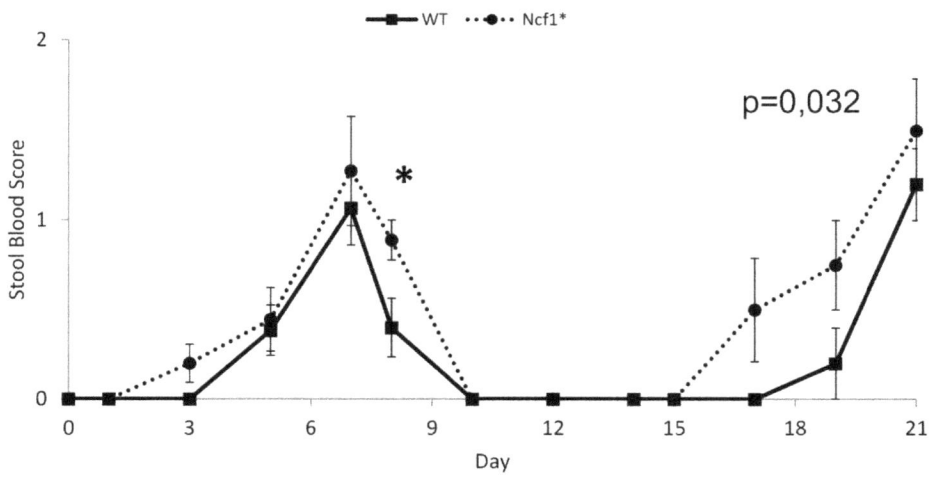

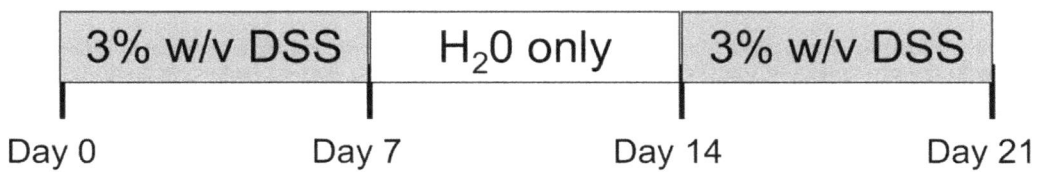

Figure 1. Clinical scores of colitis are more severe in Ncf1* mice. A) Changes in average weight ± SE, (baseline weight: WT = 25.8±0.5 g, Ncf1* = 26.5±0.8 g). B) Changes in stools consistency ± SE. C) Presence of blood in stools ± SE. Asterisks indicate p<0.05, Mann-Whitney test between Ncf1* and WT. P-values on the top right corner indicate the statistical difference between curves, permutation test. D) Schematic overview of the DSS treatment plan showing the induction and recovery periods.

Immunofluorescence detection of nitrotyrosine

The presence of 3-nitrotyrosine residues, an indirect marker of peroxynitrite formation, was evaluated by immunofluorescence. After deparaffinization, antigen retrieval was performed using citrate buffer at 95°C. sections were incubated with 1% bovine serum albumin (BSA) in PBS (PBA) for 1 h, followed by incubation with 2% normal goat serum in PBA for 30 min. Sections were then incubated overnight at 4°C with anti-nitrotyrosine antibody (1:100; Merck Millipore, USA) prepared in PBA. After washing, sections were incubated for 1 h with Alexa Fluor 488 goat anti-rabbit secondary antibody (1:200, Life Technologies) prepared in PBA. After washing, nuclei were stained with DAPI. Slides were mounted with Glycergel. A negative control without primary antibody was performed. From each section, four random sections were acquired in a laser scanning confocal microscope (Zeiss LSM 710, Germany). Densitometric analysis of 3-nitrotyrosine residues fluorescence intensity was performed using ImageJ Software 1.46r (NIH, USA).

Serum cytokine quantification

Serum samples were collected at each time-point. Cytokine titers in the sera were quantified using the cytometric bead arrays, mouse Th1/Th2/Th17/Th22 13plex FlowCytomix Multiplex kit (Bender MedSystems, Austria) according to the manufacturer's instructions and analyzed with FlowCytomix Pro Software (eBioscience, San Diego, USA). Concentrations of cytokines below the limit of detection of the assay were given zero value.

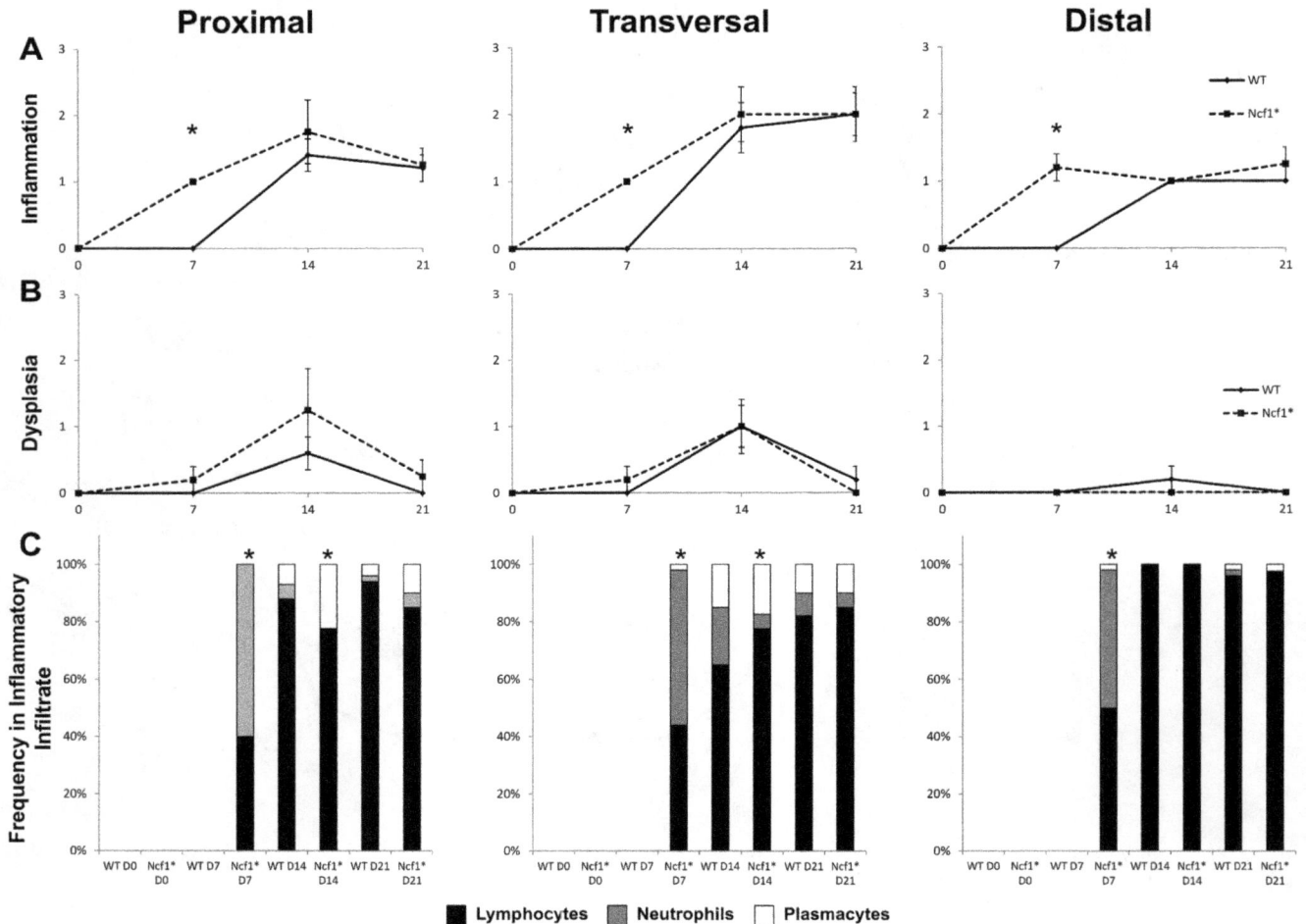

Figure 2. Histological evaluation shows that Ncf1* mice develop a severe chronic colitis with several inflammatory foci and dysplasia, particularly in the proximal and transversal sections of the colon, with a skewed leukocyte distribution. A) Inflammatory score in the different sections of the colon throughout the experimental period. B) Dysplasia score in the different sections of the colon throughout the experimental period. C) Distribution of the leukocytes subsets in the different sections of the colon throughout the experimental period. Asterisks indicate p<0.05, Mann-Whitney test between Ncf1* and WT. Inflammation and dysplasia scoring system is detailed in the methods section.

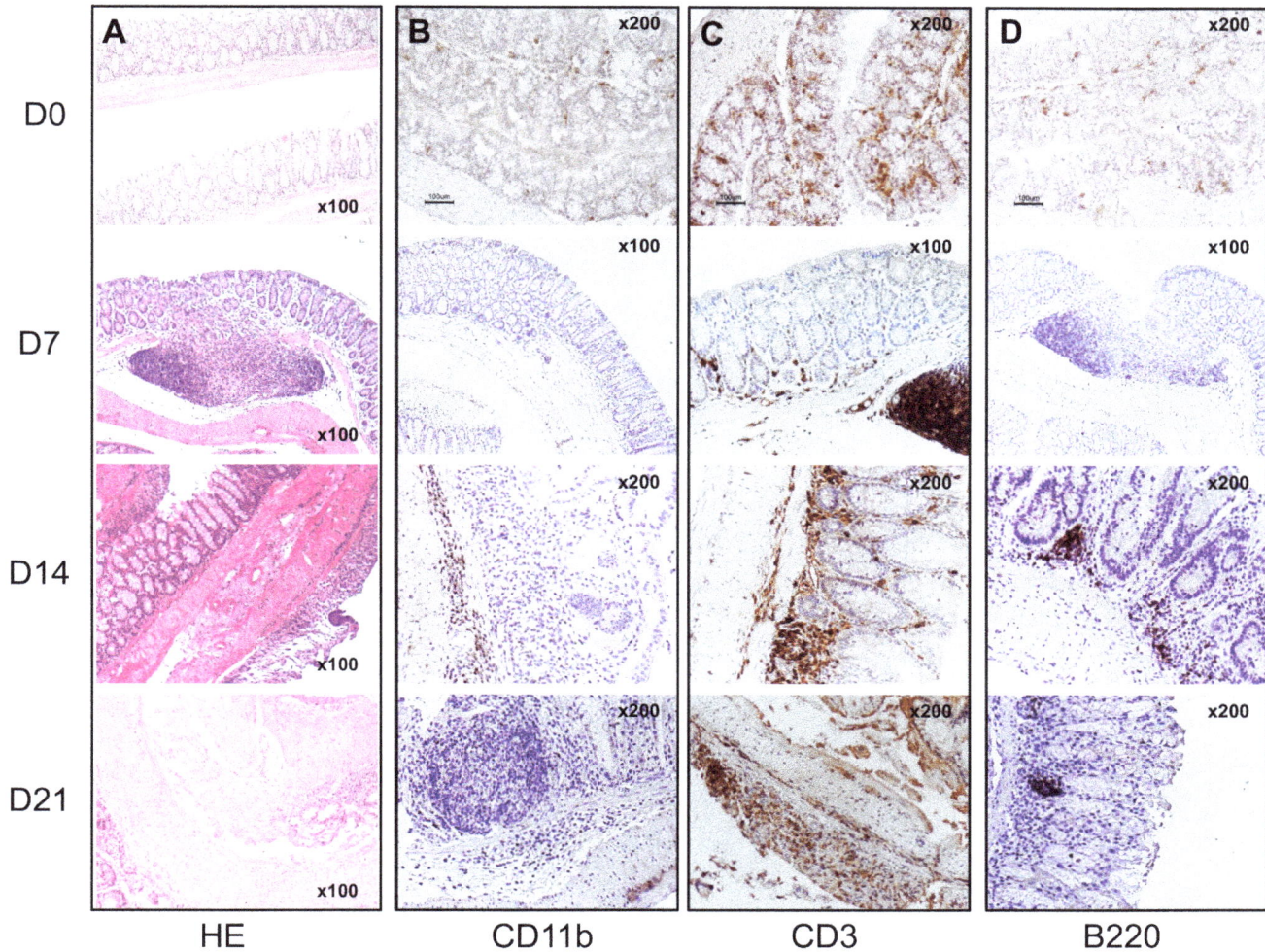

Figure 3. Histological and immunohistochemistry analyses of the WT colon show erosions, epithelial hyperplasia and low grade dysplasia, with progressive infiltration of CD3+ T and B220+ B lymphocytes and Mac-1+ cells. A) Hematoxylin-eosin (HE) staining of the colon during the different phases of the DSS-induced colitis protocol. B) Immunohistochemistry of Mac-1+ cells in the inflammatory infiltrates at days 0, 7, 14 and 21. C) Immunohistochemistry of CD3+ cells in the inflammatory infiltrates at days 0, 7, 14 and 21. D) Immunohistochemistry of B220+ cells in the inflammatory infiltrates at days 0, 7, 14 and 21. Magnification inserted in the images.

Leukocyte Phenotyping

Peripheral blood samples were collected from the base of the tail on days 0, 7, 14 and 21. Mononuclear cells were stained in a standard method using fluorochrome-conjugated anti-mouse monoclonal antibodies against: CD3, CD4, CD8, CD25, CD69, CXCR5, IgM, CD19, IgD, CD107a, CD27, CD62L, NK1.1, CD11b, and Ly-6c (all from Biolegend). Intracellular staining was done after saponin permeabilization using fluorochrome-conjugated anti-mouse FoxP3 and CD68 (all from Biolegend). Irrelevant, directly conjugated, murine IgG1 or IgG2 (Biolegend) were used to ascertain background staining. 25000 events were collected within the lymphocyte gate. After calibration with CST beads, single-fluorochrome stained cells were used for instrument compensation and PMT setup. All samples were analyzed on a BD FACSCanto II (Becton Dickinson) and data were analyzed with FlowJo 7.6.4 software (Tree Star).

Statistical Analysis

All data were tested for normal distribution with Levene's test. Since data did not follow a normal distribution the non-parametric

Kruskal-Wallis test followed by a non-parametric Mann-Whitney test were used to compare values between groups and time-points, using Statview 5.0.1 software (SAS Institute Inc, USA). Statistical differences between curves were determined using a 2-sided hypothesis permutation test with 10000 permutations [18] (http://bioinf.wehi.edu.au/software/russell/perm/). Differences were considered significant for $p < 0.05$.

Results

Clinical signs of DSS-induced colitis

Throughout the whole observation period the Ncf1* mice lost significantly more weight than the WT (p = 0.001, between curves, Fig. 1A). On day 8, after the first treatment cycle with DSS, both animal groups presented significant ($p < 0.05$) weight loss ranging from 10–15% as compared to baseline (baseline weight: WT = 25.8±0.5 g, Ncf1* = 26.5±0.8 g). For the WT group the weight-loss continued until day 10, after which they recovered, reaching their baseline weight by day 15, which was kept until the end of the study. In contrast, Ncf1* mice continued to lose weight

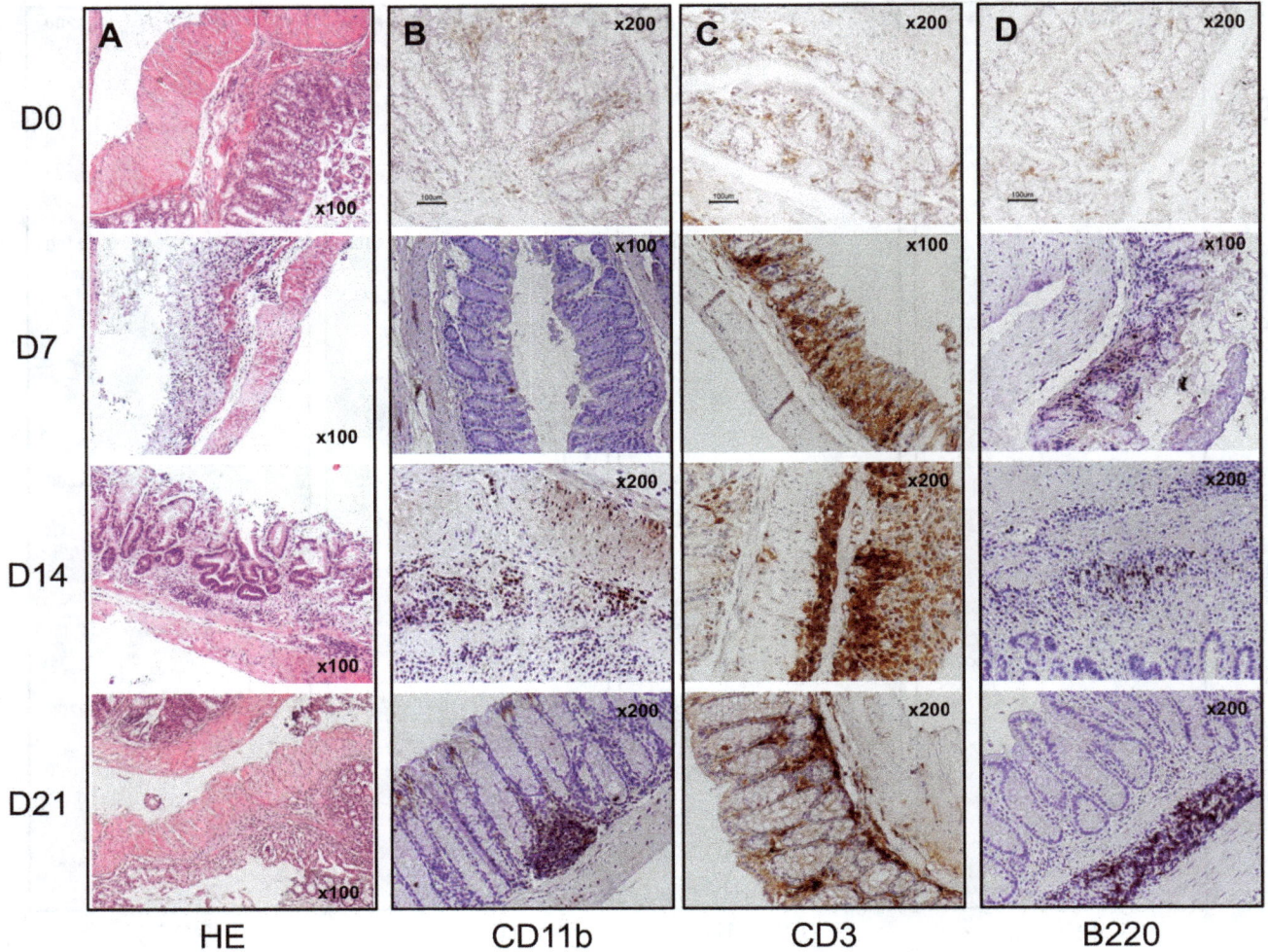

Figure 4. Histological and immunohistochemistry analyses of the Ncf1* colon show ulcers, epithelial hyperplasia and severe dysplasia, with massive infiltration of CD3$^+$ lymphocytes, and subsequently of B220$^+$ B lymphocytes and Mac-1$^+$ cells in the later time-points. A) Hematoxylin-eosin (HE) staining of the colon during the different phases of the DSS-induced colitis protocol. B) Immunohistochemistry of Mac-1$^+$ cells in the inflammatory infiltrates at days 0, 7, 14 and 21. C) Immunohistochemistry of CD3$^+$ cells in the inflammatory infiltrates at days 0, 7, 14 and 21. D) Immunohistochemistry of B220$^+$ cells in the inflammatory infiltrates at days 0, 7, 14 and 21. Magnification inserted in the images.

until day 12, recovered up till 95% of their initial weight between days 14 and 17, and started to lose again thereafter, thus having only in average 90% of their initial body-weight at the end of the second cycle of DSS administration.

The presence of blood in stools and the consistency of the feces are two further clinical signs of DSS-induced colitis. Throughout the various phases of the study, Ncf1* mice presented significantly worst clinical scores for the presence of blood (p = 0.032, between curves) and consistency (p = 0.043, between curves) of stools than WT (Fig. 1B and 1C). Throughout the resting period the Ncf1* group scored worst for the presence of blood in stools and stool consistency, and their recovery was delayed when compared to the WT animals.

Histopathological assessment of DSS-Induced Colitis

The baseline (D0) HE staining from colon sections shows that the *Ncf1*-mutation alone does not induce alterations in the colon architecture nor detectable inflammatory spots when compared to WT animals (D0 in Fig. 2A, 3A, 4A). In both groups there were

scattered resident CD3$^+$ (score: 0) and B220$^+$ lymphocytes (score: 0), and CD11b$^+$ macrophages (score: 0) (D0 in Fig. 3B–D and 4B–D). By the time the first cycle of DSS-administration was over (D7) evident differences could be seen in the colonic morphology of both groups when compared to D0. In WT mice neither inflammation (Fig. 2A) nor dysplasia (Fig. 2B) could be observed, even though there was low grade erosion of the colonic mucosa (Fig. 3A), and a significant increase in local ROS production (Fig. 5A, B). This contrasted to the findings in Ncf1* mice, which in addition to erosion and immature fibroblasts presented significantly more inflammation (Fig. 2A) in all colon sections. This inflammatory infiltrate was mainly composed of neutrophils and CD3$^+$ T lymphocytes (score: +++), though some plasmocytes were equally present (Fig. 2C, Fig. 4D). Additionally, at D7 the Ncf1* mice had a significantly higher local production of peroxynitrites in the colonic inflammatory infiltrates than at D0 or comparing to the WT group (Fig. 5C, D). After the resting period at D14, the colon tissue of the WT mice presented erosion, epithelial hyperplasia with mitosis and nuclear atypia (Fig. 3A),

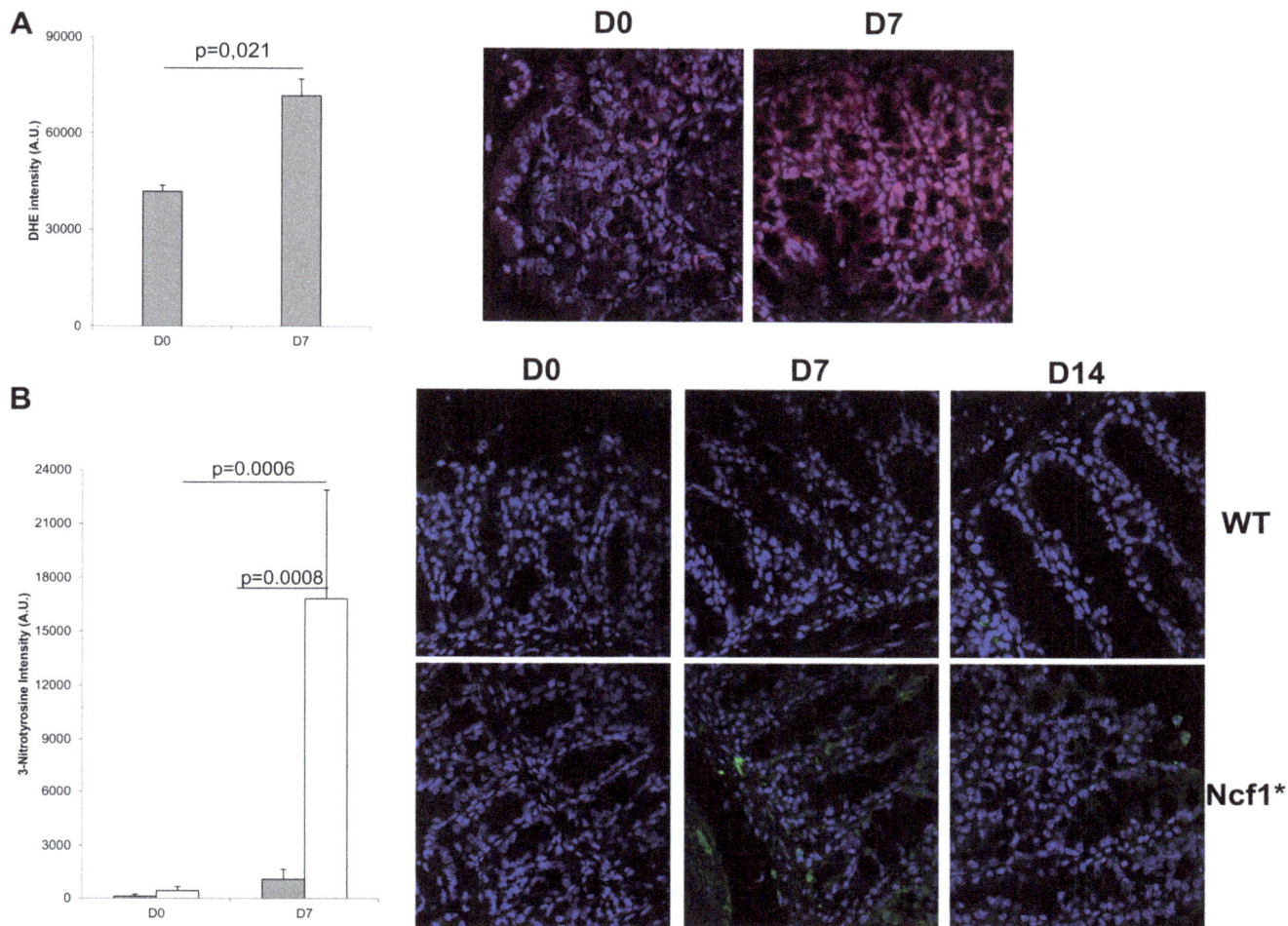

Figure 5. ROS levels increase in WT mice colonic inflammatory infiltrates after colitis induction, whereas Ncf1* mice increase the local production of peroxynitrites, which remains high after the recovery period. A) Relative DHE fluorescence intensity in colon sections of WT mice, Mann-Whitney test. B) Representative fluorescence immunohistochemistry of local ROS (red) production in WT mice before and after colitis induction (magnification 400×). C) Relative 3-nitrotyrosin residues fluorescence intensity in colon sections of WT (grey bars) and Ncf1* mice (white bars), Mann-Whitney test. D) Representative fluorescence immunohistochemistry of peroxynitrites (green) production in the colonic inflammatory infiltrates in WT and Ncf1* mice (magnification 400×).

low grade dysplasia (Fig. 2B) and an inflammatory infiltrate mainly composed of CD3$^+$ (score: +++) and B220$^+$ lymphocytes (score: ++), a few CD11b$^+$ macrophages (score: +), granulocytes (score: +) and plasmocytes (score: +) (Figs. 2A & C, 3B–E). The Ncf1* mice presented a more severe injury of the colonic tissue, with ulcers reaching the *muscularis propria* (Fig. 4A), severe dysplasia with small back to back glandules with atypical mitoses and anisocarioses (Figs. 2B, 4A), and the composition of the inflammatory infiltrate was mainly CD3$^+$ (score: +++) and B220$^+$ lymphocytes (score: ++), CD11b$^+$ macrophages (score: ++), plasmocytes (score: +), and a reduced amount of granulocytes (less than 5%) (Figs. 2C, 4B–E). The local production of peroxynitrites in Ncf1* colon inflammatory infiltrates remained higher than in the WT animals (Fig. 5D). After the second cycle of colitis induction, D21, the colon of WT mice had ulcers, and epithelial regeneration with glandular hyperplasia without nuclear atypia (Fig. 3), and the inflammatory infiltrate was mostly comprised of CD3$^+$ lymphocytes (score: +++), a few CD11b$^+$ macrophages (score: +), and less than 10% granulocytes and plasmocytes (score: 0 to +) (Figs. 2C, 3B, C & D). The Ncf1* mice equally presented ulcers with re-epithelialization

(Fig. 4A), however the epithelial regeneration showed nuclear atypia and low focal dysplasia (Fig. 2B). Moreover, the inflammatory infiltrate was mainly composed of CD3$^+$ lymphocytes (score: +++) and CD11b$^+$ macrophages (score: ++), plasmocytes (score: +) and less than 5% granulocytes (Figs. 2C, 4B, C & E). The presence of FoxP3$^+$ T cells was equivalent for both groups in all time points (data not shown).

Systemic changes in functional leukocyte subsets

In order to establish whether there were systemic disease-related and Ncf1-mutation-related alterations in the frequency of different functional subsets of T cells (CD4$^+$ and CD8$^+$), NK cells, B cells and monocytes, these populations were characterized in the peripheral blood (Fig. 6).

At D0 the only significant differences between both groups observed in the blood were in CXCR4$^+$ B cells and CD25$^+$FoxP3$^-$CD4$^+$ effector T cells. At D7 Ncf1* and WT presented significant differences in the frequency of circulating activated CD11b^{++}CD68$^+$ monocytes, CXCR4$^+$ and total CD19$^+$ B cells. When comparing D7 to D0, there were significant

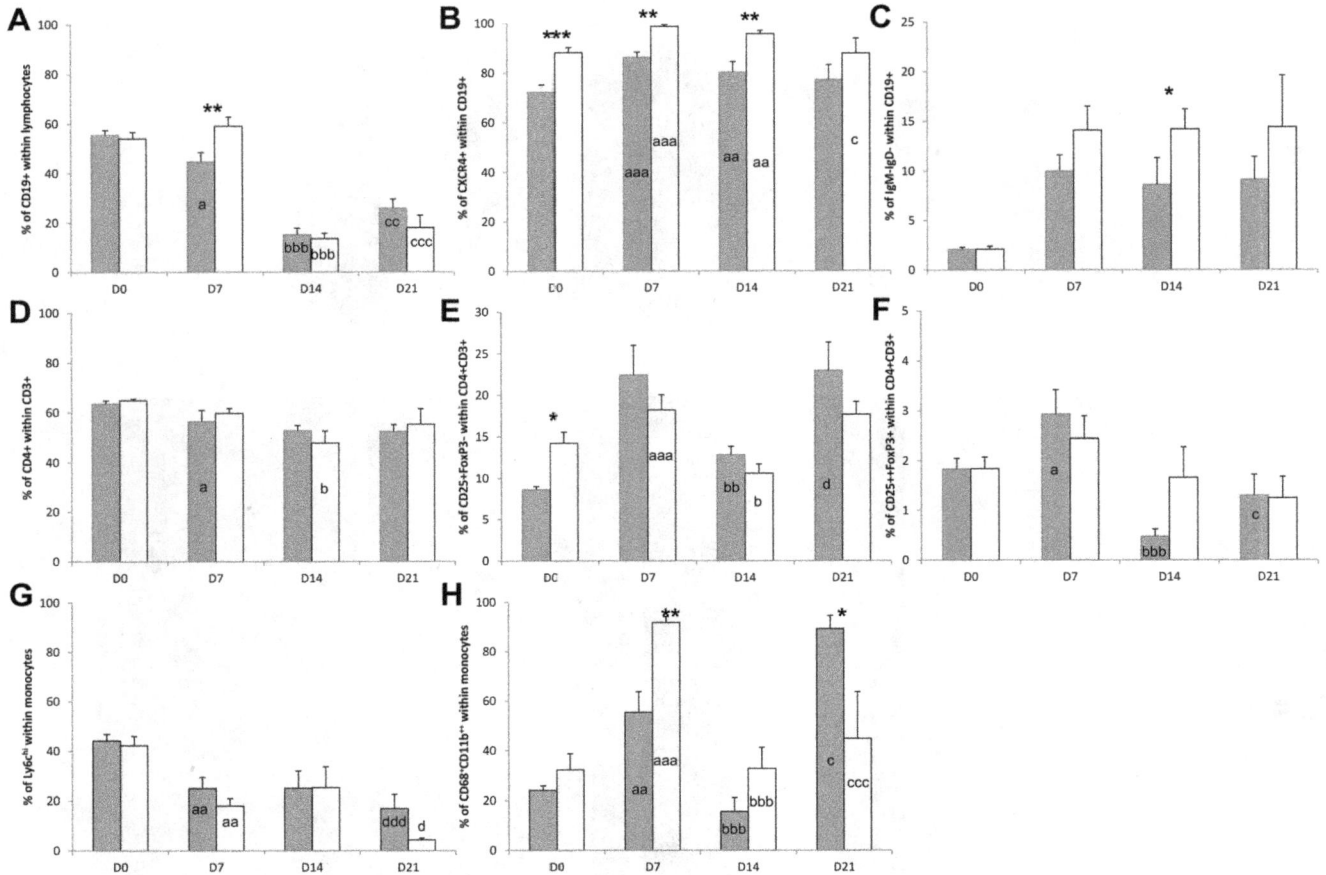

Figure 6. Analysis of peripheral blood functional leukocyte subsets at the different phases of DSS-colitis induction shows altered frequencies of circulating B and CD4+ T lymphocytes and CD11b+ monocytes between Ncf1* and WT mice. A) Frequency of CD19+ B lymphocytes within total lymphocytes. B) Frequency of CXCR4+ cells within CD19+ B lymphocytes. C) Frequency of IgM−IgD− cells within CD19+ B lymphocytes. D) Frequency of CD4+ T lymphocytes within CD3+ T lymphocytes. E) Frequency of CD25+FoxP3− cells within CD4+ T lymphocytes. F) Frequency of CD25+FoxP3+ cells within CD4+ T lymphocytes. G) Frequency of Ly6chi cells within CD11b+ monocytes. H) Frequency of CD68+CD11b++ cells within CD11b+ monocytes. * indicates p<0.05 and ** indicates p<0.01, Mann-Whitney test between Ncf1* and WT; differences between days 0 and 7 are indicated by a: p<0.05, aa: p<0.01, aaa: p<0.001; differences between days 7 and 14 are indicated by b: p<0.05, bb: p<0.01, bbb: p<0.001; differences between days 7 and 21 are indicated by c: p<0.05, cc: p<0.01, ccc: p<0.001; differences between days 14 and 21 are indicated by d: p<0.05, dd: p<0.01, ddd: p<0.001, all Mann-Whitney test. White bars Ncf1*, gray bars WT.

differences in both groups for Ly6chi monocytes and total activated monocytes, and for IgM−IgD−CD19+ post-switch and CXCR4+ B cells. The WT blood at D7 had significantly more effector and total CD4+ T cells, CD25++FoxP3+CD4+ regulatory T cells (Treg), and total CD19+ B cells than at D0. At D14 the only significant differences between WT and Ncf1* mice were in the frequency of blood post-switch and CXCR4+ B cells. However, when comparing D14 to D7, the frequencies of activated monocytes, total B cells and effector CD4+ T cells in the blood of Ncf1* and WT were significantly different, whereas WT had significantly less Treg cells than at D7 and the Ncf1* had significantly less circulating total CD4+ T cells.

When comparing the leukocyte subsets between Ncf1* and WT mice at D21 there was a significant alteration in the frequency of activated monocytes. When comparing between D7 and D21 the Ncf1* mice presented significant changes in activated monocytes, CXCR4+ B cells and total B cells. The WT counterparts presented significant changes in activated monocytes, total B cells and Treg cells. Significant differences could also be seen between D14 and D21 in WT and Ncf1* Ly6chi monocytes and WT effector CD4+ T cells. Another important observation was that CD68+CD11b+

cells in Ncf1 mice did not increment after the second DSS treatment, as in WT mice.

No significant changes were observed for CD69+CD4+ and CD69+CD8+ T cells, CXCR5+CD4+ and CXCR5+CD8+ T cells, neither for the NK cell subsets.

Quantification of cytokines and pLRRK2 production by colonic inflammatory infiltrates

In order to evaluate whether local cytokine production could be involved in the higher disease severity in Ncf1* mice, we quantified the relative expression of IL-6, IL-10, IL-17A, IFN-γ and TNF-α in the inflammatory infiltrates of the colon after disease induction (Fig. 7). Since LRRK2 has been reported to be part of the susceptibility locus for CD [19], we equally quantified the relative expression of its phosphorylated form (pLRRK2) in the inflammatory infiltrates of the colonic mucosa on days 7, 14 and 21 in both groups (Fig. 7). No quantification was made for day 0 as there were no inflammatory infiltrates present.

At D7 TNF-α and pLRRK2 expression were significantly different between Ncf1* and WT mice (p = 0.002 and p = 0.016,

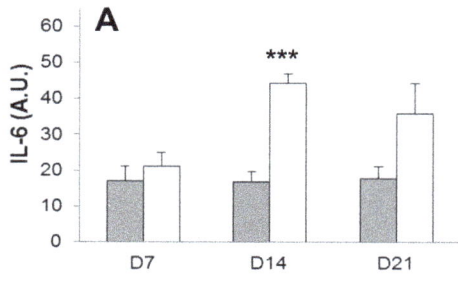

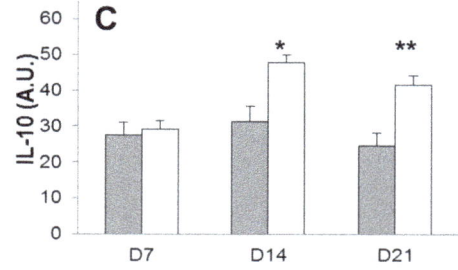

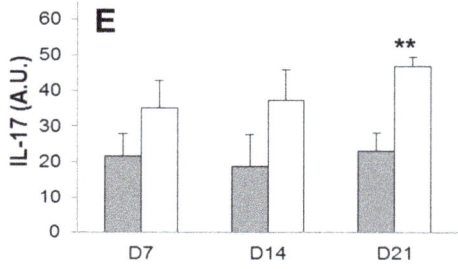

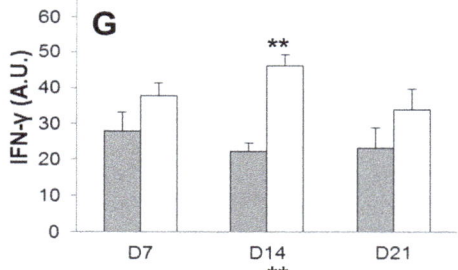

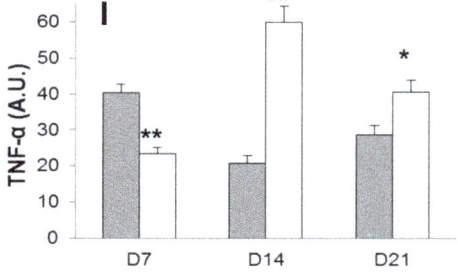

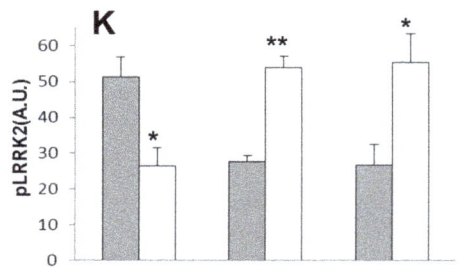

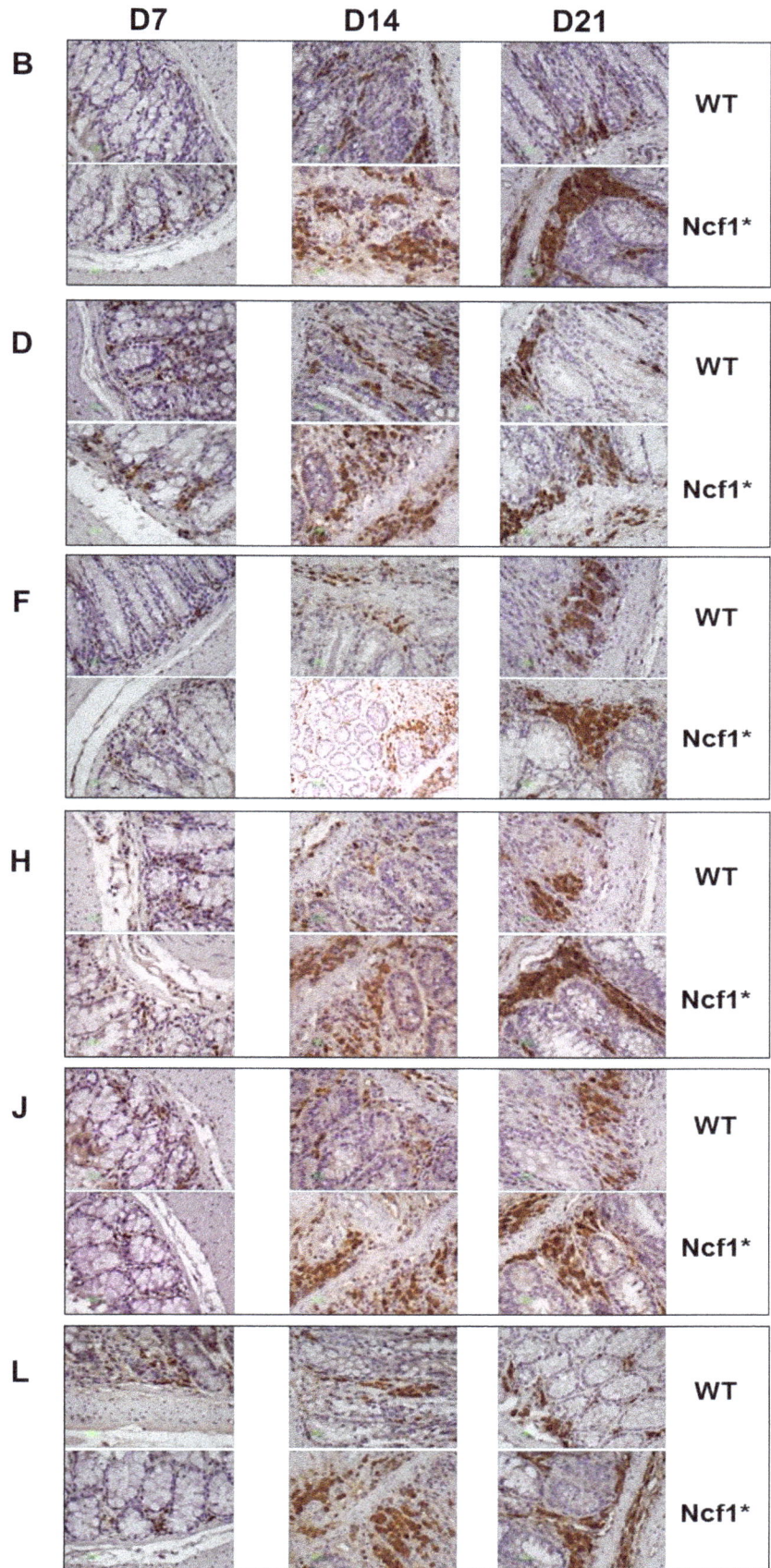

Figure 7. Colitis severity in Ncf1* mice results from increased local production of pro-inflammatory cytokines and LRRK2 phosphorilation. A) Relative expression of IL-6 in the inflammatory infiltrates of the colon mucosa at days 7, 14 and 21. B) Representative immunohistochemistry staining for IL-6 in the colon of WT and Ncf1* at days 7, 14 and 21. C) Relative expression of IL-10 in the inflammatory infiltrates of the colon mucosa at days 7, 14 and 21. D) Representative immunohistochemistry staining for IL-10 in the colon of WT and Ncf1* at days 7, 14 and 21. E) Relative expression of IL-17A in the inflammatory infiltrates of the colon mucosa at days 7, 14 and 21. F) Representative immunohistochemistry staining for IL-17A in the colon of WT and Ncf1* at days 7, 14 and 21. G) Relative expression of IFN-γ in the inflammatory infiltrates of the colon mucosa at days 7, 14 and 21. H) Representative immunohistochemistry staining for IFN-γ in the colon of WT and Ncf1* at days 7, 14 and 21. I) Relative expression of TNF-α in the inflammatory infiltrates of the colon mucosa at days 7, 14 and 21. J) Representative immunohistochemistry staining for TNF-α in the colon of WT and Ncf1* at days 7, 14 and 21. K) Relative expression of pLRRK2 in the inflammatory infiltrates of the colon mucosa at days 7, 14 and 21. L) Representative immunohistochemistry staining for pLRRK2 in the colon of WT and Ncf1* at days 7, 14 and 21. * indicates p<0.05, ** indicates p<0.01, *** indicates p<0.001 between Ncf1* and WT mice, Mann-Whitney test. White bars Ncf1*, gray bars WT. Magnification for all images 400×.

respectively). Both groups differed significantly on D14 on the expression levels of IL-6 (p = 0.0005), IL-10 (p = 0.021), IFN-γ (p = 0.001), TNF-α (p = 0.002) and pLRRK2 (p = 0.008). Finally, at D21 expression levels between groups were significantly different for IL-10 (p = 0.011), IL-17A (p = 0.011), TNF-α (p = 0.036) and pLRRK2 (p = 0.030). To assess whether cytokine and pLRRK2 production in the colonic inflammatory infiltrates varied through the different induction and rest cycles within each group, their expression was compared between time-points. Thus, when comparing to D7, at D14 the Ncf1* colons expressed significantly more IL-6 (p = 0.004), IL-10 (p = 0.002) and TNF-α (p = 0.002). Comparing to D7, on D21 the colon infiltrates in Ncf1* mice expressed significantly more IL-10 (p = 0.013), TNF-α (p = 0.008) and pLRRK2 (p = 0.028); and comparing to D14 TNF-α (p = 0.014) and IFN-γ (p = 0.022) expression was significantly lower. On days D14 and D21, when comparing to D7, inflammatory infiltrates in WT colons expressed significantly less TNF-α (D14: p = 0.001; D21: p = 0.017) and pLRRK2 (D14: p = 0.02 and D21: p = 0.021).

Serum cytokine quantification

The serological levels of pro-inflammatory and anti-inflammatory cytokines were measured at different time-points, to assess whether the changes observed in the tissue had a systemic impact (Fig. 8).

At D0 cytokines titers were similar between the two groups, indicating that the *Ncf1*-mutation *per se* does not lead to aberrant cytokine production in naïve animals. For D7 the serum concentrations of IL-6, IL-17A, IL-22 and INF-γ significantly (p<0.05) increased in both groups when compared to D0 values, whereas Ncf1* mice also presented a significant (p<0.05) increase of IL-2 and IL-21. However, when comparing between both groups, Ncf1* mice had significantly higher titers of circulating IL-2, IL-6, IL-17A; IL-21 and INF-γ. At D14 the titers of IL-6, IL-17A, IL-21 and INF-γ in both groups still remained significantly (p<0.05) higher than the baseline values. Significant differences could be detected between both groups, namely Ncf1* mice had higher titers of IL-6, IL-10 and INF-γ than WT. At D21 the titers of IL-6 and IL-2 were still significantly (p<0.05) higher than baseline values in both Ncf1* and WT. IL-17A, IL-21 and INF-γ titers returned to baseline levels in both groups. WT mice had a significant increase in serum IL-22 when compared to Ncf1* mice, and IL-10 titers in the Ncf1* serum returned to baseline concentration.

Discussion

Colitis is a major complication in CGD patients. However, existing experimental data linking defective ROS production and colitis development and severity are conflicting [16,20,21]. In particular, a suitable model to study how the deficient ROS-

production by a defective NOX2 contributes to colitis severity is still missing. In the present study, we show, for the first time, that Ncf1* treated with repeated DSS-cycles intercalated by a resting period develop an earlier and severer colitis, contrasting to the milder colitis developed by oxidative-burst competent wild-type animals. This severe colitis in Ncf1* mice was mediated by increased local production of peroxynitrites, pro-inflammatory cytokines and phosphorylated LRRK2.

In wild-type mice from several strains, diarrhea and blood in stools are the consequence of crypt loss and mucosal erosions followed by inflammation in acute DSS-induced colitis, whereas repeated cycles of DSS administration intercalated by H2O result in chronic colitis, with areas of disease activity (inflammation) and inactivity, dysplasia, and epithelial hyperplasia [22,23]. Thus, the clinical symptoms and histopathologic signs we observed in Ncf1* mice point towards a severe DSS-induced colitis. This Ncf1* colitis is characterized by the presence of inflammatory cells without epithelioid granulomata, and with dysplasia often with the criteria of severe dysplasia and intra-epithelial adenocarcinoma, in particular in the transversal region of the colon. This contrasted to the WT colitis which presented less severe morphological alterations considering both inflammation and epithelial dysplasia. Our data on Ncf1* mice are in accordance with what has been found in a systematic analysis of colon biopsies of CGD children –including p47phox-deficient- with chronic colitis: the inflammatory infiltrate present in the CGD colon and the extent of the disruption of the crypts, leading to functional changes, were less severe than in UC controls [24]. Moreover, since DSS is a chemically induced inflammation of the large bowel, which damages the mucosa and allows the fecal matter and therefore enteric bacteria across the mucosal barrier, it is possible that, similarly to CD and CGD, the Ncf1* mice have a failure in bacterial clearance leading to persistent bacterial/luminal contents in the bowel wall which may drive the chronic bowel inflammation. However, in CGD patients this incapacity to remove bacterial debris due to deficient phagocytosis leads to the formation of granulomata. In our study we did not find any granulomata in the colon mucosa, most probably because the colitis was not induced for long enough to form granulomata.

The time point at which T cells can be detected in the colon mucosa of DSS-induced colitis varies between studies and mouse strains [25–27]. The histological data we obtained at D7 suggest that the deficient ROS-production accelerates T cell infiltration of the colon mucosa in Ncf1* mice, which was accompanied by neutrophilic infiltration and a surge in local peroxynitrite production. Even though NO-production is one of the major pro-inflammatory effector mechanisms of myeloid cells, T cells –specially activated CD4+ T cells- are equally able of producing NO upon expression of inducible nitric oxide synthase (iNOS) [28]. Similarly to what has been reported for several experimental models of acute and chronic colitis, local NO-production drives an

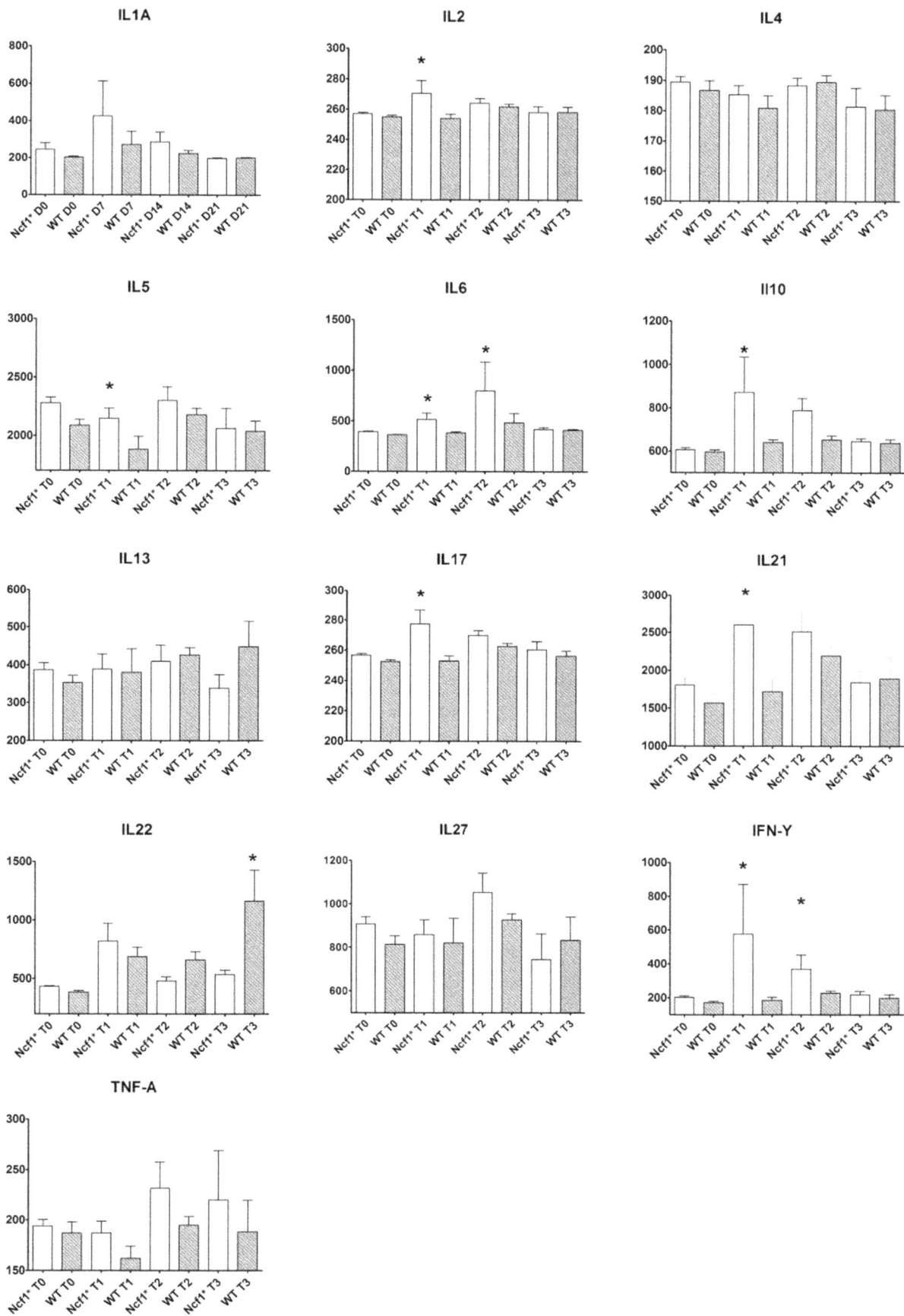

Figure 8. Variation of the serological cytokine titers in Ncf1* and WT mice during the different cycles. Data are presented as box-plots, where the boxes represent the 25th to 75th percentiles, the lines within the boxes represent the median, and the lines outside the boxes represent the 10th and 90th percentiles. For each group at D0 (n = 15), D7 (n = 15), D14 (n = 10) and D21 (n = 5); Asterisk indicates p<0.05, Mann-Whitney test between Ncf1* and WT. White bars Ncf1*, gray bars WT.

increased expression of TNF-α, IFN-γ and IL-6 [29–31]. Moreover, the inhibition of iNOS in $p47^{phox-/-}$ mice with DSS-induced colitis reduces disease severity by down-modulating the over-production of peroxynitrites [20]. In our study the exacerbated production of peroxynitrites in the colon mucosa of Ncf1* mice during the acute phase of disease might be responsible for the subsequent increase in local TNF-α, IFN-γ and IL-6 observed at D14 and continuing through D21. It has been previously shown that IL-10 production is needed to abrogate Th1 cells–mediated colitis serving as a mediator of regulatory T cell functions [32]. In our model we observed that the local and systemic levels of IL-10 were significantly higher in Ncf1* mice then in WT. However, this was not accompanied by an increased presence of Treg in the colon. Thus the observed surge in IL-10 might derive from other cells in an effort to down-modulate the markedly pro-inflammatory local and systemic cytokine profile, which is usually observed in the chronic phase of DSS-induced colitis [33]. Actually, we hypothesize that the higher B cell recruitment after the resting period relates to a peroxynitrite-induced IL-6 production by dentritic cells from the mucosa-associated lymphoid tissue, which triggers T cell-independent B cell migration [34].

The presence of significantly more CXCR4+ B cells in the peripheral blood of Ncf1* mice at baseline, D7 and D14 stresses that our animal model reproduces data obtained from IBD patients, in which circulating CXCR4+ B and plasma cells correlated with disease activity [35]. The absence of Mac-1+ macrophages at D7 in the colon of Ncf1* mice resembles what has been described for CGD patients, who present less CD68+ macrophages in their colon than CD patients and healthy individuals [36]. However, as they start infiltrating the colon mucosa after the acute phase –eventually facilitated by the vasodilatatory effect of NO-, these macrophages may become active players in the pro-inflammatory process by producing TNF-α and IFN-γ, which are hallmark cytokines of pro-inflammatory macrophages in colitis [25,37]. Albeit no double immunohistological staining was done, we hypothesize that the exacerbated local TNF-α production in the Ncf1* colon mucosa results from the infiltrating macrophages.

The LRRK2 gene is located within the risk region associated with CD-susceptibility [19] and IFN-γ-induced LRRK2 expression in CD patients increases in the inflamed colonic mucosa. In our DSS-induced colitis model we observe that between D14 and D21 Ncf1* mice had a higher IFN-γ expression in the colon mucosa, which was paralleled by a higher expression of pLRRK2. Since LRRK2 induces NFAT expression [38], and exacerbated NFAT-expression associated with IL-17A production has been observed in human and mouse colitis [39,40], we suggest that the surge of IL-17A in Ncf1* mice may be the result of a poor regulation of LRRK2-activity in the absence of ROS, thus stressing LRRK2-role in colitis susceptibility. Contrasting to previous reports [41], the increased local and systemic IL-17A-titers were not accompanied by higher systemic IL-1β-titers, but could be partially associated with the higher IL-21 serological concentration in Ncf1*, which stresses an abnormal T cell-activation.

Overall, our data present evidence that a normal production of ROS by a functional NOX2 is essential for the prevention of chronic inflammation leading to severe chronic colitis. The absence of ROS-production appears to promote peroxynitrites formation. The vasodilatatory properties of NO and its capacity to induce pro-inflammatory cytokines (and concomitant LRRK2 phosphorilation), seem to favor the infiltration and activation of leukocytes in the colon mucosa and feed a chronic inflammatory process. Since CGD is caused by point mutations in the NOX2 genes and the disease-associated colitis has a chronic profile, inducing two cycles of colitis with DSS intercalated by a resting period in mice with a point mutation in the *Ncf1* gene, the proposed colitis model presents an excellent model to study how the lack of oxidative burst can lead to the development of IBD with features reminiscent of CGD colitis.

Author Contributions

Conceived and designed the experiments: TRS LC MMSC. Performed the experiments: TRS ARS AFL HC BR AA AC LC. Analyzed the data: TRS ARS BR AC LC MMSC. Contributed reagents/materials/analysis tools: AC LC RH MMSC. Wrote the paper: TRS ARS AA BR RH LC MMSC.

References

1. Deffert C, Carnesecchi S, Yuan H, Rougemont A-L, Kelkka T, et al. (2012) Hyperinflammation of chronic granulomatous disease is abolished by NOX2 reconstitution in macrophages and dendritic cells. The Journal of Pathology: n/a–n/a.
2. Smeekens SP, Henriet SS, Gresnigt MS, Joosten LA, Hermans PW, et al. (2012) Low interleukin-17A production in response to fungal pathogens in patients with chronic granulomatous disease. J Interferon Cytokine Res 32: 159–168.
3. Bleesing JJ, Souto-Carneiro MM, Savage WJ, Brown MR, Martinez C, et al. (2006) Patients with chronic granulomatous disease have a reduced peripheral blood memory B cell compartment. J Immunol 176: 7096–7103.
4. Meissner F, Seger RA, Moshous D, Fischer A, Reichenbach J, et al. (2010) Inflammasome activation in NADPH oxidase defective mononuclear phagocytes from patients with chronic granulomatous disease. Blood 116: 1570–1573.
5. Falcone EL, Holland SM (2012) Invasive fungal infection in chronic granulomatous disease: insights into pathogenesis and management. Curr Opin Infect Dis.
6. Lewis CJ, Cobb BA (2011) Adaptive immune defects against glycoantigens in chronic granulomatous disease via dysregulated nitric oxide production. Eur J Immunol 41: 2562–2572.
7. Vasilevsky S, Liu Q, Koontz SM, Kastenmayer R, Shea K, et al. (2011) Role of p47phox in antigen-presenting cell-mediated regulation of humoral immunity in mice. Am J Pathol 178: 2774–2782.
8. Fernandez-Boyanapalli R, McPhillips KA, Frasch SC, Janssen WJ, Dinauer MC, et al. (2010) Impaired phagocytosis of apoptotic cells by macrophages in chronic granulomatous disease is reversed by IFN-gamma in a nitric oxide-dependent manner. J Immunol 185: 4030–4041.
9. Romani L, Fallarino F, De Luca A, Montagnoli C, D'Angelo C, et al. (2008) Defective tryptophan catabolism underlies inflammation in mouse chronic granulomatous disease. Nature 451: 211–215.
10. Pizzolla A, Hultqvist M, Nilson B, Grimm MJ, Eneljung T, et al. (2012) Reactive oxygen species produced by the NADPH oxidase 2 complex in monocytes protect mice from bacterial infections. J Immunol 188: 5003–5011.
11. Kraaij MD, Savage ND, van der Kooij SW, Koekkoek K, Wang J, et al. (2010) Induction of regulatory T cells by macrophages is dependent on production of reactive oxygen species. Proc Natl Acad Sci U S A 107: 17686–17691.
12. D'Angelo C, De Luca A, Zelante T, Bonifazi P, Moretti S, et al. (2009) Exogenous pentraxin 3 restores antifungal resistance and restrains inflammation in murine chronic granulomatous disease. J Immunol 183: 4609–4618.
13. Gelderman KA, Hultqvist M, Pizzolla A, Zhao M, Nandakumar KS, et al. (2007) Macrophages suppress T cell responses and arthritis development in mice by producing reactive oxygen species. J Clin Invest 117: 3020–3028.
14. Gelderman KA, Hultqvist M, Holmberg J, Olofsson P, Holmdahl R (2006) T cell surface redox levels determine T cell reactivity and arthritis susceptibility. Proc Natl Acad Sci U S A 103: 12831–12836.

15. Yu JE, De Ravin SS, Uzel G, Landers C, Targan S, et al. (2011) High levels of Crohn's disease-associated anti-microbial antibodies are present and independent of colitis in chronic granulomatous disease. Clin Immunol 138: 14–22.

16. Bao S, Carr ED, Xu YH, Hunt NH (2011) Gp91(phox) contributes to the development of experimental inflammatory bowel disease. Immunol Cell Biol 89: 853–860.

17. Conway KL, Goel G, Sokol H, Manocha M, Mizoguchi E, et al. (2012) p40phox expression regulates neutrophil recruitment and function during the resolution phase of intestinal inflammation. J Immunol 189: 3631–3640.

18. Elso CM, Roberts LJ, Smyth GK, Thomson RJ, Baldwin TM, et al. (2004) Leishmaniasis host response loci (lmr1-3) modify disease severity through a Th1/Th2-independent pathway. Genes Immun 5: 93–100.

19. Barrett JC, Hansoul S, Nicolae DL, Cho JH, Duerr RH, et al. (2008) Genome-wide association defines more than 30 distinct susceptibility loci for Crohn's disease. Nat Genet 40: 955–962.

20. Krieglstein CF, Cerwinka WH, Laroux FS, Salter JW, Russell JM, et al. (2001) Regulation of murine intestinal inflammation by reactive metabolites of oxygen and nitrogen: divergent roles of superoxide and nitric oxide. J Exp Med 194: 1207–1218.

21. Mori M, Stokes KY, Vowinkel T, Watanabe N, Elrod JW, et al. (2005) Colonic blood flow responses in experimental colitis: time course and underlying mechanisms. Am J Physiol Gastrointest Liver Physiol 289: G1024–1029.

22. Cooper HS, Murthy SN, Shah RS, Sedergran DJ (1993) Clinicopathologic study of dextran sulfate sodium experimental murine colitis. Lab Invest 69: 238–249.

23. Perse M, Cerar A (2012) Dextran sodium sulphate colitis mouse model: traps and tricks. J Biomed Biotechnol 2012: 718617.

24. Schappi MG, Klein NJ, Lindley KJ, Rampling D, Smith VV, et al. (2003) The nature of colitis in chronic granulomatous disease. J Pediatr Gastroenterol Nutr 36: 623–631.

25. Bento AF, Leite DF, Marcon R, Claudino RF, Dutra RC, et al. (2012) Evaluation of chemical mediators and cellular response during acute and chronic gut inflammatory response induced by dextran sodium sulfate in mice. Biochem Pharmacol.

26. Hall LJ, Faivre E, Quinlan A, Shanahan F, Nally K, et al. (2011) Induction and activation of adaptive immune populations during acute and chronic phases of a murine model of experimental colitis. Dig Dis Sci 56: 79–89.

27. Dieleman LA, Palmen MJ, Akol H, Bloemena E, Pena AS, et al. (1998) Chronic experimental colitis induced by dextran sulphate sodium (DSS) is characterized by Th1 and Th2 cytokines. Clin Exp Immunol 114: 385–391.

28. Jianjun Y, Zhang R, Lu G, Shen Y, Peng L, et al. (2013) T cell-derived inducible nitric oxide synthase switches off Th17 cell differentiation. J Exp Med 210: 1447–1462.

29. Naito Y, Takagi T, Uchiyama K, Kuroda M, Kokura S, et al. (2004) Reduced intestinal inflammation induced by dextran sodium sulfate in interleukin-6-deficient mice. Int J Mol Med 14: 191–196.

30. Yasukawa K, Tokuda H, Tun X, Utsumi H, Yamada K (2012) The detrimental effect of nitric oxide on tissue is associated with inflammatory events in the vascular endothelium and neutrophils in mice with dextran sodium sulfate-induced colitis. Free Radic Res 46: 1427–1436.

31. Talero E, Sanchez-Fidalgo S, Villegas I, de la Lastra CA, Illanes M, et al. (2011) Role of different inflammatory and tumor biomarkers in the development of ulcerative colitis-associated carcinogenesis. Inflamm Bowel Dis 17: 696–710.

32. Asseman C, Mauze S, Leach MW, Coffman RL, Powrie F (1999) An essential role for interleukin 10 in the function of regulatory T cells that inhibit intestinal inflammation. J Exp Med 190: 995–1004.

33. Alex P, Zachos NC, Nguyen T, Gonzales L, Chen TE, et al. (2009) Distinct cytokine patterns identified from multiplex profiles of murine DSS and TNBS-induced colitis. Inflamm Bowel Dis 15: 341–352.

34. Mora JR, Iwata M, Eksteen B, Song SY, Junt T, et al. (2006) Generation of gut-homing IgA-secreting B cells by intestinal dendritic cells. Science 314: 1157–1160.

35. Hosomi S, Oshitani N, Kamata N, Sogawa M, Okazaki H, et al. (2011) Increased numbers of immature plasma cells in peripheral blood specifically overexpress chemokine receptor CXCR3 and CXCR4 in patients with ulcerative colitis. Clin Exp Immunol 163: 215–224.

36. Liu S, Russo PA, Baldassano RN, Sullivan KE (2009) CD68 expression is markedly different in Crohn's disease and the colitis associated with chronic granulomatous disease. Inflamm Bowel Dis 15: 1213–1217.

37. Rivollier A, He J, Kole A, Valatas V, Kelsall BL (2012) Inflammation switches the differentiation program of Ly6Chi monocytes from antiinflammatory macrophages to inflammatory dendritic cells in the colon. J Exp Med 209: 139–155.

38. Liu Z, Lee J, Krummey S, Lu W, Cai H, et al. (2011) The kinase LRRK2 is a regulator of the transcription factor NFAT that modulates the severity of inflammatory bowel disease. Nat Immunol 12: 1063–1070.

39. Weigmann B, Lehr HA, Yancopoulos G, Valenzuela D, Murphy A, et al. (2008) The transcription factor NFATc2 controls IL-6-dependent T cell activation in experimental colitis. J Exp Med 205: 2099–2110.

40. Shih TC, Hsieh SY, Hsieh YY, Chen TC, Yeh CY, et al. (2008) Aberrant activation of nuclear factor of activated T cell 2 in lamina propria mononuclear cells in ulcerative colitis. World J Gastroenterol 14: 1759–1767.

41. Coccia M, Harrison OJ, Schiering C, Asquith MJ, Becher B, et al. (2012) IL-1beta mediates chronic intestinal inflammation by promoting the accumulation of IL-17A secreting innate lymphoid cells and CD4+ Th17 cells. J Exp Med 209: 1595–1609.

PTPN2 Gene Variants are Associated with Susceptibility to Both Crohn's Disease and Ulcerative Colitis Supporting a Common Genetic Disease Background

Jürgen Glas[1,2,3⦵], Johanna Wagner[1,2⦵], Julia Seiderer[1], Torsten Olszak[1,4], Martin Wetzke[1,2,5], Florian Beigel[1], Cornelia Tillack[1], Johannes Stallhofer[1], Matthias Friedrich[1,2], Christian Steib[1], Burkhard Göke[1], Thomas Ochsenkühn[1], Nazanin Karbalai[6], Julia Diegelmann[1,2], Darina Czamara[6], Stephan Brand[1]*

1 Department of Medicine II - Grosshadern, Ludwig-Maximilians-University, Munich, Germany, 2 Department of Preventive Dentistry and Periodontology, Ludwig-Maximilians-University, Munich, Germany, 3 Department of Human Genetics, Rheinisch-Westfälische Technische Hochschule (RWTH), Aachen, Germany, 4 Gastrointestinal Division, Brigham & Women's Hospital, Harvard Medical School, Boston, Massachusetts, United States of America, 5 Department of Pediatrics, Hannover Medical School, Germany, 6 Max-Planck-Institute of Psychiatry, Munich, Germany

Abstract

Background: Genome-wide association studies identified *PTPN2* (protein tyrosine phosphatase, non-receptor type 2) as susceptibility gene for inflammatory bowel diseases (IBD). However, the exact role of *PTPN2* in Crohn's disease (CD) and ulcerative colitis (UC) and its phenotypic effect are unclear. We therefore performed a detailed genotype-phenotype and epistasis analysis of *PTPN2* gene variants.

Methodology/Principal Findings: Genomic DNA from 2131 individuals of Caucasian origin (905 patients with CD, 318 patients with UC, and 908 healthy, unrelated controls) was analyzed for two SNPs in the *PTPN2* region (rs2542151, rs7234029) for which associations with IBD were found in previous studies in other cohorts. Our analysis revealed a significant association of *PTPN2* SNP rs2542151 with both susceptibility to CD ($p = 1.95 \times 10^{-5}$; OR 1.49 [1.34–1.79]) and UC ($p = 3.87 \times 10^{-2}$, OR 1.31 [1.02–1.68]). Moreover, *PTPN2* SNP rs7234029 demonstrated a significant association with susceptibility to CD ($p = 1.30 \times 10^{-3}$; OR 1.35 [1.13–1.62]) and a trend towards association with UC ($p = 7.53 \times 10^{-2}$; OR 1.26 [0.98–1.62]). Genotype-phenotype analysis revealed an association of *PTPN2* SNP rs7234029 with a stricturing disease phenotype (B2) in CD patients ($p = 6.62 \times 10^{-3}$). Epistasis analysis showed weak epistasis between the *ATG16L1* SNP rs2241879 and *PTPN2* SNP rs2542151 ($p = 0.024$) in CD and between *ATG16L1* SNP rs4663396 and *PTPN2* SNP rs7234029 ($p = 4.68 \times 10^{-3}$) in UC. There was no evidence of epistasis between *PTPN2* and *NOD2* and *PTPN2* and *IL23R*. In silico analysis revealed that the SNP rs7234029 modulates potentially the binding sites of several transcription factors involved in inflammation including GATA-3, NF-κB, C/EBP, and E4BP4.

Conclusions/Significance: Our data confirm the association of *PTPN2* variants with susceptibility to both CD and UC, suggesting a common disease pathomechanism for these diseases. Given recent evidence that *PTPN2* regulates autophagosome formation in intestinal epithelial cells, the potential link between *PTPN2* and *ATG16L1* should be further investigated.

Editor: Dominik Hartl, University of Tübingen, Germany

Funding: Dr. Glas was supported by a grant from the Broad Medical Foundation (IBD-0126R2). Dr. Seiderer and Dr. Diegelmann were supported by grants from the Ludwig-Maximilians-University Munich (FöFoLe Nr. 422; Habilitationsstipendium, LMUExcellent to Dr. Stallhofer and Promotionsstipendium to Dr. Diegelmann); Dr. Seiderer was also supported by the Robert-Bosch-Foundation and the Else Kröner-Fresenius-Stiftung (81/08//EKMS08/01). Dr. Brand was supported by grants from the DFG German research Foundation (BR 1912/6-1), the Else Kröner-Fresenius-Stiftung (Else Kröner Exzellenzstipendium 2010; 2010_EKES.32), and by grants of Ludwig-Maximilians-University Munich (Excellence Initiative, Investment Funds 2008 and FöFoLe program). This work contains parts of the unpublished doctoral theses of Dr. Wagner. The funders had no role in study design, data collection and analysis, decision to publish, or preparation of the manuscript.

Competing Interests: The authors have declared that no competing interests exist.

* E-mail: stephan.brand@med.uni-muenchen.de

⦵ These authors contributed equally to this work.

Introduction

Inflammatory bowel diseases (IBD), encompassing Crohn's disease (CD) and ulcerative colitis (UC), are characterized by chronic intestinal inflammation caused by a dysregulated interac-tion with bacterial antigens, resulting in an exaggerated immune response in a genetically predisposed host [1,2]. Genome-wide association studies (GWAS) have substantially improved our understanding of the molecular pathways leading to CD or UC and have so far identified almost 100 distinct genetic loci that confer

Table 1. Demographic characteristics of the IBD study population.

	Crohn's disease	Ulcerative colitis	Controls
	n = 905	n = 318	n = 908
Gender			
Male (%)	48.8	52.2	62.7
Female (%)	51.2	47.8	37.3
Age (yrs)			
Mean ± SD	40.9±13.3	44.2±14.8	45.8±10.3
Range	15–83	17–88	19–68
Body mass index			
Mean ± SD	23.0±4.2	23.9±4.5	
Range	13–41	15–54	
Age at diagnosis (yrs)			
Mean ± SD	26.1±12.4	28.9±14.5	
Range	1–78	2–81	
Disease duration (yrs)			
Mean ± SD	13.4±8.9	12.2±8.3	
Range	0–47	1–50	
Positive family history of IBD (%)	16.7	17.4	

Table 3. Haplotype analysis for the PTPN2 SNPs rs2542151 and rs7234029 in the CD case-control cohort.

PTPN2 SNP1	PTPN2 SNP2	Haplotype	OR	95% CI	p-value
rs2542151	rs7234029	GG	1.42	1.04–1.93	1.46×10^{-3}
rs2542151	rs7234029	TG	1.18	0.82–1.71	2.93×10^{-1}
rs2542151	rs7234029	GA	1.45	0.92–2.32	1.88×10^{-2}
rs2542151	rs7234029	TA	0.70	0.62–0.80	2.37×10^{-5}

OR = odds ratio; 95% CI = 95% confidence interval.

Table 4. Haplotype analysis for the PTPN2 SNPs rs2542151 and rs7234029 in the UC case-control cohort.

PTPN2 SNP1	PTPN2 SNP2	Haplotype	OR	95% CI	p-value
rs2542151	rs7234029	GG	1.21	0.83–1.77	0.220
rs2542151	rs7234029	TG	1.34	0.77–2.33	0.147
rs2542151	rs7234029	GA	1.37	0.76–2.47	0.151
rs2542151	rs7234029	TA	0.76	0.63–0.91	0.015

OR = odds ratio; 95% CI = 95% confidence interval.

IBD susceptibility including novel pathways involved in autophagy, innate immune response and proinflammatory IL-23/Th17 cell activation [3,4,5,6,7,8,9]. However, for many of the gene regions identified by GWAS, there is still lack of functional data and limited knowledge how these gene variants modify the IBD phenotype.

One of the recent candidate genes identified by GWAS is protein tyrosine phosphatase non-receptor type 2 (PTPN2), encoding the enzyme tyrosine-protein phosphatase non-receptor type 2, a member of the protein tyrosine kinases (PTP) superfamily. So far, two isoforms of PTPN2 generated from alternative splicing have been identified: a major TC45 isoform (45 kDa) containing a nuclear localization sequence and a less abundant TC48 isoform (48 kDa) anchored to the endoplasmic reticulum [10]. For TC45, various targets including Janus kinases (JAKs), signal transducer and activator of transcription (STAT) 1 and 3, p42/44 mitogen-activated protein kinase (MAPK) (extracellular signal–related kinase [ERK]), epidermal growth factor receptor (EGFR) as well as insulin receptor β (IRβ) [11,12,13,14] have been identified. So far, PTPN2 has been shown to be a susceptibility gene for celiac disease and for diabetes modifying

beta-cell responses to viral RNA and apoptosis [15,16,17]. Recent GWAS identified PTPN2 as susceptibility gene for CD [18,19,20,21], while a GWAS meta-analyses in UC patients showed also an association with UC [22]. Interestingly, an analysis in a Dutch-Belgian cohort [23] revealed that the PTPN2 SNP rs2542151 was only moderately CD-associated in a CD subcohort of smokers (p = 0.04), but not in the entire cohort or in the non-smoking CD cohort, implicating additional modifying factors requiring further functional analysis and replication studies.

Given the overall lack of detailed phenotype analyses of PTPN2 in IBD, we initiated an extensive genotype-phenotype analysis in a large German cohort of IBD patients including 905 patients with CD, 318 patients with UC, and 908 healthy, unrelated controls which were genotyped for the two SNPs rs2542151 and rs7234029 in the PTPN2 region. Based on a pathway analysis of gene relationships across implicated loci (GRAIL) of a recent GWAS meta-analysis in CD demonstrating a potential interaction between the PTPN2-related gene PTPN22 and NOD2 [19], we also performed analysis for gene-gene interaction between PTPN2 and NOD2 regarding CD susceptibility. Moreover, considering that PTPN2 gene variants are - similar to IL23R gene variants -

Table 2. Associations of PTPN2 gene markers in the CD and UC case-control cohorts.

PTPN2 SNP	Minor allele	Crohn's disease			Ulcerative colitis			Controls
		n = 905			n = 318			n = 908
		MAF	p value	OR [95% CI]	MAF	p value	OR [95% CI]	MAF
rs2542151	G	0.182	1.95×10^{-5}	1.49 [1.34–1.79]	0.164	3.87×10^{-2}	1.31 [1.02–1.68]	0.130
rs7234029	G	0.177	1.30×10^{-3}	1.35 [1.13–1.62]	0.167	7.53×10^{-2}	1.26 [0.98–1.62]	0.137

Minor allele frequencies (MAF), allelic test P-values, and odds ratios (OR, shown for the minor allele) with 95% confidence intervals (CI) are depicted for both the CD and UC case-control cohorts.

Table 5. Genotype-phenotype associations of the *PTPN2* SNP rs2542151 in CD patients.

PTPN2 SNP rs2542151	TT (*n=611*)	TG (*n=258*)	GG (*n=36*)	P_G	OR_G [95% CI]
Age at diagnosis (yr) (*n=817*)					
Mean ± SD	25.32±11.91	28.06±13.48	25.19±9.61	5.96×10^{-2}	0.75
Range	1–71	2–78	15–49		[0.56–1.01]
Age at diagnosis (*n=817*)					
<=16 years (A1)	126 (22.7%)	38 (16.1%)	4 (14.8%)	4.53×10^{-2}	0.67 [0.45–0.99]
(*n=168*)					(A1 vs. A2)
17–40 years (A2)	368 (66.4%)	161 (68.2%)	22 (81.5%)	0.285	0.79 [0.50–1.22]
(*n=551*)					(A2 vs. A3)
>40 years (A3)	60 (10.8%)	37 (15.7%)	1 (3.7%)	1.89×10^{-2}	0.53 [0.31–0.90]
(*n=98*)					(A1 vs. A3)
Location (*n=770*)					
Terminal ileum (L1) (*n=113*)	73 (14.3%)	33 (14.4%)	7 (21.9%)	0.715	1.08 [0.71–1.64]
Colon (L2)	62 (12.2%)	31 (13.5%)	4 (12.5%)	0.627	1.17
(*n=97*)					[0.72–1.74]
Ileocolon (L3)	366 (71.9%)	163 (71.2%)	21 (65.6%)	0.682	0.93
(*n=550*)					[0.67–1.30]
Upper GI (L4)	8 (1.6%)	2 (0.9%)	0 (0%)	0.360	0.48
(*n=10*)					[0.10–2.29]
Behaviour (*n=747*)					
Non-stricturing/Non-penetrating (B1)	111 (24.3%)	49 (23.6%)	12 (42.9%)	0.645	1.08
(*n=172*)					[0.76–1.55]
Stricturing (B2)	123 (27.0%)	57 (27.4%)	7 (25.0%)	0.941	1.01
(*n=187*)					[0.71–1.44]
Penetrating	222 (48.7%)	102 (49.0%)	9 (32.1%)	0.729	0.95
(B3) (*n=333*)					[0.70–1.29]
Use of immunosuppressive agents	no: 65 (16.6%)	35 (20.3%)	5 (22.7%)	0.237	0.77
(*n=585*)	yes: 326 (83.4%)	137 (79.7%)	17 (77.3%)		[0.50–1.19]
Surgery because of CD	no: 265 (48.7%)	106 (44.7%)	19 (59.4%)	0.547	1.09
(*n=813*)	yes: 279 (51.3%)	131 (55.3%)	13 (40.6%)		[0.82–1.47]
Fistulas	no: 290 (52.3%)	121 (50.2%)	18 (56.3%)	0.699	1.06
(*n=827*)	yes: 264 (47.7%)	120 (49.8%)	14 (43.8%)		[0.79–1.42]
Stenosis	no: 234 (42.0%)	90 (37.5%)	16 (50.0%)	0.404	1.13
(*n=829*)	yes: 323 (58.0%)	150 (62.5%)	16 (50.0%)		[0.84–1.53]

PG: p-value for association comparing carriers of the G-allele to individuals homozygous for T. Association results for age at diagnosis are based on median split. Uncorrected p-values<0.05 are depicted in bold. None of the p-values remained significant after Bonferroni correction for multiple testing (number of hypothesis tested: n=15, resulting in a significance threshold of $p<3.33 \times 10^{-3}$).

associated with a number of autoimmune diseases such as juvenile idiopathic arthritis [24] or type 1 diabetes [17], we also analysed for epistasis between *PTPN2* and *IL23R*. In addition, a very recent study suggests that *PTPN2* regulates autophagosome formation in intestinal epithelial cells [25]. We therefore analyzed also for potential epistasis with the CD susceptibility gene *ATG16L1*.

Methods

Ethics statement

Before participating in the study, all patients gave written, informed consent. In case of minors, patients' parents gave written consent. The Ethics committee of the Medical Faculty of Ludwig-Maximilians-University Munich approved this study. The study

protocol was in accordance with the ethical principles for medical research involving human subjects of the Helsinki Declaration.

Study population and genotype-phenotype analysis

Overall, 2131 individuals of Caucasian origin including 905 CD patients, 318 UC patients, and 908 healthy, unrelated controls were included in the study population. Patients with indeterminate colitis were excluded from the study. For phenotype analysis, the demographic and clinical data (behaviour and location of IBD, disease-related complications, surgical history or immunosuppressive therapy) of the patients were recorded by patient chart analysis and a detailed questionnaire including an interview at time of enrolment. The demographic characteristics of the IBD study population were collected blind to the results of the genotype

Table 6. Genotype-phenotype associations of the *PTPN2* SNP rs7234029 in CD patients.

PTPN2 SNP rs7234029	AA (n = 612)	AG (n = 253)	GG (n = 32)	P$_G$	OR$_G$ [95% CI]
Age at diagnosis (yr) (n = 811)					
Mean ± SD	25.80±12.36	26.77±12.40	25.73±12.52	0.197	0.82
Range	1–71	6–78	12–64		[0.61–1.11]
Age at diagnosis (n = 811)					
<= 16 years (A1) (n = 168)	124 (22.5%)	36 (15.3%)	8 (30.8%)	**4.25×10^{-2}**	0.67 [0.46–0.99] (A1 vs. A2)
17–40 years (A2) (n = 546)	357 (64.9%)	173 (73.6%)	16 (61.5%)	0.271	1.30 [0.81–2.09] (A2 vs. A3)
>40 years (A3) (n = 97)	69 (12.5%)	26 (11.1%)	2 (7.7%)	0.637	0.87 [0.50–1.53] (A1 vs. A3)
Location (n = 764)					
Term. ileum (L1) (n = 113)	76 (14.8%)	29 (12.6%)	8 (38.1%)	0.978	0.99 [0.65–1.52]
Colon (L2) (n = 96)	64 (12.5%)	30 (13.0%)	2 (9.5%)	0.915	1.03 [0.65–1.61]
Ileocolon (L3) (n = 545)	364 (71.0%)	170 (73.9%)	11 (52.4%)	0.740	1.06 [0.76–1.48]
Upper GI (L4) (n = 10)	9 (1.8%)	1 (0.4%)	0 (0%)	0.157	0.22 [0.03–1.78]
Behaviour (n = 686)					
Non-stricturing -Non-penetrating (B1) (n = 170)	116 (25.4%)	49 (23.0%)	8 (42.1%)	0.682	0.93 [0.64–1.34]
Stricturing (B2) (n = 187)	110 (24.1%)	72 (33.8%)	5 (26.3%)	**6.62×10^{-3}**	1.61 [1.14–2.27]
Penetrating (B3) (n = 329)	231 (50.5%)	92 (43.2%)	6 (31.6%)	9.06×10^{-2}	0.76 [0.56–1.04]
Use of immuno-suppressive agents (n = 580)	no: 67 (17.2%)	33 (18.8%)	5 (33.3%)	0.433	0.84 [0.54–1.30]
	yes: 322 (82.8%)	143 (81.3%)	10 (66.7%)		
Surgery because of CD (n = 807)	no: 260 (47.6%)	111 (47.2%)	16 (61.5%)	0.782	0.96 [0.71–1.29]
	yes: 286 (52.4%)	124 (52.8%)	10 (38.5%)		
Fistulas (n = 821)	no: 281 (50.4%)	128 (54.2%)	18 (66.7%)	0.168	0.81 [0.61–1.09]
	yes: 277 (49.6%)	108 (45.8%)	9 (33.3%)		
Stenosis (n = 823)	no: 239 (42.8%)	82 (34.3%)	16 (61.5%)	0.111	1.28
	yes: 319 (57.2%)	157 (65.7%)	10 (38.5%)		[0.95–1.72]

PG: p-value for association comparing carriers of the G-allele to individuals homozygous for A. Association results for age at diagnosis are based on median split. Uncorrected p-values<0.05 are depicted in bold. None of the p-values remained significant after Bonferroni correction for multiple testing (number of hypothesis tested: n = 15, resulting in a significance threshold of p<3.33×10^{-3}).

analyses (Table 1). The diagnosis of CD or UC was determined according to established guidelines based on endoscopic, radiological, and histopathological criteria [26]. In CD patients, the Montreal classification based on the age at diagnosis (A), location (L), and behaviour (B) of disease [27] was used for assessment. In patients with UC, anatomic location was also based on the Montreal classification using the criteria ulcerative proctitis (E1), left-sided UC (distal UC; E2), and extensive UC (pancolitis; E3).

DNA extraction and genotyping of the PTPN2 variants

From all study participants, blood samples were taken and genomic DNA was isolated from peripheral blood leukocytes using the DNA blood mini kit from Qiagen (Hilden, Germany) according to the manufacturer's guidelines. The two *PTPN2* SNPs rs2542151 and rs7234029 were genotyped by PCR and melting curve analysis using a pair of fluorescence resonance energy transfer (FRET) probes in a LightCycler® 480 Instrument (Roche Diagnostics, Mannheim, Germany) as described in detail in previous studies [28,29,30, 31,32,33]. The *PTPN2* SNP rs2542151 was selected from the GWAS by Parkes et al. [18] and the Wellcome Trust Case Control Consortium (WTCCC) [20], while the rs7234029 was chosen from the study of Thompson et al. [24]. All sequences of primers and FRET probes and primer annealing temperatures used for genotyping and for sequence analysis are given in tables S1 and S2.

Genotyping of NOD2, IL23R and ATG16L1 variants

Genotyping data of the three main CD-associated *NOD2* variants p.Arg702Trp (rs2066844), p.Gly908Arg (rs2066845), and p.Leu1007fsX1008 (rs2066847) as well as genotyping data of 10 *IL23R* SNPs (rs1004819, rs7517847, rs10489629, rs2201841, rs11465804, rs11209026 = p.Arg381Gln, rs1343151, rs10889677, rs11209032, rs1495965) were available from previous studies [28],[34,35,36] Nine *ATG16L1* variants (rs13412102, rs12471449, rs6431660, rs1441090, rs2289472, rs2241880 [= p.Thr300Ala], rs2241879, rs3792106, rs4663396) have also been genotyped in a previous study [29]. For all genotyping protocols, primer and probe sequences are available on request.

In silico analysis of transcription factor binding sites

We performed an *in silico* analysis for potential changes in transcription factor binding sites caused by the *PTPN2* SNPs rs2542151 and rs7234029 using the online tool TFSEARCH (http://www.cbrc.jp/research/db/TFSEARCH.html). This tool is based on the TRANSFAC database which was developed at GBF Braunschweig, Germany [37]. We used a threshold score for binding sites of 75.0 (score = 100.0 * ('weighted sum' - min)/(max - min); max. score = 100). For both *PTPN2* SNPs, major and minor alleles including the flanking sequences 10 bp upstream and downstream were investigated for potential changes of binding sites of human transcription factors.

Table 7. Genotype-phenotype associations of the *PTPN2* SNP rs2542151 in UC patients.

PTPN2 SNP rs2542151	TT (*n = 226*)	TG (*n = 80*)	GG (*n = 12*)	P$_G$	OR$_G$ [95% CI]
Gender *(n = 318)*					
Male	125 (55.3%)	36 (45.0%)	5 (41.7%)	8.03×10^{-2}	1.54 [0.95–2.51]
Female	101 (44.7%)	44 (55.0%)	7 (58.3%)		
Age at diagnosis (yrs) *(n = 302)*					
Mean ± SD	29.45±14.60	27.95±14.13	25.08±15.54	0.253	1.34 [0.81–2.21]
Range	2–81	4–73	9–68		
Age at diagnosis *(n = 302)*					
<= 16 years (A1) *(n = 59)*	41 (19.1%)	16 (21.3%)	2 (16.7%)	0.926	0.97 [0.51–1.83] (A1 vs. A2)
17–40 years (A2) *(n = 183)*	126 (58.6%)	49 (65.3%)	8 (66.7%)	9.95×10^{-2}	1.81 [0.89–3.67] (A2 vs. A3)
>40 years (A3) *(n = 60)*	48 (22.3%)	10 (13.3%)	2 (16.7%)	0.189	1.76 [0.76–4.07] (A1 vs. A3)
BMI (kg/m²) *(n = 209)*					
Mean ± SD	23.92±4.74	23.87±3.83	23.67±4.71	0.995	1.00 [0.55–1.82]
Range	15–54	16–36	15–30		
Location *(n = 200)*					
Proctitis (E1) *(n = 24)*	15 (12.0%)	7 (10.6%)	2 (22.2%)	0.329	1.55 [0.64–3.70]
Left-sided UC (E2) *(n = 96)*	73 (58.4%)	20 (30.3%)	3 (33.3%)	0.184	0.68 [0.38–1.20]
Extensive UC (E3) *(n = 80)*	37 (29.6%)	39 (59.1%)	4 (44.4%)	0.473	1.22 [0.83–1.80]
Extra-intestinal manifestations *(n = 191)*	no: 87 (64.4%)	33 (68.8%)	5 (62.5%)	0.652	0.86 [0.44–1.66]
	yes:48 (35.6%)	15 (31.3%)	3 (37.5%)		
Use of immuno-suppressive agents	no: 50 (26.0%)	14 (20.9%)	2 (22.2%)	0.394	1.32 [0.70–2.50]
(n = 268)	yes: 142 (74.0%)	53 (79.1%)	7 (77.8%)		
Abscesses *(n = 240)*	no: 160 (96.4%)	61 (93.8%)	7 (77.8%)	0.151	2.35 [0.73–7.56]
	yes: 6 (3.6%)	4 (6.2%)	2 (22.2%)		

PG: p-value for association comparing carriers of the G-allele to individuals homozygous for A. Association results for age at diagnosis and BMI are based on median split. None of the p-values remained significant after Bonferroni correction for multiple testing (number of hypothesis tested: n = 12, resulting in a significance threshold of p<4.167×10^{-3}).

Statistical analyses

For data evaluation, we used the SPSS 13.0 software (SPSS Inc., Chicago, IL, U.S.A.) and R-2.13.1. (http://cran.r-project.org). Each genetic marker was tested for Hardy-Weinberg equilibrium in the control population. Fisher's exact test was used for comparison between categorical variables. All tests were two-tailed, considering p-values<0.05 as significant. Odds ratios were calculated for the minor allele at each SNP. Bonferroni correction was applied by calculating the threshold for statistically significant p-values as follows: p = 0.05/n, in which n gives the number of hypotheses tested. The number of tests applied (n) and the threshold for statistically significant p-values are given in the legends for all tables in which Bonferroni correction was applied. Epistasis between different SNPs was tested using the –epistasis option in PLINK (http://pngu.mgh.harvard.edu/~purcell/plink/). Haplotype based association analysis was done with PLINK using the –hap-logistic option. The two significant SNPs (rs2542151 and rs7234029) of the single-marker association study were taken into a logistic regression model for haplotype specific associations. Genotype-phenotype associations were assessed using logistic regression analysis in R.

Results

PTPN2 gene variants are associated with the susceptibility to both CD and UC

In all three subgroups (CD, UC, and controls), the allele frequencies of the *PTPN2* SNPs (rs2542151 and rs7234029) were in accordance with the predicted Hardy-Weinberg equilibrium (Table 2). Our analysis revealed a significant association of the *PTPN2* SNP rs2542151 with both susceptibility to CD (p = 1.95×10^{-5}; OR 1.49 [1.34–1.79]) and UC (p = 3.87×10^{-2}, OR 1.31 [1.02–1.68]). Moreover, the *PTPN2* SNP rs7234029 demonstrated a significant association with susceptibility to CD (p = 1.30×10^{-3}; OR 1.35 [1.13–1.62]) and a trend towards association with UC (p = 7.53×10^{-2}; OR 1.26 [0.98–1.62]), suggesting *PTPN2* as common susceptibility gene for both CD and UC in the German population.

Haplotype analysis

Next, we analyzed haplotypes formed by the *PTPN2* SNPs rs2542151 and rs7234029 using a logistic regression model for haplotype-specific associations. The results in table 3 indicate the strongest association with CD for the TA haplotype with p = 2.37×10^{-5}. There were similar results for UC with a p-value of p = 1.52×10^{-2} for the TA haplotype (Table 4).

Genotype-phenotype analysis

Genotype-phenotype analysis (Tables 5, 6, 7, 8) revealed an association of *PTPN2* SNP rs7234029 with a stricturing disease phenotype (B2) in CD patients (p = 6.62×10^{-3}; Table 6). In addition, there were weak associations of the same SNP with an early onset (A1) of CD (p = 4.25×10^{-2}; Table 6). Similarly, *PTPN2* SNP rs7234029 modulates disease onset of UC (for A2: p = 3.47×10^{-2}; for A3: p = 2.51×10^{-2}; Table 8). In addition, we found an association of this SNP with the risk for abscess

Table 8. Genotype-phenotype associations of the *PTPN2* SNP rs7234029 in UC patients.

PTPN2 SNP rs7234029	AA *(n = 220)*	AG *(n = 83)*	GG *(n = 11)*	P$_G$	OR$_G$ [95% CI]
Gender *(n = 314)*					
Male	119 (54.1%)	42 (50.6%)	5 (45.5%)	0.506	1.18 [0.73–1.91]
Female	101 (45.9%)	41 (49.4%)	6 (54.5%)		
Age at diagnosis (yrs) *(n = 298)*					
Mean ± SD	29.95±14.90	26.32±13.49	30.50±12.70	0.401	1.24 [0.75–2.05]
Range	3–81	2–73	14–57		
Age at diagnosis *(n = 298)*					
<16 years (A1) *(n = 57)*	37 (17.5%)	19 (25.0%)	1 (10.0%)	0.558	1.21 [0.64–2.26] (A1 vs. A2)
17–40 years (A2) *(n = 181)*	125 (59.0%)	49 (64.5%)	7 (70.0%)	**3.47×10^{-2}**	2.24 [1.06–4.73] (A2 vs. A3)
>40 years (A3) *(n = 60)*	50 (23.6%)	8 (10.5%)	2 (20.0%)	**2.51×10^{-2}**	2.70 [1.13–6.45] (A1 vs. A3)
BMI (kg/m²) *(n = 207)*					
Mean ± SD	23.97±4.66	24.10±4.26	22.90±3.18	0.975	0.99 [0.54–1.82]
Range	15–54	15–36	20–29		
Location *(n = 258)*					
Proctitis (E1) *(n = 24)*	13 (7.2%)	11 (16.4%)	0 (0%)	7.75×10^{-2}	2.15 [0.92–5.05]
Left-sided UC (E2) *(n = 96)*	71 (39.2%)	20 (29.9%)	5 (50.0%)	0.305	0.74 [0.42–1.31]
Extensive UC (E3) *(n = 138)*	97 (53.6%)	36 (53.7%)	5 (50.0%)	0.960	0.99 [0.58–1.68]
Extra-intestinal manifestations *(n = 188)*	no: 87 (66.4%)	33 (63.5%)	3 (60.0%)	0.666	1.15 [0.60–2.21]
	yes: 44 (33.6%)	19 (36.5%)	2 (40.0%)		
Use of immunosuppressive agents *(n = 266)*	no: 50 (26.5%)	15 (22.4%)	1 (10.0%)	0.332	1.37 [0.72–2.60]
	yes: 139 (73.5%)	52 (77.6%)	9 (90.0%)		
Abscesses *(n = 238)*	no: 161 (97.0%)	58 (92.1%)	7 (77.8%)	**3.94×10^{-2}**	3.47 [1.06–11.32]
	yes: 5 (3.0%)	5 (7.9%)	2 (22.2%)		

PG: p-value for association comparing carriers of the G-allele to individuals homozygous for A. Association results for age at diagnosis and BMI are based on median split. Uncorrected p-values<0.05 are depicted in bold. None of the p-values remained significant after Bonferroni correction for multiple testing (number of hypothesis tested: n = 12, resulting in a significance threshold of p<4.167×10^{-3}).

formation (p = 3.94×10^{-2}) in UC (Table 8). However, none of these associations remained significant after Bonferroni correction.

Analysis for epistasis between PTPN2 and the main CD susceptibility genes NOD2, IL23R and ATG16L1

In addition, we analyzed for potential epistasis between *PTPN2* and the three main CD susceptibility genes *NOD2*, *IL23R* and *ATG16L1*, given recent evidence for a potential functional interaction between these genes. For example, GRAIL analysis identified a link between the *PTPN2*-related gene *PTPN22* and *NOD2* [19]. In addition, *PTPN2* regulates autophagosome formation in human intestinal epithelials cells, suggesting a potential link to *ATG16L1* [25]. Epistasis analysis demonstrated weak epistasis between the *ATG16L1* SNP rs2241879 and *PTPN2* SNP rs2542151 (p = 0.024) in the CD cohort (Table 9) and between *ATG16L1* SNP rs4663396 and *PTPN2* SNP rs7234029 (p = 4.68×10^{-3}) in the UC cohort (Table 10). However, significance of these associations was lost after correcting for multiple testing (Bonferroni correction). In addition, there was no evidence for epistasis between *PTPN2* and CD-associated variants in the *NOD2* and *IL23R* genes.

In silico analysis of PTPN2 SNPs identifies differences in potential transcription factor binding sites caused by SNP rs7234029

Finally, we investigated if the two *PTPN2* SNPs (including the surrounding sequences as detailed in the Methods section) result in

changes of transcription factor binding sites. This *in silico* analysis demonstrated for SNP rs7234029 differences between major and minor allele regarding the binding probability of several transcription factors including GATA-1, GATA-2, GATA-3, HSF2, NF-κB, C/EBP, E4BP4, SREBP, and HLF. While the transcription factors GATA-1, GATA-2, GATA-3 and HSF2 were predicted to bind with very high probability to the sequence comprising the major A allele, predicted binding to the minor G allele was substantially lower (Table 11). In contrast, the binding score for the transcription factors NF- κB, C/EBP, E4BP4, SREBP, and HLF were higher for the minor G allele. The details of this analysis are shown in table 11. In contrast, no major changes regarding transcription factor binding sites were found for SNP rs2542151 which is located approximately 5.5 kb downstream of *PTPN2* (data not shown).

Discussion

Our detailed analysis of a large IBD cohort demonstrates that *PTPN2* is a common susceptibility gene for both CD and UC, adding *PTPN2* to the growing list of common susceptibility genes of CD and UC. So far, 99 IBD susceptibility genes have been identified (n = 71 in CD and n = 47 in UC) [19,22]. At least 28 susceptibility loci, including *PTPN2*, are shared between CD and UC [19,22]. Our results confirm previous studies in which *PTPN2* has been shown to be associated with CD [18,19,20,21]. A very recent meta-analysis of UC susceptibility genes by Anderson et al.

Table 9. Analysis for epistasis between *PTPN2* SNPs and gene markers located in *NOD2, IL23R* and *ATG16L1* in the CD-case control population.

Epistasis between	*PTPN2* SNP rs2542151	*PTPN2* SNP rs7234029
NOD2 SNPs		
rs2066844 (p.Arg702Trp)	0.607	0.498
rs2066845 (p.Gly908Arg	0.219	0.916
rs2066847(p.Leu1007fsX1008)	0.208	0.276
IL23R SNPs		
rs1004819	0.556	0.244
rs7517847	0.723	0.916
rs10489629	0.395	0.642
rs2201841	0.303	0.414
rs11465804	0.485	0.887
rs11209026 (p.Arg381Gln)	0.943	0.754
rs1343151	0.277	0.978
rs10889677	0.508	0.417
rs11209032	0.213	0.290
rs1495965	9.86×10^{-2}	0.258
ATG16L1 SNPs		
rs13412102	0.620	0.358
rs12471449	0.419	0.383
rs6431660	5.73×10^{-2}	0.394
rs1441090	0.389	0.437
rs2289472	0.102	0.404
rs2241880 (p.Thr300Ala)	8.07×10^{-2}	0.570
rs2241879	**2.37×10^{-2}**	0.382
rs3792106	0.303	0.930
rs4663396	9.76×10^{-2}	0.109

Uncorrected p-values<0.05 are depicted in bold. None of the p-values remained significant after Bonferroni correction for multiple testing (number of hypothesis tested: n = 44, resulting in a significance threshold of $p < 1.136 \times 10^{-3}$).

Table 10. Epistasis between *PTPN2* SNPs and gene markers located in *NOD2, IL23R* and *ATG16L1* in the UC-case control population.

Epistasis between	*PTPN2* SNP rs2542151	*PTPN2* SNP rs7234029
NOD2 SNPs		
rs2066844 (p.Arg702Trp)	0.611	0.219
rs2066845 (p.Gly908Arg	0.385	0.555
rs2066847(p.Leu1007fsX1008)	0.137	0.522
IL23R SNPs		
rs1004819	0.869	0.425
rs7517847	0.561	0.972
rs10489629	0.177	0.844
rs2201841	0.711	0.421
rs11465804	0.465	0.265
rs11209026 (p.Arg381Gln)	0.471	0.831
rs1343151	0.525	0.331
rs10889677	0.889	0.303
rs11209032	0.649	0.330
rs1495965	0.847	0.740
ATG16L1 SNPs		
rs13412102	0.553	0.749
rs12471449	0.762	8.21×10^{-2}
rs6431660	0.298	0.104
rs1441090	0.455	0.544
rs2289472	0.392	0.100
rs2241880 (p.Thr300Ala)	0.536	0.615
rs2241879	0.345	0.423
rs3792106	0.787	0.714
rs4663396	0.217	**4.68×10^{-3}**

Uncorrected p-values<0.05 are depicted in bold. None of the p-values remained significant after Bonferroni correction for multiple testing (number of hypothesis tested: n = 44, resulting in a significance threshold of $p < 1.136 \times 10^{-3}$).

reported also an association of *PTPN2* (rs1893217) with UC [22], suggesting that *PTPN2* is a susceptibility gene for both UC and CD which is in complete agreement with the results of our study. The *PTPN2* variant rs1893217, which has been shown to be associated with IBD in several studies [19,22], is in complete linkage disequilibrium with the *PTPN2* SNP rs2542151, which was investigated in our study. In a smaller analysis from New Zealand, an association of *PTPN2* with CD but not of *PTPN22* could be shown [38]. Studies in an Italian cohort [39] and in a Dutch-Belgian cohort [40] also reported *PTPN2* to be a susceptibility gene for CD.

In addition, we performed a detailed genotype-phenotype analysis. Genotype-phenotype analysis revealed an association of *PTPN2* SNP rs7234029 with a stricturing disease phenotype in CD patients. In addition, we found evidence for weak associations of rs7234029 and rs2542151 with the age of IBD onset. However, after Bonferroni correction, most of these associations lost significance arguing against a strong disease-modifying role for *PTPN2* such as shown for *NOD2*. Considering that *PTPN2* predisposes to both CD and UC, someone may hypothesize that it would be associated with a predominant colonic disease location;

however, we were unable to show such an association in our detailed genotype-phenotype analysis.

Moreover, we performed epistasis analysis investigating potential gene-gene interactions between *PTPN2* and the three main CD susceptibility genes *NOD2, IL23R* and *ATG16L1*. A recent GWAS meta-analysis demonstrated for these three genes the strongest association of all 71 identified CD risk genes with CD susceptibility [19]. However, there was no epistasis between *PTPN2* and *IL23R*, although both genes predispose to autoimmune diseases. For example, associations of *IL23R* could be shown for CD and UC [3,19], psoriasis [41] and ankylosing spondylitis [42]. *PTPN2* is associated with juvenile idiopathic arthritis [24], rheumatoid arthritis, celiac disease [19,43], type 1 diabetes [20,44] and Graves' disease [44], providing an explanation for the increased incidence of several of these diseases in IBD patients.

In contrast, epistasis analysis demonstrated evidence for weak epistasis between the *ATG16L1* SNP rs2241879 and *PTPN2* SNP rs2542151 (p = 0.024) in the CD cohort and between *ATG16L1* SNP rs4663396 and *PTPN2* SNP rs7234029 (p = 4.68×10^{-3}) in the UC cohort, which, however, was lost after Bonferroni correction. Previous studies, including work from our own group

Table 11. Potential transcription factor binding sites in the genomic region harboring the *PTPN2* SNP rs7234029.

Transcription factor	Binding score major allele (A)	Binding score minor allele (G)	Consensus sequence	Position relative to SNP
GATA-X	**95.2**	**80.1**	NGATAAGNMNN	−2 to +8
GATA-1	94.8	80.2	NNCWGATARNNNN	−5 to +7
GATA-2	85.8	65.8	NNNGATRNNN	−4 to +5
GATA-3	83.4	64.1	NNGATARNG	−3 to +5
HSF2	75.0	62.2	NGAANNWTCK	−3 to +6
NF-κB	**68.5**	**79.4**	GGGAMTTYCC	−1 to +8
C/EBP	69.5	78.5	NGWNTKNKGYAAKNSAYA	−8 to +9
E4BP4	**65.7**	**76.0**	NRTTAYGTAAYN	−6 to +5
SREBP	67.2	75.0	NATCACGTGAY	−6 to +4
HLF	66.9	75.0	RTTACTYAAT	−5 to +4

The potential transcription factor binding sites were analyzed *in silico* with the program TFSEARCH (http://www.cbrc.jp/research/db/TFSEARCH.html.). Only binding sites with binding score differing more that 5 points between the two alleles are presented. Scores differing more than 10 points are depicted in bold. The binding score threshold for each allele was set to 75.0.
Nucleotide codes: K = G or T, M = A or C, R = A or G, S = C or G, W = A or T, N = A, G, C or T.

[29], indicate that autophagy genes such as *ATG16L1* and *IRGM* play an important role in CD susceptibility and not UC susceptibility. Given the epistasis between the *ATG16L1* SNP rs4663396 and the *PTPN2* SNP rs7234029 in the UC cohort, our study suggests that autophagy genes may have – in combination with "true" UC susceptibility genes such as *PTPN2* - also a role in UC susceptibility. However, the rather weak epistasis between these two genes needs further confirmation in large replication studies.

The potential epistasis between *PTPN2* and *ATG16L1* would be highly interesting, given very recent evidence that PTPN2 regulates autophagosome formation in human intestinal epithelial cells [25]. Scharl *et al.* showed that knockdown of *PTPN2* causes impaired autophagosome formation and dysfunctional autophagy [25]. This resulted in increased levels of intracellular *Listeria monocytogenes* and enhanced apoptosis of intestinal epithelial cells in response to TNF-α and IFN-γ [25]. Similar results were found in primary colonic lamina propria fibroblasts isolated from CD patients who were carriers of the CD-associated *PTPN2* SNP rs2542151 [25] which was the most strongly CD-associated SNP in our study. In the study by Scharl *et al.*, presence of the CD-associated *ATG16L1* SNP rs2241880 prevented the TNF-α/IFN-γ-mediated increase in PTPN2 protein expression which resulted in impaired autophagosome formation [25]. Interestingly, intestinal biopsies from CD patients with either CD-associated *ATG16L1* or *PTPN2* SNPs showed aberrant expression patterns of LC3B, a marker for autophagic membranes [25]. Scharl *et al.* therefore hypothesized that the combined dysfunction of the CD susceptibility genes *PTPN2* and *ATG16L1* may contribute to the pathogenesis of CD [25]. Our results demonstrating epistasis between CD-associated *PTPN2* and *ATG16L1* gene variants support this hypothesis. In addition, it has been shown that *PTPN2* regulates muramyl dipeptide (MDP)-induced autophagosome formation [45]. These experiments also demonstrated that the CD-associated *PTPN2* variant rs1893217 impairs autophagy [45]. Given the physical interaction of ATG16L1 and the MDP receptor NOD2 during autophagy [46], CD-associated *PTPN2* variants may increase the CD risk by interfering with ATG16L1-/NOD2-mediated autophagy. In addition, GRAIL analysis identified a link between the *PTPN2*-related gene *PTPN22* and *NOD2* [19]. However, we were unable to demonstrate epistasis between

PTPN2 and the three main CD-associated *NOD2* variants p.Arg702Trp (rs2066844), p.Gly908Arg (rs2066845), and p.Leu1007fsX1008 (rs2066847) on a genetic level. Additional studies suggest that PTPN2 plays an overall protective role in the intestine, particularly by limiting IFN-γ-induced signaling and consequent barrier defects [47] as well as by modulating TNF-α responses [48].

To further elucidate the potential functional consequences by which *PTPN2* SNPs modulate IBD susceptibility, we performed an *in silico* analysis regarding potential changes in binding sites for transcription factors. This analysis revealed that the SNP rs7234029 modulates potentially the binding sites of several transcription factors including GATA-3, NF-κB, C/EBP, and E4BP4 which were all shown to be involved in inflammatory processes. GATA-3 is a major transcription factor involved in differentiation of Th2 cells [49] which play a fundamental role in the pathogenesis of UC. NF-κB up-regulates the gene expression of many proinflammatory cytokines including IL-12 [50]. Together with NF-κB, C/EBP is activated by signaling via pattern recognition receptors (PRRs) which respond to pathogen-associated molecular patterns (PAMPs) or host-derived damage-associated molecular patterns (DAMPs). Both transcription factors play therefore a pivotal role in inflammatory disorders. E4BP4 is essential for the development of natural killer (NK) cells and CD8α+ conventional dendritic cells; it plays also a role in macrophage activation, polarisation of CD4+ T cell responses and B cell class switching to IgE [51]. Interestingly, E4BP4 may also modulate IL-12 expression [52] which plays a key role in the pathogenesis of CD. The predicted binding of the transcription factors NF-κB, C/EBP and E4BP4 was stronger to the CD-associated minor allele of SNP rs7234029 than to the protective major allele, suggesting that the increased CD risk may be partially modulated via the stronger activation of these proinflammatory transcription factors.

In summary, we confirm *PTPN2* as common susceptibility gene for CD and UC. Genotype-phenotype analysis could not identify a clear phenotype associated with these variants. A potential association of *PTPN2* SNP rs7234029 with a stricturing disease phenotype in CD patients (p = 6.62×10^{-3}) needs further confirmation in larger cohorts or meta-analyses which are currently organized by the subphenotyping committee of the International

IBD Genetics Consortium. Our *in silico* analysis predicted that the increased CD risk mediated by rs7234029 may be related to a stronger activation of proinflammatory transcription factors such as NF-κB, C/EBP and E4BP4. This study revealed a potential interaction between *PTPN2* and *ATG16L1* regarding susceptibility of CD and UC. However, given the rather weak interaction, this has to be further investigated. Interestingly, this finding supports the results of a very recent functional study demonstrating a major role for PTPN2 in the autophagosome formation in human intestinal epithelial cells [25]. This suggests that different IBD-related pathways may converge in common functional "end-points" such as autophagy resulting in increased IBD susceptibility in affected patients.

Supporting Information

Table S1 Primer sequences (F: forward primer, R: reverse Primer), FRET probe sequences, and primer annealing temperatures used for genotyping of *PTPN2*

variants. Note: FL: Fluorescein, LC610: LightCycler-Red 610; LC640: LightCycler-Red 640. The polymorphic position within the sensor probe is underlined. A phosphate is linked to the 3'-end of the acceptor probe to prevent elongation by the DNA polymerase in the PCR.

Table S2 Primer sequences used for the sequence analysis of the *PTPN2* variants.

Author Contributions

Conceived and designed the experiments: JG SB. Performed the experiments: JW JG MW. Analyzed the data: DC JG NK SB. Contributed reagents/materials/analysis tools: J. Seiderer T. Olszak MW FB CT MF CS BG T. Ochsenkühn J. Stallhofer JD SB. Wrote the paper: SB J. Seiderer JG JW. Interviewed patients: JW J. Seiderer T. Olszak FB CT T. Ochsenkühn J. Stallhofer SB.

References

1. Xavier RJ, Podolsky DK (2007) Unravelling the pathogenesis of inflammatory bowel disease. Nature 448: 427–434.
2. Podolsky DK (2002) Inflammatory bowel disease. N Engl J Med 347: 417–429.
3. Duerr RH, Taylor KD, Brant SR, Rioux JD, Silverberg MS, et al. (2006) A genome-wide association study identifies IL23R as an inflammatory bowel disease gene. Science 314: 1461–1463.
4. Hampe J, Franke A, Rosenstiel P, Till A, Teuber M, et al. (2007) A genome-wide association scan of nonsynonymous SNPs identifies a susceptibility variant for Crohn disease in ATG16L1. Nat Genet 39: 207–211.
5. Libioulle C, Louis E, Hansoul S, Sandor C, Farnir F, et al. (2007) Novel Crohn disease locus identified by genome-wide association maps to a gene desert on 5p13.1 and modulates expression of PTGER4. PLoS Genet 3: e58.
6. Massey DC, Parkes M (2007) Genome-wide association scanning highlights two autophagy genes, ATG16L1 and IRGM, as being significantly associated with Crohn's disease. Autophagy 3: 649–651.
7. Prescott NJ, Fisher SA, Franke A, Hampe J, Onnie CM, et al. (2007) A nonsynonymous SNP in ATG16L1 predisposes to ileal Crohn's disease and is independent of CARD15 and IBD5. Gastroenterology 132: 1665–1671.
8. Rioux JD, Xavier RJ, Taylor KD, Silverberg MS, Goyette P, et al. (2007) Genome-wide association study identifies new susceptibility loci for Crohn disease and implicates autophagy in disease pathogenesis. Nat Genet 39: 596–604.
9. Wang K, Zhang H, Kugathasan S, Annese V, Bradfield JP, et al. (2009) Diverse genome-wide association studies associate the IL12/IL23 pathway with Crohn Disease. Am J Hum Genet 84: 399–405.
10. Simoncic PD, McGlade CJ, Tremblay ML (2006) PTP1B and TC-PTP: novel roles in immune-cell signaling. Can J Physiol Pharmacol 84: 667–675.
11. Galic S, Klingler-Hoffmann M, Fodero-Tavoletti MT, Puryer MA, Meng TC, et al. (2003) Regulation of insulin receptor signaling by the protein tyrosine phosphatase TCPTP. Mol Cell Biol 23: 2096–2108.
12. ten Hoeve J, de Jesus Ibarra-Sanchez MJ, Fu Y, Zhu W, Tremblay M, et al. (2002) Identification of a nuclear Stat1 protein tyrosine phosphatase. Mol Cell Biol 22: 5662–5668.
13. Tiganis T, Bennett AM, Ravichandran KS, Tonks NK (1998) Epidermal growth factor receptor and the adaptor protein p52Shc are specific substrates of T-cell protein tyrosine phosphatase. Mol Cell Biol 18: 1622–1634.
14. Walchli S, Curchod ML, Gobert RP, Arkinstall S, Hooft van Huijsduijnen R (2000) Identification of tyrosine phosphatases that dephosphorylate the insulin receptor. A brute force approach based on "substrate-trapping" mutants. J Biol Chem 275: 9792–9796.
15. Colli ML, Moore F, Gurzov EN, Ortis F, Eizirik DL (2010) MDA5 and PTPN2, two candidate genes for type 1 diabetes, modify pancreatic beta-cell responses to the viral by-product double stranded RNA. Hum Mol Genet 19: 135–146.
16. Moore F, Colli ML, Cnop M, Esteve MI, Cardozo AK, et al. (2009) PTPN2, a candidate gene for type 1 diabetes, modulates interferon-gamma-induced pancreatic beta-cell apoptosis. Diabetes 58: 1283–1291.
17. Smyth DJ, Plagnol V, Walker NM, Cooper JD, Downes K, et al. (2008) Shared and distinct genetic variants in type 1 diabetes and celiac disease. N Engl J Med 359: 2767–2777.
18. Parkes M, Barrett JC, Prescott NJ, Tremelling M, Anderson CA, et al. (2007) Sequence variants in the autophagy gene IRGM and multiple other replicating loci contribute to Crohn's disease susceptibility. Nat Genet 39: 830–832.
19. Franke A, McGovern DP, Barrett JC, Wang K, Radford-Smith GL, et al. (2010) Genome-wide meta-analysis increases to 71 the number of confirmed Crohn's disease susceptibility loci. Nat Genet 42: 1118–1125.
20. Wellcome Trust Case Control Consortium (2007) Genome-wide association study of 14,000 cases of seven common diseases and 3,000 shared controls. Nature 447: 661–678.
21. Barrett JC, Hansoul S, Nicolae DL, Cho JH, Duerr RH, et al. (2008) Genome-wide association defines more than 30 distinct susceptibility loci for Crohn's disease. Nat Genet 40: 955–962.
22. Anderson CA, Boucher G, Lees CW, Franke A, D'Amato M, et al. (2011) Meta-analysis identifies 29 additional ulcerative colitis risk loci, increasing the number of confirmed associations to 47. Nat Genet 43: 246–252.
23. van der Heide F, Nolte IM, Kleibeuker JH, Wijmenga C, Dijkstra G, et al. (2010) Differences in genetic background between active smokers, passive smokers, and non-smokers with Crohn's disease. Am J Gastroenterol 105: 1165–1172.
24. Thompson SD, Sudman M, Ramos PS, Marion MC, Ryan M, et al. (2010) The susceptibility loci juvenile idiopathic arthritis shares with other autoimmune diseases extend to PTPN2, COG6, and ANGPT1. Arthritis Rheum 62: 3265–3276.
25. Scharl M, Wojtal KA, Becker HM, Fischbeck A, Frei P, et al. (2011) Protein tyrosine phosphatase nonreceptor type 2 regulates autophagosome formation in human intestinal cells. Inflamm Bowel Disdoi: 10.1002/ibd.21891. [Epub ahead of print].
26. Lennard-Jones JE (1989) Classification of inflammatory bowel disease. Scand J Gastroenterol Suppl 170: 2–6; discussion 16–19.
27. Silverberg MS, Satsangi J, Ahmad T, Arnott ID, Bernstein CN, et al. (2005) Toward an integrated clinical, molecular and serological classification of inflammatory bowel disease: Report of a Working Party of the 2005 Montreal World Congress of Gastroenterology. Can J Gastroenterol 19 Suppl A: 5–36.
28. Glas J, Seiderer J, Wetzke M, Konrad A, Torok HP, et al. (2007) rs1004819 is the main disease-associated IL23R variant in German Crohn's disease patients: combined analysis of IL23R, CARD15, and OCTN1/2 variants. PLoS ONE 2: e819.
29. Glas J, Konrad A, Schmechel S, Dambacher J, Seiderer J, et al. (2008) The ATG16L1 gene variants rs2241879 and rs2241880 (T300A) are strongly associated with susceptibility to Crohn's disease in the German population. Am J Gastroenterol 103: 682–691.
30. Glas J, Stallhofer J, Ripke S, Wetzke M, Pfennig S, et al. (2009) Novel genetic risk markers for ulcerative colitis in the IL2/IL21 region are in epistasis with IL23R and suggest a common genetic background for ulcerative colitis and celiac disease. Am J Gastroenterol 104: 1737–1744.
31. Glas J, Seiderer J, Bayrle C, Wetzke M, Fries C, et al. (2011) The role of osteopontin (OPN/SPP1) haplotypes in the susceptibility to Crohn's disease. PLoS One 6: e29309.
32. Glas J, Seiderer J, Fries C, Tillack C, Pfennig S, et al. (2011) CEACAM6 gene variants in inflammatory bowel disease. PLoS One 6: e19319.
33. Torok HP, Glas J, Endres I, Tonenchi L, Teshome MY, et al. (2009) Epistasis between Toll-like receptor-9 polymorphisms and variants in NOD2 and IL23R modulates susceptibility to Crohn's disease. Am J Gastroenterol 104: 1723–1733.
34. Seiderer J, Brand S, Herrmann KA, Schnitzler F, Hatz R, et al. (2006) Predictive value of the CARD15 variant 1007fs for the diagnosis of intestinal stenoses and the need for surgery in Crohn's disease in clinical practice: results of a prospective study. Inflamm Bowel Dis 12: 1114–1121.
35. Schnitzler F, Brand S, Staudinger T, Pfennig S, Hofbauer K, et al. (2006) Eight novel CARD15 variants detected by DNA sequence analysis of the CARD15 gene in 111 patients with inflammatory bowel disease. Immunogenetics 58: 99–106.
36. Glas J, Seiderer J, Tillack C, Pfennig S, Beigel F, et al. (2010) The NOD2 single nucleotide polymorphisms rs2066843 and rs2076756 are novel and common Crohn's disease susceptibility gene variants. PLoS One 5: e14466.

37. Heinemeyer T, Wingender E, Reuter I, Hermjakob H, Kel AE, et al. (1998) Databases on transcriptional regulation: TRANSFAC, TRRD and COMPEL. Nucleic Acids Res 26: 362–367.

38. Morgan AR, Han DY, Huebner C, Lam WJ, Fraser AG, et al. (2010) PTPN2 but not PTPN22 is associated with Crohn's disease in a New Zealand population. Tissue Antigens 76: 119–125.

39. Latiano A, Palmieri O, Latiano T, Corritore G, Bossa F, et al. (2011) Investigation of multiple susceptibility loci for inflammatory bowel disease in an Italian cohort of patients. PLoS One 6: e22688.

40. Weersma RK, Stokkers PC, Cleynen I, Wolfkamp SC, Henckaerts L, et al. (2009) Confirmation of multiple Crohn's disease susceptibility loci in a large Dutch-Belgian cohort. Am J Gastroenterol 104: 630–638.

41. Cargill M, Schrodi SJ, Chang M, Garcia VE, Brandon R, et al. (2007) A large-scale genetic association study confirms IL12B and leads to the identification of IL23R as psoriasis-risk genes. Am J Hum Genet 80: 273–290.

42. Lees CW, Barrett JC, Parkes M, Satsangi J (2011) New IBD genetics: common pathways with other diseases. Gut 60: 1739–1753.

43. Festen EA, Goyette P, Green T, Boucher G, Beauchamp C, et al. (2011) A meta-analysis of genome-wide association scans identifies IL18RAP, PTPN2, TAGAP, and PUS10 as shared risk loci for Crohn's disease and celiac disease. PLoS Genet 7: e1001283.

44. Todd JA, Walker NM, Cooper JD, Smyth DJ, Downes K, et al. (2007) Robust associations of four new chromosome regions from genome-wide analyses of type 1 diabetes. Nat Genet 39: 857–864.

45. Scharl M, Mwinyi J, Fischbeck A, Leucht K, Eloranta JJ, et al. (2011) Crohn's disease-associated polymorphism within the PTPN2 gene affects muramyl-dipeptide-induced cytokine secretion and autophagy. Inflamm Bowel Disdoi: 10.1002/ibd.21913. [Epub ahead of print].

46. Travassos LH, Carneiro LA, Ramjeet M, Hussey S, Kim YG, et al. (2010) Nod1 and Nod2 direct autophagy by recruiting ATG16L1 to the plasma membrane at the site of bacterial entry. Nat Immunol 11: 55–62.

47. Scharl M, Paul G, Weber A, Jung BC, Docherty MJ, et al. (2009) Protection of epithelial barrier function by the Crohn's disease associated gene protein tyrosine phosphatase N2. Gastroenterology 137: 2030–2040.

48. Scharl M, McCole DF, Weber A, Vavricka SR, Frei P, et al. (2011) Protein tyrosine phosphatase N2 regulates TNFalpha-induced signalling and cytokine secretion in human intestinal epithelial cells. Gut 60: 189–197.

49. Zheng W, Flavell RA (1997) The transcription factor GATA-3 is necessary and sufficient for Th2 cytokine gene expression in CD4 T cells. Cell 89: 587–596.

50. Murphy TL, Cleveland MG, Kulesza P, Magram J, Murphy KM (1995) Regulation of interleukin 12 p40 expression through an NF-kappa B half-site. Mol Cell Biol 15: 5258–5267.

51. Male V, Nisoli I, Gascoyne DM, Brady HJ (2012) E4BP4: an unexpected player in the immune response. Trends Immunol 33: 98–102.

52. Kobayashi T, Matsuoka K, Sheikh SZ, Elloumi HZ, Kamada N, et al. (2011) NFIL3 is a regulator of IL-12 p40 in macrophages and mucosal immunity. J Immunol 186: 4649–4655.

3

Inflammasome-Independent Modulation of Cytokine Response by Autophagy in Human Cells

Tania O. Crişan[1,2], **Theo S. Plantinga**[1,2], **Frank L. van de Veerdonk**[1,2], **Marius F. Farcaş**[1,2], **Monique Stoffels**[1,2], **Bart-Jan Kullberg**[1,2], **Jos W. M. van der Meer**[1,2], **Leo A. B. Joosten**[1,2], **Mihai G. Netea**[1,2]*

1 Department of Medicine, Radboud University Nijmegen Medical Center, Nijmegen, The Netherlands, 2 Nijmegen Institute for Infection, Inflammation and Immunity (N4i), Radboud University Nijmegen Medical Center, Nijmegen, The Netherlands

Abstract

Autophagy is a cell housekeeping mechanism that has recently received attention in relation to its effects on the immune response. Genetic studies have identified candidate loci for Crohn's disease susceptibility among autophagy genes, while experiments in murine macrophages from *ATG16L1* deficient mice have shown that disruption of autophagy increases processing of IL-1β and IL-18 through an inflammasome-dependent manner. Using complementary approaches either inducing or inhibiting autophagy, we describe modulatory effects of autophagy on proinflammatory cytokine production in human cells. Inhibition of basal autophagy in human peripheral blood mononuclear cells (PBMCs) significantly enhances IL-1β after stimulation with TLR2 or TLR4 ligands, while at the same time reducing the production of TNFα. In line with this, induction of autophagy by starvation inhibited IL-1β production. These effects of autophagy were not exerted at the processing step, as inflammasome activation was not influenced. In contrast, the effect of autophagy on cytokine production was on transcription level, and possibly involving the inhibition of p38 mitogen activated protein kinase (MAPK) phosphorylation. In conclusion, autophagy modulates the secretion of proinflammatory cytokines in human cells through an inflammasome-independent pathway, and this is a novel mechanism that may be targeted in inflammatory diseases.

Editor: Kathleen A. Kelly, University of California Los Angeles, United States of America

Funding: The study was financed by the Vici grant of the Netherlands Organization for Scientific Research. The funders had no role in study design, data collection and analysis, decision to publish, or preparation of the manuscript.

Competing Interests: The authors have declared that no competing interests exist.

* E-mail: m.netea@aig.umcn.nl

Introduction

Autophagy is a conserved mechanism for degradation of defective organelles and long-lived proteins, that plays an important role in the homeostasis of the cell by recycling cytoplasmic cargo for aminoacid and energy re-use [1]. Autophagy comprises three main processes – chaperone-mediated autophagy, microautophagy and macroautophagy. The latter, henceforth referred to as autophagy, is characterized by the sequestration of cytosolic proteins and organelles into double-membrane vesicles called autophagosomes. These autophagosomes maturate through fusion with lysosomes, a process that will eventually lead to the breakdown of the protein content [2]. Through these effects, autophagy has been demonstrated to be a biological response of the cell in stressful situations, traditionally during starvation and growth factor deprivation, ensuring the degradation of old structures with the purpose of sustaining the essential anabolic processes of the cell [3]. Consequently, through its main roles in survival and housekeeping, the process of autophagy has gained relevance in the context of human pathologies like neurodegenerative diseases [4], cancer [5], lysosomal diseases [6], and ageing [1].

In addition to its role in cell survival, autophagy is emerging as a process of high importance for the host defense, influencing both the innate and adaptive immune responses [7]. This role is exerted at three levels [8]: direct involvement in engulfment and removal of intracellular pathogens [9,10], facilitation of the MHC class II antigen presentation [11], and support of the T-lymphocyte development and survival for optimal protective immune responses [12,13]. Whether the involvement of autophagy in the immune processes is due to the autophagic mechanism itself or to independent effects of autophagy-related genes [14], is still a matter of debate.

Genetic studies [15–17] have identified allelic variants of the autophagy genes *ATG16L1* (autophagy related 16-like 1) and *IRGM* (immunity related GTP-ases, M) as important risk factors for Crohn's disease, an autoinflammatory disease characterized by severe chronic inflammation of the gut mucosa [18,19]. One possible explanation for the involvement of defective autophagy in Crohn's disease inflammation couples the risk alleles in *ATG16L1* and *NOD2* (nucleotide-binding oligomerization domain containing 2) to an impaired clearance of microorganisms [20,21]. The persistence of bacteria in the mucosa could induce an inflammatory reaction, leading to the clinical features of Crohn's disease. An alternative explanation has also been proposed by Saitoh *et al.*, who demonstrated that the disruption of autophagy in *ATG16L1*-deficient murine macrophages enhances the LPS-induced IL-1β production through an inflammasome-dependent pathway [22]. However, whether autophagy has similar inhibitory effects in human cells is not known.

In the present study, we assessed the effect of autophagy on the production of proinflammatory cytokines in human cells. By stimulating human peripheral blood mononuclear cells (PBMCs), we show that the inhibition of autophagy increases IL-1β production after stimulation with TLR2 or TLR4 ligands. These effects were specific for the modulation of IL-1β secretion, while TNFα production was significantly reduced by agents that inhibited autophagy. In contrast to murine macrophages, these effects on human cells were exerted at the transcriptional level, rather than at the level of the inflammasome.

Results

Western blot assessment of autophagy marker LC3-II shows that starvation induces, whereas 3MA treatment inhibits, the autophagic process

Microtubule associated protein 1 light chain 3 (LC3) is one of the autophagy-related proteins involved in the direct formation of the autophagosome. Through conjugation with phosphatidylethanolamine, the cytosolic LC3-I is transformed to LC3-II which is then bound to the autophagosome membrane, being indicative of autophagic activity inside the cell [23]. In order to verify the modulation of autophagy using the typical induction method by starvation and the inhibition method using the pharmacological inhibitor 3-Methyl Adenine (3MA) in the human PBMCs system used in this study, Western blotting of the two LC3 fractions was performed. Freshly isolated human PBMCs treated with the starvation medium EBSS (Earle's Balanced Salt Solution) showed a markedly increased level of LC3-II compared to RPMI controls. Moreover, when 3MA was added, the LC3-II fraction was decreased (Figure 1), attesting to the validity of the classical autophagy methodologies in human PBMCs.

Inhibition of autophagy enhances IL-1β production while decreasing TNFα in human PBMCs

To assess its effect on the cytokine production, autophagy was inhibited using 3MA, a blocker of the Beclin-1 complex that regulates the initiation of autophagy. PBMCs treated with 3MA showed a significant higher IL-1β secretion after stimulations with TLR2 or TLR4 ligands (Figure 2A). In contrast, TNFα production was diminished in cells conditioned with 3MA compared to controls (Figure 2B). No specific trend for the effect of 3MA on IL-10 production was observed (Figure 2C).

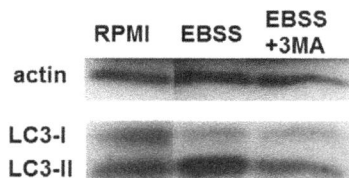

Figure 1. Assessment of LC3 I and II levels in PBMCs under starving conditions or pharmacological treatment with 3MA. Human PBMCs were pre-incubated for 1 hour at 37°C in either RPMI, starvation medium (EBSS) or EBSS with 3MA (10 mM) in which inhibitors of lysosomal fusion have been added: Ammonium chloride 20 mM and Leupeptine 100 μM. This was followed by 3 hours stimulation with culture medium, LPS (10 ng/ml) or Pam3Cys (10 μg/ml) prepared in the corresponding media (RPMI or EBSS). Cells were lysed and western blot of LC3 fractions I and II has been performed.

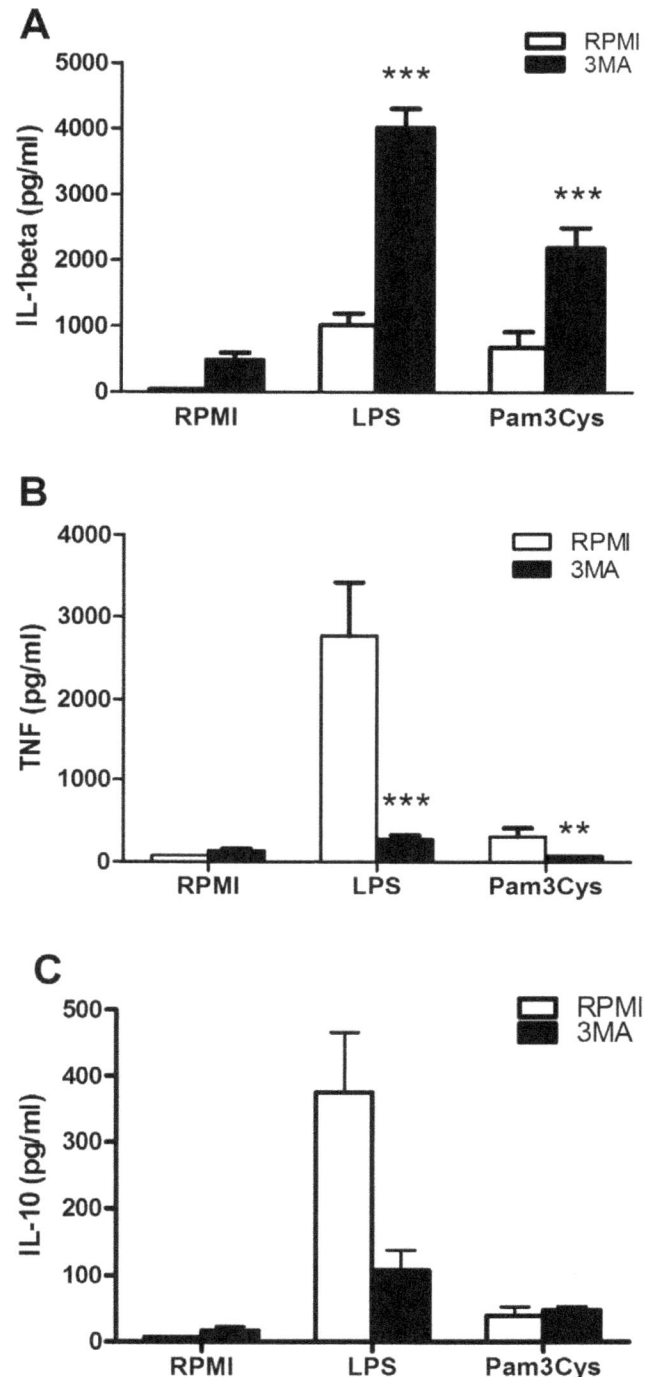

Figure 2. Modulation of inflammatory cytokine production by autophagy inhibition. Freshly isolated human PBMCs were pre-incubated for 1 hour at 37°C in culture medium in the presence or absence of 3MA (10 mM) and afterwards stimulated with culture medium, LPS (10 ng/ml) or Pam3Cys (10 μg/ml). After 24 hours incubation, IL-1β (A), TNFα (B) and IL-10 (C) were measured in the supernatant by specific ELISA. Data are presented as means ± SEM of cells harvested from 15 volunteers, **p<0.01, ***p<0.001.

The modulation of IL-1β and TNFα production is regulated at the transcriptional level

To identify the level in the cytokine production which is modulated by 3MA, we assessed its effect on transcription and processing of IL-1β. IL-1β mRNA levels were increased in human PBMCs in the presence of 3MA (Figure 3A). Similarly, RT-PCR for TNFα mRNA revealed that the inhibitory effect of 3MA on TNFα production starts with the decrease of the TNFα transcription rate (Figure 3B). On the other hand, western blot analysis of caspase-1 did not show an increased caspase-1 activation (p35 fragment) by 3MA compared to controls (Figure 3C).

3MA has an inhibitory effect on the ATP-dependent release of IL-1β

It is known that the inflammasome activator ATP (adenosine triphosphate) is a potent stimulator of IL-1β processing and release [24]. In experiments aiming to assess how this effect is influenced in the circumstances of autophagy inhibition, control PBMCs showed a significantly higher increase (5.73 fold) of secreted IL-1β when exposed to ATP then in samples treated with 3MA (2.25 fold increase) (Figure 4).

Induction of autophagy by starvation inhibits IL-1β transcription

In an additional set of experiments, we pursued to verify whether consistent findings with those revealed when inhibiting autophagy could be seen in the context of autophagy induction, typically obtained during starvation. In line with the effects observed by the experiments using 3MA, starvation reduced the transcription of IL-1β after LPS or Pam3Cys stimulation of cells (Figure 5A). Furthermore, these effects of starvation were reversed by 3MA, demonstrating the involvement of autophagy in the effects of starvation (Figure 5B). In contrast to its effect on IL-1β, starvation inhibited TNFα mRNA, but 3MA decreased even further TNFα transcription. This observation is consistent with the experiments showed earlier that 3MA reduces the TNFα gene transcription.

The role of MAP kinases for the modulatory effects of autophagy inhibition by 3MA

Mitogen-activated protein kinases (MAPKs) such as ERK1/2 (activated by MEK), JNK or p38 are important intracellular mediators of the stimulation of pro-inflammatory cytokine production during innate immune responses [25]. In order to decipher the mechanism through which autophagy inhibition modulates cytokine transcription, we investigated the effects of MAPK inhibition on the 3MA-dependent variation of cytokine production. Cells pre-treated with inhibitors of MEK, JNK or p38 in the presence or absence of 3MA have further been stimulated with LPS and Pam3Cys and cytokine production is depicted in Figure 6 (panels A and B for IL-1β; C and D for TNFα). With all inhibitors, except p38i, 3MA had similar consequences on the cytokine production, consisting in increasing IL-1β and decreasing TNFα secretion after both LPS and Pam3Cys stimulation. Nevertheless, when using p38i, lower IL-1β concentrations were measured in samples treated with 3MA after Pam3Cys stimulation than in controls. Consequently, in order to test the hypothesis of p38 being involved in the effects of 3MA, we performed Western blots of total and phosphorylated (active) p38 which revealed that in samples treated with the autophagy inhibitor, the phosphorylated fraction of p38 is lower than in controls, after TLR4 or TLR2 stimulations (Figure 6E). Furthermore, the slight induction of TNFα and IL-1β by 3MA alone was shown to be dependent on

p38 MAPK signaling (3MA: IL-1β 665±135 pg/ml, TNFα 215±45 pg/ml and 3MA+p38i: IL-1β 20±10 pg/ml, TNFα 40±15 pg/ml; p<0.05 for both IL-1β and TNFα).

Discussion

Earlier studies linked autophagy to innate immunity as a defense system against invading pathogens in nonphagocytic cells [26]. Later it has been also demonstrated that autophagy regulates pathogen-associated molecular pattern (PAMP) recognition by facilitating TLR stimulation in response to viral antigens [27]. Subsequently, it has been discovered that components of the autophagy machinery are used for intracellular degradation of bacteria and MHC-II dependent activation of specific immunity [9]. These effects could prove very relevant, as genetic polymorphisms of the autophagy genes ATG16L1 and IRGM are associated with Crohn's disease [15–17]. In addition, deletion of the autophagy gene ATG16L1 in mice resulted in inflammasome activation and more severe experimental colitis [22]. However, the effect of autophagy on IL-1β production was demonstrated only in murine cells, and no information was available whether similar effects may be exerted in human cells.

In the present study, using a complementary approach by both inhibition and induction of autophagy as verified using the LC3-II marker, we show that autophagy has strong inhibitory effects on IL-1β production. These results add to the increasing body of evidence showing that basal autophagy in physiological conditions has important modulatory effects on inflammation [22,28]. However, in contrast to murine cells, autophagy did not inhibit inflammasome activation in human PBMCs, and its effects were the consequence of the modulatory effect on transcription of cytokine genes. These data point out once again that inflammasome activation and regulation differs greatly in human PBMCs and murine macrophages, as inflammasome activation is constitutive in human monocytes, but not in mouse macrophages [29]. Subsequently, in human PBMCs, caspase-1 activation is not increased by autophagy inhibition. In addition, the assessment of ATP/inflammasome-dependent release of IL-1β shows that this is not increased in the presence of 3MA compared to controls. This would suggest that although the cytokine release appears to be slightly inhibited on the short term (15 minutes after ATP addition), transcriptional regulation is sufficient to determine the higher levels obtained in longer stimulations. These findings confirm that the increase of IL-1β production during autophagy inhibition is determined by the activation of transcription and is not due to the influence on the subsequent steps of processing by caspase-1 or secretion from the intracellular compartment.

In the attempt to point out to the mechanism underlying the effect of autophagy on gene transcription, we have tested the importance of several MAPK-dependent mechanisms and observed that the only condition that reversed the stimulatory effects of 3MA was the p38 inhibitor SB202190. As there is evidence of this inhibitor also influencing Rip2 activation [30], the observed effect might also be involving other p38-related MAP kinases in addition to p38. However, while these results have led us to the hypothesis that p38 activation might be important for the effect of 3MA on IL-1β, this was not confirmed by Western blot analysis, as phosphorylated p38 (active form) was decreased in 3MA treated samples. However, in line with earlier evidence showing that p38 phosphorylation is positively linked to the process of autophagy [31,32], 3MA treatment led to inhibition of p38 phosphorylation and this could, at least in part, represent a pathway of autophagy effect on TNFα release. In summary, while the inhibitory effects of 3MA on p38 phosphorylation can explain its effect on TNFα

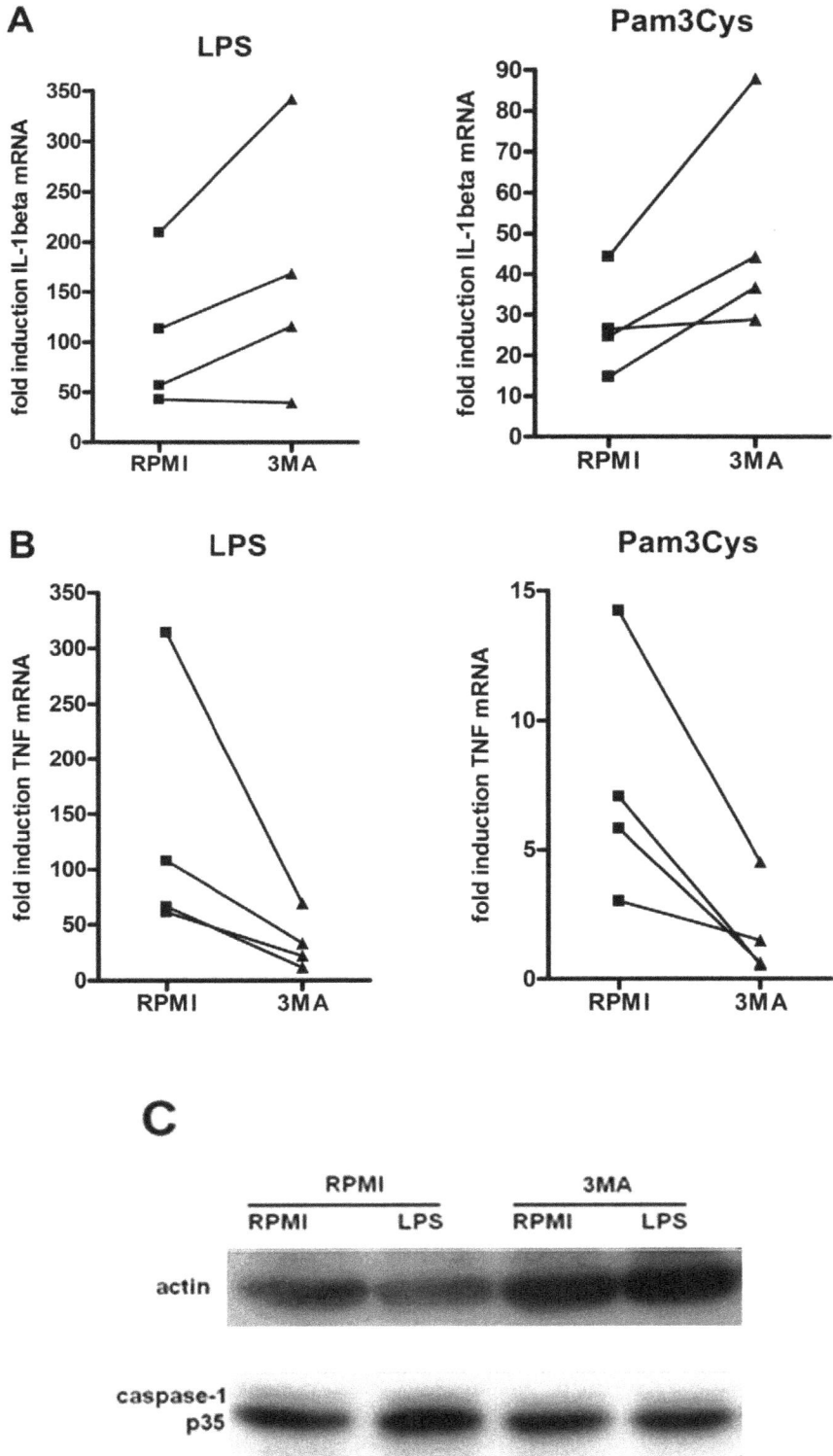

Figure 3. The effects of 3MA on transcription and processing of inflammatory cytokines. Cells pre-treated for 1 hour with culture medium with or without 3MA (10 mM) were stimulated for 4 hours with RPMI, LPS (10 ng/ml) or Pam3Cys (10 μg/ml). RT-PCR was performed and relative levels of IL-1β and TNFα (B) mRNA were determined in 4 volunteers. (C) Western blot of p35 caspase-1 after 1 hour pre-incubation with or without 3MA (10 mM in RPMI), followed by 2 hours stimulation with LPS (10 ng/ml). The picture is representative for results obtained from 6 volunteers.

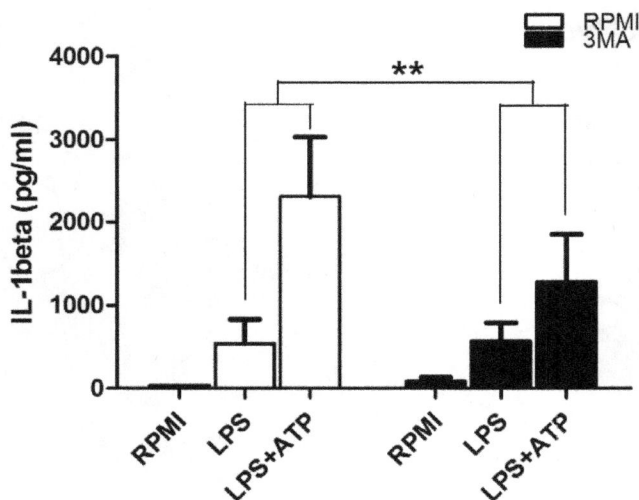

Figure 4. The influence of 3MA on the ATP-dependent release of IL-1β. PBMCs were pre-incubated for 1 hour in the presence or absence of 3MA and were stimulated for 4 hours with LPS (10 ng/ml). After the stimulation, supernatants were discarded and refreshed with RPMI or with RPMI containing 1 mM ATP and cells were incubated for another 15 min. Data are shown as mean ± SEM of supernatant IL-1β levels obtained in 8 volunteers, **p<0.01.

production, this cannot be the cause of the potentiation of IL-1β transcription, and further studies are needed to decipher this aspect.

Recently, two new studies have also reported that the peptidoglycan receptor NOD2, whose gene is considered a susceptibility locus for Crohn's disease, is linked to autophagy by recruiting ATG16L1 at the site of the microbial entry within the infected cell [21], directing microbial engulfment in the autophagosome and inducing antigen presentation [20]. These latest two studies represent the connection between the two genetic pathways that induce susceptibility to Crohn's disease: NOD2 and autophagy. Crohn's disease is a chronic inflammatory reaction in the gut mucosa, and recent studies strongly suggested a role of autophagy in this process. On the one hand, autophagy seems to be crucial for the homeostasis of Paneth cells. Mice with a defective ATG16L1 display abnormal Paneth cells with a lower amount of granules containing antibacterial defensins, while in turn displaying an increased IL-1β production [28]. These effects could lead to bacterial persistence in the mucosa and overwhelming inflammation. The studies by Cooney et al. [20] and Travassos et al. [21] show for the first time that a decreased autophagy in humans can lead to decreased bacterial clearance, while our study provides evidence that diminished autophagy in human cells (e.g. through pharmacological inhibition as shown here, or through genetic mutations in Crohn's disease) could lead to uncontrolled IL-1β production.

The differential findings in mice and humans concerning the modulation of IL-1β by autophagy, transcription in humans and caspase-1 activation in mice, remains to be elucidated. One possible explanation lies in the different cell populations studied: monocytes in our study in humans versus macrophages in the mouse studies. We have previously shown clear differential regulation of the caspase-1 inflammasome in monocytes (constitutive activation) versus macrophages (inducible activation) [29]. Another source of difference could be species specificity, an aspect which in terms of the autophagy-inflammation interaction is still

largely unknown. This is an aspect which certainly deserves attention in future studies, and the present study represents an important first step in this direction.

In conclusion, this study is the first attempt to investigate the modulation of inflammatory cytokines by the process of autophagy in humans. We have shown that disruption of autophagy has an important impact on inflammatory cytokine modulation, determining a remarkable and specific increase of IL-1β secretion, while decreasing TNFα production. We demonstrate that the inflammasome activation is not influenced in human PBMCs and that the changes are exerted at the gene transcription level. Although the p38 MAPK pathway seems to be linked to the autophagy process and our findings may explain the effects on TNFα production through modulation of p38 phosphorylation, this is probably not the mechanism of the observed higher IL-1β mRNA levels in the circumstances of autophagy inhibition. Further assessment of the mechanisms through which inflammation is regulated by autophagy may bring new opportunities for the understanding and treatment of autoinflammatory disorders such as Crohn's disease.

Materials and Methods

Reagents

3-Methyl Adenine (3MA) was purchased from Sigma (St. Louis, MO). LPS (E. coli serotype 055:B5) was purchased from Sigma. Synthetic Pam3Cys was purchased from EMC Microcollections (Tubingen, Germany). Anti-actin (A2066) antibody was purchased from Sigma; anti-human caspase-1 p10 (sc515) antibody was purchased from Santa Cruz Biotechnologies (Santa Cruz, CA); anti-human/mouse LC3B antibody (NB600-1384) was purchased from Novus Biologicals (Cambridge, UK); anti-human total p38 antibody (CS9212) and phosphorylated p38 antibody (Phospho p38 MAPK Thr180/Tyr182 Antibody, CS4511) were purchased from Cell Signaling (Danvers, MA). oxATP was purchased from Sigma. SB202190 p38/Rip2 MAPK inhibitor (p38i); SP600125, JNK1/2/3 inhibitor (JNKi) and U0126 MEK1/2 inhibitor (MEKi) were purchased from Superarray Bioscience Corporation (Bethesda, MD). In experiments using pharmacological inhibitors, control cells were treated with an equivalent concentration of vehicle (0.1% DMSO).

PBMC isolation and stimulation

Peripheral blood was harvested from the antecubital vein of healthy volunteers, after obtaining informed consent. The PBMC fraction was obtained by differential centrifugation over Ficoll-Paque (Sigma). Cells adjusted to 5×10^6 cells/ml were suspended in culture medium RPMI (Roswell Park Memorial Institute) 1640, supplemented with 50 µg/ml gentamicin, 2 mM L-glutamine and 1 mM pyruvate. All cytokine induction experiments were performed in duplicate wells. Cells were pre-incubated for 1 hour at 37°C in culture medium or in the presence of 3MA (10 mM). After the pre-treatment, RPMI (negative controls), purified LPS (10 ng/ml) or Pam3Cys (10 µg/ml) was added to the cells. In separate experiments, cells were first incubated for 1 h with RPMI, MEK inhibitor (5 µM), JNK inhibitor (20 µM) or p38 inhibitor (1 µM) before performing the steps described above. After 24 hours, the supernatants were collected and stored at −20°C until assayed.

To investigate the effect of 3MA on the ATP-dependent IL-1β release, cells pre-treated for 1 hour with RPMI with or without 10 mM 3MA were stimulated for 4 hours with LPS (10 ng/ml or 1 µg/ml). After the stimulation, supernatants were discarded and refreshed with RPMI containing 1mM ATP, after which the cells

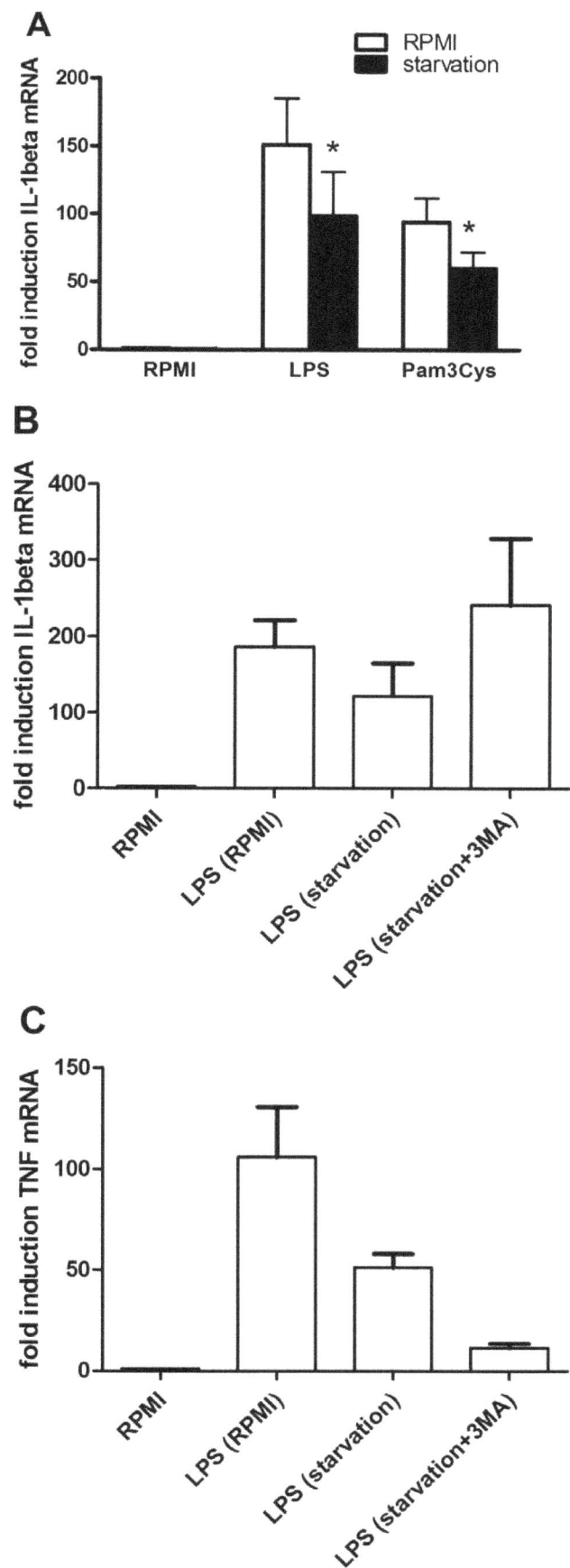

Figure 5. The effects of starvation on mRNA levels of inflammatory cytokines. Cells pre-incubated for 2 hours in either starvation medium (Earle's Balanced Salt Solution) or RPMI were stimulated for 4 hours with medium, LPS (10 ng/ml) or Pam3Cys (10 μg/ml) prepared respectively in starvation medium or RPMI. Subsequently, RT-PCR was performed and IL-1β mRNA levels are depicted as mean ± SEM of cells harvested from 6 volunteers, *p<0.05 (A). RT-PCR results of IL-1β (B) and TNFα (C) mRNA levels in cells pre-incubated for 2 hours with RPMI, starvation medium or starvation medium and 3MA (10 mM) followed by 4 hours stimulation with RPMI or LPS (10 ng/ml). Results are shown as mean ± SEM of data obtained in 4 volunteers.

were incubated for another 15 min. The LPS-dependent IL-1β production during the first 4 hours, and the ATP-dependent IL-1β secretion after the additional 15 minutes, was assessed in the supernatant.

Autophagy induction was performed in adherent monocytes using starvation medium, Earle's Balanced Salt Solution, EBSS (Invitrogen, Carlsbad, California). PBMCs were incubated for 1 hour after which the supernatant containing the non-adherent lymphocytes was discarded. Adherent cells were pre-treated for 2 hours with starvation medium. Subsequently, cells were stimulated for 4 hours with LPS or Pam3Cys prepared in starvation medium. In parallel, controls were given the same treatment using RPMI. After 4 hours, supernatants were discarded and TRIzol Reagent was added to the cells which were subsequently frozen and stored at −80°C until assayed. In different experiments, 3MA was also used in combination with starvation medium to investigate whether the effects of starvation are reversed by 3MA.

Both experiments involving stimulation or inhibition of autophagy were performed with cells isolated from the same healthy volunteers. However, in some experiments in which not all experiments could be performed with blood collected from the same volunteers, studies were done in cells collected from additional healthy volunteers.

Cytokine measurements

Cytokine concentrations were determined using specific sandwich ELISA kits for IL-1β, TNFα (R&D Systems), and IL-10 (Sanquin).

RT-PCR

Samples stimulated for 4 hours at 37°C were treated with TRIzol Reagent (Invitrogen) and total RNA purification was performed according to manufacturer's instructions. Isolated RNA was subsequently transcribed into complementary DNA using iScript cDNA Synthesis Kit (Bio-Rad) followed by quantitative PCR using the Sybr Green method. The following primers were used in the reaction: IL-1β forward 5′-GCCCTAAACAGAT GAAGTGCTC-3′ and reverse 5′-GAACCAGCATCTTCCT CAG-3′, TNFα forward 5′-TGGCCCAGGCAGTCAGA-3′ and reverse 5′-GGTTTGCTACAACATGGGCTACA-3′, β2-microglobulin forward 5′-ATGAGTATGCCTGCCGTGTG-3′ and reverse 5′-CCAAATGCGGCATCTTCAAAC-3′ (Biolegio). Results are shown as fold increases in mRNA levels in stimulated samples compared to controls. Quantitative PCR for cytokines was used especially in short-term induction of autophagy experiments using starvation medium, in which long-term incubation led to a high percentage of cell death, and in which ELISA cytokine measurements in the supernatants were not able to provide an appropriate assessment of cytokine stimulation.

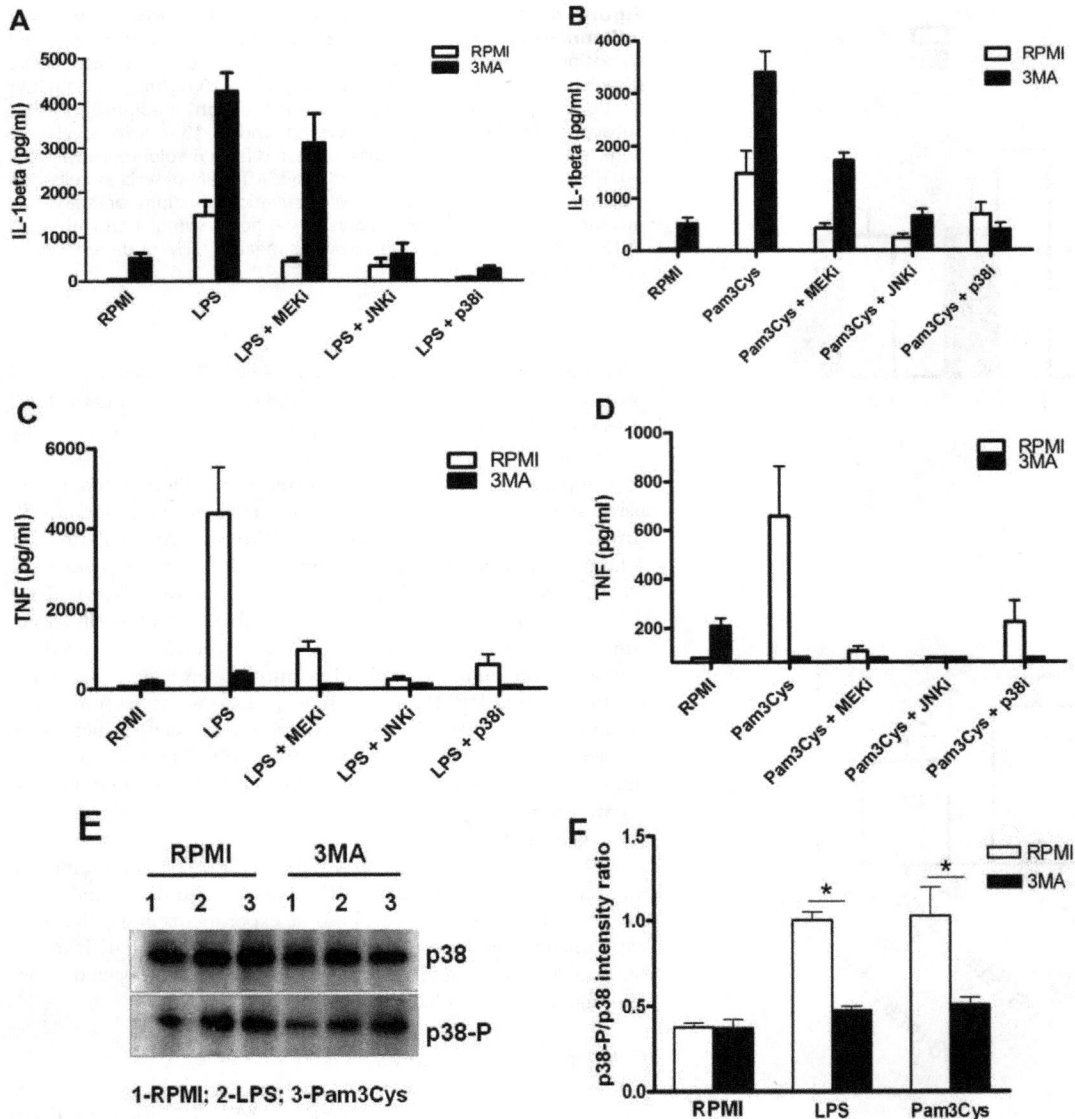

Figure 6. MAPK influence on the 3MA-dependent modulation of IL-1β and TNFα production. PBMC samples conditioned for 1 hour in either medium or in the presence of MAPK inhibitors: MEK inhibitor (5 μM), JNK inhibitor (20 μM) or p38 inhibitor (1 μM) were subjected to 1 hour treatment with RPMI or 3MA (10 mM), followed by stimulation with RPMI, LPS (10 ng/ml) or Pam3Cys (10 μg/ml). After 24 hours incubation, specific ELISA was performed to determine the level of IL-1β in response to LPS (A) and Pam3Cys (B) stimulations, same as for TNFα (panels C and D, respectively). Data from 6 volunteers are shown as mean ± SEM. (E) Western blot of total and phosphorylated p38 in cells pre-treated for 1 hour with RPMI or 3MA (10 mM) and subjected to 1 hour stimulation with RPMI, LPS (10 ng/ml) or Pam3Cys (10 μg/ml). (F) Quantification of the effect of 3MA on the phosphorylation of p38.

Western blot

For western blotting of actin, caspase-1 and p38 MAPK (total and phosphorylated), 5×10^6 cells were lysed in 100 μl lysis buffer (50 mM Tris, pH 7.4, 150 mM NaCl, 2 mM EDTA, 2 mM EGTA, 10% glycerol, 1% Triton X-100, 40 mM β-glycerophosphate, 50 mM sodium fluoride, 200 μM sodium orthovanadate, complete mini EDTA-free protease inhibitor cocktail (Roche) and PhosSTOP Phosphatase Inhibitor Cocktail (Roche)). The homogenate was stored at −20°C. When needed, samples were thawed, then centrifuged for 10 min at 14,000 rpm, and the supernatant was taken for western blotting. Equal amounts of protein were subjected to SDS-PAGE electrophoresis using 12% polyacrylamide gels at a voltage of 100V. After separation, proteins were transferred to polyvinylidene fluoride (PVDF) membrane using the dry blotting method (iBlot™, Invitrogen). The membrane was blocked with 5% (w/v) milk powder in Tris-buffered saline/Tween 20 (TBST) for 1 hour at room temperature followed by incubation over night at 4°C with the primary antibody 1:500 in 5% (w/v) BSA/TBST (5% bovine serum albumin/TBST). After overnight incubation the blots were washed three times with TBST and incubated with HRP-conjugated anti-rabbit antibody at a dilution of 1:5000 in 5% (w/v) milk powder in TBST for 1 hour at room temperature. After washing three times with TBST the blots were developed using ECL Plus Western Blot Detection Reagents (Amersham Biosciences, Buckinghamshire, UK). For western blotting of LC3, an amount of 10×10^6 cells were lysed after being cultured in media containing the inhibitors of lysosomal fusion, ammonium chloride,20 mM, and leupeptine,100 µM. After protein electrophoresis in 15% polyacrylamide gel, the transfer was performed on nitroglycerine membranes using the wet blotting method (Bio-Rad) and was followed by blocking, incubation with first and then second antibody, each time using 5% (w/v) milk powder in Tris-buffered saline/Tween 20 (TBS-T). After washing 3 times with TBS-T, blots were developed using the Super Signal® West Femto Maximum Sensitivity Substrate (Thermo Scientific, Rockford, IL, USA) according to the manufacturer's instructions. Quantitative assessment of band intensity was performed by Image Lab statistical software (Bio-Rad, CA, USA).

Statistical analysis

The differences were analysed using Wilcoxon signed rank test and were considered statistically significant at a p-value<0.05. Data are shown as cumulative results of levels obtained in all volunteers (means ± SEM).

Author Contributions

Conceived and designed the experiments: FLV BK JWMM LABJ MGN. Performed the experiments: TOC TSP MFF MS. Analyzed the data: TOC. Contributed reagents/materials/analysis tools: MS BK. Wrote the paper: TOC MGN.

References

1. Todde V, Veenhuis M, van der Klei IJ (2009) Autophagy: Principles and significance in health and disease. Biochim Biophys Acta 1792: 3–13.
2. Kundu M, Thompson CB (2008) Autophagy: Basic Principles and Relevance to Disease. Annu Rev Pathol Mech Dis 3: 427–55.
3. Hsieh YC, Athar M Chaudry IH (2009) When apoptosis meets autophagy: deciding cell fate after trauma and sepsis. Trends Mol Med 15: 129–138.
4. Alirezaei M, Kiosses WB, Flynn CT, Brady NR, Fox HS (2008) Disruption of Neuronal Autophagy by Infected Microglia Results in Neurodegeneration. PLoS ONE DOI:10.1371/journal.pone.0002906.
5. Chen N, Karantza-Wadsworth V (2009) Role and regulation of autophagy in cancer. Biochim Biophys Acta;DOI:10.1016/j.bbamcr.2008.12.013.
6. Tessitore A, Pirozzi M, Auricchio A (2008) Abnormal autophagy, ubiquitination, inflammation and apoptosis are dependent upon lysosomal storage and are useful biomarkers of mucopolysaccharidosis VI. PathoGenetics DOI:10.1186/1755-8417-2-4.
7. Deretic V, Levine B (2009) Autophagy, Immunity and Microbial Adaptations. Cell Host Microbe 5: 527–549.
8. Münz C (2009) Enhancing Immunity Through Autophagy. Annu Rev Immunol 27: 423–49.
9. Jagannath C, Lindsey DR, Dhandayuthapani S, Xu Y, Hunter Jr. RL, et al. (2009) Autophagy enhances the efficacy of BCG vaccine by increasing peptide presentation in mouse dendritic cells. Nat Med 15: 267–276.
10. Gutierrez MG, Master CC, Singh SB, Taylor GA, Colombo MI, et al. (2004) Autophagy is a defense mechanism inhibiting BCG and Mycobacterium tuberculosis survival in infected macrophages. Cell 119: 753–766.
11. Schmid D, Pypaert M, Münz C (2007) MHC class II antigen loading compartments continuously receive input from autophagosomes. Immunity 26: 79–92.
12. Nedjic J, Aichinger M, Emmerich J, Mizushima N, Klein L (2008) Autophagy in thymic epithelium shapes the T-cell repertoire and is essential for tolerance. Nature 455: 396–400.
13. Pua HH, Dzhgalov I, Chuck M, Mizushima N, He Y-W (2006) A critical role for the autophagy gene Atg5 in T cell survival and proliferation. J Exp Med 204: 25–31.
14. Virgin HW, Levine B (2009) Autophagy genes in immunity. Nat Immunol 10: 461–470.
15. Massey DCO, Parkes M (2007) Genome-Wide Association Scanning Highlights Two Autophagy Genes, ATG16L1 and IRGM, as Being Significantly Associated with Crohn's Disease. Autophagy 3: 649–651.
16. Márquez A, Núñez C, Martínez A, Mendoza JL, Taxonera C, et al. (2009) Role of ATG16L1 Thr300Ala Polymorphism in Inflammatory Bowel Disease: A Study in the Spanish Population. Inflamm Bowel Dis DOI:10.1002/ibd.21001.
17. Zhang HF, Qiu LX, Chen Y, Zhu WL, Mao C, et al. (2009) ATG16L1 T300A polymorphism and Crohn's disease susceptibility: evidence from 13,022 cases and 17,532 controls. Hum Genet 125: 627–631.
18. Kaser A, Blumberg RS (2008) Paneth cells and inflammation dance together in Crohn's disease. Cell Res 18: 1160–1162.
19. Deretic V, Master S, Singh S (2008) Autophagy Gives a Nod and a Wink to the Inflammasome and Paneth Cells in Crohn's Disease. Dev Cell 15: 641–642.
20. Cooney R, Baker J, Brain O, Danis B, Pichulik T, et al. (2009) NOD2 stimulation induces autophagy in DCs influencing bacterial handling and antigen presentation. Nat Med 16: 90–97.
21. Travassos LH, Carneiro LAM, Ramjeet M, Hussey S, Kim Y-G, et al. (2010) Nod1 and Nod2 direct autophagy by recruiting ATG16L1 to the plasma membrane at the site of bacterial entry. Nat Immunol 11: 55–62.
22. Saitoh T, Fujita N, Jang MH, Uematsu S, Yang BG, et al. (2008) Loss of the autophagy protein Atg16L1 enhances endotoxin-induced IL-1b production. Nature 456: 264–269.
23. Kabeya Y, Mizushima N, Ueno T, Yamamoto A, Kirisako T, et al. (2000) LC3, a mammalian homologue of yeast Apg8p, is localized in autophagosome membranes after processing. EMBO J 19: 5720–5728.
24. Laliberte RE, Perregaux DG, McNift P, Gabel CA (1997) Human monocyte ATP-induced IL-1 β posttranslational processing is a dynamic process dependent on in vitro growth conditions. J Leukoc Biol 62: 227–239.
25. Cobb MH (1999) MAP kinase pathways. Prog Biophys Mol Biol 71: 479–500.
26. Nagakawa I, Amano A, Mizushima N, Yamamoto A, Yamaguchi H, et al. (2004) Autophagy Defends Cells Against Invading Group A Streptococcus. Science 306: 1037–1040.
27. Jounai N, Takeshita F, Kobiyama K, Sawano A, Miyawaki A, et al. (2007) The Atg5-Atg12 conjugate associates with innate antiviral immune responses. Proc Natl Acad Sci U S A 104: 14050–14055.
28. Cadwell K, Liu JY, Brown SL, Miyoshi H, Loh J, et al. (2008) A key role for autophagy and the autophagy gene Atg16l1 in mouse and human intestinal Paneth cells. Nature 456: 259–263.
29. Netea MG, Nold-Petry CA, Nold MF, Joosten LA, Opitz B, et al. (2009) Differential requirement for the activation of the inflammasome for processing and release of IL-1β in monocytes and macrophages. Blood 113: 2324–2335.
30. Bain J, Plater L, Elliott M, Shpiro N, Hastie CJ, et al. (2007) The selectivity of protein kinase inhibitors: a further update. Biochem J 408: 297–315.
31. Yuan H, Perry CN, Huang C, Iwai-Kanai E, Carreira RS, et al. (2009) LPS-induced autophagy is mediated by oxidative signaling in cardiomyocytes and is associated with cytoprotection. Am J Physiol Heart Circ Physiol 296: H470–H479.
32. Cheng Y, Qiu F, Ye Y-C, Guo Z-M, Tashiro S-I, et al. (2009) Autophagy inhibits reactive oxygen species-mediated apoptosis via activating p38-nuclear factor-kappa B survival pathways in oridonin-treated murine fibrosarcoma L929 cells. FEBS J 276: 1291–1306.

4

Probiotics Modulate Intestinal Expression of Nuclear Receptor and Provide Counter-Regulatory Signals to Inflammation-Driven Adipose Tissue Activation

Andrea Mencarelli[1], Eleonora Distrutti[2], Barbara Renga[1], Claudio D'Amore[1], Sabrina Cipriani[1], Giuseppe Palladino[1], Annibale Donini[3], Patrizia Ricci[3], Stefano Fiorucci[1]*

1 Dipartimento di Medicina Clinica e Sperimentale, University of Perugia, Facoltà di Medicina e Chirurgia, Via Gerardo Dottori n° 1 S. Andrea delle Fratte, Perugia, Italy, 2 Azienda Ospedaliera di Perugia, Ospedale Santa Maria della Misericordia, S. Andrea delle Fratte, Perugia, Italy, 3 Dipartimento di Scienze Chirurgiche, Radiologiche e Odontostomatologiche, Nuova Facoltà di Medicina e Chirurgia Sant' Andrea delle Fratte, Perugia, Italy

Abstract

Background: Adipocytes from mesenteric white adipose tissue amplify the inflammatory response and participate in inflammation-driven immune dysfunction in Crohn's disease by releasing proinflammatory mediators. Peroxisome proliferator-activated receptors (PPAR)-α and -γ, pregnane x receptor (PXR), farnesoid x receptor (FXR) and liver x-receptor (LXR) are ligand-activated nuclear receptor that provide counter-regulatory signals to dysregulated immunity and modulates adipose tissue.

Aims: To investigate the expression and function of nuclear receptors in intestinal and adipose tissues in a rodent model of colitis and mesenteric fat from Crohn's patients and to investigate their modulation by probiotics.

Methods: Colitis was induced by TNBS administration. Mice were administered vehicle or VSL#3, daily for 10 days. Abdominal fat explants obtained at surgery from five Crohn's disease patients and five patients with colon cancer were cultured with VSL#3 medium.

Results: Probiotic administration attenuated development of signs and symptoms of colitis, reduced colonic expression of TNFα, IL-6 and IFNγ and reserved colonic downregulation of PPARγ, PXR and FXR caused by TNBS. Mesenteric fat depots isolated from TNBS-treated animals had increased expression of inflammatory mediators along with PPARγ, FXR, leptin and adiponectin. These changes were prevented by VSL#3. Creeping fat and mesenteric adipose tissue from Crohn's patients showed a differential expression of PPARγ and FXR with both tissue expressing high levels of leptin. Exposure of these tissues to VSL#3 medium abrogates leptin release.

Conclusions: Mesenteric adipose tissue from rodent colitis and Crohn's disease is metabolically active and shows inflammation-driven regulation of PPARγ, FXR and leptin. Probiotics correct the inflammation-driven metabolic dysfunction.

Editor: Raffaella Bonecchi, Università degli Studi di Milano, Italy

Funding: The authors have no support or funding to report.

Competing Interests: The authors have declared that no competing interests exist.

* E-mail: fiorucci@unipg.it

Introduction

Crohn's disease is a chronic and progressive inflammatory disorder of gastrointestinal tract. Transmural inflammation is the histological hallmark of Crohn's disease with inflammation extending beyond the intestinal wall. An involvement of mesenteric adipose tissue (MAT) is increasingly thought to provide a mechanistic contribution to disease progression. This contention is supported by the fact that at the onset of disease, although patients show a weight loss, [1] a specific hypertrophy of MAT is frequently identified [1–3]. Fat wrapping extending from the mesenteric attachment and partially covering the intestinal circumference, is common in both the small and large intestine and is also considered a hallmark of Crohn's disease [1]. This ectopic tissue is referred to as "creeping fat" and is encroached at the antimesenteric surface of the bowel. Surgeons are familiar with creeping fat and use it as an anatomical marker to delineate the extent of active disease [4]. Adipose tissue is increasingly identified as a major endocrine organ from which either metabolic and inflammatory signals propagate systemically, potentially modulating clinical features of Crohn's disease. In Crohn's disease patients creeping fat is infiltrated by activated macrophages and releases high amount of TNF-α and leptin, a proinflammatory adipokine, indicating that this tissue could play a mechanistic role in maintaining local and systemic inflammation [5,6]. In chronic disorders such as diabetes and obesity MAT hypertrophy is governed by the activation of a family of nuclear receptors-peroxisome proliferator-activated receptor (PPAR) α and γ, farnesoid-x-receptor (FXR) and liver–x-receptor (LXR)- and adipokynes that are well identified targets for medical interventions. In contrast it is still unknown whether MAT could be modulated by pharmacological interventions in Crohn's disease [7]. The commensal gut microbiota has profound effects on the physiology of the host [8]. The intestinal microbiota may be exerting effects beyond the intestine and patients with chronic inflammatory disorders such as obesity and Type I diabetes display an altered gut flora that may have a pathogenetic readout on the phenotype of these disorders [8–10]. It is increasingly appreciated that circulating levels of xeno- and endo-biotics including bile acids, lipids and metabolism intermediates are regulated by gut microbiota [11–13]. Nutrients and metabolites are transported from the intestine to the liver via the afferent pathways, the i.e. the portal vein and the lymphatic system exerting a wide range of regulatory functions in abdominal tissues beyond the intestinal wall. Decoding the interactions between metabolic intermediates and endogenous receptors has lead to understanding that some of these metabolites act as ligands or activators for nuclear receptors, a large family of ligand activated regulatory factors that exert their homeostatic functions at the interface between nutrients metabolism and innate immunity. Thus, activation of PPAR-α and γ, FXR and LXR by lipid mediators, bile acids and oxysterols modulates lipid/cholesterol metabolism but also provides counter-regulatory signals for cells of innate immunity [14-18]. Probiotics which deliver some of the beneficial immunomodulatory effects of the commensal gut microbiota and induce immune homeostasis have been proposed as a suitable treatment for mild to moderate IBD. Probiotics intervention results in a site-specific reduction of inflammatory pathways with an increased expression of mediators involved in PPAR signalling, a pathway that is counter-regulatory for NF-κB [19]. The beneficial effects of probiotics extend outside the intestine and probiotics have been shown to exert a beneficial effects in obesity, NASH and diabetes despite the mechanisms mediating these effects have not been elucidated [20]. In this study we have investigated whether intestinal inflammation modulates the expression of nuclear receptors in the intestine and MAT in a rodent model of colitis and whether this pattern could be regulated by administration of probiotics. In addition, we have investigated whether this findings might have a translational relevance by examining the expression of nuclear receptors and adipokines in explants of creeping fat and MAT from Crohn's disease patients. Finally, by culturing creeping fat and MAT explants from Crohn's disease patients with conditioned medium from probiotics cultures we have provided evidence that probiotics modulate leptin release.

Results

Anti-Inflammatory effects of VSL#3 the TNBS model of colitis

Colon inflammation that develops in mice administered TNBS is thought to be a model of Th1-mediated disease with dense infiltrations of lymphocytes/macrophages in the *lamina propria* and thickening of the colon wall [18,21]. The TNBS colitis is therefore characterized by typical sign and symptoms of colitis, including weight loss, diarrhea, macroscopic inflammation and prototypical histological and biochemical intestinal changes including increased levels of myeloperoxidase (MPO) activity, a biochemical marker of neutrophils infiltration. No changes in body weight were recorded in mice administered ethanol alone and followed for 7 days after TNBS administration (data not shown). In order to assess whether VSL#3 would exert immune-modulatory activity, mice administered TNBS were treated with VSL#3 (50×10^9 colony-forming units (cfu)/day) for 5 days before induction of colitis. VSL#3 pretreatment effectively attenuated colitis development as measured by assessing local and systemic signs of inflammation.

VSL#3 administration protected against the development of wasting disease measured by the weight loss and the diarrhea score (Figure 1A and 1B; n = 8–10, #p<0.05 versus naive group; *p<0.05 versus TNBS group) and reduced the macroscopic score of colitis (Figure 1 C; #p<0.05 versus control group; *p<0.05 versus TNBS group); moreover, it attenuated colon neutrophils infiltration, as measured by assessing the colonic activity of MPO (Figure 1 D #p<0.05 versus naive group; *p<0.05 versus TNBS group). Mortality was 10% per group and was related to TNBS inoculation. Indeed, mice deaths occurred mostly on day 7, i.e. one day after TNBS inoculation (data not shown). Figure 2 (panel A,D and G) illustrates a representative image of histopathological analysis of colons obtained from each treatment group. Compared with colons of naïve mice, colons obtained from mice administered with TNBS showed an extensive cellular infiltrate, submucosal edema and large areas of epithelial erosions. These changes were robustly attenuated by VSL#3 treatment. To gain insights on the immune-phenotype of colon lamina propria mononuclear cells (LPMC), the phenotype of LPMC cells isolated from animals administered TNBS alone or in combination with VSL#3 was compared to LPMC isolated from naïve mice. The immune-phenotypic characterization of these cells by CD3, CD19, CD14 and NK1.1 antibodies reveled that, in comparison to TNBS treated mice, VSL#3 co-administration caused a slight, thought significant, reduction in the percentage of CD14+ and CD3 +cells (see Figure S1). This effect associates with a robust attenuation of colonic expression of inflammatory and immune mediators including IL-6, TNFα, IL-1β and INFγ caused by TNBS (Figure 3 Panel 1A, B, C and D ; n = 5; #p<0.05 versus naïve; *p<0.05 versus TNBS), while failed to change the mRNA levels of IL-10 and TGF-β (Figure 3 Panel 1 E and F).

A growing body of evidence supports the notion that a mutual inhibition between pro-inflammatory mediators and nuclear receptors does exist in inflammatory bowel diseases (IBDs). [22,23]. Consistent with this view, we found that acute TNBS-colitis causes a robust decrease in the expression of several nuclear receptor including PPARγ, PXR and FXR. These changes were antagonized by VSL#3 cotreatment (Figure 3, Panel 2; n = 5; #p<0.05 versus naïve; *p<0.05 versus TNBS). These changes in gene product expression are mirrored by changes at the protein levels, as demonstrated by the analysis of the colonic expression of FXR protein (see Figure S2).

Effects of VSL#3 administration on the mesenteric adipose tissue in mouse colitis

TNBS administration resulted in robust inflammatory changes in the abdominal fat. Histophatlogy analysis of abdominal fat isolated from TNBS treated mice revealed extensive venular congestion, neutrophil margination and diapedesis and perivascular accumulation of neutrophils in the adipose tissue indicating that TNBS-induced inflammatory changes in the colonic mucosa are reflected in the surrounding fat (Figure 2, panel B,E,H). The mesenteric fat depots from the TNBS treated mice were characterized by an increased levels of the proinflammatory cytokines, including TNF-α, IL-6 and MCP-1 compared to naive mice (Figure 4, panel 1 A, B and C respectively n = 5; #p<0.05 versus naïve). In addition we observed an induction in the expression of leptin and adiponectin mRNAs (Figure 4 D and E respectively n = 5; #p<0.05 versus naïve) in mesenteric fat of colitic mice. These changes were abrogated by VSL#3 administration (Figure 4 and Figure 3; n = 5; #p<0.05 versus naïve; *p<0.05 versus TNBS).

In contrast to the colon, we found that in comparison with fat tissue from naive mice, the expression of PPARγ and FXR was

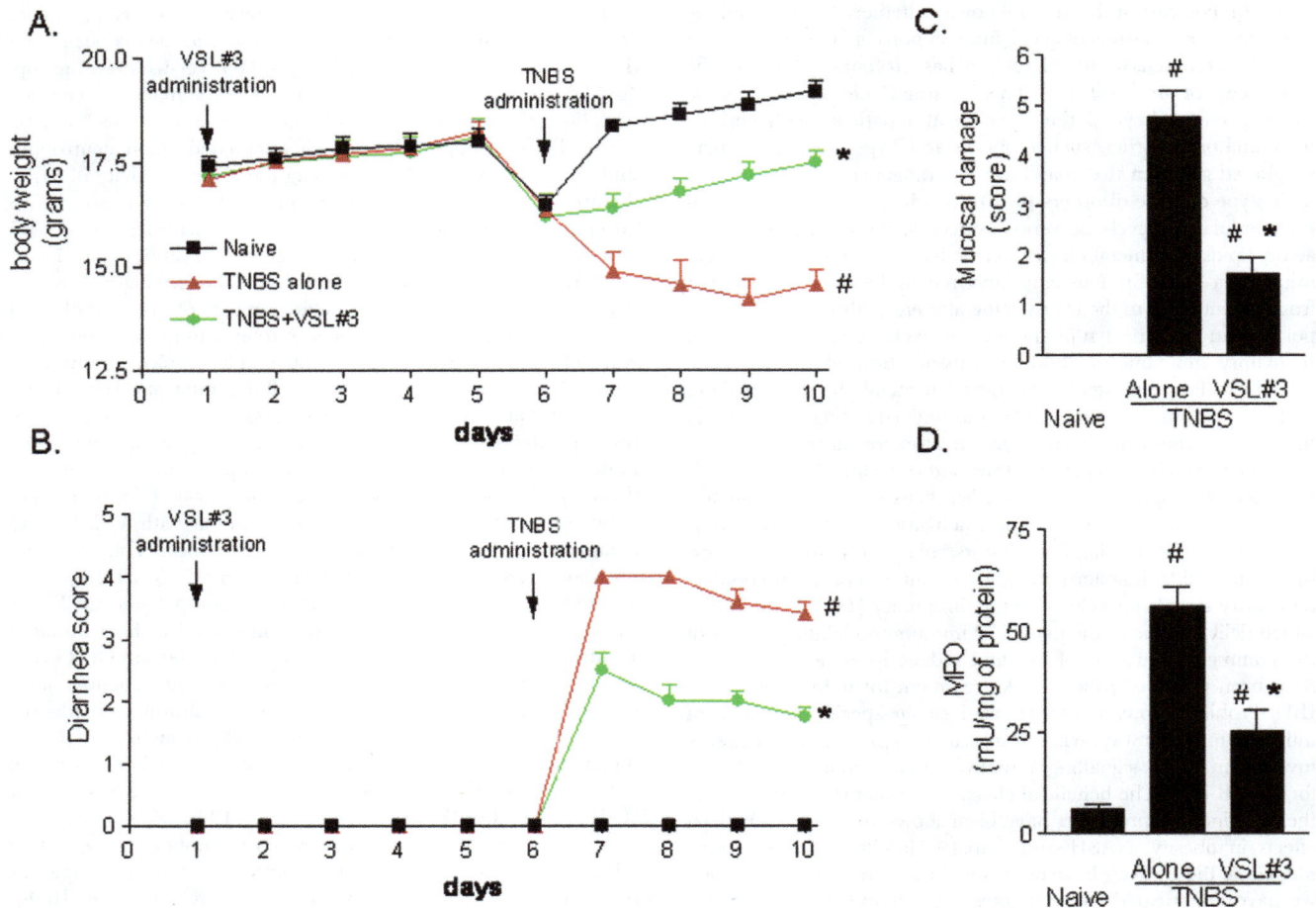

Figure 1. Anti-inflammatory activity of VSL#3 in TNBS colitis. Preteatment with VSL#3 (50×10^9 colony-forming units (cfu)/kg/day) protects against the development of TNBS-induced colitis in mice. Colitis was induced by intrarectal instillation of 1.5 mg of TNBS per mouse. Mice were sacrificed 5 days after TNBS administration. (**A** and **B**) The severity of TNBS-induced inflammation (weight loss and fecal score) is reduced by VSL#3 administration. Data represent the mean ± SE of 8–10 mice per group. (#$p<0.05$ versus naïve; *$p<0.05$ versus TNBS). (**C** and **D**) VSL#3 reduces local signs of inflammation and inhibits the increase of macroscopic-score and neutrophil infiltration (MPO activity) induced by TNBS. Data represent the mean ± SE of 8–10 mice per group. (#$p<0.05$ versus naïve; *$p<0.05$ versus TNBS).

increased in the adipose tissue of colitic mice while LXR and PPARα were unchanged and PXR was downregulated (Figure 4, Panel 2; n = 5; #$p<0.05$ versus naïve). VSL#3 coadmistration restored the PPARγ and FXR mRNA levels (Figure 4, Panel 2; n = 5; *$p<0.05$ versus TNBS) while reduced drastically the LXR expression (Figure 4, Panel 2; n = 5; #$p<0.05$; *$p<0.05$ versus TNBS). The expression of PXR was upregulated (Figure 4, Panel 2; n = 5; #$p<0.05$ versus naïve; *$p<0.05$ versus TNBS).

Finally, we have investigated whether VSL#3 treatment could attenuate signs and symptoms of an established colitis. For this purpose animals were administered with VSL#3 (50^9 cfu/day) starting one day after TNBS inoculation. As illustrated in Figure S3, this treatment attenuated colitis development as evaluated by assessing body weight changes, the macroscopic damage score and the MPO activity (n = 8-10. #$p<0.05$ versus naïve; *$p<0.05$ versus TNBS).

Expression of nuclear receptors, adipokines in creeping fat and MAT explants from Crohn's disease patients

Histopathological examination of mesenteric fat explants form Crohn's disease patient demonstrate a large number of inflammatory cells in creeping adipose tissue (Figure 5 A). In contrast,

very few inflammatory cells were detected in distal mesenteric adipose tissue (Figure 5 B). Consistent with these changes creeping fat explants were characterised by increased mRNA levels of the proinflammatory cytokines such as TNFα, IL-6, MCP-1 and leptin and adiponectin (Figure 6, panel 1 B, C, D and E respectively n = 5; * $p<0.05$). However, MAT explants obtained from Crohn's disease patients had a significant higher level of expression of inflammatory mediators (IL-6, MCP-1) and leptin and adiponectin when compared to MAT obtained from patients with colon carcinomas (Figure 6, panel 1; n = 5; # $p<0.05$). The creeping fat was also characterized by a decreased expression of PPAR α and γ and FXR compared to MAT from Crohn's disease patients and control subjects (Figure 6, panel 2).

To determine whether VSL#3's bacteria secrete factors possessing anti-inflammatory activity, creeping fat and MAT explants from Crohn's disease were cultured with increasing concentrations of VSL#3 CM for 48h. A shown in Figure 7, explants from creeping fat released significant higher levels of leptin, IL-6 and TNFα compared to MAT (#$p<0.05$; n = 25). Interestingly, treatment with VSL#3-CM (all doses) reduced drastically the leptin production by creeping adipose tissue (Figure 7 B; *$p<0.05$; n = 25). In addition VSL#3-CM reduced

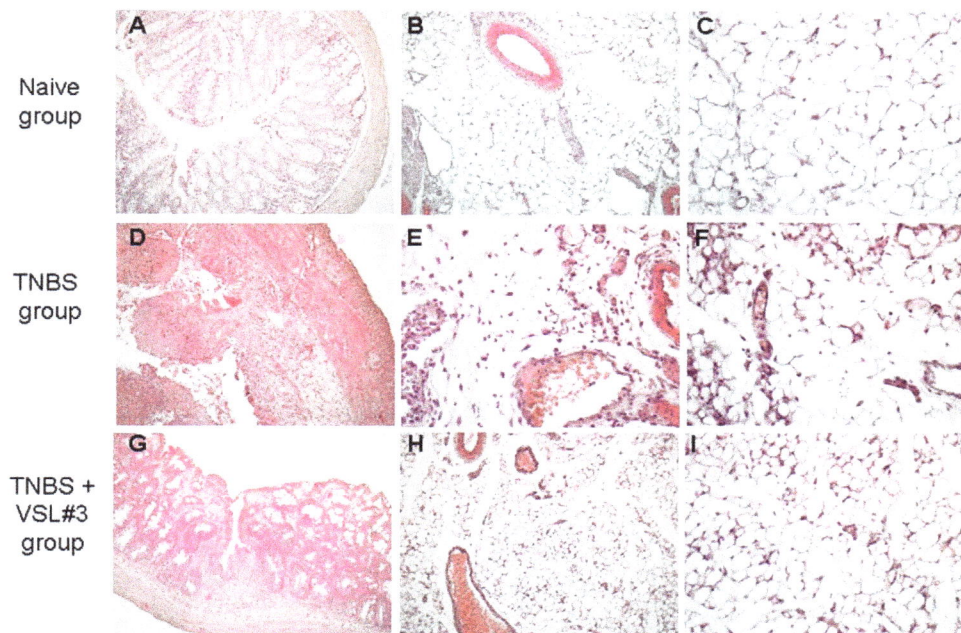

Figure 2. Histological analysis of colon and mesenteric adipose tissue of mice treated with TNBS alone or in combination with VSL#3. (A, D and G) Histopathology analysis of colon samples, original magnification 10×; H&E staining. **(A)** naïve mice; **(D)** TNBS administration causes colon wall thickening and massive inflammatory infiltration in the *lamina propria* and mucosal erosions; **(G)** VSL#3 attenuates colon thickening and inflammatory infiltration of the mucosa and submucosa. **(B,C,E,F,H and I)** Histologic analysis of mesenteric adipose tissue, H&E staining. **(B and C)** Naïve mice, original magnification 10× and 20×; **(E and F)** TNBS group mice, original magnification 10× and 20×; **(H and I)** VSL#3 treated mice, original magnification 10× and 20x.

the production of IL-6 and TNFα (Figure 7 C and D; *p<0.05; n = 25).

Discussion

Probiotics which deliver some of the beneficial immunomodulatory effects of the commensal gut microbiota and induce immune homeostasis are an effective treatment for mild to moderate IBD [24–29]. Here we report that VSL#3 administration is effective in preventing development of an acute colitis induced by TNBS and found that protection correlates with a robust attenuation of inflammation as measured by assessing the colitis macroscopic score, neutrophil infiltration and the mRNA levels of TNFα, IL-1β, IL-6 and IFNγ.

Nuclear receptors are a superfamily of regulatory factors that exert homeostatic functions in the intestine at the interface between nutrients metabolism and immunity. Activation of PPARá and ã, PXR, FXR and LXR by lipid mediators, bile acids and oxysterols modulates lipid/cholesterol metabolism, provides counter-regulatory signals for macrophages and protection in rodent models of dysregulated innate immunity [18,30]. A confirmation of the inverse correlation existing between nuclear receptors expression/activity and host susceptibility to inflammation in the intestinal compartment, comes from the observation that acute exposure to TNBS results in a downregulation of colonic expression of PPARã, PXR, and FXR. Of relevance, VSL#3 counter-reacts the effect of TNBS on inflammation and preserves the intestinal expression of these nuclear receptors.

The adipose tissue is an important source of hormones and cytokines [31]. Patients with Crohn's disease accumulate adipokine-releasing intra-abdominal fat from the onset of the disease [32,33] indicating that expansion of mesenteric fat depots may be an important source of inflammatory mediators in IBDs [34]. Here we have shown that acute colitis induced by TNBS in mice associates with inflammatory changes in the mesenteric fat depots sampled proximally to the inflamed intestine. These changes are characterised by infiltration of mesenteric fat by leucocytes and increased expression of TNFα, IL–6, MCP-1, that have a mechanistic relevance in the development of systemic manifestations of IBDs [35].

The key finding of the present study, however, is that this inflammation-driven metabolic activation of adipose tissue is mediated by a differential regulation in the expression and several nuclear receptors. An abnormal expression of PPARγ, a nuclear receptor which is predominantly expressed in adipocytes and involved in adipogenesis, has been reported in the MAT of Crohn's patients [32]. Activation of PPARγ has important functionl consequences. Indeed PPARγ is a potent inducer of adipocytes growth and differentiation promoting their transition from small, quiescent, adipocytes to large, activated, adipocytes [36–38]. The fact that TNBS induced acute inflammation exerts different effects on PPARγ, with a reduced expression in the colon and an increased expression in the mesenteric fact, seems to support a role for this nuclear receptor in promoting the acquisition of a pro-inflammatory phenotype by mesenteric adipocytes. A similar pattern of expression was observed with FXR. Indeed, while colitis associates with a reduced expression of FXR in the colon, the expression of this nuclear receptor was robustly increased in the mesenteric fat of TNBS-treated mice. We and other have shown that FXR is involved in adipocytes differentiation, adipogenesis, and lipid storage in *vivo* and in *vitro* increasing the adiponectin through a mechanism that is partially mediated by PPARγ [39–40].

Panel 1: Colon cytokines

Panel 2: Colon nuclear receptors

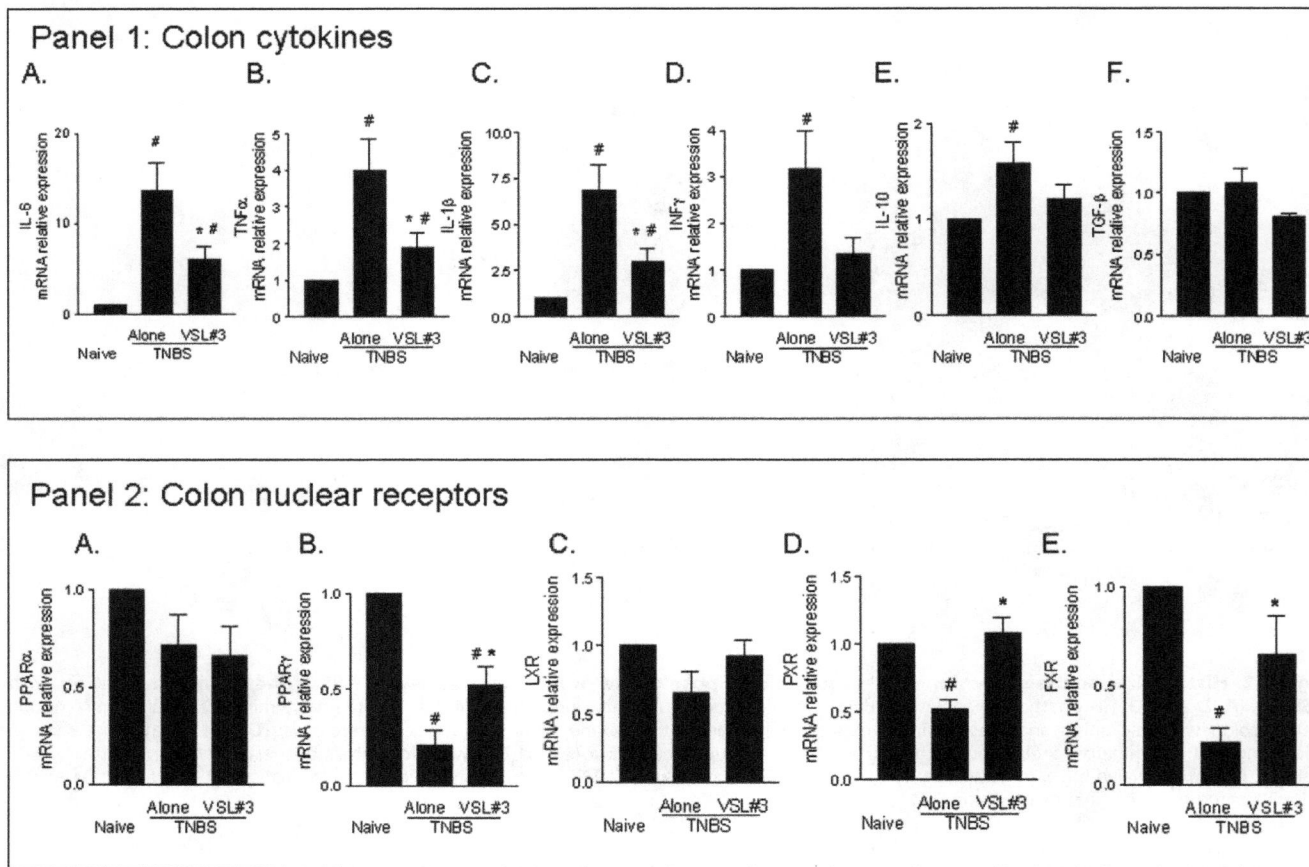

Figure 3. VSL#3 attenuates inflammatory changes in the colon and restores nuclear receptors expression in mice administered TNBS. (Panel 1. A–F) RT-PCR analysis of the expression of inflammatory cytokines (IL-6, TNFα, IL-1β, and INFγ) and anti-inflammatory cytokines (IL-10 and TGF-β) in colons obtained 5 days after TNBS. Data represent the mean ± SE of 5 mice per group. (#p<0.05 versus naïve; *p<0.05 versus TNBS). **(Panel 2 A–E)** RT-PCR analysis of the expression of PPARα, PPARγ, FXR, LXR, PXR and CAR in colons removed 5 days after administration of TNBS alone or in combination with VSL#3. Data represent the mean ± SE of 5 mice per group. (#p<0.05 versus naïve; *p<0.05 versus TNBS).

In contrast to mesenteric fat depots obtained from TNBS mice, we have observed that in comparison to MAT obtained from control subjects and Crohn's patients, creeping fat tissue obtained from Crohn's disease patients is characterized by an increased expression of IL-6, MCP-1 and leptin but has a reduced expression of PPARα, PPARγ and FXR. In contrast, in comparison to MAT from control subjects, MAT tissue from Crohn's patients was characterised by an increased expression of IL-6, MCP-1, leptin and adiponectin, as well as an increased expression of PPARγ and FXR. These changes seem to support a different biological roles of creeping fat and MAT in Crohn's disease. However, it is noteworthy that even MAT was characterized by the expression of a subset of genes known to support an active adipocytes differentiation, i.e.PPARγ and FXR [39,40,41]. In aggregate these data seems to suggest that activation of mesenteric adipose tissue is common in Crohn's patients and might contribute to development of local and systemic signs of disease.

IBDs, including Crohn's disease, are characterized by an increase in mucosal permeability allowing luminal molecules to travel through the intestinal wall or from lymphatic vessel to surrounding tissues. Thus we have investigated whether probiotics release factors that might drive the inflammatory response in the adipose tissue. Interestingly we found that, while creeping fat

releases higher levels of leptin, IL-6 and TNFα compared to the MAT explants obtained from Crohn's disease patients, incubation with VSL#3-CM conter-regulates the production of these inflammatory mediators and abrogates the generation of leptin. Leptin is an adipocyte-secreted hormone that regulates the size of adipose tissue mass [42], reduces food intake and increases the metabolic rate [42]. Despite the correlation between body mass index and plasma leptin is usually preserved in IBDs [43], the mechanistic role of hyperleptinaemia in the onset of anorexia and weight loss associated with IBDs remains unclear [44]. However, it well recognized that circulating levels of leptin does not accurately reflect the local production of this hormone. Indeed a lack of correlation between leptin mRNA levels and plasma levels in IBDs has already been reported [45], reinforcing the notion that leptin produced by MAT might not contribute significantly to the plasma level of the hormone, but rather contributes to a local paracrine effect in the intestine and mesenteric fat. In fact, leptin increases TNFα secretion [45] and promotes changes in the balance between Th1 and Th2 cytokines increasing the generation of Th1 cytokines (IFN-γ and IL-2) and repressing IL-4 [45]. It is also well recognized, that in the other tissue, such as the liver, leptin promotes the activation of locally resident fibroblasts and leptin production associates with liver fibrosis [46]. Because activation of intestinal fibroblasts by locally released mediators and enhanced

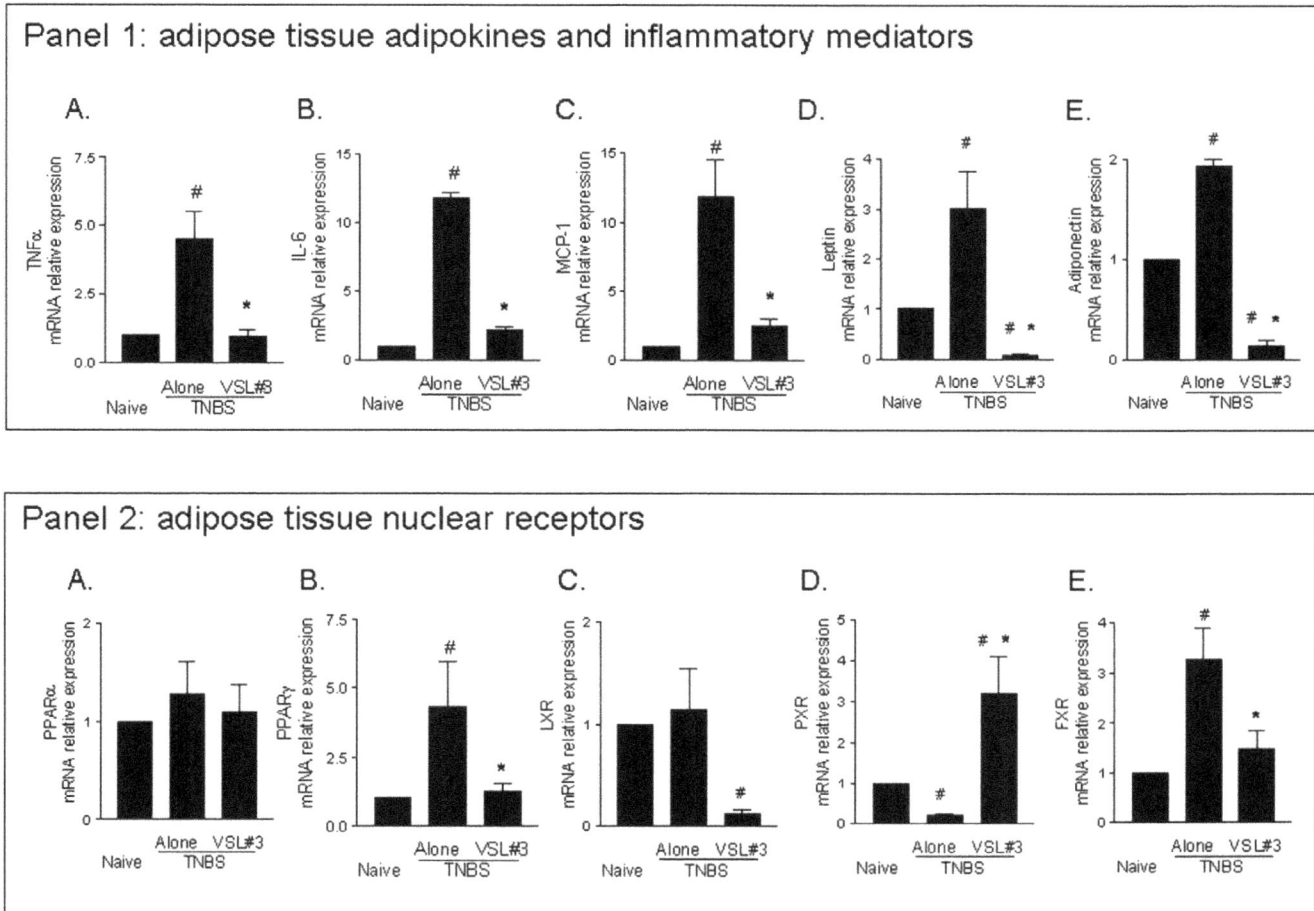

Figure 4. VSL#3 attenuates inflammation-driven metabolic dysfunction in the mesenteric adipose tissue. (Panel 1 A-E) RT-PCR analysis of expression of inflammatory cytokines (TNFα, IL-6, and MCP1) and adipokines (leptin and adiponectin) in mesenteric adipose tissues. Data represent the mean ± SE of 5 mice per group. (#p<0.05 versus naïve; *p<0.05 versus TNBS). **(Panel 2 A-E)** RT-PCR analysis of the expression of PPARα, PPARγ, LXR, PXR and FXR in mesenteric adipose tissues obtained 5 days after administration of TNBS alone or in combination with VSL#3. Data represent the mean ± SE of 5 mice per group. (#p<0.05 versus naïve; *p<0.05 versus TNBS).

deposition of extracellular matrix is a prototypical features in Crohn's disease, is could be speculated that the uncheked leptin production we documented by creping fat and MAT might contribute to intestinal fibrosis in Crohn's patients. The demonstration that VSL#3-CM attenuates leptin production from MAT and creeping fat explants might have therefore a role in explaining the clinical effects of this agent, and paves the way to develop specific therapies.

The increasing awareness that mesenteric and creeping fat might contribute to inflammation and perhaps, to fibrosis, in Crohn's disease and that activity of these tissues could be regulated through a differential expression of nuclear receptors, raises the possibility to target these tissues with selective ligands for these transcription factors. Selective PPARγ agonists exerts anti-inflammatory effects while regulating major metabolic pathways in the abdominal fat and have been demonstrated useful in reducing intestinal inflammation in IBDs [47]. However, the use of PPARγ ligands associates with an increased risk of cardiovascular ischemic events, at least in the case of rosiglitazone [48]. Present results and previous data demonstrate that FXR exerts an anti-inflammatory activity in rodent models of colitis [18] while promoting a less activated phenotype in the adipose tissue [39],

suggesting a potential therapeutic role for ligands of this nuclear receptor in the treatment of inflammation-driven activation of adipose tissue in Crohn's disease. However, further investigations are required to better define interactions between intestinal inflammation and mesenteric fat activation and whether mesenteric fat could be targeted by nuclear receptor modulators.

In conclusion, we have shown that colonic inflammation regulates the expression of several nuclear receptor in MAT in a model of colitis and in Crohn's disease patients. MAT activation could contribute to inflammation-driven immune and metabolic dysfunction in these patients by generating a subset of pro-inflammatory mediators and modulating the expression of several nuclear receptors. These effects are counter-regulated by changing the composition of enteric flora with a probiotic.

Materials and Methods

Animals

CD1 mice, 8 weeks of age, were obtained from Harlan Nossan (Udine, Italy). Mice were housed under controlled temperatures (22°C) and photoperiods (12:12-hour light/dark cycle), allowed unrestricted access to standard mouse chow and tap water and

HUMAN

A) creeping adipose tissue
20 X   40 X

B) distal mesenteric adipose tissue
20 X   40 X

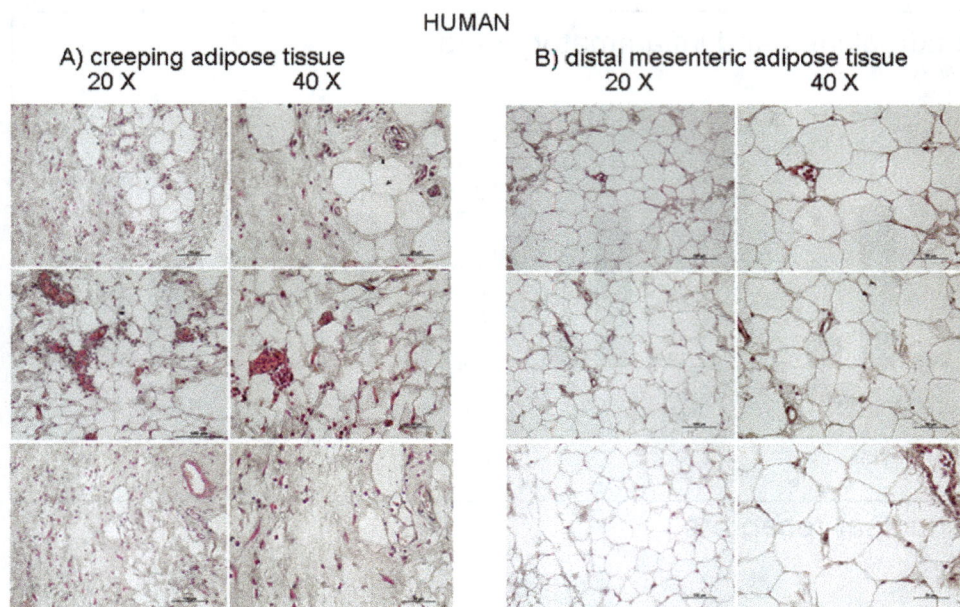

Figure 5. Distinctive histologic features the creeping fat and mesenteric adipose tissue in Crohn's disease patients. Rappresentative haematoxylin-eosin (H&E) staining of mesenteric adipose tissue of Crohn's patients. Creeping fat original magnification 10× and 20×, respectively (A) adipose tissue distal to intestinal mucosa of Crohn's disease patients, original magnification 20× (Bars: 100 μm) and 40×(Bars: 50 μm), respectively (B). Paired samples from three patients are shown.

allowed to acclimate to these conditions for at least 5 days before inclusion in an experiment. Protocols were approved by the University of Perugia Animal Care Committee according to the Italian guideline for care and use of laboratory animals. The ID for this project is #98/2010-B. The authorization was released to Prof. Stefano Fiorucci, as a principal investigator, on May 19, 2010.

Reagents

Purified myeloperoxidase (MPO) and tri-methylbenzidine, trinitro-benzene sulfonic acid (TNBS) were obtained from Sigma-Aldrich (Milan, Italy). The probiotics compound VSL3, consisting of 8 strains of bacteria (*L. acidophilus* MB 443, *L. delbrueckii* subsp. *bulgaricus* MB 453, *L. casei* MB 451, *L. plantarum* MB 452, *B. longum* Y10, *B. infantis* Y1, *B. breve* Y8, and *S. salivarius* subsp. *thermophilus* MB 455), was obtained from VSL Pharmaceuticals.

Experimental Procedures

Mice were lightly anesthetized by intraperitoneal injection of 100 μl of ketamine/xylazine solution [18,21] per 10 g body weight and then administered intrarectally (i.r.) with the haptenating agent TNBS (1.5 mg/mouse) dissolved in ethanol 50%, via a 3.5 French (F) catheter equipped with a 1-ml syringe. The catheter was advanced into the rectum for 4 cm and then the haptenating agent was administered in a total volume of 150 μl. To ensure distribution of the agent within the entire colon and cecum, mice were held in a vertical position for 30 seconds. An additional control group was obtained by administering mice with ethanol alone on day 6. Animals (n = 5) were followed for body weight changes for 7 days.

Treated animals received, orally, saline or probiotics, daily, at dose of 50×10^9 colony-forming units (cfu)/kg/day (1.25×10^9/mouse) (n = 10–8 for each group), 5 days before induction of

colitis. Mice were sacrificed 5 days after TNBS administration. The mice were monitored daily for weigh loss and fecal score. Probitics were dissolved each day in physiologic solution and administrated orally at the final volume of 200 μL/mouse. The TNBS group mice received the vehicle alone every day. Five days after TNBS administration, surviving mice were sacrificed, colons and mesenteric adipose tissue were removed and immediately snap-frozen in liquid nitrogen and stored at −80°C until use. The macroscopic appearance was analyzed under a dissecting microscope (× 5) and graded for macroscopic lesions on a scale from 0 to 10 based on criteria reflecting inflammation, such as hyperemia, thickening of the bowel, and the extent of ulceration. Neutrophil infiltration in the colon was monitored by measuring MPO activity using a spectrophotometric assay with tri-methyl-benzidine (TMB) as a substrate. Activity is expressed as mU per mg protein.

Patients

MAT and creeping fat explants were obtained from five patients affected by Crohn's disease (2 women; mean age 36±8 years old). All patients underwent right ileocolonic resection because of symptomatic ileal stenosis with transmural inflammation. All patients had a stenotic disease complicated buy by ileocolonic abscesses in 3 patients and an intestinal fistula, 2 patients. All were treated with antibiotic (ciprofloxacin and metronidazole) for before surgery. Anti-TNFα therapy was the main therapy in two patients. All had been treated with azathioprine in the weeks before the surgery. Five subjects with carcinoma of the right colon (2 women ; mean age 47±8 years old) served as controls. None of these control subjects was obese. In patients with colon carcinoma mesenteric fat samples were obtained in front of normal intestine at a sufficient minimal distance from tumour. Adipose tissue samples were immediately frozen in liquid nitrogen and stored at −80°C for subsequent mRNA analysis or processed to tissue culture biopsy. An informed written consent on the use of removed

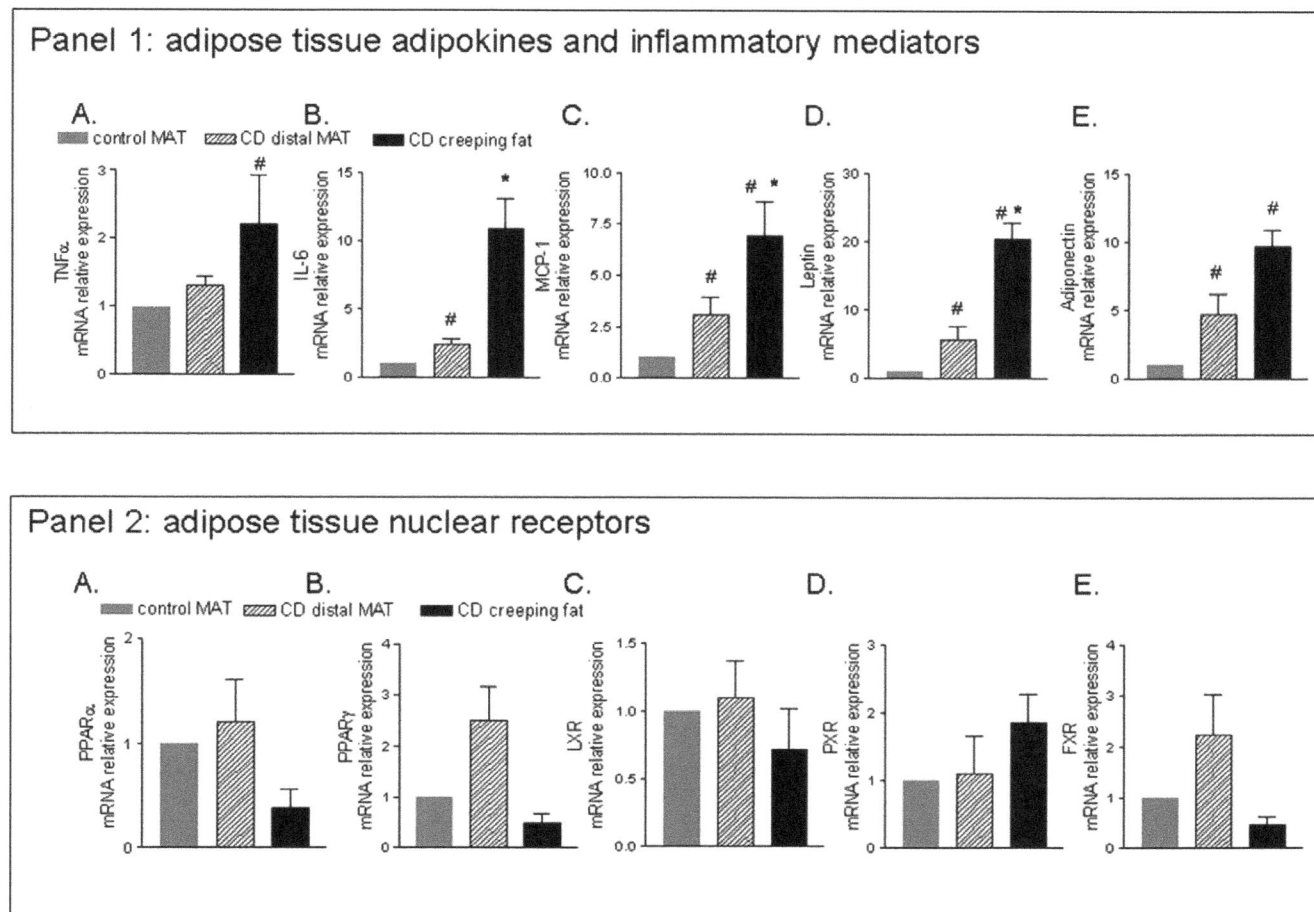

Figure 6. Expression of inflammatory mediators, adipokines and selected nuclear receptors in mesenteric adipose tissues from Crohn's patients. RT-PC analysis of expression of inflammatory TNFα, IL-6, MCP1, leptin and adiponectin **(Panel 1 A-E)** and nuclear receptors (PPARα, PPARγ, LXR, PXR and FXR) **(Panel 2 A-E)** in mesenteric adipose tissue (MAT) obtained from control subjects (N = 5) (colon carcinoma) and in Crohn's patients (creeping fat and distal MAT) (N = 5). Data represent the mean ± SE of 5 different subjects per group. (#p<0.05 versus MAT of control subjects ; *p<0.05 versus distal MAT obtained from Crohn's disease patients).

surgical samples was obtained by each patient. The authorization of an ethical committee was not requested because for small exploratory studies, by internal hospital guidelines, only the informed consent by the patient is requested.

VSL#3 conditioned media preparations and human adipose tissue cultures

To prepare conditioned medium (CM), 10 mg of VSL#3 probiotics formula was reconstituted in 10 ml of serum/antibiotic-free Dulbeccos Modified Eagle's cell culture medium and was grown overnight in medium at 37°C without shaking. The CM was centrifuged at 4,100 rpm for 10 min to separate the bacteria, and the resulting supernatant was filtered two times through a 0.22- µm membrane (Millipore) to remove any insoluble particles and diluted with DMEM cell culture medium free of serum and supplemented with to have a final concentration of 10 mg/ml bovine serum albumin, 5 µg/ml ethanolamine, 0.1 ng/ml sodium selenite, 100 U/mL penicillin and 100 µg/mL streptomycin, 50 µg/ml gentamicin and 55 µM ascorbic acid. The pH of the buffer was adjusted to 7.4 and then filtered through a 0.22- µm filter (100-50-30-10%). The fat tissue samples were surgically removed and placed in Hanks' Balanced Salt Solution, (HBSS)

supplemented with 100 U/mL penicillin and 100 µg/mL streptomycin. Fat tissue lobules were prepared under sterile conditions by microdissection. Vessels and adjacent soft tissue were carefully removed. After preparation, the fat tissue samples were washed four time with HBSS supplemented with 300 U/mL penicillin and 300 µg/mL streptomycin. At least 25 fat tissue specimens, creeping and distal, were cultured from each patient and secretion of Leptin, Adiponectin, IL-6 (Orgenium Laboratories) and TNFα (SABioscence) was determined. Based on this procedure, a total number of n = 25 tissue samples was incubated from 5 CD patients, alone or in combination VSL#3 CM (100-50-30-10%). The tissue samples were incubated in 1 mL medium for 48 h at 37°C in a 95% O2 and 5% CO2 incubator. Supernatants were collected and stored at−20°C. The wet weight of fat tissue was measured (60–80 mg) in order to express the cytokine secretion as pg/mg fat per 48 h.

Histological Analysis

For histological examination, tissues were fixed in 10% buffered formalin phosphate, embedded in paraffin, sectioned, and stained with hematoxylin and eosin (H&E). Histology images were captured by a digital camera (Digital Microscope Camera

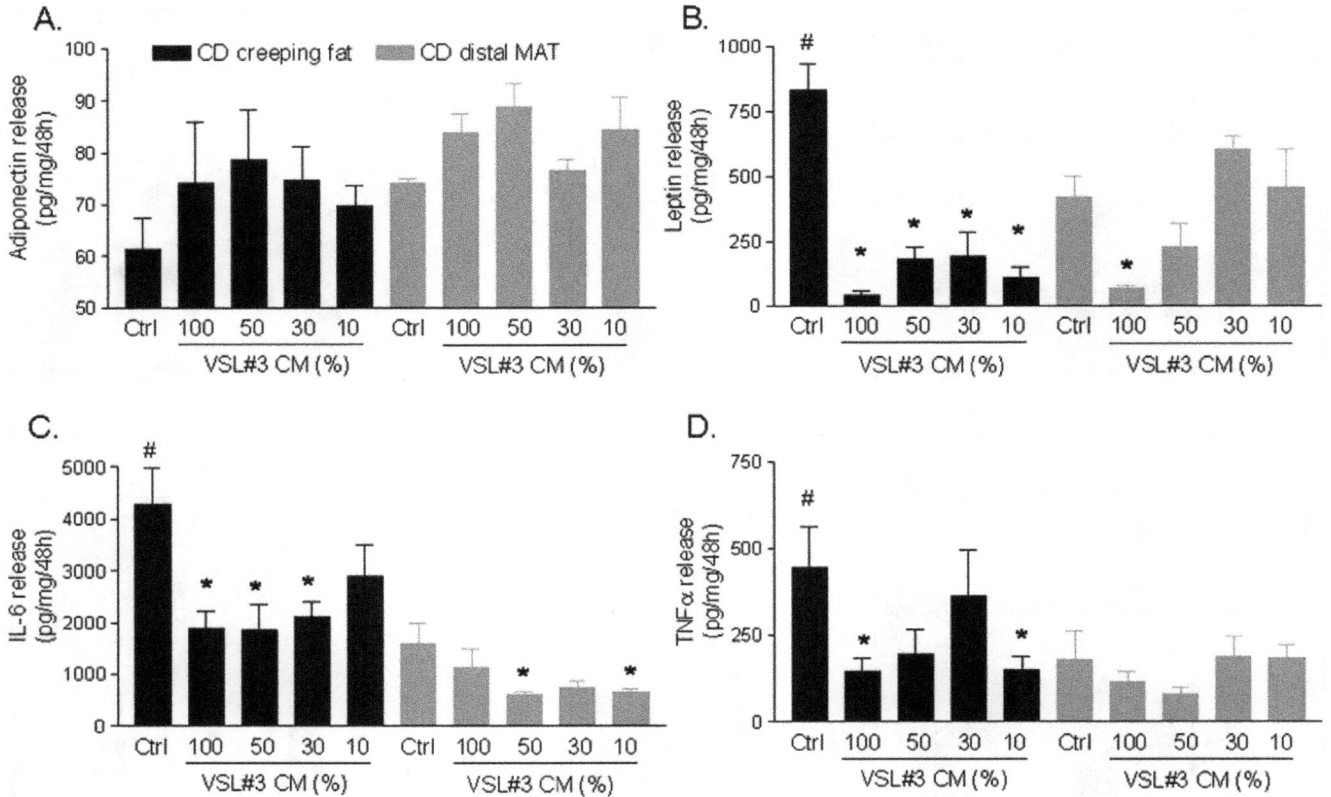

Figure 7. VSL#3 CM modulates the production of mesenteric adipose tissue factors. Release of adiponectin, leptin, IL-6 and TNFα by adipose tissue explants. Release by proximal (creeping fat) and distal MAT explants from 5 Crhon's patients is shown. Creeping fat and MAT explants were cultured alone or in combination with different concentrations of VSL#3 CM for 48 h. (#$p<0.05$ basal production (Ctrl) creeping versus MAT; n = 25; * $p<0.05$ verus control group, n = 25).

ProgResC14, Jenoptik, Germany) and analyzed by specific software (Delta Sistemi, Rome, Italy).

Real-Time PCR

Quantization of the expression level of selected genes was performed by quantitative real-time PCR (qRT-PCR). Total RNA were obtained from colon and adipose tissue pieces (100–50 mg) and isolated with TRIzol reagent (Invitrogen, Milan, Italy), incubated with DNase I and reverse-transcribed with Superscript II (Invitrogen) according to manufacturer specifications. For real-time PCR, 50–25 ng of template was used in a 25- μl reaction containing a 0.3 μM concentration of each primer and 12.5 μl of 2x SYBR Green PCR Master Mix (Bio-Rad Laboratories, Hercules, CA). All reactions were performed in triplicate using the following cycling conditions: 2 min at 95°C, followed by 50 cycles of 95°C for 10 s and 60°C for 30 s using an iCycler iQ instrument (Bio-Rad Laboratories). The mean value of the replicates for each sample was calculated and expressed as cycle threshold (C_T). The amount of gene expression was then calculated as the difference (ΔC_T) between the C_T value of the sample for the target gene and the mean C_T value of that sample for the endogenous control (GAPDH). Relative expression was calculated as the difference ($\Delta\Delta C_T$) between the ΔC_T values of the test and control samples for each target gene. The relative level of expression was measured as $2^{-\Delta\Delta CT}$. All PCR primers were designed using the software PRIMER3-OUTPUT using published sequence data obtained from the NCBI database.

Mouse and Human primers were as follows:

mGAPDH: CTGAGTATGTCGTGGAGTCTAC and GTT-GGTGGTGCAGGATGCATTG;

mIL1β: TCACAGCAGCACATCAACAA and TGTCCTCA-TCCTCGAAGGTC;

mIL-6: CCGGAGAGGAGACTTCACAG and TCCACGAT-TTCCCAGAGAAC;

mIL-10: GCTGGACAACATACTGCTAACC and CTGGG-GCATCACTTCTACCA;

mINFγ: GCGTCATTGAATCACACCTG and GACCTGT-GGGTTGTTGACTC;

mMCP-1: CCCAATGAGTAGGCTGGAGA and TCTGGA-CCCATTCCTTCTTG;

mTNFα: ACGGCATGGATCTCAAAGAC and GTGGGT-GAGGAGCACGTAGT;

mTGFβ: TGGCTTCAGCTCCACAGAGA and TGGTTGT-AGAGGGCAAGGAC;

mLeptin: TTCACACACGCAGTCGGTAT and TCATTGG-CTATCTGCAGCAC;

mAdiponectin: ACAATGGCACACCAGGCCGT and CCC-TTAGGACCAAGAAGACCTGCA;

mPPARα: CAGAGGTCCGATTCTTCCAC and GATCAG-CATCCCGTCTTTGT;

mPPARγ: GCCAGTTTCGATCCGTAGAA and AATCC-TTGGCCCTCTGAGAT;

mLXR: GCAGGACCAGCTCCAAGTAG and GGCTCAC-CAGCTTCATTAGC;

mPXR: ACGGCAGCATCTGGAACTAC and TGGTCC-TCAATAGGCAGGTC;

mFXR: TGTGAGGGCTGCAAAGGTTT and ACATCCC-CATCTCTCTGCAC.

hPPARa: ACGATTCGACTCAAGCTGGT and GTTGTG-TGACATCCCGACAG;

hPPARg: GCTGGCCTCCTTGATGAATA and TTGGG-CTCCATAAAGTCACC;

hPXR: AGCTGGAACCATGCTGACTT and CACATA-CACGGCAGATTTGG;

hFXR: TACATGCGAAGAAAGTGTCAAGA and ACTGT-CTTCATTCACGGTCTGAT;

hTNFa: AACCTCCTCTCTGCCATCAA and GGAAGAC-CCCTCCCAGATAG;

hIL6: AGGAGACTTGCCTGGTGAAA and CAGGGGTG-GTTATTGCATCT;

hMCP1: CCCCAGTCACCTGCTGTTAT and TCCTGA-ACCCACTTCTGCTT;

HLXR: CGCACTACATCTGCCACAGT and TCAGGCG-GATCTGTTCTTCT;

hLeptin: GGCTTTGGCCCTATCTTTTC and GCCAGT-TCTGGTCCATCTT;

hAdiponectin: CCTGGTGAGAAGGGTGAGAA and GTAA-AGCGAATGGGCATGTT.

Statistical analysis

All values are expressed as the mean ± SE of n mice per group. Comparisons of more than 2 groups were made with a one-way analysis of variance with post hoc Tukey tests. Differences were considered statistically significant if p was <0.05.

Supporting Information

Figure S1 LPMC were isolated from freshly obtained colonic specimens. After excision of all visible lymphoid follicles, colons were digested with type IV collagenase (Sigma) for 20 min in a shaking incubator at 37°C; this step was repeated twice. The released cells were then layered on a 40%-100% Percoll gradient (Pharmacia, Upsala, Sweden) and spun at 1,800 rpm to obtain the lymphocyte-enriched populations at the 40–100% interface. For flow cytometry analysis 0.8×10^6 LPMC obtained from naïve and TNBS (1.5 mg/mouse) treated mice (4 after colitis induction) alone or in combination with VSL#3 (50×109 colony-forming units (cfu)/kg/day) for 5 days before induction of colitis. Cells were stained (20 min at 4°), with specific mAbs against CD3, CD14, CD19, and NK-1.1 (phycoerythrin (PE) or fluorescein isothiocyanate (FITC)--conjugated) (BD Biosciences). At the end of incubation, cells were washed two times with phosphate buffered saline (PBS) buffer and resuspended in PBS containing formaldehyde (4%) prior to flow cytometric analysis (Epics XL-2; Beckman Coulter, USA).

Figure S2 Total lysates from colon were prepared by E1A-buffer. Protein levels in tissue extract were quantified with Bradford reagent. Proteins, 30 µgrams, (a pool of 5 different animals, 6 µgrams each) were separated by polyacrylamide gel electrophoresis, transferred to nitrocellulose membranes (Bio-Rad, Hercules, CA) and than probed with primary anti-FXR antibody (0.5 µg/ml) (Ab 28676, Abcam). The anti-immunoglobulin G Rabbit (Bio-Rad) was used as a secondary antibody, and specific protein bands were visualized by chemoluminescence using Supersignal West Dura reagent (Pierce, Rockford, IL).

Figure S3 Colitis was induced in Balb/c by intrarectal administration of TNBS (0.5 mg/mouse) in 50% ethanol. To assess whether administration of VSL#3 would protect against development of colitis, TNBS-treated mice were randomized to receive vehicle or probiotics, daily, (the day after TNBS administration) at dose of 50×10^9 colony-forming units (cfu) (n = 10 for each group). The mice were monitored daily for weigh loss and fecal score (A and B). The macroscopic appearance was analyzed under a dissecting microscope (x 5) and graded for macroscopic lesions on a scale from 0 to 10 based on criteria reflecting inflammation, such as hyperemia, thickening of the bowel, and the extent of ulceration (C). Neutrophil infiltration in the colon was monitored by measuring MPO activity using a spectrophotometric assay with tri-methylbenzidine (TMB) as a substrate (D). Activity is expressed as mU per mg protein. *P value <.05 was considered significant vs Naive group. #P value <.05 was considered significant vs TNBS group. The ANOVA test was used for statistical comparisons.

Author Contributions

Conceived and designed the experiments: AM SF. Performed the experiments: AM BR CD SC GP. Analyzed the data: ED AM PR SF. Contributed reagents/materials/analysis tools: AD PR. Wrote the paper: AM ED SF.

References

1. Sheehan AL, Warren BF, Gear MW, Shepherd NA (1992) Fat-wrapping in Crohn's disease: pathological basis and relevance to surgical practice. Br J Surg 79: 955–958.
2. Smedh K, Olaison G, Nyström PO, Sjödahl R (1993) Intraoperative enteroscopy in Crohn's disease. Br J Surg 80: 897–900.
3. Borley NR, Mortensen NJ, Jewell DP, Warren BF (2000) The relationship between inflammatory and serosal connective tissue changes in ileal Crohn's disease: evidence for a possible causative link. J Pathol 190: 196–202.
4. Fazio VW, Jones IT (1987) Standard surgical treatment of Crohn's disease of the small intestine and ileocolitis. In: Lee ECG, Nolan DJ, eds. Surgery of inflammatory bowel disorders. Edinburgh: Churchill Livingstone 147–56.
5. Paul G, Schäffler A, Neumeier M, Fürst A, Bataillle F, et al. (2006) Profiling adipocytokine secretion from creeping fat in Crohn's disease. Inflamm Bowel Dis 12: 471–477.
6. Schaffler A, Herfarth H (2005) Creeping fat in Crohn's disease: travelling in a creeper lane of research? Gut 54: 742–744.
7. Boss O, Bergenhem N (2006) Adipose targets for obesity drug development. Expert Opin Ther Targets 10: 119–134.
8. Bäckhed F, Ding H, Wang T, Hooper LV, Koh GY, et al. (2004) The gut microbiota as an environmental factor that regulates fat storage. Proc Natl Acad Sci U S A 101: 15718–15723.
9. Bäckhed F, Manchester JK, Semenkovich CF, Gordon JI (2007) Mechanisms underlying the resistance to diet-induced obesity in germ-free mice. Proc Natl Acad Sci U S A 104: 979–984.
10. Wen L, Ley RE, Volchkov PY, Stranges PB, Avanesyan L, et al. (2008) Innate immunity and intestinal microbiota in the development of Type 1 diabetes. Nature 455: 1109–1113.
11. Einarsson K, Gustafsson JA, Gustafsson BE (1973) Differences between germfree and conventional rats in liver microsomal metabolism of steroids. J Biol Chem 248: 3623–3630.
12. Gustafsson BE, Angelin B, Einarsson K, Gustafsson JA (1977) Effects of cholesterol feeding on synthesis and metabolism of cholesterol and bile acids in germfree rats. J Lipid Res 18: 717–721.
13. Einarsson K, Gustafsson JA, Gustafsson BE (1977) Hepatic 3-hydroxy-3-methylglutaryl CoA reductase activity in germfree rats. Proc Soc Exp Biol Med 154: 319–321.
14. Desreumaux P, Dubuquoy L, Nutten S, Peuchmaur M, Englaro W, et al. (2001) Attenuation of colon inflammation through activators of the retinoid X receptor (RXR)/peroxisome proliferator-activated receptor γ (PPARγ) heterodimer. A basis for new therapeutic strategies. J Exp Med 193: 827–838.
15. Ricote M, Li AC, Willson TM, Kelly CJ, Glass CK (1998) The peroxisome proliferator-activated receptor-γ is a negative regulator of macrophage function. Nature 391: 79–82.

16. Jiang C, Ting AT, Seed B (1998) PPAR-γ agonists inhibit production of monocyte inflammatory cytokines. Nature 391: 82–86.

17. Chawla A, Barak Y, Nagy L, Liao D, Tontonoz P, et al. (2001) PPAR-γ dependent and independent effects on macrophage-gene expression in lipid metabolism and inflammation. Nature Med 7: 48–52.

18. Vavassori P, Mencarelli A, Renga B, Distrutti E, Fiorucci S (2009) The bile acid receptor FXR is a modulator of intestinal innate immunity. J Immunol 183: 6251–6261.

19. Reiff C, Delday M, Rucklidge G, Reid M, Duncan G, et al. (2009) Balancing inflammatory, lipid, and xenobiotic signaling pathways by VSL#3, a biotherapeutic agent, in the treatment of inflammatory bowel disease. Inflamm Bowel Dis 15: 1721–1736.

20. Lam B, Younossi ZM (2010) Treatment options for nonalcoholic fatty liver disease. Therap Adv Gastroenterol 3: 121–137.

21. Fiorucci S, Mencarelli A, Palazzetti B, Sprague AG, Distrutti E, et al. (2002) Importance of innate immunity and collagen binding integrin alpha1beta1 in TNBS-induced colitis. Immunity 17: 769–780.

22. Joseph SB, Castrillo A, Laffitte BA, Mangelsdorf DJ, Tontonoz P (2003) Reciprocal regulation of inflammation and lipid metabolism by liver X receptors. Nature Med 9: 213–219.

23. Fiorucci S, Cipriani S, Mencarelli A, Renga B, Distrutti E, et al. (2010) Counter-regulatory role of bile acid activated receptors in immunity and inflammation. Curr Mol Med 10: 579–595.

24. Chapman TM, Plosker GL, Figgit DP (2006) VSL#3 probiotics mixture. A review of its use in chronic inflammatory bowel disease. Drugs 66: 1371–1387.

25. Madsen K, Cornish A, Soper P, McKaigney C, Jijon H, et al. (2001) Probiotics bacteria enhance murine and human intestinal epithelial barrier function. Gastroenterology 121: 580–591.

26. Kühbacher T, Ott SJ, Helwig U, Mimura T, Rizzello F, et al. (2006) Bacterial and fungal microbiota in relation to probiotics therapy (VSL#3) in pouchitis. Gut 55: 833–841.

27. Gaudier E, Michel C, Segain JP, Cherbut C, Hoebler C (2005) The VSL#3 probiotics mixture modifies microflora but does not heal chronic dextran-sodium sulphate induced colitis or reinforce the mucosal barrier in mice. J Nutr 135: 2753–2761.

28. Pronio A, Montesani C, Butteroni C, Vecchione S, Mumolo G, et al. (2008) Probiotics administration in patients with ileal pouch-anal anastomosis for ulcerative colitis is associated with expansion of mucosal regulatory cells. Inflamm Bowel Dis 14: 662–668.

29. Di Giacinto C, Marinaro M, Sanchez M, Strober W, Boirivant M (2005) Probiotics ameliorate recurrent Th1-mediated murine colitis by inducing IL-10 and IL-10-dependent TGF-beta-bearing regulatory cells. J Immunol 174: 3237–3246.

30. Langmann T, Moehle C, Mauerer R, Scharl M, Liebisch G, et al. (2004) Loss of detoxification in inflammatory bowel disease: dysregulation of pregnane X receptor target genes. Gastroenterology 127: 26–40.

31. Kershaw EE, Flier JS (2004) Adipose tissue as an endocrine organ. J Clin Endocrinol Metab 89: 2548–2556.

32. Desreumaux P, Ernst O, Geboes K, Gambiez L, Berrebi D, et al. (1999) Inflammatory alterations in mesenteric adipose tissue in Crohn's disease. Gastroenterology 117: 73–81.

33. Schaffler A, Scholmerich J, Buchler C (2005) Mechanisms of disease: Adipocytokines and visceral adipose tissue—emerging role in nonalcoholic fatty liver disease. Nat Clin Pract Gastroenterol Hepatol 2: 273–280.

34. Karagiannides I, Kokkotou E, Tansky M, Tchkonia T, Giorgadze N, et al. (2006) Induction of colitis causes inflammatory responses in fat depots: Evidence for substance P pathways in human mesenteric preadipocytes. Proc Natl Acad Sci U S A 103: 5207–5212.

35. Fernandez-Real JM, Ricart W (2003) Insulin resistance and chronic cardiovascular inflammatory syndrome. Endocr Rev 24: 278–301.

36. Brun RP, Kim JB, Hu E, Spiegelman BM (1997) Peroxisome proliferator-activated receptor gamma and the control of adipogenesis. Curr Opin Lipidol 8: 212–218.

37. Buechler C, Wanninger J, Neumeier M (2010) Adiponectin receptor binding proteins--recent advances in elucidating adiponectin signalling pathways. FEBS Lett 584: 4280–4286.

38. Paul G, Schäffler A, Neumeier M, Fürst A, Bataillle F, et al. (2006) Profiling adipocytokine secretion from creeping fat in Crohn's disease. Inflamm Bowel Dis 12: 471–477.

39. Rizzo G, Disante M, Mencarelli A, Renga B, Gioiello A, et al. (2006) The farnesoid X receptor promotes adipocyte differentiation and regulates adipose cell function in vivo. Mol Pharmacol 70: 1164–11673.

40. Abdelkarim M, Caron S, Duhem C, Prawitt J, Dumont J, et al. (2010) The farnesoid X receptor regulates adipocyte differentiation and function by promoting peroxisome proliferator-activated receptor-gamma and interfering with the Wnt/beta-catenin pathways. J Biol Chem 285: 36759–36767.

41. Yoshinari K, Sato T, Okino N, Sugatani J, Miwa M (2004) Expression and induction of cytochromes p450 in rat white adipose tissue. J Pharmacol Exp Ther 311: 147–154.

42. Campfield LA, Smith FJ, Guisez Y, Devos R, Burn P (1995) Recombinant mouse OB protein: evidence for a peripheral signal linking adiposity and central neural networks. Science 269: 546–549.

43. Maffei M, Halaas J, Ravussin E, Pratley RE, Lee GH, et al. (1995) Leptin levels in human and rodent: measurement of plasma leptin and ob RNA in obese and weight-reduced subjects. Nat Med 1: 1155–1161.

44. Ballinger A, Kelly P, Hallyburton E, Besser R, Farthing M (1998) Plasma leptin in chronic inflammatory bowel disease and HIV: implications for the pathogenesis of anorexia and weight loss. Clinical Science 94: 479–483.

45. von der Weid PY, Rainey KJ (2010) Review article: lymphatic system and associated adipose tissue in the development of inflammatory bowel disease. Aliment Pharmacol Ther 32: 697–711.

46. Marra F, Bertolani C (2009) Adipokines in liver diseases. Hepatology 50: 957–69.

47. Wu GD (2003) Is there a role for PPAR gamma in IBD? Yes, no, maybe. Gastroenterology 124: 1538–42.

48. Nesto RW, Bell D, Bonow RO, Fonseca V, Grundy SM, et al. (2004) Thiazolidinedione use, fluid retention, and congestive heart failure: a consensus statement from the *American Heart Association and American Diabetes Association*, *Diabetes Care* 27: 256–263.

5

Tumor Necrosis Factor-α and Muc2 Mucin Play Major Roles in Disease Onset and Progression in Dextran Sodium Sulphate-Induced Colitis

Poonam Dharmani, Pearl Leung, Kris Chadee*

Department of Microbiology, Immunology and Infectious Diseases, Gastrointestinal Research Group, Health Sciences Centre, University of Calgary, Calgary, Alberta, Canada

Abstract

The sequential events and the inflammatory mediators that characterize disease onset and progression of ulcerative colitis (UC) are not well known. In this study, we evaluated the early pathologic events in the pathogenesis of colonic ulcers in rats treated with dextran sodium sulfate (DSS). Following a lag phase, day 5 of DSS treatment was found clinically most critical as disease activity index (DAI) exhibited an exponential rise with severe weight loss and rectal bleeding. Surprisingly, on days 1-2, colonic TNF-α expression (70-80-fold) and tissue protein (50-fold) were increased, whereas IL-1β only increased on days 7-9 (60-90-fold). Days 3-6 of DSS treatment were characterized by a prominent down regulation in the expression of regulatory cytokines (40-fold for IL-10 and TGFβ) and mucin genes (15-18 fold for Muc2 and Muc3) concomitant with depletion of goblet cell and adherent mucin. Remarkably, treatment with TNF-α neutralizing antibody markedly altered DSS injury with reduced DAI, restoration of the adherent and goblet cell mucin and IL-1β and mucin gene expression. We conclude that early onset colitis is dependent on TNF-α that preceded depletion of adherent and goblet cell mucin prior to epithelial cell damage and these biomarkers can be used as therapeutic targets for UC.

Editor: Irun R. Cohen, Weizmann Institute of Science, Israel

Funding: This work was supported by a grant from the Canadian Institute for Health Research (CIHR, KC). PD is funded by a Canadian Association of Gastroenterology-AstraZeneca-CIHR Research and Fellowship Award. The funders had no role in study design, data collection and analysis, decision to publish, or preparation of the manuscript.

Competing Interests: The authors have declared that no competing interests exist.

* E-mail: kchadee@ucalgary.ca

Introduction

Inflammatory bowel disease (IBD), an umbrella term that includes Crohn's disease and ulcerative colitis (UC), are chronic relapsing inflammatory disorders of the gut that are believed to occur in genetically predisposed individuals due to exposure of unknown environmental and microbial agents [1]. A normal healthy intestine exhibits homeostasis where the mucosal immune system escalates an immune response against pathogens but remains tolerant to antigens derived from food and commensal microbes. Loss of mucosal tolerance is due to an uncontrolled inflammatory cascade resulting from a number of mutual and probably sequential events involving both immune (gut associated lymphoid tissues, GALT and professional antigen presenting cells, APC) and non-immune cells/molecules (epithelial cells of gut and resident microflora) [1,2]. However, the precise etiology of the pathogenesis of UC is still not known.

To date, studies to unravel the pathogenesis of UC have been focused on various mucosal models of inflammation that closely resembles human colitis. One of the most comprehensively illustrated models of experimental colitis is Dextran Sodium Sulphate (DSS) induced colitis which mimics the clinical and histological features of human UC as the colonic lesions exhibits high homogeneity and reproducibility [3]. Acute and chronic colitis induced by DSS has been used to study changes in metabolically labeled and tissue mucin content [4] and/or changes in epithelial permeability, MPO and pro-inflammatory cytokines [4].

However, the inflammatory mediators that play a role in disease onset and progression of colitis are poorly defined. Clinical and experimental studies using DSS models of colitis suggests that the key contributors in disease pathogenesis include: (i) an alteration in the mucosal barrier integrity and function; (ii) reallocation in the role of pathogen recognition receptors (PRRs) of APCs and, (iii) an immune response skewed towards effector cell function (Th1 and probably Th2) [2,5]. Despite these advances, it is still not clear which mediator(s) play a central role in disease onset and/or progression of colitis.

As TNF-α and adherent and goblet cell mucin are two major components that are altered in UC, we reasoned that both of these components play major roles in epithelial barrier function and may be selectively altered prior to epithelial cell damage in DSS-induced colitis. In the present study, we used a protocol-treating animal for 9 consecutive days with DSS to characterize the earliest events in disease onset and progression to acute colitis. In particular, we focused on the contribution of TNF-α and colonic mucin in innate host defense prior to epithelial cell damage and investigated whether TNF-α neutralizing antibody can alter disease onset and/or progression in DSS-induced colitis in rats.

Results

Disease Activity Index (DAI) and Tissue damage

DAI is a cumulative index of body weight loss, rectal bleeding and stool malformation and is considered as the best measure of clinical activity of colitis [6]. DAI during the first 4 days was not associated with significant change in the body weight of control and DSS treated animals. However, on day 5 there was an exponential increase in DAI that continued up to day 9 (Fig. 1A). Clinically, day 5 of DSS treatment was a critical turning point as DAI strongly correlated with weight loss (Fig. 1B) in comparison to control animals. An approximate reduction of 18–20% total body weight was observed in DSS treated animals on day 9. After 9 days of continuous 5% DSS treatment, animals suffered severe rectal bleeding (30%) and/or deaths (10% of animals).

To determine the earliest histological alterations during DSS-induced colitis, serial sections of the distal colon predicted to develop ulcers were evaluated on a daily basis. On days 2–4, no histological alterations were observed (Fig. 2B), but as early as day 5, focal erosions of the epithelium with acute inflammatory infiltrate (Fig. 2C) including lymphocyte and polymorphonuclear lymphocytes were seen in DSS treated animals. In particular, crypt dysplasia (Fig. 2D) was evident during the development of colitis from days 5–9. Notably, moderate to severe submucosal edema, hyperemia and erosions were observed in the colon in DSS treated animals on day 9 (Fig. 2E). Typical histological alteration in the mucosa resembled active UC with severe mucosal and submucosal lesions.

DSS Alters Colonic Mucin and Muc2/3 Expression

Mucin is the first line of host defense and its alteration severely affects epithelial barrier function [7]. Defects in mucosal cell barrier function are related to permeability to macromolecules, increased bacterial invasion and/or translocation which primarily depends upon depletion of the thick viscous mucin layer due to severe mucus secretagogues activity, depletion of mucin by goblet cells and mucin wash out due to mucosal inflammation and diarrhea [8]. As loss of the protective mucus barrier and goblet cell mucin may be the initial

inciting event that underlies injury and inflammation in UC, we quantified randomly the number of goblet cells in the crypts that were filled/empty or releasing mucin in DSS-treated rats. In control animals there was a thick adherent mucus layer on the epithelium and well-organized long crypts with dense mucin-filled goblet cells (Fig. 3A). Morphologically, in control animals, 84% of goblet cells were filled with mucin and only 4% of empty goblet cells were seen. However, in DSS-treated animals a significant temporal change in the number and morphology of mucin secreting activity of goblet cells were observed. On day 2 of DSS treatment, goblet cells were filled with mucin (87%) accompanied by a thick adherent and loose mucus exudate in the lumen in the absence of tissue injury or abnormal cellular infiltrate (Fig. 3B and Table 1). However, on day 5, intense mucus secretagogue activity resulted in goblet cells depleted of mucin and in other areas mucus streaming for goblet cells with a thick none adherent mucus layer on the surface epithelium (Fig. 3C). As shown in Table 1, there was a significant decrease in the number of filled goblet cells (21% in comparison to 84% of control) with a corresponding rise in number of empty goblet cells (49% in comparison to 4% of control) and goblet cells releasing mucin (31% in comparison to 12% of control). The mucus cap was layered on the injured surface focal lesions. A curious finding was that goblet cells in the lower half of the crypts were devoid of mucin (Fig. 3C). This time point of high mucin secretagogue activity also coincided with a sharp increase in DAI (day 5). On day 7 of DSS treatment, few goblet cells were seen at the site of well-developed ulcers formation, the mucus cap was completely lost and goblet cells in areas adjacent to the ulcers had very little mucin (Fig. 3D). In particular, there was a significant increase in the number of empty goblet cells (77% in comparison to 4% of control, Table 1). On the day 9 of DSS treatment, goblet cells were almost absent with a paucity of PAS positive proteins in the ulcerated site. In the adjacent areas to the ulcers, crypts were

A

B

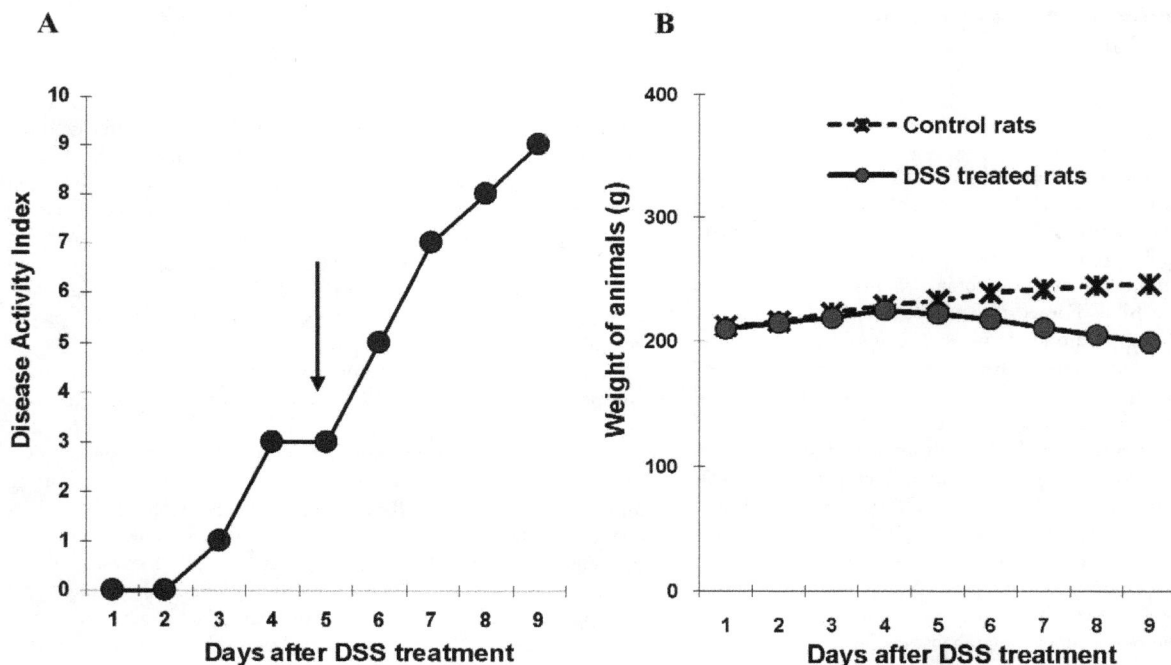

Figure 1. Disease Activity Index (A, DAI) and change in body weight (B) during the progressive development of DSS-induced colitis in rats. Animals received 5% DSS in drinking water for 1–9 days. Note, a striking difference in DAI (A) was observed from day 5 onwards (*arrow*). Changes in the body weight (B) of control (*asterisk*) and DSS treated animals (*circles*). Loss in the body weight coincides well with increase in DAI. Data represents the means ± SEM from 6 animals per day.

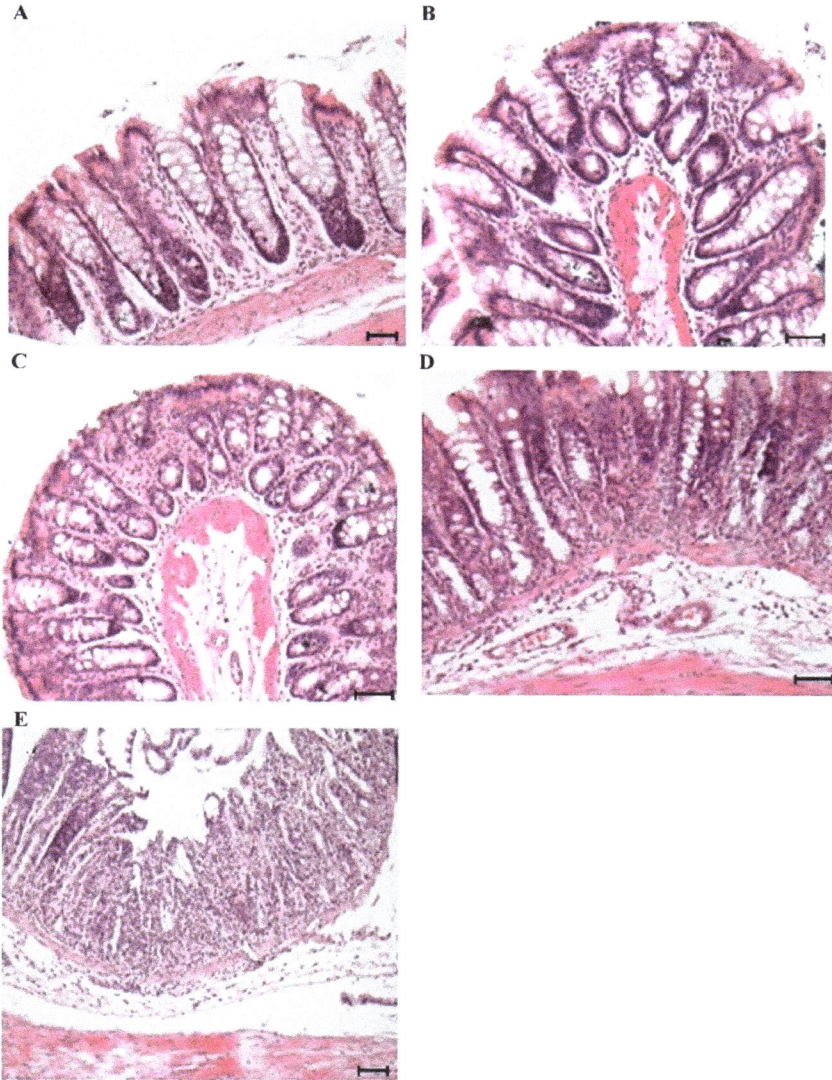

Figure 2. Histopathological characterization of DSS-induced colitis. *A*: Normal control rat colon on day 9 showing well organized crypts and lamina propria and submucosal structures. *B*: DSS treatment on day 2 showing intact mucosal and sub-mucosal structures. *C*: DSS treatment on day 5 showing focal erosions of the epithelium with an acute inflammatory infiltrate. *D*: DSS treatment on day 7 showing crypt dysplasia and edema of the submucosa. *E*: DSS treatment on day 9 showing complete denuding of the surface epithelium, dense cellular inflammatory infiltrate in the lamina propria and loss of crypt structures (Scale bar represents 25 μm; all sections were stained with H&E).

damaged and the few goblet cells contained insignificant amount of mucin (Fig. 3E).

As a decrease in luminal mucin content may reflect a differential expression of mucin genes, we determine whether the expression of secretory (Muc2) and membrane bound (Muc3) mucin were also altered during the onset of ulcer formation. As shown in Fig. 3F, following a significant increase in Muc2 (~22 fold) and Muc3 (~8 fold) gene expression between days 1–2, there was a marked down regulation of Muc2/3 from day 4 onwards (15- and 18-fold lower respectively). No significant difference in the expression of Muc1 was observed in DSS treated and control animals.

DSS Treatment Alters the Expression Pattern of TLRs

TLRs are sensors on epithelial cells/APCs that identify and respond to microbes by eliciting effector, regulatory or cytoprotective responses [7]. As changes in TLR expression pattern are

critical for the induction of both mucosal effector and regulatory cell responses, the expression of TLR2, TLR4, TLR5 and TLR9 genes involved in microbial recognition was examined. Surprisingly, the expression profiles for TLR2/4 (Fig. 4A) and TLR5/9 (Fig. 4B) genes in DSS treated animals increased 60–80-fold and 10–20-fold, respectively, on days 1–3. The increase in TLR2/4 expression was evidenced through all 9 days of DSS treatment, albeit was not as prominent as during the first three days (Fig. 4A). TLR5/9 expression levels returned to normal on day 5 and remained low up to day 9 (Fig. 4B). DSS was a potent inflammatory insult for TLR expression in the onset of disease.

DSS Stimulates the Production of Pro-inflammatory and Regulatory Cytokines

A break in tolerance to enteric bacteria and an aberrant response to normal luminal flora leading to an immunological imbalance is

Table 1. Morphology of goblet cells from rat tissue treated with DSS for different time point.

DSS Treatment	Percentage of total goblet cells		
	Filled	Releasing Mucus	Empty
Control	84.0±1.3	12.0±0.4	4.0±0.2
Day 2	86.5±0.5	10.4±0.4	3.1±0.5
Day 5	20.9±0.6***	30.5±0.5*	48.6±0.9**
Day 7	17.1±0.64***	5.7±0.4	77.1±1.4***
Day 9	ND	ND	ND

Data are presented as % of goblet cells ± SEM. *P<0.05, **P<0.01, ***P<0.0001 compared to control group. Goblet cell morphology was quantified from randomly selected crypts of PAS stained sections. A minimum number of 100 (100–110) goblet cells were counted under 40 X magnification from each section. Goblet cell morphology was designated as adapted as previously described [28]. Filled goblet cells: goblet cells with intact mucus granules; Releasing mucus: cells releasing mucus with PAS-stained mucus emerging as a thick stream; Empty goblet cells with PAS stained mucus absent from cells exhibiting a deep concave cavitation of the apical surface. ND: Not determined as the epithelial layer and crypts on day 9 DSS treatment was destroyed or too damaged in the ulcerated site.

the hallmark of UC pathogenesis. This imbalance represents both effector and regulatory mucosal immune responses. We therefore next considered the impact of DSS treatment on production of the important pro-inflammatory (TNF-α and IL-1β, Fig. 5A) and regulatory cytokines (IL-10 and TGFβ, Fig. 5B). Pro-inflammatory cytokine expression exhibited a bimodal expression profile (Fig. 5A), which was initially led by a significant increase in TNF-α (~70–80-fold increase on days 1–2), while acute disease was dominated by significant high expression of IL-1β (~60–90-fold increase on days 6–9). Even though TNF-α expression decreased to 30-fold on day 3, its expression remained significantly high up to day 9 (Fig. 5A). Predictable, colonic tissues also showed high levels of TNF-α protein (Fig. 5C) and mirrored the TNF-α gene expression profile. Interestingly, the regulatory cytokines IL-10 and TGFβ were significant up regulated during the onset of disease (days 2–4) but at day 5, there was a sharp decline in the expression of both regulatory cytokines that stayed low up to day 9 (Fig. 5B). Early onset and acute colitis was dominated by a marked up-regulation of TNF-α, whereas, IL-1β was prominent in acute disease.

DSS Treatment Affected MPO Activity and Chemokine Expression

Colonic myeloperoxidase (MPO) activity is an indicator of neutrophil infiltration and inflammation. DSS treated animals showed a significant rise in MPO activity from day 6 onwards that peaked on day 8–9 (Fig. 6A). This rise in MPO activity during later stages of DSS-induced colitis were further corroborated by the alteration in the gene expression of CINC-1, an analogue of human IL-8 and a rat chemokine that has potent chemo attractant effects on neutrophils [9]. Gene expression analysis of CINC-1 depicted a baseline profile during the onset of disease (days 1–5) but between days 6–9 of acute phase of the disease, a 4–5-fold increase in expression of CINC-1 was observed (Fig. 6B). As expected, MPO activity and CINC-1 expression were highly correlated with DAI.

The Effect of TNF-α Neutralizing Antibody on Disease Onset and Progression

As TNF-α mRNA expression and colonic tissue protein were markedly up regulated in disease onset (Days 2–3, Fig. 5)

associated with alterations in Muc2 expression (Fig. 3F) which preceded goblet and luminal mucin alterations, we determined if TNF-α neutralizing antibody could alter the course of the disease. As shown in Fig. 7A, TNF-α neutralizing antibody significant decreased DAI on day 5 and 9 as compared to untreated controls. Notably, the TNF-α neutralizing antibody treated group had significantly lower DAI (Fig. 7A) and higher body weight (Fig. 7B) at the critical day 5 time point associated with the exponential rise in the DAI observed in the DSS treated group. As expected, there was a significant reduction in the levels of TNF-α protein in colonic tissues on days 2, 5 and 9 in the TNF-α neutralizing antibody treated groups as compared to DSS untreated treated animals (Fig. 7C). Consistent with the protein level, TNF-α neutralizing antibody treatment significantly inhibited the up regulation of TNF-α mRNA expression seen in the DSS treated rats (Fig. 7D). The most prominent effect of TNF-α neutralizing antibody treatment was observed on the expression of IL-1β gene expression. IL-1β gene expression was 32-fold higher on day 9 in the TNF-α neutralizing antibody treated group compared to controls (Fig. 7E). In comparison, DSS-treated rats showed 85-fold increase in IL-1β gene expression on day 9 of DSS treatment as compared to controls (Fig. 7E). These results suggest a TNF-α dependent cytokine network in the pathogenesis of DSS-induced colitis.

In addition to the effect on pro-inflammatory cytokine production, TNF-α neutralizing antibody also showed significant cessation in the alteration of mucin expression and mucus production triggered by DSS-treatment. Muc2 gene expression was only 12-fold higher on day 2 and 6-fold lower on day 9 in the TNF-α neutralizing antibody treated group as compared to controls (Fig. 7F). In comparison, DSS-treated rats showed a 22-fold increase in the Muc2 gene expression on day 2 and a 10-fold decrease on day 9 when compared to controls. H&E and PAS staining showed less focal erosions and inflammatory cellular infiltrate (Fig. 8 and Fig. 9), more adherent mucus in the lumen and organized long crypts containing mucin-filled goblet cells on day 2 and 5 in the TNF-α neutralizing antibody treated group. Even on day 9, mucins filled goblet cells were seen in the colonic tissue of the TNF-α neutralizing antibody treated group whereas untreated DSS treated rats showed mucin-devoid goblet cells from day 5 onwards (Fig. 9F). In particular, on day 5 there were more filled goblet cells (60% in comparison to 37% of DSS treated group) and less numbers of empty goblet cells (29% in comparison to 40% of DSS treated group) in the TNF-α neutralizing antibody treated group compared to the DSS only treated group (Table 2). Even on day 9, there were goblet cells in ulcerated area, whereas in the DSS only treated group we were no goblet cells in the ulcerated areas. The ulcerated areas in the TNF-α neutralizing antibody treated group on day 9 seem restricted to the surface epithelium (Fig. 9F) with well-organized crypts with mucin filled goblet cells. These data suggest that neutralizing TNF-α markedly affected mucin release, mucus depletion and crypt inflammation to restrict the mucosal damaging effects of DSS.

Discussion

This is the first comprehensive study to quantify the salient features of early onset and acute progressive events in the pathogenesis of DSS induced colitis. Onset of disease (days 1–5) was characterized by elevated levels of TNF-α mRNA expression, protein production, depletion of luminal adherent mucin and goblet cell mucin stores prior to the appearance of focal erosions on mucosal epithelial cells. These early events resulted in a progressive increase in DAI (from day 5 onwards) and weight loss

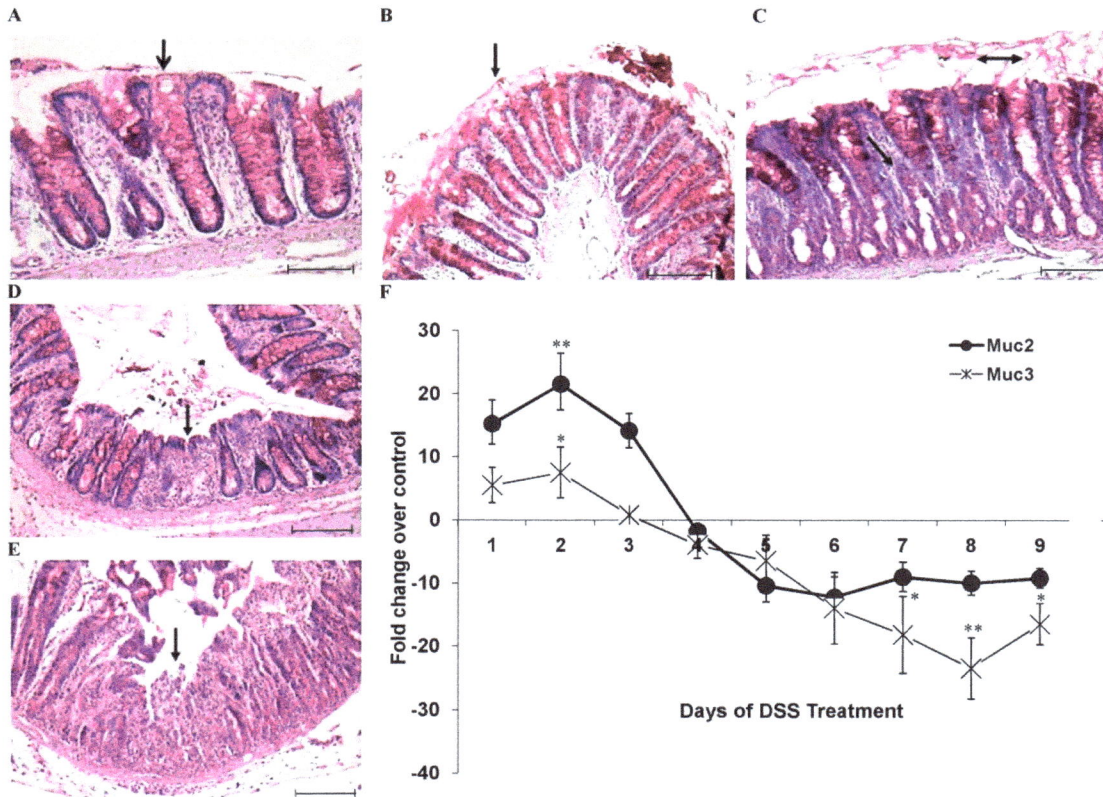

Figure 3. The effect of DSS treatment on adherent and goblet cell mucin content and mucin gene expression. Colonic tissues sections were stained with Periodic acid Schiff reagent to visualize adherent and goblet cell mucin content. *A*: Control rat colon on day 0 showing goblet cells with high mucin content from the base to the tip of the crypts (magenta color). *B*: DSS treatment on day 2 showing mucin filled goblet cells as well as large amount of secreted adherent mucus (single head arrow) in the lumen. *C*: DSS treatment on day 5 showing disrupted elongated basal crypts with little mucin. Goblet cells at the tips of the crypts show intense mucus secretagogue activity with loose disorganized luminal mucus (double head arrow). *D*: DSS treatment on day 7 demonstrating loss of goblet cells at the site of ulcer formation (single head arrow), dense cellular infiltrate and loss of the adherent mucus barrier. *E*: DSS treated rat on day 9 showing ruptured mucosa (single head arrow) with no evident of goblet cells at the site of damage or in the adjacent areas. Scale bar represents 25 µm. *F*: The effect of DSS treatment on Muc2 and Muc3 gene expression. The relative gene expression levels were determined by real time PCR for using mRNA extracted from control and DSS treated rats during the 9 consecutive days of DSS treatment. Expression levels were normalized using GAPDH as housekeeping gene and the mRNA levels plotted as fold change over control. Data shown are the means ± SEM of 6 animals/day. *$P<0.05$ and **$P<0.001$ compared to control colon.

associated with rectal bleeding and organized ulcers in the distal colon. Treatment with TNF-α neutralizing antibody significantly decreased DAI, delayed the acute phase of colitis and effectively curtailed alterations in the expression and production of TNF-α and mucins. These results suggest that both increased TNF-α and mucin depletion was a prerequisite for the development of focal erosions. The acute phase of disease was dominated by loss of luminal and cellular mucin stores, down regulation of regulatory cytokines, elevated levels of MPO, CINC-1 and IL-1β expression.

The most dominant biomarker in the onset of disease was the pro-inflammatory cytokine-TNF-α, which was increased 70–80-fold suggesting that it played a major role in innate host defense. TNF-α is a 17-kda pro-inflammatory cytokine produced by monocytes, macrophages, and T cells. Our data suggests that TNF-α target epithelial cells (and perhaps lymphocytes) during the initial phase of colitis to trigger a cytokine network as well as to enhance mucin production. Treatment with TNF-α neutralizing antibody significantly reduced both DAI and IL-1β and Muc2 gene expression induced by DSS treatment. Our findings are in contrast with a report that shows an exacerbated DSS-induced colitis in TNF-α knockout mice [10]. We speculate that this might be due to the partial blockage of TNF-α achieved with TNF-α

neutralizing antibody in our study and that complete knocking out of the TNF-α gene may have triggered other pro-inflammatory responses [10]. Another critical characteristic of this phase is high mucin content in goblet cells and a significant up regulation Muc2 and Muc3 gene expression. This is contradictory to the view that impairment of mucosal barriers via depletion of mucin layer and/or downregulation of mucin producing genes may be an early event of pathogenesis. The up regulation of mucin genes could also be an early event of inflammation triggered by pro-inflammatory cytokines including TNF-α [11]. Perhaps mucin production is a component of the inflammatory responses of epithelial tissue [12,13]. Several studies have shown that mucin secretion is increased upon IL-1β, IL-4, IL-13 or TNF-α stimulation [14–16]. Other noteworthy changes during the first 1-3 days are an extensive up regulation of TLR2 and 4 and controlled up regulation of TLR5 and TLR9. *In vivo* and *in vitro* studies have shown an exaggerated TLR expression (especially TLR4) that leads to an uncontrolled immune response (Th1 or Th17 mediated) against resident microflora [17]. It could be noted that no significant change in DAI or histological damage of colonic mucosa was seen in the early phase of colitis suggesting that the clinical sign of colitis are not evident unless there is complete

A

B

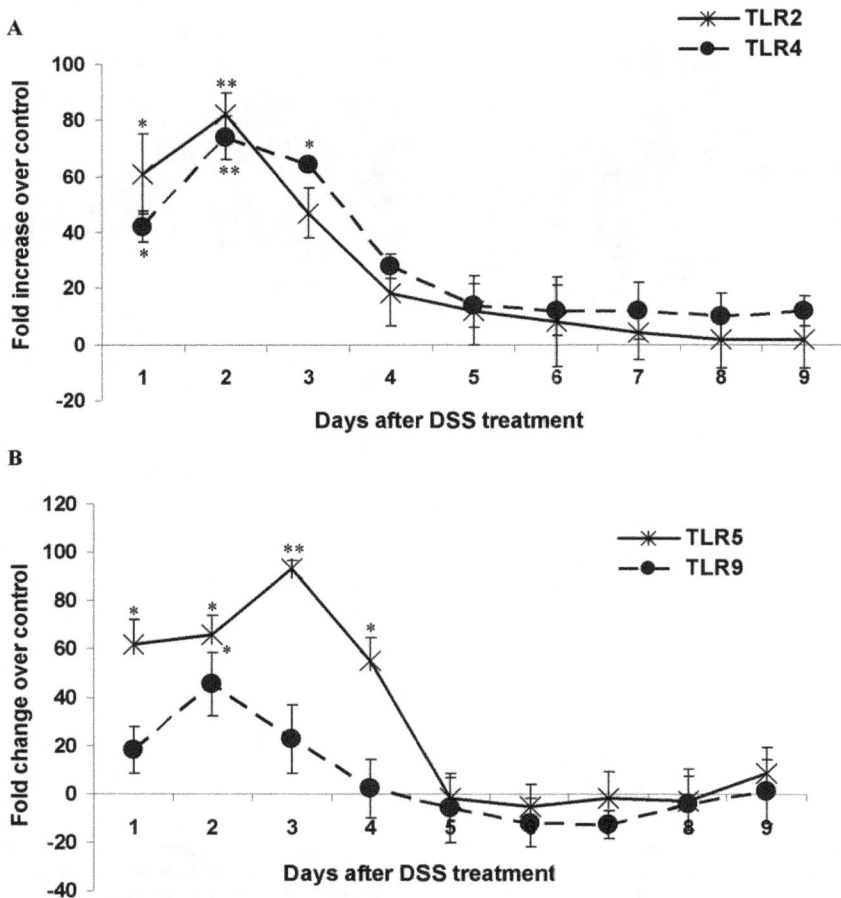

Figure 4. The effect of DSS treatment on the TLR gene expression. Relative gene expression of (A) TLR2 (asterisks) and TLR4 (circles) and (B) TLR5 (asterisks) and TLR9 (circles) genes in DSS treated rats over controls during 9 days of DSS treatment. The expression levels of TLR genes were determined by real time PCR and normalized using GAPDH as housekeeping gene. The mRNA levels are plotted as fold change over control. Data shown are the means ± SEM of 6 animals/day. *$P<0.05$ and **$P<0.001$ compared to control colon.

destruction of mucosal homeostasis. Importantly, this phase with no significant DAI was prolonged in rats treated with TNF-α neutralizing antibody. The pro-inflammatory cytokine TNF-α was the most prominent early biomarker of DSS-induced colitis based on its extensive up regulation during the onset of colitis induction and the fact that treatment of TNF-α neutralizing antibody significantly reduced DSS induced DAI.

Our data suggests that days 4–6 are the most crucial in the induction of DSS induced colitis. Unlike a universal up-regulation of different genes seen in the onset of disease, days 4–6 showed a differential expression profile of various genes suggesting an alteration in factors responsible for mucosal homeostasis. For example, there was exponential rise in DAI (mainly due to extensive drop in the body weight) and the presence of focal lesions from day 5 onwards in DSS animals. Curiously, this phase was dominated by the down regulation of regulatory and cytoprotective factors. In particular, the regulatory cytokines IL-10 and TGFβ were significant down regulated in DSS treatment (40-fold less than controls). Down regulation of regulatory T cell activation including Treg and Th3 cells (secreting TGFβ and IL-10) is a major predisposing factor in the pathogenesis of IBD [18,19]. Decrease in TGFβ leads to diminished regulation of Th1, Th2 and Th17 effector T cell activation and also more epithelial cell apoptosis, while lowered IL-10 expression leads to more aggressive

macrophage activity. An initial upregulation of mucin genes was replaced by sudden down regulation of both Muc2 and Muc3 genes supporting the fact impairment of the intestinal mucosal barrier may lead to high mucosal permeability and diminished epithelial protection [20] that probably leads to later immune assault. A number of reports have documented that inflamed and non-inflamed intestinal tissues in UC and CD have impaired and permeable mucosal barriers [20,21]. Another critical aspect is the change in the expression profile of various TLR genes. TLR2 and 4 continued to be up regulated though not as extensive as in the first phase, but TLR5 and 9 showed 5–15 fold down regulation from day 5 onward. The results points toward the putative tolerogenic role for the two PRRs. It has been reported earlier that low expression of TLR5 is seen in both forms of IBD [22]. The pro-inflammatory cytokines continued to be up-regulated but in more controlled fashion than the initial phase. Significant delay in reaching the acute phase, relatively intact mucosal architecture, significant mucin content in the goblet cells and limited down regulation of Muc2 gene in TNF-α neutralizing antibody treated rats on day 5 and 9 of DSS treatment further suggests that depletion of mucosal barrier is a key event during transition of initial to acute phase. Together these results reinforces that day 5 of DSS treatment is a critical time point exhibiting a sharp rise in DAI complemented by extensive change of trend for the

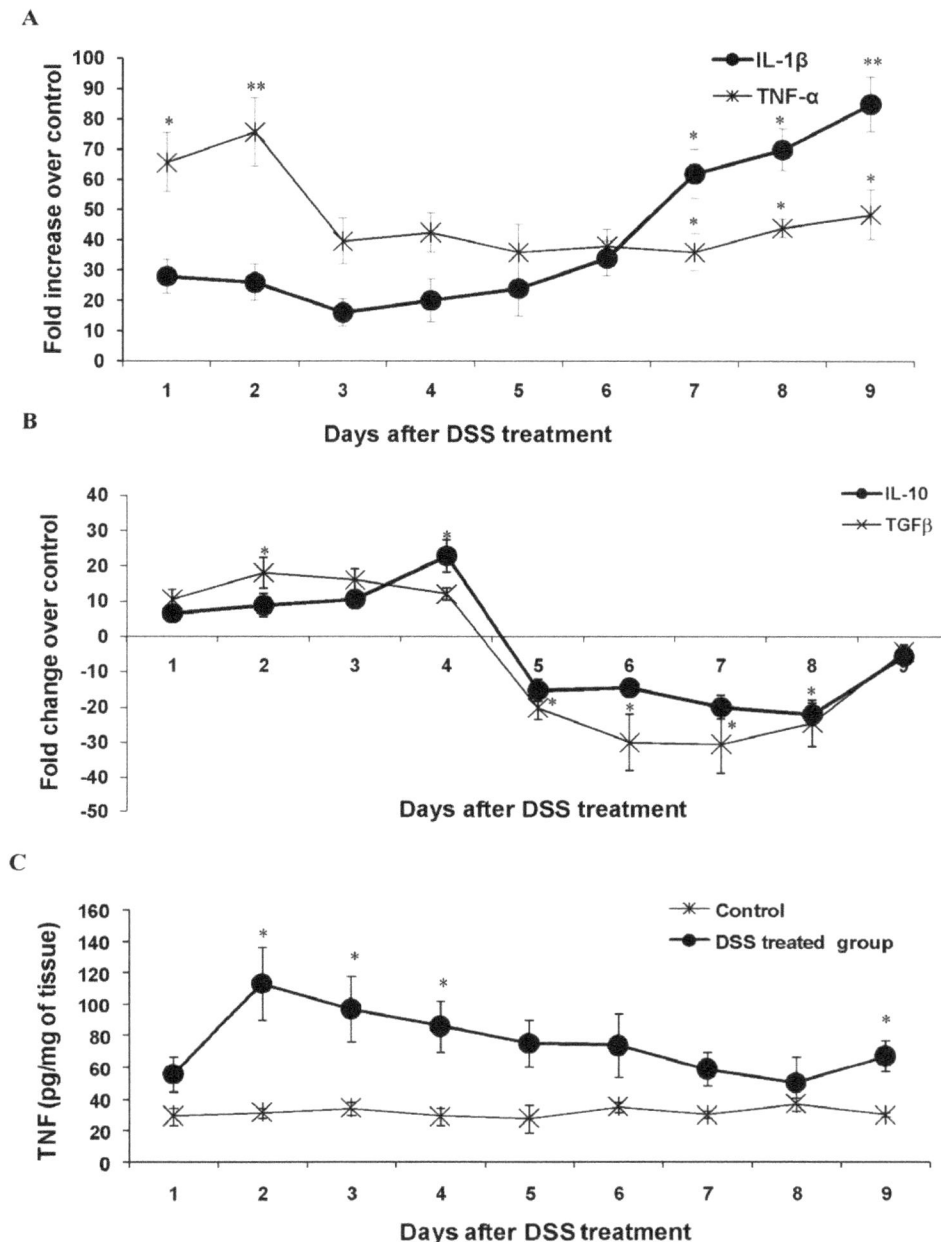

Figure 5. The effect of DSS treatment on pro-inflammatory and regulatory cytokine gene expression. The relative gene expression levels were determined by real time PCR for (A) TNF-α (circle) and IL-1β (asterisks) and (B) TGFβ (circle) and IL-10 (asterisks) genes using mRNA extracted from control and DSS treated rats during 9 days of DSS treatment. Expression levels of all genes were normalized using GAPDH as housekeeping gene. The mRNA levels are plotted as fold change over control. Data shown are the means ± SEM of 6 animals/day. *P<0.05 and **P<0.001 compared to control colon. C: The effect of DSS treatment on the TNF-α protein secretion as measured by ELISA. TNF-α protein in DSS treated rats (circle) and controls (asterisks) are plotted as pg/mg of tissue. Data shown are the means ± SEM of 6 animals/day. *P<0.05 and **P<0.001 compared to control colon.

expression/production of TLR, cytokine and mucin genes. DAI, mucosal depletion and regulatory cytokines, by virtue of their prominent down-regulation appears to be the most prominent and indicative biomarker at this stage in the pathogenesis of DSS-induced colitis.

Acute inflammation on days 7–9 was dominated by an extensive increase in the expression of pro-inflammatory cytokines with IL-1β taking up the center stage (an increase of 80-fold higher

expression than controls on day 9) and TNF-α showing second most prominent change in expression (50-fold higher expression than controls on day 9). The results are suggestive of the predominating role of T cells in the later stages of colitis. Genes encoding mucin, IL-10, TGFβ, TLR5 and TLR9 continued to be down regulated during this phase. Colitis was well documented at this stage with the highest DAI score on day 9 and histological analysis showed crypt damage, dysplasia, inflammatory infiltrates

A

B

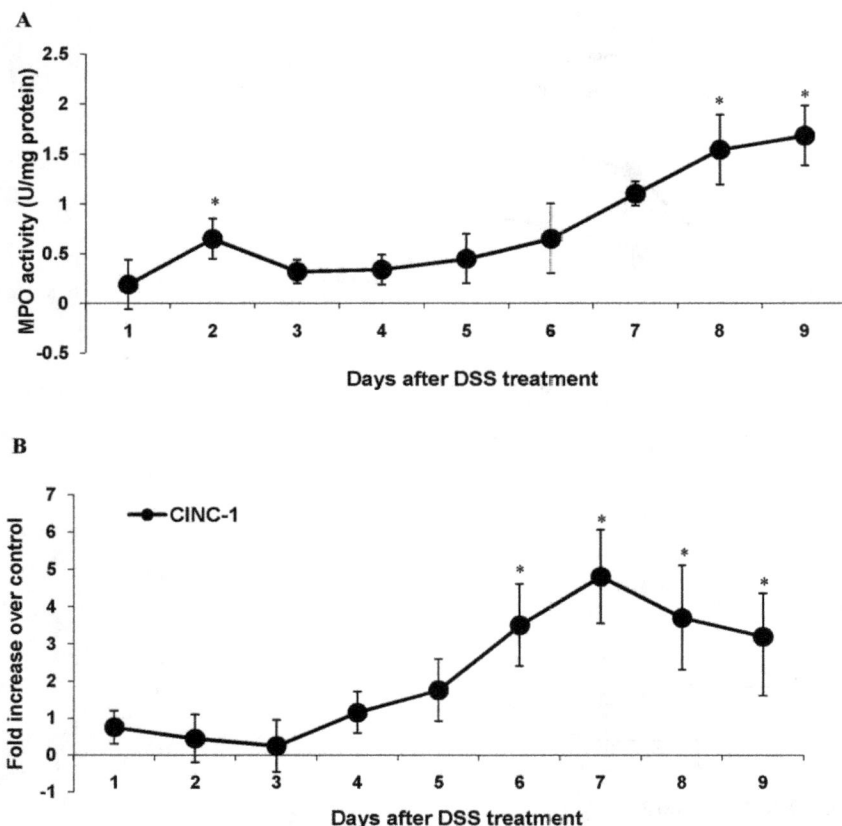

Figure 6. The effect of DSS treatment on the expression and activity of pro-inflammatory mediators. *A*: Myeloperoxidase activity (MPO) was measured in the colonic mucosa of rats administered 5% DSS in drinking water for 1–9 days. MPO activity is expressed as unit per mg tissue and all values are the means ± SEM of 6 animals/day. *P<0.05 compared with normal control groups. *B*: The effect of DSS treatment on CINC expressions. The relative gene expression levels were determined by real time PCR for CINC gene using mRNA extracted from control and DSS treated rats during 9 days of DSS treatment. Expression levels of all genes were normalized using GAPDH as housekeeping gene. The mRNA levels are plotted as fold change over control. Data shown are the means ± SEM of 6-animals/day. *P<0.05 and **P<0.001 compared to control colon.

and ulcerations in the mucosa of the DSS treated group. In UC, leucocytes numbers are increased associated with high migration from the vasculature into the intestinal mucosa mediated by several chemokines including IL-6, RANTES, MCP1 and MCP2 mediated by various adhesion molecules [23,24]. This is followed by high release of tissue damaging deleterious metabolites and mediators including nitric oxide, free oxygen radicals, PGs, leukotrienes, histamine, proteases and MMPs by macrophages and other immune cells [25,26], which cause extensive mucosal damage analogous to what is observed in DSS colitis.

In conclusion, this study demonstrates for the first time that mucosal TNF-α and alteration of the adherent mucus barrier are predisposing factors for early onset epithelial cells damage in DSS colitis. In contrast, high-sustained levels of TNF-α and depletion of adherent and goblet cell mucin are necessary for maintenance of acute colitis. Treatment with TNF-α neutralizing antibody significant altered the onset and severity of disease and prevented the loss of the adherent mucus layer and goblet cell mucin.

Materials and Methods

Animals

Six-week-old male Sprague–Dawley rats weighing between 250 and 300 g (Charles River, St. Constant, Quebec) were housed in cages 2 per group at a constant room temperature, with 12-h light

and dark cycles, and fed standard rodent chow and water *ad libitum*. Following a 7-day acclimation period, rats were randomized into experimental and control groups for induction of colitis. The Animal Experiment Ethics Committee of the University of Calgary, Canada approved this study (ID MO8123).

Experimental Design and Induction of Colitis

To study the earliest events in disease onset and progression of DSS induced colitis rats were divided into two groups, controls which had free access to water and the DSS colitis group which had free access to a water containing 5% DSS (wt/vol; molecular weight 50 KDa; Fisher Biotech, Canada) for 9 consecutive days. Animals were sacrificed on all consecutive days of DSS treatment from day 0 to day 9. A total of 18 animals were utilized for each time point (*N*=6 for each trial/day). To study the effect of anti-TNF-α neutralizing antibody on disease onset and progression of colitis a third group of rats were treated with neutralizing TNF-α antibody in addition to the above-mentioned control and DSS colitis group. The TNF-α antibody treated group were administered the antibody at a dose of 100 μg/animal/day (for rationale, see the section on TNF-α neutralizing antibody treatment) and had free access to water containing 5% DSS for 9 consecutive days. A total of 18 animals were utilized for each time point (*N*=6 for each trial/day). On the day of sacrifice, animals were given sodium pentobarbital anesthesia (35 mg/kg body weight). Blood specimens were collected

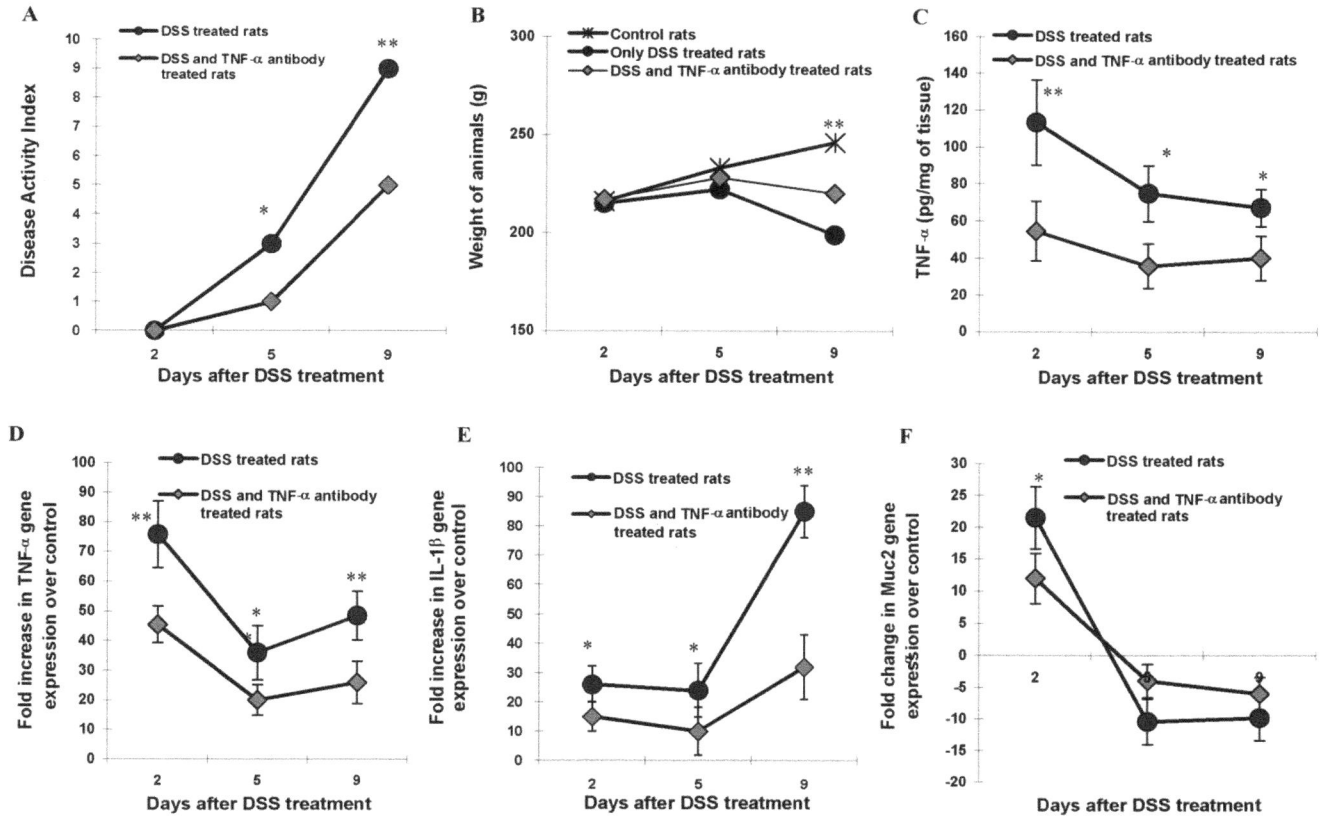

Figure 7. The effect of TNF-α neutralizing antibody treatment on disease onset and progression in DSS induced colitis. *A:* Comparison of disease activity index (DAI) on day 2, 5 and 9 of DSS treatment in animals that received 5% DSS in drinking water alone (black circles) or with TNF-α neutralizing antibody (grey diamonds). *B:* Body weight change plotted for control (asterisks), DSS only (black circles) or DSS + TNF-α neutralizing antibody treatment (grey diamonds). Data represents the means ± SEM from 6 animals per day. *C:* TNF-α protein secretion measured by ELISA on days 2, 5 and 9 of DSS treatment in animals that received 5% DSS in drinking water alone (black circles) or with TNF-α neutralizing antibody (grey diamonds). Data shown are the means ± SEM of 6-animals/day. *$P<0.05$ and **$P<0.001$ compared to control colon. *D–F:* The relative gene expression levels determined by real time PCR for TNF-α (*D*), IL-1β (*E*) and Muc2 (*F*) genes on day 2, 5 and 9 of DSS treatment in animals that received 5% DSS in drinking water alone (black circles) or with TNF-α neutralizing antibody (grey diamonds). The expression levels of all genes were normalized using GAPDH as housekeeping gene and mRNA levels are as fold change over control. Data shown are the means ± SEM of 6-animals/day. *$P<0.05$ and **$P<0.001$ compared to control colon.

by cardiac puncture for flow cytometric enumeration of circulating leukocyte and T cell subset counts. Colons were immediately excised, rinsed with ice-cold phosphate-buffered saline, and placed on ice and four cross sections of the each proximal, middle and distal colon (50–100 mg) were collected. Three cross sections were snap-frozen in liquid nitrogen and stored at −70°C for RNA isolation, protein preparation and analysis of myeloperoxidase activity. The fourth cross section was immediately fixed in 10% neutral buffered formalin for histological analysis.

Disease Activity Index and Pathological Evaluation of Colitis

Disease Activity Index (DAI) was quantified using the parameters of animal weight loss, stool consistency, and gross blood in the feces, which were recorded daily for each animal. These parameters were each assigned a score, which was utilized to calculate an average daily (DAI) for each animal, as previously described [27].

Macroscopic and Histological Examination

The proximal, middle and distal colon were examined macroscopically and reported as showing: no mucosal lesions,

hyperemia, edema or small area of erosion/ulceration and extensive, marked erosion/ulceration. Assessment of body weight and evaluation of stool consistency (diarrhea) and rectal bleeding were performed on a daily basis. Body weight was assessed at baseline and every day for the duration of the experiment in the control and DSS-treated groups. Weight change was calculated as percentage change in weight compared with baseline. Animals were monitored for rectal bleeding, diarrhea and general signs of morbidity. In three separate preliminary experiments, we consistently observed that most ulcers developed in the distal colon 1–2 cm from the anus. We therefore designated this area for tissues examination for all subsequent experiments listed below.

Tissue sections from the distal colon were fixed in 10% buffered formalin, embedded in paraffin and 6 μm sections were stained with hematoxylin and eosin (H&E) and Periodic acid-Schiff (PAS). Microscopically, H&E tissues were reported as showing: a normal appearance, mild infiltrates of small round cells and polymorphonuclear leukocytes into the lamina propria mucosa, with either no or only shallow erosion, or deep erosion, ulceration and marked infiltration with small round cells and polymorphonuclear leukocytes, often including crypt abscess formation. PAS was used to visualize pre-formed mucin in goblet cells and mucin that were

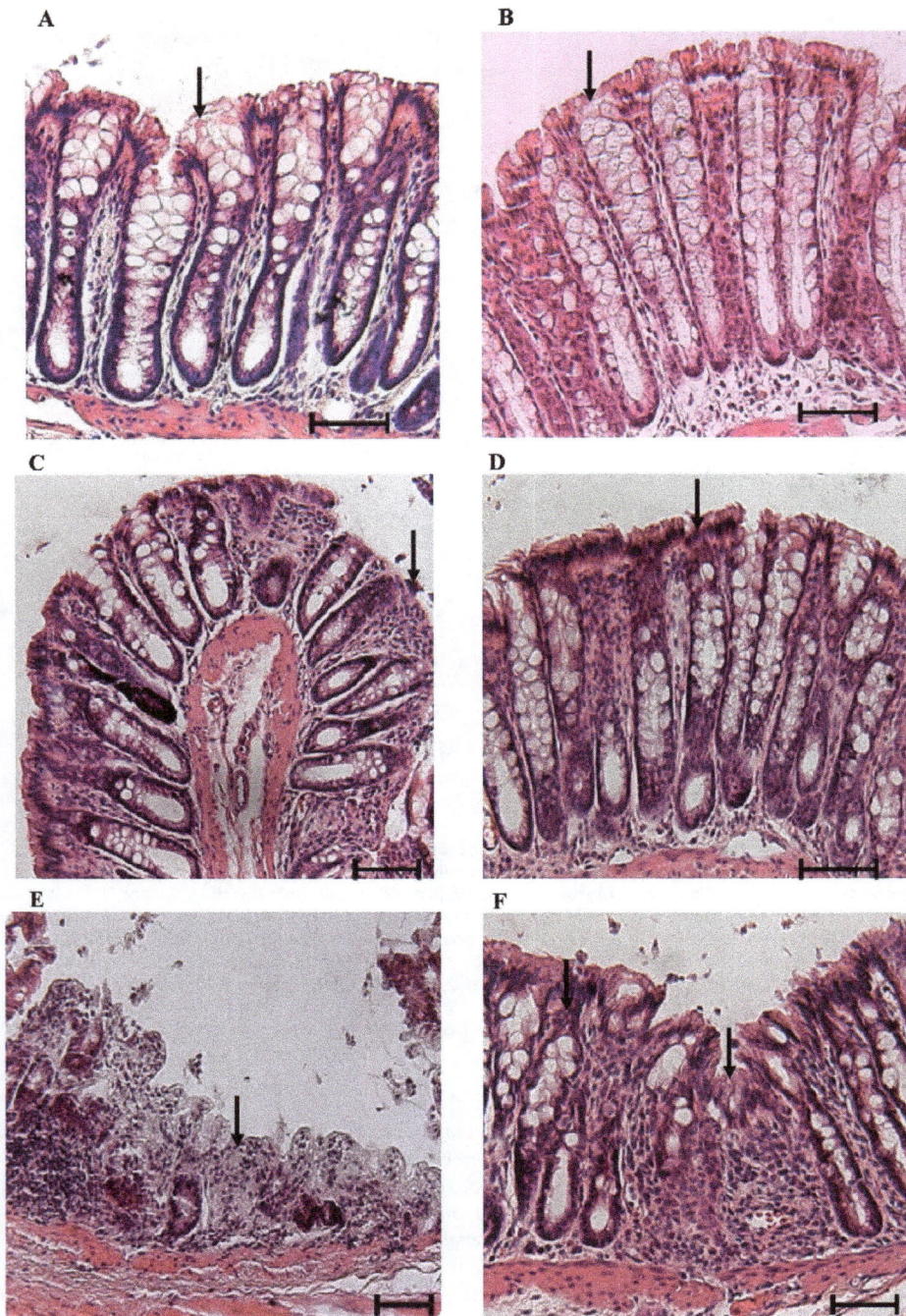

Figure 8. The effect of TNF-α neutralizing antibody on the development of colonic lesions in DSS treated rats. *A*: DSS treatment alone on day 2 showing intact mucosal (arrow) and sub-mucosal structures. *B*: TNF-α neutralizing antibody plus DSS treatment on day 2 showing intact crypts and mucosal (arrow) and submucosal structure. *C*: DSS treatment alone on day 5 showing focal erosions of the epithelium (arrow) with acute inflammatory infiltrate. *D*: The effect of TNF-α neutralizing antibody plus DSS treatment on day 5 showing well developed crypts with no abnormal cellular infiltrate with intact mucosa (arrow). *E*: DSS treatment alone on day 9 showing extensive mucosal damage and deep ulceration (arrow) with large numbers of inflammatory cellular infiltrates. *F*: The effect of TNF-α neutralizing antibody plus DSS treatment on day 9 showing focal erosions (arrow) with less damaged and cellular infiltrate in the mucosal architecture adjacent to the lesion. (All sections were stained with H&E; scale bar represents 25 μm).

secreted and/or in the mucus gel in the lumen. Mucins in goblet cells were quantified as previously described [28]. Filled goblet cells: goblet cells with intact mucus granules; Releasing mucus: cells releasing mucus with PAS-stained mucus emerging as a thick stream; Empty goblet cells with PAS stained mucus absent from cells exhibiting a deep concave cavitation of the apical surface.

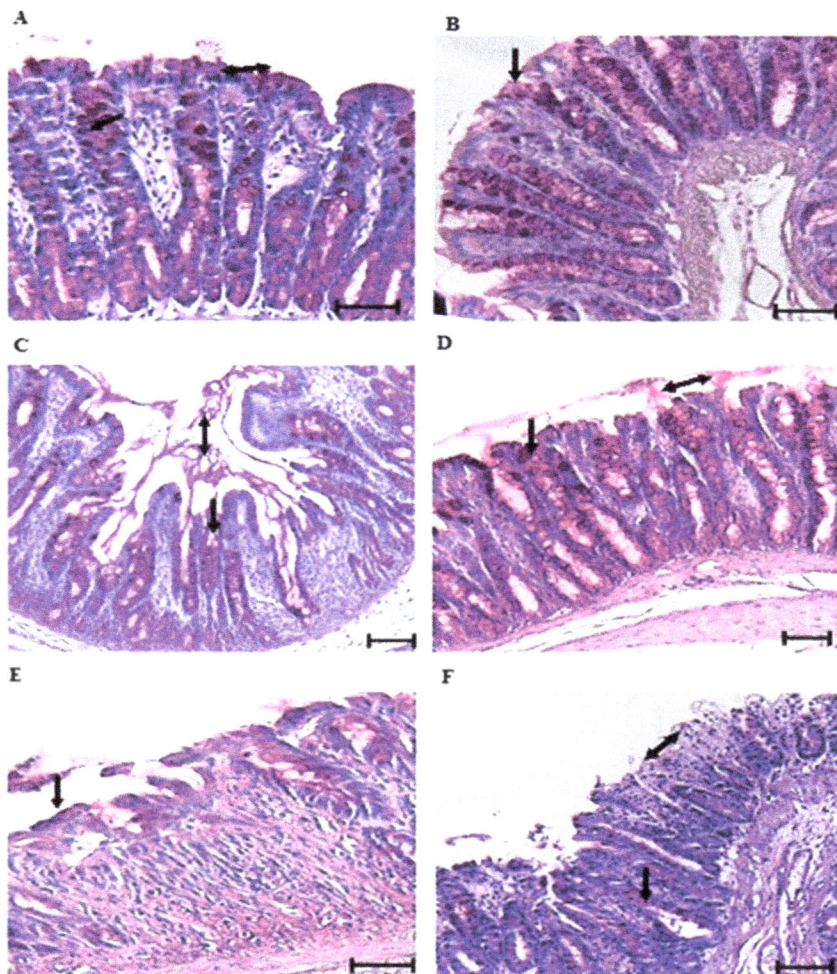

Figure 9. The effect of TNF-α neutralizing antibody on the adherent mucus layer and goblet cell mucin in DSS-induced colitis. Rat colonic tissues sections were stained with Periodic acid Schiff reagent to visualize adherent and goblet cell mucin content. *A*: DSS treatment alone on day 2 showing mucin filled goblet cells (magenta color) and secreted mucin in the lumen (double head arrow) with a modest inflammatory infiltrate. *B*: TNF-α neutralizing antibody plus DSS treatment on day 2, showing mucus secretion from crypt goblet cells. *C*: DSS treatment only rat on day 5 showing disrupted crypts, intense inflammatory cellular infiltrate and intense mucus secretion from crypt goblet cells (single head arrow) with loss of the adherent mucus layer (double head arrow). *D*: TNF-α neutralizing antibody plus DSS treatment on day 5 showing well organized crypts filled with mucin (single head arrow) and an adherent mucus layer (double head arrow) on the surface epithelium. *E*: DSS treatment on day 9 showing an ulcerated region with a ruptured mucosa with complete loss of crypts. The residual goblet cells adjacent to the ulcer show remnants of mucin. *F*: TNF-α neutralizing antibody plus DSS treatment on day 9 demonstrating only to the surface mucosa (double head arrow) and the deep crypts show evidence of mucin in goblet cells beneath the lesions (single head arrow). Scale bar represents 25 μm.

MPO Activity in Colonic Tissues

For measurement of MPO activity tissues were weighed and homogenized in 10 volume of 50 mM phosphate buffer (pH 6.0) at 4°C, and centrifuged at $30,000\times$ g for 30 min at 4°C. The pellet was extracted with 0.5% hexadecyltrimethylammonium bromide (HTAB; Sigma Chemical Co.) in 50 mM phosphate buffer (pH 6.0) at 25°C(23). Samples were sonicated for 10–15 sec and then centrifuged at $30,000\times$ g for 30 min. Supernatants were reacted with o-dianisidine dihydrochloride (Sigma Chemical Co.) containing 1 μL/mL of 3% H2O2, and MPO activity was assayed in a 96-well microtiter plate by mixing 20 μl of the supernatant. The change in absorbance was measured spectrophotometrically. Bradford assay was used to measure protein content in the supernatant and results are expressed as MPO activity (mU/mg).

Quantitative Real-Time PCR Analysis

Quantitative real time PCR analysis was performed to assess changes in the expression of genes encoding for the major secretory and membrane bound mucins (Muc2, Muc1 and Muc3), Toll-like receptors (TLR2, TLR4, TLR5 and TLR9), Cytokine-induced neutrophils chemoattractant (CINC) and various pro-inflammatory (TNF-α and IL-1β) and regulatory (IL-10 and TGFβ) cytokines. Total RNA was extracted with TriZol reagent (Invitrogen). The yield and purity of the RNA was determined by spectroscopic analysis. 2 μg of RNA was reverse transcribed using M-MLV reverse transcriptase (Invitrogen) as per manufacturer's instructions. One microlitre of cDNA was used for real-time PCR (Corbett Research). Real-time primers used with the specific annealing temperatures are shown in Table 3. Amplifications were carried out with Qiagen's Quantitect SYBR Green PCR kit by

Table 2. Goblet cell morphology in DSS + TNF-α neutralizing antibody treated group in comparison to only DSS treatment.

Groups		Percentage of total goblet cells		
		Filled	Releasing Mucus	Empty
Day 2	DSS only	77.4±3.6	16.5±1.2	6.1±0.6
	DSS + anti-TNF-α	67.9±1.2	22±0.7	10.1±0.5
Day 5	DSS only	37.1±0.9	22.6±0.5	40.2±0.7
	DSS + anti-TNF-α	59.6±1.3*	22.8±0.7	29.4±1.6*
Day 9	DSS only	ND	ND	ND
	DSS + anti-TNF-α	19.6±0.4	21.6±0.3	58.8±1.0

Data are presented as % of goblet cells ± SEM. *P<0.05 when compared to DSS treated group of the respective day. Goblet cell morphology was quantified from randomly selected crypts of PAS stained sections. A minimum number of 100 (100–110) goblet cells were counted under 40 X magnification from each section. Only in the DSS + anti-TNFα treated group we were able to count 51 goblet cells. Goblet cell morphology was designated as previously described [28]. Filled goblet cells: goblet cells with intact mucus granules; Releasing mucus: cells releasing mucus with PAS-stained mucus emerging as a thick stream; Empty goblet cells with PAS stained mucus absent from cells exhibiting a deep concave cavitation of the apical surface. ND: Not determined as the epithelial layer and crypts on day 9 of DSS treatment was destroyed or too damaged in the ulcerated site.

Table 3. Rat primers sequences and their annealing temperature.

Gene		Primer Sequence	Annealing temperature
Muc1:	Forward	GAGTGAATATCCTACCTACCAC	58°C
	Reverse	TTCACCAGGCTAACGTGGTGAC	
Muc2:	Forward	GCCAGATCCCGAAACCA	55°C
	Reverse	TATAGGAGTCTCGGCAGTCA	
Muc3:	Forward	AACTTCCAGCCCTCCCTAAG	50°C
	Reverse	GCTTCCAGCATCGTCTCTCT	
TLR2:	Forward	GAGTCTGCTGTGCCCTTCTC	50°C
	Reverse	CATGAGGTTCTCCACCCAAT	
TLR4:	Forward	GTTGGATGGAAAAGCCTTGA	50°C
	Reverse	CCTGTGAGGTCGTTGAGGTT	
TLR5:	Forward	GAAGGCTGTGAATCTCGTTGG	50°C
	Reverse	CTGCCCAACCTCAGGATCTTA	
TLR9:	Forward	CCTGGCACACAATGACATTCA	50°C
	Reverse	TAAGGTCCTCCTCGTCCCA	
IL-1β:	Forward	CACCTCTCAAGCAGAGCACAG	59°C
	Reverse	GGGTTCCATGGTGAAGTCAAC	
TNFα:	Forward	AAATGGGCTCCCTCTCATCAGTT	59°C
	Reverse	TCTGCTTGGTGGTTTGCTACGAC	
IL-10	Forward	GGCTCAGCACTGCTATGTTGCC	65°C

using the following cycling conditions: 94°C hold for 15 min, followed by 40 cycles of denaturation at 94°C for 20 s, annealing at different temperatures for 30 s and extension at 72°C for 30 s following the manufacturer's instructions. Specificity of amplification was checked by melt curve analysis. mRNA expression for the different genes was normalized against GAPDH and fold change over control was determined according to the ddCt method [29].

Protein Level of TNF-α in Colonic Tissues

TNF-α in homogenized intestinal tissues was measured using an ELISA kit according to the manufacturer's protocol (rat TNF-α ELISA Kit, Abcam, Canada). Colonic tissues (20 mg) were homogenized in cold phosphate buffer saline (PBS) using a Polytron homogenizer and centrifuged at 20,000 g for 20 min to 4°C to obtain the supernatant. Total protein concentration of the tissue supernatant was measured using a BCA kit. TNF-α is expressed as pg/mg of tissue.

Assessment of Administration of Anti TNF-α Neutralizing Antibody on the Onset and Progression of DSS-Induced Colitis

In preliminary experiments, three doses of anti TNF-α antibody (50, 100 and 200 μg/animal/day; ip) were administered to animals for 9 consecutive days with free access to water containing 5% DSS. A dose of 100 μg/animal/day was found most optimal in significantly reducing DAI (data not shown) and was used for all the further experiments. DAI was quantified and histological examination was performed for colitis as described above. A quantitative real time PCR analysis was performed using RNA

isolated form colonic tissue to assess the changes in the gene expression of TNF-α in addition to other genes (Muc2, TLR4, TLR5, IL-1β, IL-10 and TGFβ) that have shown alteration on DSS treatment in the first set of experiments (see results). TNF-α protein in homogenized intestinal tissues was also measured using ELISA as described above.

Statistical Analysis

Results are expressed as means ± SD. Significance differences between control and the other strains were determined using Kruskal-Wallis test with Dunns post-test to compare specific groups. The choice of a non-parametric test (Kruskal-Wallis test) instead of a parametric test (Analysis of Variance, ANOVA) was based on the fact that at least one of the groups in all but two of the comparisons was non-Gaussian. To maintain consistency, Kruskal-Wallis test was used for all comparisons. All statistical analyses were performed using Graph Pad Instat software. P values >0.05 were considered significant.

Author Contributions

Conceived and designed the experiments: KC PD. Performed the experiments: PD PL. Analyzed the data: PD PL. Contributed reagents/materials/analysis tools: PD KC PL. Wrote the paper: PD KC.

References

1. Dharmani P, Chadee K (2008) Biologic therapies against inflammatory bowel disease: a dysregulated immune system and the cross talk with gastrointestinal mucosa hold the key. Curr Mol Pharmacol 1: 195–212.
2. Hendrickson BA, Gokhale R, Cho JH (2002) Clinical aspects and pathophysiology of inflammatory bowel disease. Clin Microbiol Rev 15: 79–94.
3. Yan Y, Kolachala V, Dalmasso G, Nguyen H, Laroui H, et al. (2009) Temporal and spatial analysis of clinical and molecular parameters in dextran sodium sulfate induced colitis. PLoS One 4: e6073.
4. Renes IB, Boshuizen JA, Van Nispen DJ, Bulsing NP, Buller HA, et al. (2002) Alterations in Muc2 biosynthesis and secretion during dextran sulfate sodium-

induced colitis. Am J Physiol Gastrointest Liver Physiol 282: G382–389.

5. Baumgart DC, Sandborn WJ (2007) Inflammatory bowel disease: clinical aspects and established and evolving therapies. Lancet 369: 1641–1657.

6. Dieleman LA, Pena AS, Meuwissen SG, van Rees EP (1997) Role of animal models for the pathogenesis and treatment of inflammatory bowel disease. Scand J Gastroenterol Suppl 223: 99–104.

7. Moncada DM, Kammanadiminti SJ, Chadee K (2003) Mucin and Toll-like receptors in host defense against intestinal parasites. Trends Parasitol 19: 305–311.

8. Clayburgh DR, Shen L, Turner JR (2004) A porous defense: the leaky epithelial barrier in intestinal disease. Lab Invest 84: 282–291.

9. Toshina K, Hirata I, Maemura K, Sasaki S, Murano M, et al. (2000) Enprostil, a prostaglandin-E(2) analogue, inhibits interleukin-8 production of human colonic epithelial cell lines. Scand J Immunol 52: 570–575.

10. Xu Y, Hunt NH, Bao S (2007) The correlation between pro-inflammatory cytokines, MAdCAM-1 and cellular infiltration in the inflamed colon from TNF-alpha gene knockout mice. Immunol Cell Biol 85: 633–639.

11. Dharmani P, Srivastava V, Kissoon-Singh V, Chadee K (2009) Role of intestinal mucins in innate host defense mechanisms against pathogens. J Innate Immun 1: 123–135.

12. Andrianifahanana M, Moniaux N, Batra SK (2006) Regulation of mucin expression: mechanistic aspects and implications for cancer and inflammatory diseases. Biochim Biophys Acta 1765: 189–222.

13. Shekels LL, Anway RE, Lin J, Kennedy MW, Garside P, et al. (2001) Coordinated Muc2 and Muc3 mucin gene expression in Trichinella spiralis infection in wild-type and cytokine-deficient mice. Dig Dis Sci 46: 1757–1764.

14. Enss ML, Cornberg M, Wagner S, Gebert A, Henrichs M, et al. (2000) Pro-inflammatory cytokines trigger MUC gene expression and mucin release in the intestinal cancer cell line LS180. Inflamm Res 49: 162–169.

15. Iwashita J, Sato Y, Sugaya H, Takahashi N, Sasaki H, et al. (2003) mRNA of MUC2 is stimulated by IL-4, IL-13 or TNF-alpha through a mitogen-activated protein kinase pathway in human colon cancer cells. Immunol Cell Biol 81: 275–282.

16. Kim YD, Jeon JY, Woo HJ, Lee JC, Chung JH, et al. (2002) Interleukin-1beta induces MUC2 gene expression and mucin secretion via activation of PKC-MEK/ERK, and PI3K in human airway epithelial cells. J Korean Med Sci 17: 765–771.

17. Franchimont D, Vermeire S, El Housni H, Pierik M, Van Steen K, et al. (2004) Deficient host-bacteria interactions in inflammatory bowel disease? The toll-like receptor (TLR)-4 Asp299gly polymorphism is associated with Crohn's disease and ulcerative colitis. Gut 53: 987–992.

18. Hahm KB, Im YH, Parks TW, Park SH, Markowitz S, et al. (2001) Loss of transforming growth factor beta signalling in the intestine contributes to tissue injury in inflammatory bowel disease. Gut 49: 190–198.

19. Kuhn R, Lohler J, Rennick D, Rajewsky K, Muller W (1993) Interleukin-10-deficient mice develop chronic enterocolitis. Cell 75: 263–274.

20. Soderholm JD, Olaison G, Peterson KH, Franzen LE, Lindmark T, et al. (2002) Augmented increase in tight junction permeability by luminal stimuli in the non-inflamed ileum of Crohn's disease. Gut 50: 307–313.

21. Sun Y, Fihn BM, Sjovall H, Jodal M (2004) Enteric neurones modulate the colonic permeability response to luminal bile acids in rat colon in vivo. Gut 53: 362–367.

22. Cario E, Podolsky DK (2000) Differential alteration in intestinal epithelial cell expression of toll-like receptor 3 (TLR3) and TLR4 in inflammatory bowel disease. Infect Immun 68: 7010–7017.

23. Charo IF, Ransohoff RM (2006) The many roles of chemokines and chemokine receptors in inflammation. N Engl J Med 354: 610–621.

24. Goebel S, Huang M, Davis WC, Jennings M, Siahaan TJ, et al. (2006) VEGF-A stimulation of leukocyte adhesion to colonic microvascular endothelium: implications for inflammatory bowel disease. Am J Physiol Gastrointest Liver Physiol 290: G648–654.

25. Keshavarzian A, Choudhary S, Holmes EW, Yong S, Banan A, et al. (2001) Preventing gut leakiness by oats supplementation ameliorates alcohol-induced liver damage in rats. J Pharmacol Exp Ther 299: 442–448.

26. Leeb SN, Vogl D, Gunckel M, Kiessling S, Falk W, et al. (2003) Reduced migration of fibroblasts in inflammatory bowel disease: role of inflammatory mediators and focal adhesion kinase. Gastroenterology 125: 1341–1354.

27. Hogan SP, Seidu L, Blanchard C, Groschwitz K, Mishra A, et al. (2006) Resistin-like molecule beta regulates innate colonic function: barrier integrity and inflammation susceptibility. J Allergy Clin Immunol 118: 257–268.

28. Chadee K, Keller K, Forstner J, Innes DJ, Ravdin JI (1991) Mucin and nonmucin secretagogue activity of Entamoeba histolytica and cholera toxin in rat colon. Gastroenterology 100: 986–997.

29. Livak KJ, Schmittgen TD (2001) Analysis of relative gene expression data using real-time quantitative PCR and the 2(-Delta Delta C(T)) Method. Methods 25: 402–408.

6

Evidence for *STAT4* as a Common Autoimmune Gene: rs7574865 is Associated with Colonic Crohn's Disease and Early Disease Onset

Jürgen Glas[1,2,3⑨], Julia Seiderer[1⑨], Melinda Nagy[1], Christoph Fries[1], Florian Beigel[1], Maria Weidinger[1], Simone Pfennig[1], Wolfram Klein[4], Jörg T. Epplen[4], Peter Lohse[5], Matthias Folwaczny[2], Burkhard Göke[1], Thomas Ochsenkühn[1], Julia Diegelmann[1,2], Bertram Müller-Myhsok[6], Darina Roeske[6], Stephan Brand[1*]

1 Department of Medicine II - Grosshadern, University of Munich, Munich, Germany, 2 Department of Preventive Dentistry and Periodontology, University of Munich, Munich, Germany, 3 Institute of Human Genetics, RWTH Aachen, Aachen, Germany, 4 Department of Human Genetics, Ruhr-University Bochum, Bochum, Germany, 5 Institute of Clinical Chemistry - Grosshadern, University of Munich, Munich, Germany, 6 Max-Planck-Institute of Psychiatry, Munich, Germany

Abstract

Background: Recent studies demonstrated an association of *STAT4* variants with systemic lupus erythematosus (SLE) and rheumatoid arthritis (RA), indicating that multiple autoimmune diseases share common susceptibility genes. We therefore investigated the influence of *STAT4* variants on the susceptibility and phenotype of inflammatory bowel diseases (IBD) in a large patient and control cohort.

Methodology/Principal Findings: Genomic DNA from 2704 individuals of Caucasian origin including 857 patients with Crohn's disease (CD), 464 patients with ulcerative colitis (UC), and 1383 healthy, unrelated controls was analyzed for seven SNPs in the *STAT4* gene (rs11889341, rs7574865, rs7568275, rs8179673, rs10181656, rs7582694, rs10174238). In addition, a detailed genotype-phenotype analysis was performed. Our analysis revealed an association of the *STAT4* SNP rs7574865 with overall decreased susceptibility to CD (p = 0.047, OR 0.86 [95% CI 0.74–0.99]). However, compared to CD patients carrying the wild type genotype, the *STAT4* SNP rs7574865 was significantly associated with early CD onset (p = 0.021) and colonic CD (p = 0.008; OR = 4.60, 95% CI 1.63–12.96). For two other *STAT4* variants, there was a trend towards protection against CD susceptibility (rs7568275, p = 0.058, OR 0.86 [95% CI 0.74–1.00]; rs10174238, p = 0.057, OR 0.86 [95% CI 0.75–1.00]). In contrast, we did not observe any association with UC susceptibility. Evidence for weak gene-gene interaction of *STAT4* with the *IL23R* SNP rs11209026 was lost after Bonferroni correction.

Conclusions/Significance: Our results identified the *STAT4* SNP rs7574865 as a disease-modifying gene variant in colonic CD. However, in contrast to SLE and RA, the effect of rs7574865 on CD susceptibility is only weak.

Editor: Derya Unutmaz, New York University, United States of America

Funding: J. Glas was supported by a grant from the Broad Medical Foundation (IBD-0126R2). J. Seiderer and J. Diegelmann were supported by grants from the Ludwig-Maximilians-University Munich (FöFoLe Nr. 422; Habilitationsstipendium, LMUExcellent to J.S. and Promotionsstipendium to J.D.); J. Seiderer was also supported by the Robert-Bosch-Foundation and the Else Kröner-Fresenius-Stiftung (81/08//EKMS08/01). S. Brand was supported by grants from the DFG (BR 1912/5-1), the Else Kröner-Fresenius-Stiftung (Else Kröner Fresenius Memorial Stipendium 2005; P50/05/EKMS05/62), by the Ludwig-Demling Grant 2007 from DCCV e.V., and by grants of Ludwig-Maximilians-University Munich (Excellence Initiative, Investment Funds 2008 and FöFoLe program). The funders had no role in study design, data collection and analysis, decision to publish, or preparation of the manuscript.

Competing Interests: The authors have declared that no competing interests exist.

* E-mail: stephan.brand@med.uni-muenchen.de

⑨ These authors contributed equally to this work.

Introduction

The precise etiology of inflammatory bowel disease (IBD) is not completely understood but accumulating data on genetic risk factors, including genome-wide association studies, have significantly advanced our understanding of its pathogenesis. [1,2] During the last decade, substantial progress has been made in identifying susceptibility genes for Crohn's disease (CD) involved in innate immunity (particularly genetic variants in the *NOD2/CARD15* region) [3–7] and autophagy (variants in the *ATG16L1* [8–11] and *IRGM* region) [12] as well as in the proinflammatory IL-23 [13,14] and T-helper cell type 17 (Th17) pathway, [15,16]

highlighting the complex interaction between gut homeostasis, bacterial recognition and proinflammatory mucosal immune response in IBD. Moreover, it is now clear that adaptive immune responses involved in the IBD pathogenesis are more complex than the traditional dichotomous Th1/Th2 paradigm. Particularly the identification of the IL-23-Th17 pathway highlights the importance of T-cell differentiation in maintaining intestinal immune homeostasis in the pathogenesis of both CD and ulcerative colitis (UC). [16–18]

STAT4 (signal transducers and activators of transcription-4) represents a transcription factor transducing IL-12-, IL-23-, and type 1 interferon-mediated signals into Th1 and Th17 differentiation, monocyte activation, and interferon-gamma production. [19–23] The requirement for STAT4-dependent cytokine regulation has well been replicated for the pathogenesis of autoimmune encephalomyelitis, [24,25] rheumatoid arthritis, [26,27] and also IBD, [28–30] highlighting a critical role for STAT4 in autoimmune diseases. [23] Previous studies demonstrated constitutive STAT4 activation in intestinal T cells of CD patients [28] and an increased expression and activation of IL-12-induced STAT4 signaling in the mucosa of patients with UC. [29] Interestingly, STAT4 isoforms differentially regulate Th1 cytokine production and thereby the severity of IBD. [30] Using a transfer colitis model, it has been shown that particularly STAT4beta promotes colonic inflammation and tissue destruction which correlates with STAT4 isoform-dependent expression of TNF-α and GM-CSF *in vitro* and *in vivo*. [30] A recent *in vivo* study [31] demonstrated an impaired development of human Th1 cells in patients with deficient expression of STAT4.

Investigating the genetic background of STAT4 regulation, very recent studies suggested a significant association of genetic variants in the *STAT4* gene on chromosome 2q with systemic lupus erythematosus (SLE) and rheumatoid arthritis [23,27,32,33] as well as Sjögren's disease (SD), [34] systemic sclerosis, [23,35] psoriasis [36] and also type-1 diabetes, [37] thus indicating common genetic and molecular pathways in multiple autoimmune diseases. In patients with IBD, there are so far only limited data including a study on 700 Spanish IBD patients reporting a significant association of the *STAT4* variant rs7574865 with both susceptibility to CD and UC. [38] However, this association has not been replicated in larger patient cohorts of different ethnic origin and the phenotypic consequences are unknown so far. We therefore initiated a large genotype-phenotype analysis including 1321 Caucasian IBD patients (857 patients with CD, 464 patients with UC) and 1383 healthy, unrelated controls investigating genetic variants in *STAT4* as potential susceptibility genes in IBD and potential phenotypic consequences.

Methods

Study population and assessment of disease phenotype

The study population (n = 2704) consisted of 1321 Caucasian IBD patients including 857 patients with CD, 464 patients with UC, and 1383 healthy, unrelated controls. Written, informed consent was obtained from all patients prior to the study. The study was approved by the Ethics committee of the Ludwig-Maximilians-University Munich (Department of Medicine, Munich-Grosshadern) and adhered to the ethical principles for medical research involving human subjects of the Helsinki Declaration (http://www.wma.net/e/policy/b3.htm). For the diagnosis of CD or UC, established diagnostic guidelines including endoscopic, radiological, and histopathological criteria were used. [39] Patients with CD were assessed according to the Montreal classification [40] based on age at diagnosis (A), location (L), and behaviour (B) of disease. In patients with UC, anatomic location was also assessed in accordance to the Montreal classification, using the criteria ulcerative proctitis (E1), left-sided UC (distal UC; E2), and extensive UC (pancolitis; E3). Patients with indeterminate colitis were excluded from the study. Phenotypic characteristics included demographic data and clinical parameters (behaviour and anatomic location of IBD, disease-related complications, previous surgery or immunosuppressive therapy) which were recorded by investigation of patient charts and a detailed questionnaire including an interview at time of enrolment. All phenotypic data were collected blind to the results of the genotypic

data. The demographic characteristics of the IBD study population are summarized in Table 1.

DNA extraction and genotyping of the *STAT4* variants

From all study participants, blood samples were taken and genomic DNA was isolated from peripheral blood leukocytes using the DNA blood mini kit from Qiagen (Hilden, Germany) according to the manufacturer's guidelines. Seven *STAT4* SNPs (rs11889341, rs7574865, rs7568275, rs8179673, rs10181656, rs7582694, rs10174238) were genotyped by PCR and melting curve analysis using a pair of fluorescence resonance energy transfer (FRET) probes in a LightCycler® 480 Instrument (Roche Diagnostics, Mannheim, Germany). The SNP selection was based on a previous study demonstrating significant associations of these SNPs with SLE and rheumatoid arthritis. [27] The donor fluorescent molecule (fluorescein) at 3′-end of the sensor probe is excited at its specific fluorescence excitation wavelength (533 nm) and the energy is transferred to the acceptor fluorescent molecule at the 5′-end (LightCycler Red 610, 640 or 670) of the anchor probe. The specific fluorescence signal emitted by the acceptor molecule is detected by the optical unit of the LightCycler 480 Instrument. The sensor probe is exactly matching to one allele of each SNP, preferentially to the rarer allele, whereas in the case of the other allele there is a mismatch resulting in a lower melting temperature. The total volume of the PCR was 5 µl containing 25 ng of genomic DNA, 1× Light Cycler 480 Genotyping Master (Roche Diagnostics), 2.5 pmol of each primer and 0.75 pmol of each FRET probe (TIB MOLBIOL, Berlin, Germany). In the case of rs11889341, rs7574865, rs7568275 and rs8179673, the concentration of the forward primer, and in the case of rs7582694, the concentration of the reverse primer, were reduced to 1.25 pmol. For rs10181656, the concentration of the forward primer, and for rs10174238 the concentration of the reverse primer, were reduced to 0.5 pmol. The PCR comprised an initial

Table 1. Demographic characteristics of the IBD study population.

	Crohn's disease N = 857	Ulcerative colitis n = 464	Controls n = 1383
Gender			
Male (%)	45.3	47.9	62.6
Female (%)	54.7	52.5	37.4
Age (yrs)			
Mean ± SD	40.2±13.2	42.4±14.4	45.8±10.7
Range	11–81	7–86	18–71
Body mass index			
Mean ± SD	23.1±4.2	23.9±4.1	
Range	13–40	15–41	
Age at diagnosis (yrs)			
Mean ± SD	27.7±11.8	32.0±13.3	
Range	1–78	9–81	
Disease duration (yrs)			
Mean ± SD	11.9±8.6	10.5±7.7	
Range	0–44	1–40	
Positive family history of IBD (%)	16	16.1	

denaturation step (95°C for 10 min) and 45 cycles (95°C for 10°C sec, 60 for 10 sec, 72°C for 15 sec). The melting curve analysis comprised an initial denaturation step (95°C for 1 min), a step rapidly lowering the temperature to 40°C and holding for 2 min, and a heating step slowly (1 acquisition/°C) increasing the temperature up to 95°C and continuously measuring the fluorescence intensity. The results of melting curve analysis have been confirmed by analyzing two patient samples for each possible genotype using sequence analysis. For sequencing, the total volume of the PCR was 100 µl containing 250 ng of genomic DNA, 1× PCR-buffer (Qiagen, Hilden, Germany), a final MgCl₂ concentration of 1.5 mM, 0.2 mM of a dNTP-Mix (Sigma, Steinheim, Germany), 2.5 units of HotStar Plus Taq™ DNA polymerase (Qiagen) and 10 pmol of each primer (TIB MOL-BIOL). The PCR comprised an initial denaturation step (95°C for 5 min), 35 cycles (denaturation at 94°C for 30 sec, primer annealing at 60°C for 30 sec, extension at 72°C for 30 sec) and a final extension step (72°C for 10 min). The PCR products were purified using the QIAquick PCR Purification Kit (Qiagen) and sequenced by a commercial sequencing company (Sequiserve, Vaterstetten, Germany). All sequences of primers and FRET probes and primer annealing temperatures used for genotyping and for sequence analysis are given in Tables 2 and 3. The genotype data for 10 IBD-associated *IL23R* SNPs (rs1004819, rs7517847, rs10489629, rs2201841, rs11465804, rs11209026 = p.Arg381Gln, rs1343151, rs10889677, rs11209032, rs1495965) were available from a previous study. [14]

Statistical analyses

For data evaluation, we used the SPSS 13.0 software (SPSS Inc., Chicago, IL, U.S.A.) and R-2.4.1. (http://cran.r-project.org). Each genetic marker was tested for Hardy-Weinberg equilibrium in the control population. Fisher's exact test was used for comparison between categorical variables, while Student's t test was applied for quantitative variables. Single-marker allelic tests were performed with Pearson's χ^2 test. All tests were two-tailed, considering p-values<0.05 as significant. Odds ratios were calculated for the minor allele at each SNP.

Bonferroni correction was applied for multiple comparisons as indicated. LD was calculated using the library genetics implement in R (http://www.r-project.org). We also used R for interaction analysis using the allelic model. Haplotypes were calculated using a sliding-window approach varying the window size from 2 to 7 included SNPs and using the option "hap-logistic" as implemented in PLINK (http://pngu.mgh.harvard.edu/~purcell/plink/).

Results

The *STAT4* SNP rs7574865 modulates susceptibility to CD but not to UC

In all three subgroups (CD, UC, and controls), the allele frequencies of the *STAT4* SNPs rs11889341, rs7574865, rs7568275, rs8179673, rs10181656, rs7582694 and rs10174238 were in accordance with the predicted Hardy-Weinberg equilibrium (Table 4). Overall, we observed no significant differences in the frequencies of seven SNPs investigated in UC patients compared to healthy controls (Table 4). In patients with CD, the analysis revealed a significant association of the *STAT4* SNP rs7574865 with decreased susceptibility to CD (p = 0.047, OR 0.86 [95% CI 0.74–0.99]) (Table 4); however, this significance would have been lost after Bonferroni correction, which has not been applied since all seven *STAT4* SNP were in very strong linkage disequilibrium in all three subgroups of the study population (Supplemental Tables S1, S2, S3) as also described before [27]. Moreover, for two other variants there was a trend towards association with decreased CD susceptibility (rs7568275, p = 0.058, OR 0.86 [95% CI 0.74–1.00]; rs10174238, p = 0.057, OR 0.86 [95% CI 0.75–1.00]). For all other *STAT4* SNPs investigated, we could not demonstrate significant differences comparing the allele frequencies of CD patients with those of healthy controls (Table 4). Moreover, analysis of haplotypes consisting of SNPs within the *STAT4* gene did not detect any significant differences between CD and UC, respectively, when compared to the control group (Supplemental Tables S4 and S5).

Table 2. Primer sequences (F: forward primer, R: reverse primer), FRET probe sequences, and primer annealing temperatures used for *STAT4* genotyping.

Polymorphism	Primer sequences	FRET probe sequences
rs11889341	F: TCATTTTTTTCCACATGTCTAC R: GAATGGAGTCCAGAAACAAG	TGAACATCTTATTCTTTTACCACTGC-FL LC610-CTGCTGGGCCAGCTCTGTCA
rs7574865	F: TTATGGAAAATTACATGAGTGTG GCAAATCTTTGTAAAAAGTCAA	GGTGACCAAAATGTTAATAGTGGT-FL LC640-ATCTTATTTCAGTGGAATTTCAGGGGAT
rs7568275	F: CCAACAATATTTTAGCCCTAGTCTA R: AGCCCAAAATCAATAACCAG	ACTTTATATGTTCAGTTAATATTACTTGGT-FL LC670-CATACTGACCCATGAGTGTTCAATTG
rs8179673	F: GCCATAGAAGTCTTTGAAGCTGA R: GTTTTTACCAGTTGGCAGCA	AAGTATATATTAAACAAAGGTCCATAACC-FL LC610-CCATACACATCATCATCATTTTAT*
rs10181656	F: AGTTTTCAAAGTCTAACACTGTG R: GCTGCCATGTCGAGAGTA	AACTCTTCTCACCCCTTGTACC-FL LC640-CTACCCTCCTTTGTAGCCTGGCTT
rs7582694	F: AACCTTCCAATGGTTTCTCA R: AAAGAACAAGCAAACATCCATAG**	GTTGCATACTCTATGTGTCATCCC-FL LC670-TCATGAATTTGGTGTGGGTAGAACAAT
rs10174238	F: GTTGAGAGAGGAGAATCTGTTGAACC R: ATGAACAAGACTGTCACTATCGAG	AAGGTAAACAATGATAACGTCTTTTT-FL LC610-TTTTGAGATAGAGTTTCAATCTGTCACCCA

Note: FL: Fluorescein, LC610: LightCycler-Red 610; LC640: LightCycler-Red 640. The polymorphic position within the sensor probe is underlined. A phosphate is linked to the 3′-end of the acceptor probe to prevent elongation by the DNA polymerase in the PCR.
*The underlined T bases within the rs8179673 anchor probe represent LNA (locked nucleic acid) bases in.
**The underlined C base within the rs7582694 reverse primer differs from the original sequence.

Table 3. Primer sequences used for the sequence analysis of *STAT4* variants.

Polymorphism	Primer sequences
rs11889341	CAAATACCTTCTACTCTATGGCT GAATGGAGTCCAGAAACAAG
rs7574865	AAAGAAGTTTGTAATTAAAAAGCTA GCAAATCTTTGTAAAAAGTCAA
rs7568275	AAACCAACCTCATTAAATTATAGCA GAAGACAAAAAGAAAATATGGTCAC
rs8179673	TTAGTTTTTCCCACGTTTAGTTCTC TCAAATCATATGGGGAGGAGTG
rs10181656	GTGGATAAAAATACAAAATAAAAGAC GGATTTCAACAGGATCACC
rs7582694	AACCTTCCAATGGTTTCTCA CAGTGGATATGGATTTTAGTACTCTG
rs10174238	GAGGTAGAGGTTACAGTGAGCCGA AAGCAATGTTTCACCTGTCCCT

Associations between *STAT4* genotype status and the CD phenotype

Based on the significant association of the *STAT4* SNP rs7574865 with the susceptibility to CD, we next performed a detailed genotype-phenotype analysis in a subgroup of n = 622 phenotypically well-characterized CD patients carrying SNP rs7574865. CD patients homozygous for rs7574865 showed a significant younger age at disease onset (23.2 years ±7.5) compared to wildtype patients (27.9 years ±12.3; p = 0.021) and also heterozygous patients (29.0 years ±12.4; p = 0.007). In addition, we observed significantly more male patients in the subcohort of homozygous carriers of the SNP rs7574865 compared to the wildtype patients (p = 0.040) and heterozygous patients (p = 0.005; Table 5). CD patients homozygous for rs7574865 were found to have significantly more frequent colonic disease compared to wildtype patients (p = 0.008) and heterozygous carriers (p = 0.033; Table 6). Moreover, none of the homozygous carriers demonstrated isolated CD of the terminal ileum. In contrast, the analysis revealed no significant associations with other phenotypic disease characteristics such as body mass index (BMI), incidence of stenoses and fistulas, use of immunosuppressive agents, or extraintestinal manifestations (Tables 5 and 6).

Analysis for epistasis with *IL23R*

Given that IL-23, a cytokine involved in Th17 cell differentiation, activates not only *STAT3* but also to a lesser degree *STAT4*, we next investigated potential epistasis with the IBD susceptibility gene *IL23R*. Analysis for 10 SNPs in the *IL23R* region which have previously shown to significantly influence CD susceptibility [14] found weak interactions between the *STAT4* SNPs rs8179673, rs7582694 and rs10174238 with the coding *IL23R* SNP rs11209026 = p.Arg181Gln in CD (Supplemental Table S6) but significance was lost after correction for multiple comparisons. Interestingly, similar to the effect of the *STAT4* SNP rs7574865 shown in this study, the *IL23R* SNP rs11209026 is protective for CD susceptibility. However, none of the three *STAT4* SNPs with epistasis to the *IL23R* SNP rs11209026 were independently associated with CD, although there was a trend for association of CD with rs10174238 (rs10174238: p = 0.057; rs8179673: p = 0.12; rs7582694: p = 0.15; Table 4). Furthermore, no significant interaction was observed between *STAT4* and *IL23R* SNPs in UC (Supplemental Table S7).

Discussion

Here, we present the first detailed genotype-phenotype analysis of *STAT4* gene variants in a large Caucasian IBD cohort. In line with previous reports of significant associations of genetic variants in the *STAT4* gene with the risk for autoimmune diseases such as SLE, rheumatoid arthritis [23,27,32] and psoriasis, [23,36] our study could identify the *STAT4* SNP rs7574865 also to be associated with the susceptibility to CD. However, this association to CD did not reach the extent of significance or clinical relevance shown for other CD susceptibility genes such as *NOD2/CARD15* and *IL23R* [5,13,14,41–43]. For all other *STAT4* gene variants investigated (rs11889341, rs7568275, rs8179673, rs10181656, rs7582694 and rs10174238), our analysis did not reveal any significant association with CD or UC susceptibility. However, there was a trend towards an association in the case of rs7568275 and rs10174238 in CD, which can be explained by the strong linkage disequilibrium between all seven *STAT4* SNPs [27] investigated in our study. A smaller Spanish study including 700 IBD patients also reported a significant association of the *STAT4* variant rs7574865 with CD susceptibility, although rs7574865 was in this study a risk allele and not protective [38]. In contrast, a very recent Korean study found

Table 4. Associations of *STAT4* gene markers in CD and UC case-control association studies.

SNP	Minor allele	Crohn's disease n = 857			Ulcerative colitis n = 464			Controls n = 1383
		MAF	p value	OR [95% CI]	MAF	p value	OR [95% CI]	MAF
rs11889341	T	0.194	0.11	0.88 [0.76–1.03]	0.215	0.96	1.01 [0.84–1.20]	0.214
rs7574865	T	0.190	**0.047**	0.86 [0.74–0.99]	0.214	1.00	1.00 [0.83–1.20]	0.215
rs7568275	G	0.193	0.058	0.86 [0.74–1.00]	0.212	0.78	0.97 [0.81–1.17]	0.217
rs8179673	C	0.198	0.12	0.89 [0.76–1.03]	0.215	0.93	0.99 [0.82–1.18]	0.217
rs10181656	G	0.197	0.12	0.89 [0.76–1.03]	0.211	0.74	0.96 [0.80–1.16]	0.217
rs7582694	C	0.197	0.15	0.89 [0.77–1.04]	0.212	0.89	0.98 [0.82–1.18]	0.215
rs10174238	G	0.202	0.057	0.87 [0.75–1.00]	0.229	0.85	1.02 [0.85–1.22]	0.226

Minor allele frequencies (MAF), allelic test *P*-values, and odds ratios (OR, shown for the minor allele) with 95% confidence intervals (CI) are depicted for both the CD and UC case-control cohorts.

Table 5. Association between the *STAT4* rs7574865 gene variant and demographic characteristics of the CD cohort.

rs7574865 Crohn's disease	(1) GG (n = 399)	(2) GT (n = 203)	(3) TT (n = 20)	(1) vs. (2) p value OR	(1) vs. (3) p value OR	(2) vs. (3) p value OR	(1) vs. (2+3) p value OR
Male sex	203/399 (51.0%)	84/203 (41.0%)	15/20 (75.0%)	**0.031**	**0.040**	**0.005**	0.132
				0.68 CI (0.48–0.96)	2.90 CI (1.03–8.12)	4.25 (1.49–12.14)	0.77 (0.56–1.07)
Age (yr)							
Mean ± SD	40.7±13.3	42.0±12.9	34.4±7.2	0.225	**0.001**	**0.0002**	0.528
Range	16–82	18–82	21–49				
Age at diagnosis (yr)							
Mean ± SD	27.9±12.3	29.0±12.4	23.2±7.5	0.308	**0.021**	**0.007**	0.551
Range	6–71	11–78	13–37				
Disease duration (yr)							
Mean ± SD	12.7±9.1	13.1±8.4	10.8±4.3	0.643	0.103	0.067	0.823
Range	0–46	1–42	2–19				
BMI							
Mean ± SD	23.2±4.3	22.8±4.2	23.4±3.3	0.312	0.808	0.487	0.366
Range	13–41	16–34	16–29				

no association of *STAT4* SNPs with CD but a weak association of the *STAT4* SNP rs925847 with susceptibility to UC (P = 0.025; OR = 0.63). [44] Similar to the findings in CD in our study, *STAT4* was protective against UC in the Korean study. [44] In contrast, another very recent study from Spain found no association of the *STAT4* SNP rs7574865 with CD and UC [45], while an extended meta-analysis showed a disease association of this SNP with UC and not CD in the Spanish population. [45] Considering the limited data of *STAT4* gene variants in IBD patients and the conflicting results from the Spanish studies, the impact of *STAT4* on IBD susceptibility seems to be much more limited than that of *STAT3* variants.

In addition, this study demonstrated weak epistasis between the CD-protective *IL23R* variant rs11209026 with several *STAT4* SNPs (Supplementary Table S6). However, none of these gene-gene interactions remained significant after Bonferroni correction. Interestingly, similar to our findings, opposing effects of *STAT3* variants on different Th17-mediated autoimmune diseases have been reported. A very recent genome-wide association study identified *STAT3* as a new susceptibility gene for multiple sclerosis (MS), a disorder in which the Th17 pathway plays a major role. [46] Remarkably, in MS, the G allele of the *STAT3* SNP rs744166 is the risk allele, whereas in CD, the A allele has been found to increase disease susceptibility. [47] Thus, it is possible that a SNP can confer opposite effects in different disorders within the same pathway. Further genotype-phenotype studies in large patient cohorts of different ethnic origin will therefore be required before final conclusion on the influence of *STAT4* on IBD susceptibility can be drawn.

In our study, CD patients homozygous for the SNP rs7574865 were significantly younger at disease onset compared to wildtype and heterozygous patients. Moreover, CD patients homozygous for rs7574865 were found to have significantly more frequent colonic disease compared to wildtype patients (p = 0.008) and heterozygous carriers (p = 0.033). It is therefore of special interest that particularly the *STAT4* SNP rs7574865, which has previously shown to be the most significant SNP in the association studies for

other IBD-associated autoimmune diseases such as SLE, rheumatoid arthritis [23,27,32] and Sjögren's disease, [23,34] is associated with both CD susceptibility and CD phenotype. However, similar to *STAT4*, other IBD susceptibility genes such as *IL23R*, *IL2/IL21*, *STAT3*, and *PTPN2* are associated with other autoimmune diseases. [48–53]

Regarding the disease-modifying effect of genetic variants in the *STAT4* region on IBD observed in our study, one might hypothesize whether the *STAT4* risk allele has different expression levels or functional effects in different effector cells. A recent study demonstrated a significant association of the *STAT4* risk allele with overexpression of *STAT4* in primary cells of mesenchymal origin such as osteoblasts but not in B cells. [54] This might indicate the potential presence of a tissue-specific intragenic enhancer and cell-type-specific effects of different *STAT4* gene variants on STAT4 expression levels. This would be in line with previous studies demonstrating that STAT4 isoforms differentially regulate Th1 cytokine production with STAT4β promoting greater colonic inflammation and tissue destruction which correlates with STAT4 isoform-dependent expression of TNF-α and GM-CSF *in vitro* and *in vivo*, but not Th1 expression of IFN-γ or Th17 expression of IL-17. [30] Further investigations on the effect of genetic variants on the expression levels and splicing isoforms in both T cells and B cells as well as intestinal epithelial cells will therefore be necessary. Moreover, based on previous studies [55] reporting an increased sensitivity to IFN-α in lupus patients carrying the risk variant of *STAT4*, one might also speculate whether this mechanism might contribute to increased mucosal inflammation in IBD patients and to the response of immunosuppressive and immunomodulatory therapies.

In summary, our results identified the *STAT4* SNP rs7574865 as a disease-modifying gene variant in CD. Homozygous carriers of the minor allele of rs7574865 have an earlier CD onset and more often colonic disease than carriers of the major allele. Further studies on expression and regulation of STAT4 in the intestinal mucosa will be required to investigate the functional consequences of *STAT4* gene variants in more detail.

Table 6. Association between the *STAT4* rs7574865 gene variant and CD characteristics based on the Montreal classification [40].

rs7574865	(1)	(2)	(3)	(1) vs. (2)	(1) vs. (3)	(2) vs. (3)	(1) vs. (2+3)
	GG	GT	TT	p value	p value	p value	p value
Crohn's disease	(n = 399)	(n = 203)	(n = 20)	OR	OR	OR	OR
Age at diagnosis							
≤16 years (A1)	45/383 (11.7%)	21/193 (10.9%)	4/18 (22.2%)	0.890 0.92 CI (0.53–1.59)	0.256 2.15 CI (0.68–6.80)	0.241 2.34 CI (0.70–7.77)	0.896 0.95 CI (0.56–1.59)
17–40 years (A2)	286/383 (74.7%)	142/193 (73.6%)	14/18 (78.8%)	0.840 0.94 CI (0.94–1.40)	1.000	1.000	0.446 0.86 CI (0.59–1.25)
>40 years (A3)	52/383 (13.6%)	30/193 (15.5%)	0	0.248 1.33 CI (0.82–2.18)	1.19 CI (0.38–3.69) 0.146	1.26 CI (0.40–4.00) 0.083	1.000 0.99 CI (0.61–1.60)
Location							
Terminal ileum (L1)	45/385 (11.7%)	31/192 (16.1%)	0	0.151 1.45 CI (0.89–2.38)	0.242	0.082	0.305 1.31 CI (0.80–2.14)
Colon (L2)	37/385 (9.6%)	25/192 (13.0%)	6/18 (33.3%)	0.253 1.41 CI (0.82–2.42)	**0.008** 4.60 CI (1.63–12.96)	**0.033** 3.32 CI (1.14–9.64)	0.079 1.63 CI (0.98–2.71)
Ileocolon (L3)	230/385 (59.7%)	115/192 (59.9%)	8/18 (44.4%)	1.000 1.01 CI (0.71–1.43)	0.225 0.54 CI (0.21–1.40)	0.220 0.54 CI (0.20–1.42)	0.794 0.95 CI (0.68–1.34)
Upper GI (L4)	10/385 (2.6%)	0	0	**0.035**	1.000	-	-
Terminal ileum and Upper GI (L1+L4)	10/385 (2.6%)	2/192 (1.0%)	0	0.354 0.39 CI (0.09–1.82)	1.000	1.000	0.230 0.36 CI (0.08–1.66)
Colon and Upper GI (L2+L4)	4/385 (1.0%)	3/192 (1.6%)	0	0.691 1.51 CI (0.33–6.82)	1.000	1.000	0.702 1.38 CI (0.31–6.23)
Ileocolon and Upper GI (L3+L4)	49/385 (12.7%)	16/192 (8.3%)	4/18 (22.2%)	0.123 0.62 CI (0.34–1.13)	0.275 1.96 CI (0.62–6.20)	0.076 3.14 CI (0.92–10.68)	0.284 0.72 CI (0.42–1.25)
Behaviour [1]							
Non-stricturing, Non-penetrat (B1)	82/369 (22.2%)	45/184 (24.5%)	2/19 (10.5%)	0.592 1.13 CI (0.75–1.72)	0.389 0.41 CI (0.09–1.82)	0.254 0.36 CI (0.08–1.64)	0.835 1.05 CI (0.70–1.59)
with perianal f. (B1p)	8/369 (2.2%)	4/184 (2.2%)	0	1.000 1.00 CI (0.30–3.37)	1.000	1.000	1.000 0.91 CI (0.27–3.05)
Stricturing (B2)	100/369 (27.1%)	39/184 (21.2%)	6/19 (31.6%)	0.146 0.72 CI (0.47–1.10)	0.792 1.24 CI (0.46–3.35)	0.382 1.72 CI (0.61–4.81)	0.228 0.77 CI (0.51–1.15)
with perianal f. (B2p)	10/369 (2.7%)	9/184 (4.9%)	0	0.217 1.85 CI (0.74–4.63)	1.000	1.000	0.330 1.66 CI (0.67–4.17)
Penetrating (B3)	152/369 (41.2%)	81/184 (44.0%)	10/19 (52.6%)	0.584 1.12 CI (0.78–1.60)	0.348 1.59 CI (0.63–4.00)	0.480 1.41 CI (0.55–3.64)	0.427 1.16 CI (0.82–1.64)
with perianal f. (B3p)	17/369 (4.6%)	6/184 (3.3%)	1/19 (5.3%)	0.508 0.70 CI (0.27–1.80)	0.603 1.15 CI (0.14–9.13)	0.503 1.65 CI (0.19–14.45)	0.664 0.74 CI (0.30–1.81)
Use of immuno-suppressive agents	307/376 (82.0%)	154/188 (82.0%)	16/20 (80.0%)	1.000 1.01 CI (0.65–1.60)	0.772 0.90 CI (0.29–2.77)	0.767 0.88 CI (0.28–2.81)	1.000 1.00 CI (0.65–1.56)
Use of infliximab	156/397 (39.0%)	80/199 (40.0%)	9/20 (45.0%)	0.859 1.04 CI (0.73–1.47)	0.644 1.26 CI (0.51–3.12)	0.812 1.22 CI (0.48–3.07)	0.796 1.06 CI (0.75–1.48)
Fistula	187/369 (50.7%)	102/184 (55.4%)	11/19 (57.9%)	0.321 1.21 CI (0.85–1.73)	0.641 1.34 CI (0.53–3.40)	1.000 1.10 CI (0.42–2.87)	0.257 1.22 CI (0.87–1.72)
Stenosis	241/364 (66.2%)	123/182 (67.6%)	12/19 (63.2%)	0.773 1.06 CI (0.73–1.55)	0.806 0.87 CI (0.34–2.28)	0.798 0.82 CI (0.31–2.20)	0.853 1.04 CI (0.72–1.50)
Abscesses	112/335 (33.0%)	71/169 (42.0%)	7/19 (37.0%)	0.063 1.44 CI (0.99–2.11)	0.805 1.16 CI (0.44–3.03)	0.807 0.80 CI (0.30–2.14)	0.072 1.41 CI (0.98–2.04)
Surgery because of CD	219/355 (62.0%)	116/177 (66.0%)	10/18 (56.0%)	0.393 1.18 CI (0.81–1.71)	0.626 0.78 CI (0.30–2.01)	0.442 0.66 CI (0.25–1.75)	0.157 1.34 CI (0.91–1.93)
Positive family history of IBD	55/291 (18.9%)	17/139 (12.2%)	1/13 (7.7%)	0.098 0.60 CI (0.33–1.07)	0.475 0.36 CI (0.05–2.81)	1.000 0.60 CI (0.07–4.89)	0.060 0.58 CI (0.32–1.02)

For each variable, the number of patients with complete information on this particular disease variable included in the analysis is given.
[1]Disease behaviour was defined according to the Montreal classification [40]. A stricturing disease phenotype was defined as presence of stenosis without penetrating disease. The diagnosis of stenosis was made surgically, endoscopically, or radiologically (using MR enteroclysis).
[2]Immunosuppressive agents included azathioprine, 6-mercaptopurine, methotrexate, and/or infliximab.
[3]Only surgery related to CD-specific problems (e.g. fistulectomy, colectomy, ileostomy) was included.

Supporting Information

Table S1   Linkage disequilibrium (LD) between *STAT4* SNPs in controls. Values are given as D'/r^2.

Table S2   LD between *STAT4* SNPs in CD patients. Values are given as D'/r^2.

Table S3   LD between *STAT4* SNPs in UC patients. Values are given as D'/r^2.

Table S4   Haplotype analysis for *STAT4* SNPs in the CD case-control cohort.

Table S5   Haplotype analysis for *STAT4* SNPs in the UC case-control cohort.

Table S6   Epistasis between *STAT4* and *IL23R* SNPs in the CD case-control cohort.

Table S7   Epistasis between *STAT4* and *IL23R* SNPs in the UC case-control cohort.

Acknowledgments

This work contains parts of the unpublished degree thesis of M. Nagy.

Author Contributions

Conceived and designed the experiments: JG SB. Performed the experiments: JG MN CF PL. Analyzed the data: JG SP BMM DR SB. Contributed reagents/materials/analysis tools: JG FB MW SP WK JTE PL MF BG TO JD SB. Wrote the paper: JG JS SB. Obtained funding for study: SB.

References

1. Xavier RJ, Podolsky DK (2007) Unravelling the pathogenesis of inflammatory bowel disease. Nature 448: 427–434.
2. Podolsky DK (2002) Inflammatory bowel disease. N Engl J Med 347: 417–429.
3. Hugot JP, Chamaillard M, Zouali H, Lesage S, Cezard JP, et al. (2001) Association of NOD2 leucine-rich repeat variants with susceptibility to Crohn's disease. Nature 411: 599–603.
4. Ogura Y, Bonen DK, Inohara N, Nicolae DL, Chen FF, et al. (2001) A frameshift mutation in NOD2 associated with susceptibility to Crohn's disease. Nature 411: 603–606.
5. Seiderer J, Schnitzler F, Brand S, Staudinger T, Pfennig S, et al. (2006) Homozygosity for the CARD15 frameshift mutation 1007fs is predictive of early onset of Crohn's disease with ileal stenosis, entero-enteral fistulas, and frequent need for surgical intervention with high risk of re-stenosis. Scand J Gastroenterol 41: 1421–1432.
6. Seiderer J, Brand S, Herrmann KA, Schnitzler F, Hatz R, et al. (2006) Predictive value of the CARD15 variant 1007fs for the diagnosis of intestinal stenoses and the need for surgery in Crohn's disease in clinical practice: results of a prospective study. Inflamm Bowel Dis 12: 1114–1121.
7. Schnitzler F, Brand S, Staudinger T, Pfennig S, Hofbauer K, et al. (2006) Eight novel CARD15 variants detected by DNA sequence analysis of the CARD15 gene in 111 patients with inflammatory bowel disease. Immunogenetics 58: 99–106.
8. Glas J, Konrad A, Schmechel S, Dambacher J, Seiderer J, et al. (2008) The ATG16L1 gene variants rs2241879 and rs2241880 (T300A) are strongly associated with susceptibility to Crohn's disease in the German population. Am J Gastroenterol 103: 682–691.
9. Hampe J, Franke A, Rosenstiel P, Till A, Teuber M, et al. (2007) A genome-wide association scan of nonsynonymous SNPs identifies a susceptibility variant for Crohn disease in ATG16L1. Nat Genet 39: 207–211.
10. Prescott NJ, Fisher SA, Franke A, Hampe J, Onnie CM, et al. (2007) A nonsynonymous SNP in ATG16L1 predisposes to ileal Crohn's disease and is independent of CARD15 and IBD5. Gastroenterology 132: 1665–1671.
11. Rioux JD, Xavier RJ, Taylor KD, Silverberg MS, et al. (2007) Genome-wide association study identifies new susceptibility loci for Crohn disease and implicates autophagy in disease pathogenesis. Nat Genet 39: 596–604.
12. Massey DC, Parkes M (2007) Genome-wide association scanning highlights two autophagy genes, ATG16L1 and IRGM, as being significantly associated with Crohn's disease. Autophagy 3: 649–651.
13. Duerr RH, Taylor KD, Brant SR, Rioux JD, Silverberg MS, et al. (2006) A genome-wide association study identifies IL23R as an inflammatory bowel disease gene. Science 314: 1461–1463.
14. Glas J, Seiderer J, Wetzke M, Konrad A, Török HP, et al. (2007) rs1004819 is the main disease-associated IL23R variant in German Crohn's disease patients: combined analysis of IL23R, CARD15, and OCTN1/2 variants. PLoS ONE 2: e819.
15. Seiderer J, Elben I, Diegelmann J, Glas J, Stallhofer J, et al. (2008) Role of the novel Th17 cytokine IL-17F in inflammatory bowel disease (IBD): Upregulated colonic IL-17F expression in active crohn's disease and analysis of the IL17F p.His161Arg polymorphism in IBD. Inflamm Bowel Dis 14: 437–445.
16. McGovern D, Powrie F (2007) The IL23 axis plays a key role in the pathogenesis of IBD. Gut 56: 1333–1336.
17. Neurath MF (2007) IL-23: a master regulator in Crohn disease. Nat Med 13: 26–28.
18. Brand S (2009) Crohn's disease: Th1, Th17 or both? The change of a paradigm: new immunological and genetic insights implicate Th17 cells in the pathogenesis of Crohn's disease. Gut 58: 1152–1167.
19. Lankford CS, Frucht DM (2003) A unique role for IL-23 in promoting cellular immunity. J Leukoc Biol 73: 49–56.
20. Watford WT, Hissong BD, Bream JH, Kanno Y, Muul L, et al. (2004) Signaling by IL-12 and IL-23 and the immunoregulatory roles of STAT4. Immunol Rev 202: 139–156.
21. Mathur AN, Chang HC, Zisoulis DG, Stritesky GL, Yu Q, et al. (2007) Stat3 and Stat4 direct development of IL-17-secreting Th cells. J Immunol 178: 4901–4907.
22. Ciric B, El-behi M, Cabrera R, Zhang GX, Rostami A (2009) IL-23 drives pathogenic IL-17-producing CD8+ T cells. J Immunol 182: 5296–5305.
23. Korman BD, Kastner DL, Gregersen PK, Remmers EF (2008) STAT4: genetics, mechanisms, and implications for autoimmunity. Curr Allergy Asthma Rep 8: 398–403.
24. Chitnis T, Najafian N, Benou C, Salama AD, Grusby MJ, et al. (2001) Effect of targeted disruption of STAT4 and STAT6 on the induction of experimental autoimmune encephalomyelitis. J Clin Invest 108: 739–747.
25. Mo C, Chearwae W, O'Malley JT, Adams SM, Kanakasabai S, et al. (2008) Stat4 isoforms differentially regulate inflammation and demyelination in experimental allergic encephalomyelitis. J Immunol 181: 5681–5690.
26. Frucht DM, Aringer M, Galon J, Danning C, Brown M, et al. (2000) Stat4 is expressed in activated peripheral blood monocytes, dendritic cells, and macrophages at sites of Th1-mediated inflammation. J Immunol 164: 4659–4664.
27. Remmers EF, Plenge RM, Lee AT, Graham RR, Hom G, et al. (2007) STAT4 and the risk of rheumatoid arthritis and systemic lupus erythematosus. N Engl J Med 357: 977–986.
28. Mudter J, Weigmann B, Bartsch B, Kiesslich R, Strand D, et al. (2005) Activation pattern of signal transducers and activators of transcription (STAT) factors in inflammatory bowel diseases. Am J Gastroenterol 100: 64–72.
29. Pang YH, Zheng CQ, Yang XZ, Zhang WJ (2007) Increased expression and activation of IL-12-induced Stat4 signaling in the mucosa of ulcerative colitis patients. Cell Immunol 248: 115–120.
30. O'Malley JT, Eri RD, Stritesky GL, Mathur AN, Chang HC, et al. (2008) STAT4 isoforms differentially regulate Th1 cytokine production and the severity of inflammatory bowel disease. J Immunol 181: 5062–5070.
31. Chang HC, Han L, Goswami R, Nguyen ET, Pelloso D, et al. (2009) Impaired development of human Th1 cells in patients with deficient expression of STAT4. Blood 113: 5887–5890.
32. Orozco G, Alizadeh BZ, Delgado-Vega AM, Gonzalez-Gay MA, Balsa A, et al. (2008) Association of STAT4 with rheumatoid arthritis: a replication study in three European populations. Arthritis Rheum 58: 1974–1980.
33. Ji JD, Lee WJ, Kong KA, Woo JH, Choi SJ, et al. (2010) Association of STAT4 polymorphism with rheumatoid arthritis and systemic lupus erythematosus: a meta-analysis. Mol Biol Rep 37: 141–147.
34. Korman BD, Alba MI, Le JM, Alevizos I, Smith JA, et al. (2008) Variant form of STAT4 is associated with primary Sjogren's syndrome. Genes Immun 9: 267–270.

35. Rueda B, Broen J, Simeon C, Hesselstrand R, Diaz B, et al. (2009) The STAT4 gene influences the genetic predisposition to systemic sclerosis phenotype. Hum Mol Genet 18: 2071–2077.

36. Zervou MI, Goulielmos GN, Castro-Giner F, Tosca AD, Krueger-Krasagakis S (2009) STAT4 gene polymorphism is associated with psoriasis in the genetically homogeneous population of Crete, Greece. Hum Immunol 70: 738–741.

37. Lee HS, Park H, Yang S, Kim D, Park Y (2008) STAT4 polymorphism is associated with early-onset type 1 diabetes, but not with late-onset type 1 diabetes. Ann N Y Acad Sci 1150: 93–98.

38. Martinez A, Varade J, Marquez A, Cenit MC, Espino L, et al. (2008) Association of the STAT4 gene with increased susceptibility for some immune-mediated diseases. Arthritis Rheum 58: 2598–2602.

39. Lennard-Jones JE (1989) Classification of inflammatory bowel disease. Scand J Gastroenterol Suppl 170: 2–6; discussion 16–19.

40. Silverberg MS, Satsangi J, Ahmad T, Arnott ID, Bernstein CN, et al. (2005) Toward an integrated clinical, molecular and serological classification of inflammatory bowel disease: Report of a Working Party of the 2005 Montreal World Congress of Gastroenterology. Can J Gastroenterol 19 Suppl A: 5–36.

41. Seiderer J, Dambacher J, Kuhnlein B, Pfennig S, Konrad A, et al. (2007) The role of the selenoprotein S (SELS) gene −105G>A promoter polymorphism in inflammatory bowel disease and regulation of SELS gene expression in intestinal inflammation. Tissue Antigens 70: 238–246.

42. Brand S, Beigel F, Olszak T, Zitzmann K, Eichhorst ST, et al. (2006) IL-22 is increased in active Crohn's disease and promotes proinflammatory gene expression and intestinal epithelial cell migration. Am J Physiol Gastrointest Liver Physiol 90: G827–G838.

43. Begue B, Dumant C, Bambou JC, Beaulieu JF, Chamaillard M, et al. (2006) Microbial induction of CARD15 expression in intestinal epithelial cells via toll-like receptor 5 triggers an antibacterial response loop. J Cell Physiol 209: 241–252.

44. Moon CM, Cheon JH, Kim SW, Shin DJ, Kim ES, et al. Association of signal transducer and activator of transcription 4 genetic variants with extra-intestinal manifestations in inflammatory bowel disease. Life Sci, 2010 Feb 20. [Epub ahead of print].

45. Diaz-Gallo LM, Palomino-Morales RJ, Gómez-García M, Cardeña C, Rodrigo L, et al. STAT4 gene influences genetic predisposition to ulcerative colitis but not Crohn's disease in the Spanish population: A replication study. Hum Immunol, 2010 Mar 7. [Epub ahead of print].

46. Jakkula E, Leppä V, Sulonen AM, Varilo T, Kallio S, et al. (2010) Genome-wide association study in a high-risk isolate for multiple sclerosis reveals associated variants in STAT3 gene. Am J Hum Genet 86: 285–291.

47. Barrett JC, Hansoul S, Nicolae DL, Cho JH, Duerr RH, et al. (2008) Genome-wide association defines more than 30 distinct susceptibility loci for Crohn's disease. Nat Genet 40: 955–962.

48. Ban Y, Tozaki T, Taniyama M, Nakano Y, Yoneyama K, et al. (2009) Association studies of the IL-23R gene in autoimmune thyroid disease in the Japanese population. Autoimmunity 42: 126–130.

49. Huffmeier U, Lascorz J, Bohm B, Lohmann J, Wendler J, et al. (2009) Genetic variants of the IL-23R pathway: association with psoriatic arthritis and psoriasis vulgaris, but no specific risk factor for arthritis. J Invest Dermatol 129: 355–358.

50. Fedetz M, Ndagire D, Fernandez O, Leyva L, Guerrero M, et al. (2009) Multiple sclerosis association study with the TENR-IL2-IL21 region in a Spanish population. Tissue Antigens 74: 244–247.

51. Fung EY, Smyth DJ, Howson JM, Cooper JD, Walker NM, et al. (2009) Analysis of 17 autoimmune disease-associated variants in type 1 diabetes identifies 6q23/TNFAIP3 as a susceptibility locus. Genes Immun 10: 188–191.

52. Smyth DJ, Plagnol V, Walker NM, Cooper JD, Downes K, et al. (2008) Shared and distinct genetic variants in type 1 diabetes and celiac disease. N Engl J Med 359: 2767–2777.

53. Glas J, Stallhofer J, Ripke S, Wetzke M, Pfennig S, et al. (2009) Novel genetic risk markers for ulcerative colitis in the IL2/IL21 region are in epistasis with IL23R and suggest a common genetic background for ulcerative colitis and celiac disease. Am J Gastroenterol 104: 1737–1744.

54. Sigurdsson S, Nordmark G, Garnier S, Grundberg E, Kwan T, et al. (2008) A risk haplotype of STAT4 for systemic lupus erythematosus is over-expressed, correlates with anti-dsDNA and shows additive effects with two risk alleles of IRF5. Hum Mol Genet 17: 2868–2876.

55. Kariuki SN, Kirou KA, MacDermott EJ, Barillas-Arias L, Crow MK, et al. (2009) Cutting edge: autoimmune disease risk variant of STAT4 confers increased sensitivity to IFN-alpha in lupus patients in vivo. J Immunol 182: 34–38.

7

Proteasome Inhibitor Bortezomib Ameliorates Intestinal Injury in Mice

Koichi Yanaba*, Yoshihide Asano, Yayoi Tada, Makoto Sugaya, Takafumi Kadono, Shinichi Sato

Department of Dermatology, Faculty of Medicine, University of Tokyo. Tokyo, Japan

Abstract

Background: Bortezomib is a proteasome inhibitor that has shown impressive efficacy in the treatment of multiple myeloma. In mice, the addition of dextran sulfate sodium (DSS) to drinking water leads to acute colitis that can serve as an experimental animal model for human ulcerative colitis.

Methodology/Principal Findings: Bortezomib treatment was shown to potently inhibit murine DSS-induced colitis. The attenuation of DSS-induced colitis was associated with decreased inflammatory cell infiltration in the colon. Specifically, bortezomib-treated mice showed significantly decreased numbers of CD4$^+$ and CD8$^+$ T cells in the colon and mesenteric lymph nodes. Bortezomib treatment significantly diminished interferon (IFN)-γ expression in the colon and mesenteric lymph nodes. Furthermore, cytoplasmic IFN-γ production by CD4$^+$ and CD8$^+$ T cells in mesenteric lymph nodes was substantially decreased by bortezomib treatment. Notably, bortezomib enhanced T cell apoptosis by inhibiting nuclear factor-κB activation during DSS-induced colitis.

Conclusions/Significance: Bortezomib treatment is likely to induce T cell death, thereby suppressing DSS-induced colitis by reducing IFN-γ production.

Editor: Lionel G. Filion, University of Ottawa, Canada

Funding: This work was supported by a grant of Research on Intractable Diseases from the Ministry of Health, Labor and Welfare of Japan. The funders had no role in study design, data collection and analysis, decision to publish, or preparation of the manuscript.

Competing Interests: The authors have declared that no competing interests exist.

* E-mail: yanabak-der@h.u-tokyo.ac.jp

Introduction

Ulcerative colitis is an inflammatory bowel disease characterized by pathologic mucosal damage and ulceration, which can involve the rectum and extend proximally [1]. Although its etiology and pathogenesis have not yet been identified, inappropriate activation of the mucosal immune system has been found to play an important role in mucosal inflammation. At sites of intestinal inflammation, granulocytes and macrophages produce high levels of pro-inflammatory cytokines, including interleukin (IL)-1β, IL-6, and tumor necrosis factor (TNF)-α [2,3], which are directly involved in the pathogenesis of ulcerative colitis.

The oral administration of dextran sulfate sodium (DSS) solution to rodents is widely employed as a model of human ulcerative colitis, because it causes acute inflammatory reactions and ulceration in the entire colon similar to that observed in patients [4,5]. Mice exposed to DSS in drinking water develop inflammation only in the large intestine and show signs such as diarrhea, hematochezia, and body weight loss with histologic findings including inflammatory cell infiltration, erosion, ulceration, and crypt abscesses. Furthermore, increased production of pro-inflammatory cytokines, including interferon (IFN)- γ, TNF-α, IL-1, IL-6, IL-12, and IL-17, has been found in the colon of mice with DSS-induced colitis [6,7].

The major intracellular pathway for protein degradation is the ubiquitin-proteasome pathway [8]. Proteasomes are large multimeric protease complexes located in both the cytoplasm and nuclei

that selectively and timely degrade most cellular proteins [9,10]. The 26S proteasome consists of a central 20S core and two 19S regulatory complexes. Upon stimulation, the formation of immunoproteasomes is induced. The ubiquitination of target proteins is an important mechanism for the discriminatory nature of protein degradation by proteasomes [10]. Proteasome inhibitors have received much attention because of their potent anti-tumor activity [11]. In particular, bortezomib, a boronic acid dipeptide derivative, is a specific protease inhibitor that has recently been approved for the treatment of relapsed multiple myeloma, a plasma cell neoplasia, because of its direct growth-inhibitory and apoptotic effects on this cancer [11,12]. Furthermore, bortezomib is effective in the treatment of allograft rejection, graft-versus-host disease, contact hypersensitivity responses, and lupus-like disease in mice [13–16]. Proteasome inhibitors induce apoptosis in activated and proliferating, but not resting, T cells [17,18], suggesting one possible mechanism for the suppression of T cell-mediated immune responses by bortezomib. In this study, the effect of bortezomib in ulcerative colitis was examined using DSS-induced mouse colitis.

Results

Bortezomib treatment attenuates DSS-induced colitis

To assess the therapeutic effect of bortezomib in DSS-induced colitis, we treated mice with 3% DSS for 7 days and quantitatively evaluated the severity of intestinal injury by measuring body

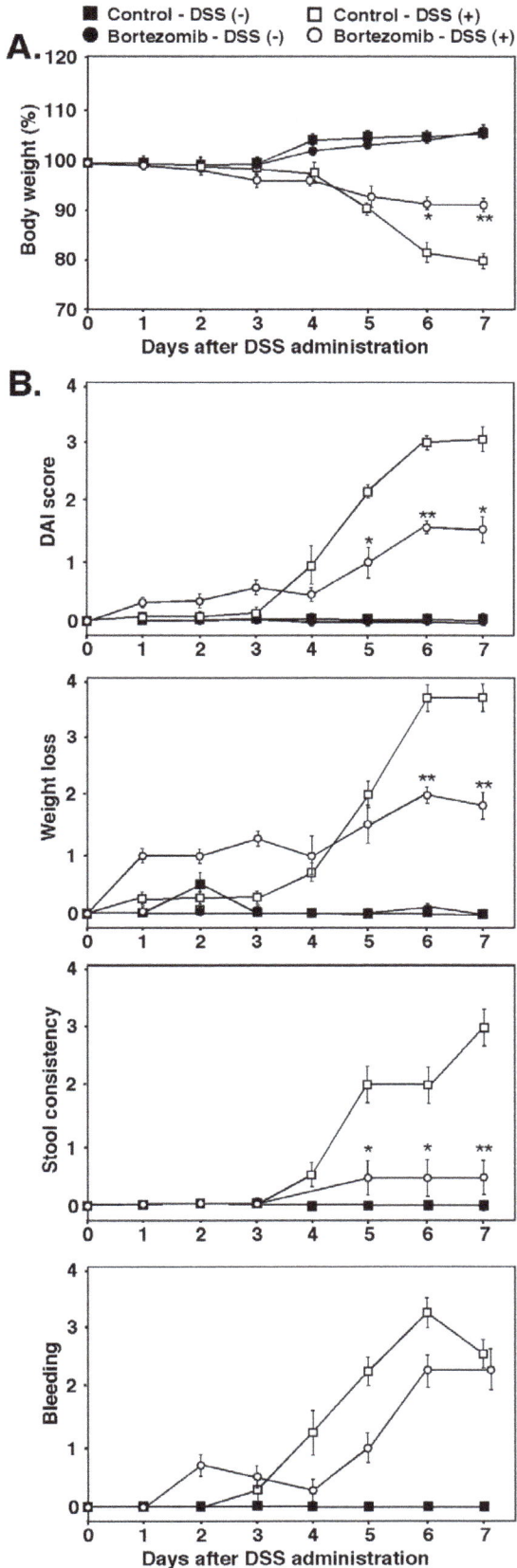

Figure 1. Bortezomib suppressed the severity of DSS-induced colitis. Mice ingested either DSS solution or normal drinking water.

Mice were treated with 200 µl of bortezomib (0.75 mg/kg) or PBS (control) intravenously twice weekly, starting 2 days prior to DSS administration. The severity of intestinal injury was evaluated by quantitatively measuring body weight (**A**) and DAI scores (**B**). DAI scores were based on weight loss, stool consistency, and bleeding. Values represent means ($\pm$SEM) from $\geq$4 mice per group. Significant differences between sample means are indicated: *$P<0.05$; **$P<0.01$. Similar results were obtained in at least two independent experiments.

weight and disease activity index (DAI) scores. We treated mice twice weekly with bortezomib or phosphate buffered saline (PBS) control starting 2 days before DSS administration. DAI scores were based on weight loss, stool consistency, and bleeding.

Statistically significant body weight loss was first observed in DSS-treated mice on day 6 (Figure 1A). Bortezomib treatment significantly attenuated body weight loss compared with control-treated mice and delayed the increase in DAI scores by 1 day from day 4 (control-treated mice) to day 5 (bortezomib-treated mice) (Figure 1B). DAI scores were also significantly higher in bortezomib-treated mice than in control-treated mice from day 5–7. Each element of the DAI score showed the same trend as the overall DAI score, suggesting that bortezomib treatment suppressed DSS-induced colitis in mice.

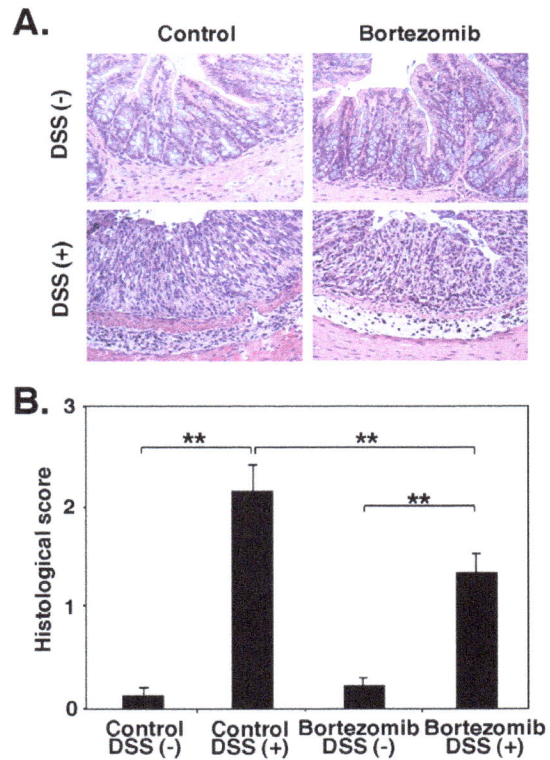

Figure 2. Bortezomib treatment reduced the severity of DSS-induced colitis. Colon sections were harvested from mice treated with bortezomib or control after ingestion of either DSS solution or normal drinking water for 7 days, and stained with hematoxylin and eosin. (**A**) Representative colon sections at 7 days after induction of colitis. (**B**) Histologic sections were blindly scored on a scale of 0–4 for severity of colitis. Values represent means ($\pm$SEM) from $\geq$4 mice per group. Significant differences between sample means are indicated: **$P<0.01$**. Results represent one of two independent experiments producing similar results.

a. Colon

b. Mesenteric lymph node

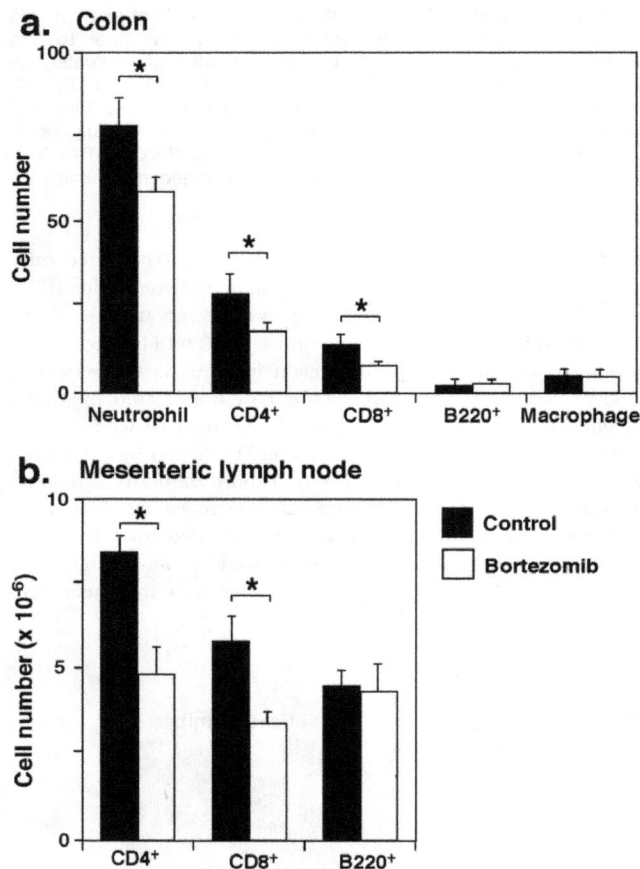

Figure 3. Profile of infiltrating cells in the colon and mesenteric lymph nodes during DSS-induced colitis in mice treated with bortezomib or control. (A) The numbers of neutrophils, CD4+ T cells, CD8+ T cells, B220+ B cells, and F4/80+ macrophages per one field of view (×200) in the colon were counted. **(B)** Bortezomib affects CD4+ and CD8+ T cell numbers in mesenteric lymph nodes during DSS-induced colitis. Bar graphs indicate CD4+ T cells, CD8+ T cells, and B220+ cells in mesenteric lymph nodes 7 days after induction of colitis. A, B) Values represent means (± SEM) from ≥4 mice per group. Significant differences between sample means are indicated: *$P<0.05$. Similar results were obtained in at least two independent experiments.

To further evaluate disease severity, the degree of intestinal injury was assessed histopathologically. Following the 7-day period of ingestion of 3% DSS or normal drinking water, colons were removed for histopathologic evaluation (Figure 2A). DSS treatment induced epithelial injury and increased mononuclear cell infiltration and inflammatory changes in submucosal tissues of control-treated mice, but these changes were less severe in bortezomib-treated mice. The pathologic scores were significantly lower in bortezomib-treated mice than in control-treated mice ($P<0.01$; Figure 2B). Thus, bortezomib treatment reduced DSS-induced colitis both clinically and histopathologically.

Bortezomib inhibits T cell accumulation during DSS-induced colitis

The profile of infiltrating cells in the colon was further examined immunohistologically. Seven days after DSS administration, neutrophil numbers were significantly decreased in bortezomib-treated mice relative to control-treated mice (23% decrease, $P<0.05$; Figure 3A). The numbers of CD4+ and CD8+ T cells

were also significantly lower in mice treated with bortezomib than in control mice (38% decrease, $P<0.05$ and 41% decrease, $P<0.05$, respectively), but there were no significant differences in numbers of B cells or macrophages. Thus, bortezomib treatment reduced both neutrophil and T cell infiltration in the colon.

To determine whether bortezomib treatment altered the populations of T cells and B cells in mesenteric lymph nodes during DSS-induced colitis, the numbers of CD4+, CD8+, and B220+ cells in mesenteric lymph nodes were assessed by flow cytometry 7 days after DSS administration. Mice treated with bortezomib had fewer CD4+ and CD8+ T cells than control mice (42% decrease, $P<0.05$ and 41% decrease, $P<0.05$, respectively; Figure 3B). Thus, bortezomib treatment decreased the numbers of both CD4+ and CD8+ T cells in mesenteric lymph nodes.

Bortezomib reduces IFN-γ production during DSS-induced colitis

The effect of bortezomib treatment on cytokine expression during DSS-induced colitis was examined by assessing the mRNA expression of several cytokines in control and bortezomib-treated mice. Colons and mesenteric lymph nodes were harvested 7 days after the induction of colitis, and the expression of IFN-γ, IL-6, IL-17, IL-4, and IL-10 mRNA was quantified by real-time PCR. Bortezomib treatment significantly decreased IFN-γ colon mRNA levels by 70% and IL-6 colon mRNA levels by 58% compared with control mice ($P<0.05$, Figure 4A). By contrast, mRNA expression of IL-17, IL-4 and IL-10 in the colons was not affected by bortezomib treatment. In mesenteric lymph nodes, IFN-γ transcripts of bortezomib-treated mice were significantly decreased relative to those of control mice (75% decrease, $P<0.01$; Figure 4B). IL-6, IL-17, IL-4 and IL-10 mRNA expression in mice treated with bortezomib was comparable to control mice. Thus, bortezomib treatment substantially decreased IFN-γ mRNA levels during DSS-induced colitis.

Bortezomib diminishes T cell IFN-γ production during DSS-induced colitis

Intracellular cytokine staining was used to assess whether bortezomib treatment affected IFN-γ production from mesenteric lymph node CD4+ and CD8+ T cells. Bortezomib treatment significantly reduced the frequency (43% decrease, $P<0.05$) and number (53% decrease, $P<0.01$) of IFN-γ-producing CD4+ T cells compared with control mice (Figure 5A). Furthermore, the frequency and number of CD8+ T cells in mice treated with bortezomib were 40% ($P<0.05$) and 66% ($P<0.01$) lower, respectively, than in control mice (Figure 5B). Thus, bortezomib treatment diminished T cell IFN-γ production during DSS-induced colitis.

Bortezomib induces T cell apoptosis by inhibiting NF-κB activation during DSS-induced colitis

To determine whether bortezomib treatment induced T cell apoptosis, thereby suppressing DSS-induced colitis, the percentages of Annexin-V/7-AAD+ CD4+ and CD8+ T cells in mesenteric lymph nodes were assessed 7 days after the induction of colitis. In mice treated with bortezomib, the numbers of Annexin-V/7-AAD+ CD4+ and CD8+ T cells were significantly increased compared with control-treated mice (2.7-fold, $P<0.05$ and 3.2-fold, $P<0.01$, respectively; Figure 6A). As proteasome inhibitors counteract NF-κB activation by interfering with the proteasomal degradation of IκB proteins, we also assessed the transcriptional activity of NF-κB using real-time PCR for NF-κB-induced IκBα mRNA. IκB mRNA levels of CD4+ and CD8+ T

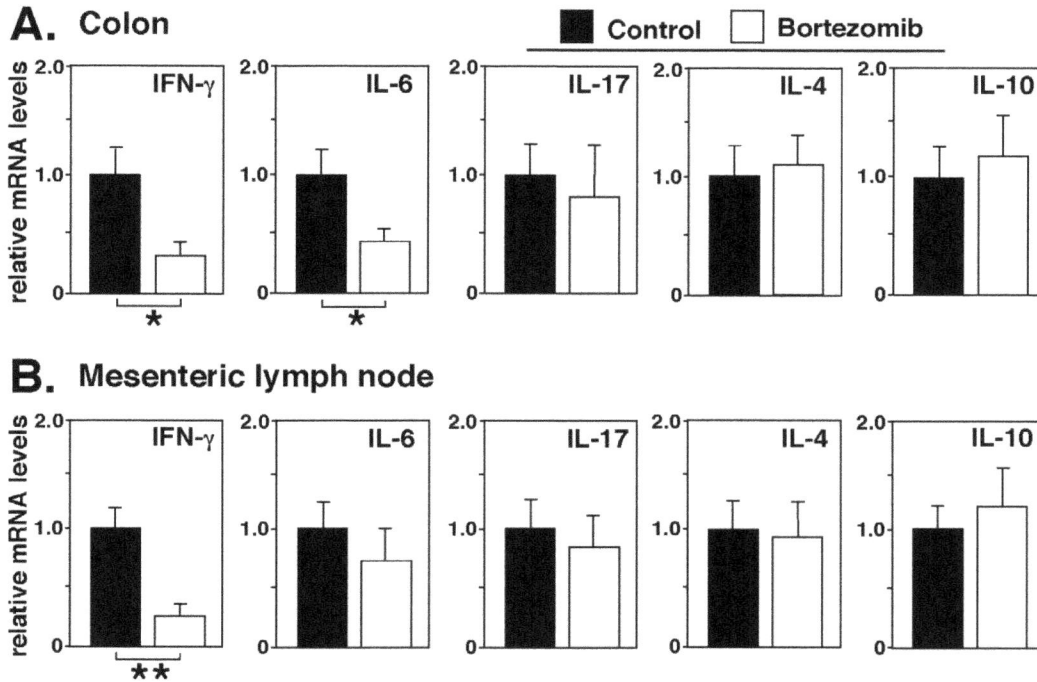

Figure 4. Bortezomib treatment affects cytokine production in DSS-induced colits. Cytokine mRNA expression in the colon (**A**) and mesenteric lymph nodes (**B**) in mice treated with bortezomib or control during DSS-induced colitis. Colon tissue and mesenteric lymph nodes were collected from control- or bortezomib-treated mice 7 days following DSS administration. Transcript levels were quantified by real-time PCR analysis and were normalized with an internal control. Values represent means (± SEM) from ≥4 mice of each group. Significant differences between sample means are indicated; *P<0.05, **P<0.01. Results represent one of two independent experiments producing similar results.

cells in mesenteric lymph nodes from bortezomib-treated mice were significantly enhanced compared with control-treated mice (2.5-fold, P<0.05 and 3.2-fold, P<0.01, respectively; Figure 6B). Thus, NF-κB inhibition is likely to contribute to bortezomib-induced cell death in T cells, thereby suppressing DSS-induced colitis.

Discussion

The results of this study demonstrate that bortezomib treatment inhibits DSS-induced colitis in mice (Figures 1 and 2). The suppression of DSS-induced colitis by bortezomib treatment correlated with a decrease in CD4+ and CD8+ T cell accumulation both in the colon and mesenteric lymph nodes (Figure 3). Remarkably, bortezomib treatment significantly reduced IFN-γ mRNA expression in the colon and mesenteric lymph nodes, while IL-17, IL-4 and IL10 mRNA expression was not affected (Figure 4). Consistently, IFN-γ production from CD4+ and CD8+ T cells in mesenteric lymph nodes was inhibited by bortezomib treatment (Figure 5). Thus, bortezomib treatment attenuated DSS-induced colitis by inhibiting excessive IFN-γ production from CD4+ and CD8+ T cells.

The immunoproteasome subunit LMP7 is critical for proteasome activity [19], and it was recently reported that LMP7-deficiency is associated with reduced severity of DSS-induced colitis in mice [20]. Patients with inflammatory bowel disease exhibit high levels of LMP7 in the inflamed gut [21], and their increased proteasome activity induced by high levels of expression of immunoproteasome subunits mediates sustained activation of NF-κB [22]. These results suggest that proteasome inhibitors may ameliorate inflammatory bowel disease. In this study, bortezomib

administration substantially reduced the severity of DSS-induced colitis as well as significantly enhancing apoptosis and IκB expression of CD4+ and CD8+ T cells during DSS-induced colitis (Figure 6). Thus, NF-κB inhibition is likely to contribute to bortezomib-induced cell death in T cells, thereby suppressing DSS-induced colitis.

Bortezomib treatment of mice with lupus-like disease significantly improves the disease severity by reducing the numbers of both CD4+ and CD8+ T cells in the spleen [14]. Bortezomib treatment also demonstrates significant protection from acute graft-versus-host disease in a murine allogeneic bone marrow transplantation model by inhibiting allogeneic T cell proliferation [16]. By contrast, bortezomib administration largely eliminates plasma cells but not T cells or B cells in murine models of human systemic lupus erythematosus [14]. In the current study, bortezomib treatment reduced the numbers of CD4+ and CD8+ T cells, but not B cells or macrophages during DSS-induced colitis. It has been reported that proliferating T cells are more sensitive to bortezomib-mediated cytotoxity than resting T cells [16,17]. Proteasome inhibitors induce endoplasmic reticulum stress-induced apoptosis in multiple myeloma cells as a result of the terminal unfolded protein response [23], while inhibition of proteasome activities by proteasome inhibitors induces apoptosis preferentially in rapid proliferating neoplastic cells [24]. Thus, bortezomib treatment is likely to eliminate only excessively proliferating immune cells, thereby suppressing harmful inflammatory responses.

Proteasome inhibition using bortezomib has recently emerged as an effective anticancer therapy [11]. Thus far, the therapeutic feasibility of protease inhibition in inflammatory and autoimmune diseases has been revealed only in murine models of human systemic lupus erythematosus [14], experimental autoimmune

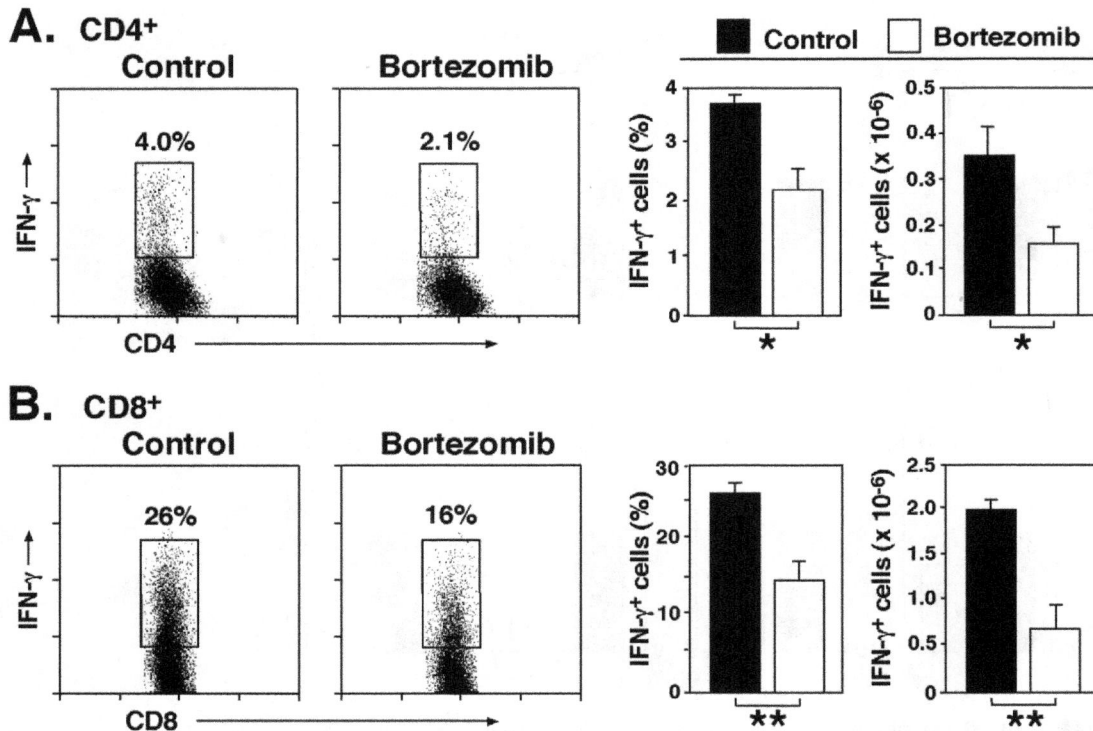

Figure 5. Bortezomib treatment reduces IFN-γ production by CD4+ and CD8+ T cells in mesenteric lymph nodes during DSS-induced colitis. IFN-γ production by mesenteric lymph node CD4+ (**A**) or CD8+ (**B**) T cells 7 days following DSS administration as determined by intracellular cytokine staining with flow cytometry analysis. Bar graphs indicate mean (± SEM) percentages and numbers of draining lymph node IFN-γ-producing CD4+ or CD8+ T cells following bortezomib or control treatment in one representative experiment with three mice per group. Significant differences between PBS-treated mice versus other group are indicated; *P<0.05, **P<0.01. Similar results were obtained in at least two independent experiments.

encephalomyelitis [25,26], rheumatoid arthritis [27], asthma [28], and contact dermatitis [13]. In the current study, bortezomib treatment in mice resulted in attenuated DSS-induced colitis, suggesting that bortezomib may also be effective for the treatment of human ulcerative colitis. Patients with this disease are generally treated with anti-inflammatory and immunosuppressive drugs, antibiotics, and biologics such as anti-tumor necrosis factor therapies and/or surgery. However, such therapies do not cure the disease and patients suffer a life-long illness. Further studies are needed to determine the precise mechanisms by which bortezomib treatment reduces the severity of DSS-induced colitis. Nonetheless, if the efficacy seen in mice translates to humans, the current results may provide new insights and therapeutic approaches for treating ulcerative colitis.

Materials and Methods

Ethics statement

All animal studies and procedures were approved by The Committee on Animal Experimentation of the University of Tokyo, Tokyo, Japan (Approval ID: P10-134).

Induction and evaluation of DSS-induced colitis

C57BL/6 mice were purchased from Clea Japan Inc. (Tokyo, Japan), bred in a pathogen-free barrier facility and used at 8–12 weeks of age. Three % (w/v) DSS (molecular mass, 36–50 kDa; Sigma, St. Louis, MO) was dissolved in purified water and administered to mice instead of normal drinking water for 7 days

[29]. The volume of water intake was measured daily to determine the amount of DSS consumed per mouse; this was comparable between treatment groups in all experiments. To analyze the therapeutic effect of bortezomib (LC Laboratories, Woburn, MA), 0.75 mg/kg was injected in 200 µl PBS through lateral tail veins twice weekly, starting 2 days before the administration of DSS. Control animals received an identical volume of PBS alone.

Clinical DAI scoring for DSS-induced colitis was based on weight loss, stool consistency, and bleeding as described previously [30]. The DAI was scored on a scale from 0–4 for each clinical parameter and then averaged for each group. Weight changes were based on the starting weight of each mouse at the initiation of DSS treatment. Weight-loss scores were determined as follows: 0, no weight loss; 1, 1–5% weight loss; 2, 6–10% weight loss; 3, 11–15% weight loss; and 4, >15% weight loss. Stool samples were collected from each mouse at all timepoints and stool scores were determined as follows: 0, normal stools; 2, loose stools; and 4, diarrhea. Fecal blood testing kits (Shionogi, Osaka, Japan) were used to check the stools for the presence of blood. Bleeding scores were determined as: 0, no bleeding; 1, guiaiac occult blood test (minimal color change to green); 2, guiaiac occult blood test (maximal color change to blue); 3, blood visibly present in the stool and no clotting on the anus; and 4, gross bleeding from the anus with clotting present.

Histologic analysis

Mice were sacrificed 5 days after the induction of intestinal injury. Colon samples were removed and segments fixed in 10%

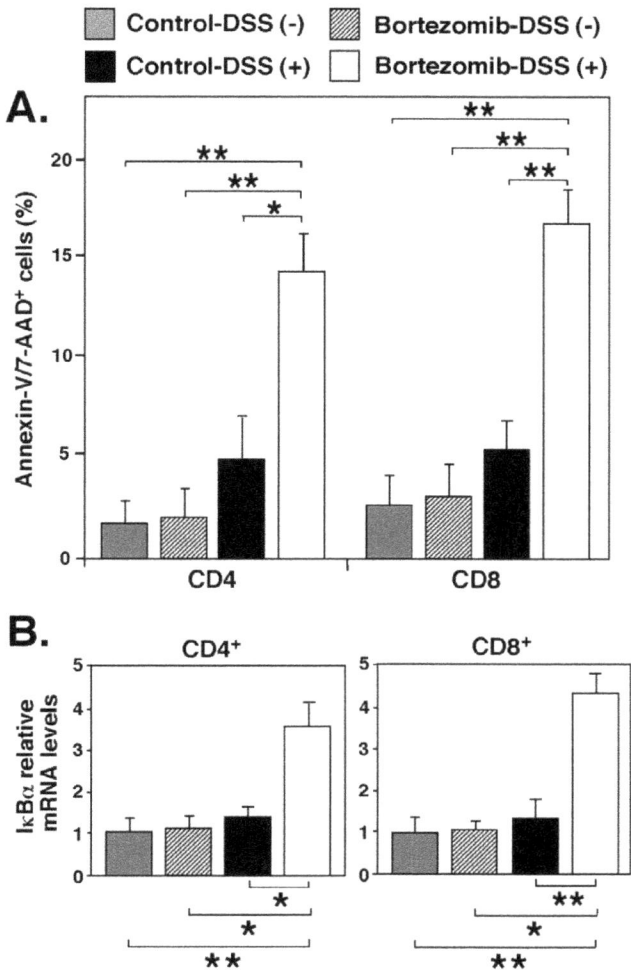

Figure 6. Bortezomib treatment enhances T cell apoptosis by inhibiting NF-κB activation. (A) The percentages of Annexin-V/7-AAD$^+$ CD4$^+$ and CD8$^+$ T cells in mesenteric lymph nodes 7 days after the administration of DSS. Bar graphs indicate mean (± SEM) percentages of mesenteric lymph node Annexin-V/7-AAD$^+$ CD4$^+$ and CD8$^+$ T cells following bortezomib or control treatment in one representative experiment with 4 mice per group. **(B)** IκBα mRNA expression in mesenteric lymph nodes CD4$^+$ and CD8$^+$ T cells. Transcript levels were quantified by real-time PCR analysis and were normalized with an internal control. Values represent means (± SEM) from ≥4 mice of each group. A, B) Significant differences between sample means are indicated; *P<0.05; **P<0.01. Similar results were obtained in at least two independent experiments.

buffered formalin. After paraffin embedding, 5-μm-thick sections were cut and stained with hematoxylin and eosin. Histologic scoring was based on a previously described method [29]. Briefly, hematoxylin and eosin-stained cross-sections of the descending colon tissue were scored microscopically in a blinded fashion on a scale from 0–4 based on the following histologic criteria: 0, no change from normal tissue; 1, low level of inflammation with scattered infiltrating mononuclear cells (1–2 foci); 2, moderate inflammation with multiple foci; 3, high level of inflammation with increased vascular density and marked wall thickening; 4, maximal severity of inflammation with transmural leukocyte infiltration and loss of goblet cells. An average of four fields of view per colon were evaluated for each mouse. These scores were averaged for each group and recorded as the histopathology score.

For immunohistochemistry, frozen tissue sections of the colon samples were acetone-fixed and incubated with 10% normal rabbit serum in PBS for 10 minutes at 37°C to block non-specific staining. Sections were then incubated with rat mAbs specific for mouse CD4, CD8, B220 (BD PharMingen; San Diego, CA), and macrophages (F4/80; American Type Culture Collection; Rockville, MD). Rat IgG (Southern Biotechnology Associates Inc., Birmingham, AL) was used as a control for non-specific staining. Sections were then incubated sequentially for 20 minutes at 37°C with a biotinylated rabbit anti-rat IgG and then horseradish peroxidase-conjugated avidin–biotin complex (Vectastain ABC kit; Vector Laboratories, Burlingame, CA). Sections were developed with 3,3'-diaminobenzidine tetrahydrochloride and hydrogen peroxide and counterstained with methyl green. Stained cells were counted in 10 random grids under high-magnification (×400) power fields of a light microscope. Each section was examined independently by two investigators in a blinded manner.

Cell isolation

Single-cell suspensions of spleen and mesenteric lymph nodes were generated by gentle dissection. Magnetic cell sorting technology (Miltenyi Biotech, Auburn, CA) was used to purify CD4$^+$ and CD8$^+$ T cell lymphocyte populations.

Antibodies and immunofluorescence analysis

Anti-mouse mAbs B220 (RA3-6B2), CD4 (H129.19), CD8 (53-6.7), and CD19 (1D3) were from BD PharMingen. Intracellular staining used mAbs reactive with IFN-γ (XMG1.2), IL-17A (eBio17B7), and IL-4 (BVD6-24G2), and the Cytofix/Cytoperm kit (BD Biosciences, San Diego, CA). Single cell suspensions of draining lymph nodes (paired axillary ad inguinal) were generated by gentle dissection. Viable cells were counted using a hemocytometer, with relative lymphocyte percentages determined by flow cytometry analysis. Single-cell leukocyte suspensions were stained on ice using predetermined optimal concentrations of each antibody for 20–60 minutes, and fixed as described [31]. For intracellular cytokine staining, lymphocytes were stimulated in vitro with phorbol 12-myristate 13-acetate (50 ng/ml; Sigma-Aldrich), ionomycin 1 μg/ml; Sigma-Aldrich) in the presence of monensin (1 μM; eBioscience) for 5 hours before staining. In certain experiments, apoptosis was measured by flow-cytometric staining for Annexin-V and 7-AAD (BD PharMingen). Cells with lymphocyte light scatter properties were analyzed by 2–4 color immunofluorescence staining and FACSCalibur flow cytometers (Becton Dickinson, San Jose, CA). Background staining was determined using unreactive isotype-matched control mAbs (Caltag Laboratories, San Francisco, CA) with gates positioned to exclude ≥98% of unreactive cells.

RNA isolation and real-time reverse transcription-PCR

Total RNA was isolated from colon specimens and mesenteric lymph node suspensions with RNeasy spin columns (Qiagen, Crawley, UK). Total RNA from each sample was reverse-transcribed into cDNA. Expression of IL-4, IL-6, IL-10, IL-17, IFN-γ and IκBα was analyzed using a real-time PCR quantification method according to the manufacturer's instructions (Applied Biosystems, Foster City, CA). Sequence-specific primers and probes were designed by Pre-Developed TaqMan assay reagents or Assay-On-Demand (Applied Biosystems). Real-time PCR (40 cycles of denaturing at 92°C for 15 seconds and annealing at 60°C for 60 seconds) was performed on an ABI Prism 7000 sequence detector (Applied Biosystems). Glyceraldehyde-3-phosphate was used to normalize mRNA. Relative expression of real-time PCR products was determined by using ΔΔCT methods [32] to compare target gene and housekeeping gene mRNA expression. One of the control samples was chosen as a calibrator sample.

Statistical analysis

All data are expressed as mean ± SEM. The Mann–Whitney U test was used to determine the level of significance of differences in sample means, and the Bonferroni test was used for multiple comparisons.

References

1. Fiocchi C (1998) Inflammatory bowel disease: etiology and pathogenesis. Gastroenterology 115: 182–205.
2. Hibi T, Ogata H (2006) Novel pathophysiological concepts of inflammatory bowel disease. J Gastroenterol 41: 10–16.
3. Sands BE (2007) Inflammatory bowel disease: past, present, and future. J Gastroenterol 42: 16–25.
4. Okayasu I, Hatakeyama S, Yamada M, Ohkusa T, Inagaki Y, et al. (1990) A novel method in the induction of reliable experimental acute and chronic ulcerative colitis in mice. Gastroenterology 98: 694–702.
5. Cooper HS, Murthy SN, Shah RS, Sedergran DJ (1993) Clinicopathologic study of dextran sulfate sodium experimental murine colitis. Lab Invest 69: 238–249.
6. Melgar S, Karlsson A, Michaelsson E (2005) Acute colitis induced by dextran sulfate sodium progresses to chronicity in C57BL/6 but not in BALB/c mice: correlation between symptoms and inflammation. Am J Physiol Gastrointest Liver Physiol 288: G1328–1338.
7. Egger B, Bajaj-Elliott M, MacDonald TT, Inglin R, Eysselein VE, et al. (2000) Characterisation of acute murine dextran sodium sulphate colitis: cytokine profile and dose dependency. Digestion 62: 240–248.
8. King RW, Deshaies RJ, Peters JM, Kirschner MW (1996) How proteolysis drives the cell cycle. Science 274: 1652–1659.
9. Ciechanover A, Schwartz AL (1998) The ubiquitin-proteasome pathway: the complexity and myriad functions of proteins death. Proc Natl Acad Sci USA 95: 2727–2730.
10. Baumeister W, Walz J, Zuhl F, Seemuller E (1998) The proteasome: paradigm of a self-compartmentalizing protease. Cell 92: 367–380.
11. Adams J (2004) The proteasome: a suitable antineoplastic target. Nat Rev Cancer 4: 349–360.
12. Richardson PG, Hideshima T, Anderson KC (2003) Bortezomib (PS-341): a novel, first-in-class proteasome inhibitor for the treatment of multiple myeloma and other cancers. Cancer Control 10: 361–369.
13. Yanaba K, Yoshizaki A, Muroi E, Hara T, Ogawa F, et al. (2010) The proteasome inhibitor bortezomib inhibits T cell-dependent inflammatory responses. J Leukoc Biol 88: 117–122.
14. Neubert K, Meister S, Moser K, Weisel F, Maseda D, et al. (2008) The proteasome inhibitor bortezomib depletes plasma cells and protects mice with lupus-like disease from nephritis. Nat Med 14: 748–755.
15. Luo H, Wu Y, Qi S, Wan X, Chen H, et al. (2001) A proteasome inhibitor effectively prevents mouse heart allograft rejection. Transplantation 72: 196–202.
16. Sun K, Welniak LA, Panoskaltsis-Mortari A, O'Shaughnessy MJ, Liu H, et al. (2004) Inhibition of acute graft-versus-host disease with retention of graft-versus-tumor effects by the proteasome inhibitor bortezomib. Proc Natl Acad Sci USA 101: 8120–8125.
17. Blanco B, Perez-Simon JA, Sanchez-Abarca LI, Carvajal-Vergara X, Mateos J, et al. (2006) Bortezomib induces selective depletion of alloreactive T lymphocytes and decreases the production of Th1 cytokines. Blood 107: 3575–3583.
18. Naujokat C, Daniel V, Bauer TM, Sadeghi M, Opelz G (2003) Cell cycle- and activation-dependent regulation of cyclosporin A-induced T cell apoptosis. Biochem Biophys Res Commun 310: 347–354.
19. Coux O, Tanaka K, Goldberg AL (1996) Structure and functions of the 20S and 26S proteasomes. Annu Rev Biochem 65: 801–847.
20. Schmidt N, Gonzalez E, Visekruna A, Kuhl AA, Loddenkemper C, et al. (2010) Targeting the proteasome: partial inhibition of the proteasome by bortezomib or deletion of the immunosubunit LMP7 attenuates experimental colitis. Gut 59: 896–906.
21. Visekruna A, Joeris T, Schmidt N, Lawrenz M, Ritz JP, et al. (2009) Comparative expression analysis and characterization of 20S proteasomes in human intestinal tissues: The proteasome pattern as diagnostic tool for IBD patients. Inflamm Bowel Dis 15: 526–533.
22. Visekruna A, Joeris T, Seidel D, Kroesen A, Loddenkemper C, et al. (2006) Proteasome-mediated degradation of IκBα and processing of p105 in Crohn disease and ulcerative colitis. J Clin Invest 116: 3195–3203.
23. Obeng EA, Carlson LM, Gutman DM, Harrington WJ, Jr., Lee KP, et al. (2006) Proteasome inhibitors induce a terminal unfolded protein response in multiple myeloma cells. Blood 107: 4907–4916.
24. Naujokat C, Hoffmann S (2002) Role and function of the 26S proteasome in proliferation and apoptosis. Lab Invest 82: 965–980.
25. Fissolo N, Kraus M, Reich M, Ayturan M, Overkleeft H, et al. (2008) Dual inhibition of proteasomal and lysosomal proteolysis ameliorates autoimmune central nervous system inflammation. Eur J Immunol 38: 2401–2411.
26. Vanderlugt CL, Rahbe SM, Elliott PJ, Dal Canto MC, Miller SD (2000) Treatment of established relapsing experimental autoimmune encephalomyelitis with the proteasome inhibitor PS-519. J Autoimmun 14: 205–211.
27. Palombella VJ, Conner EM, Fuseler JW, Destree A, Davis JM, et al. (1998) Role of the proteasome and NF-κB in streptococcal cell wall-induced polyarthritis. Proc Natl Acad Sci USA 95: 15671–15676.
28. Elliott PJ, Pien CS, McCormack TA, Chapman ID, Adams J (1999) Proteasome inhibition: A novel mechanism to combat asthma. J Allergy Clin Immunol 104: 294–300.
29. Wirtz S, Neufert C, Weigmann B, Neurath MF (2007) Chemically induced mouse models of intestinal inflammation. Nat Protoc 2: 541–546.
30. Murthy SN, Cooper HS, Shim H, Shah RS, Ibrahim SA, et al. (1993) Treatment of dextran sulfate sodium-induced murine colitis by intracolonic cyclosporin. Dig Dis Sci 38: 1722–1734.
31. Sato K, Ono N, Steeber DA, Pisetsky DS, Tedder TF (1996) CD19 regulates B lymphocyte signaling thresholds critical for the development of B-1 lineage cells and autoimmunity. J Immunol 157: 4371–4378.
32. Meijerink J, Mandigers C, van de Locht L, Tonnissen E, Goodsaid F, et al. (2001) A novel method to compensate for different amplification efficiencies between patient DNA samples in quantitative real-time PCR. J Mol Diag 3: 55–61.

Author Contributions

Conceived and designed the experiments: KY. Performed the experiments: KY. Analyzed the data: KY. Contributed reagents/materials/analysis tools: KY YA YT MS TK SS. Wrote the paper: KY.

8

Iridoid Glycosides Fraction of *Folium syringae* Leaves Modulates NF-*κ*B Signal Pathway and Intestinal Epithelial Cells Apoptosis in Experimental Colitis

Xin Liu[1]*, Jian Ming Wang[2]

1 College of Pharmaceutical Sciences, Zhejiang University, Hangzhou, China, **2** Academy of Traditional Chinese Medicine, Heilongjiang University of Chinese Medicine, Harbin, China

Abstract

Background and Aims: Iridoid glycosides (IG), the major active fraction of *F. syringae* leaves has been demonstrated to have strong anti-inflammatory properties to ulcerative colitis (UC) in our previous study. The aim of this study was to investigate whether IG modulates the inflammatory response in experimental colitis at the level of NF-*κ*B signal pathway and epithelial cell apoptosis.

Methods: UC in rats was induced by administration with dextran sulfate sodium (DSS) in drinking water. The inflammatory damage was assessed by disease activity index (DAI), macroscopic findings, histology and myeloperoxidase (MPO) activity. The effect of IG on pro-inflammatory cytokines TNF-α, IL-8, COX-2 and regulatory peptide TGF-β1 was measured. Epithelial cell apoptosis and the protein and mRNA expressions of Fas/FasL, Bcl-2/Bax, caspase-3, NF-*κ*B p65, I*κ*Bα, p-I*κ*Bα and IKKβ were detected by TUNEL method, immunohistochemistry, Western blotting and real-time quantitative PCR, respectively.

Results: IG significantly ameliorated macroscopic damage and histological changes, reduced the activity of MPO, and strongly inhibited epithelial cell apoptosis. Moreover, IG markedly depressed TNF-α, IL-8, COX-2 and TGF-β1 levels in the colon tissues in a dose-dependent manner. Furthermore, IG significantly blocked of NF-*κ*B signaling by inhibiting I*κ*Bα phosphorylation/degradation and IKKβ activity, down-regulated the protein and mRNA expressions of Fas/FasL, Bax and caspase-3, and activated Bcl-2 in intestinal epithelial cells.

Conclusions: These results demonstrated for the first time that IG possessed marked protective effects on experimental colitis through inhibition of epithelial cell apoptosis and blockade of NF-*κ*B signal pathway.

Editor: Stefan Bereswill, Charité-University Medicine Berlin, Germany

Funding: This work was supported by a grant from the Specialized Research Foundation for the Doctoral Program of Ministry of Education of China (SRFDP) (No. 20060228005). The funder had no role in study design, data collection and analysis, decision to publish, or preparation of the manuscript.

Competing Interests: The authors have declared that there are no conflicts of interest.

* E-mail: xinliu98@126.com

Introduction

Ulcerative colitis (UC), the major forms of inflammatory bowel disease (IBD), is an immunologically mediated chronic intestinal disorder. The disease commonly follows a chronic relapsing course with clinically quiescent periods followed by bouts of severe intestinal inflammation, which are characterized by abdominal pain, diarrhea, rectal bleeding and weight loss [1]. Furthermore, prolonged and chronic UC may progress to colorectal cancer [2]. Despite substantial progress has been made in the treatment of UC along the immune and inflammatory pathways, no definitive therapies with a nonrelapsing cure rate are available for this disorder until now, and limiting drug-induced toxicity is a continuous challenge [3,4]. Traditional therapeutic modalities are used for UC including anti-inflammatory therapy (5-aminosalicylic acid and corticosteroids), some immunomodulators (azathioprine, 6-mercaptopurine and cyclosporine) [5]. However, these drugs have demonstrated unsatisfactory results and the recrudescence rates of IBD are rather high. Therefore, it is challenging to develop new and specific therapies for the treatment of IBD.

Although the exact etiology and pathogenesis of IBD are not fully defined up to now, a growing body of work suggests that inflammatory response and intestinal epithelial cell (IEC) apoptosis mainly participate in the pathogenesis of IBD [1,6]. The abnormal mucosal immune and inflammation responses in IBD are predominantly characterized by increased synthesis of pro-inflammatory cytokines, the activation of neutrophils, and enhanced formation of reactive oxygen and nitrogen species. These mediators can activate the nuclear factor kappa B (NF-κB) pathway, modulating a number of different steps in the inflammatory cascade [7,8]. These include production of pro-inflammatory cytokines such as tumour necrosis factor alpha (TNF-α), interleukin-1β (IL-1β), interferon-γ (INF-γ), IL-6, IL-8, and IL-12 in different cell-types, degranulation of neutrophils, as well as the expression of important inflammatory proteins such as cyclooxygenase-2 (COX-2) and inducible nitric oxide synthase (iNOS) [9–11]. Therefore, imbalance between pro-inflammatory and anti-inflammatory cytokines and inflammatory proteins expression, plays an important role in the modulation of intestinal immune system and contributes to the inflammatory cascade in the pathological process of colitis [12]. On the other hand, the pathogenesis of UC involved in the abnormality of apoptosis. Growing evidence indicated that the nuber of apoptotic epithelial cells is increased during active UC, which may lead to an alteration of the epithelial barrier function resulting in pathogenic microorganism infiltration [6,13]. It has been reported that different mechanisms are involved in the induction of apoptosis. One pathway is mediated by the interaction between cell surface death receptor Fas and its specific ligand FasL. Such an interaction leads to the formation of the death-inducing signalling complex and activation of caspase-8 and caspase-10, two initiator caspases that in turn activate downstream effector caspase-3 [14]. Another is mediated by proapoptotic signals at the mitochondria level including members of Bcl-2 family and caspase-9 [15]. Transforming growth factor-β1 (TGF-β1) counteracts TNF-α and regulates cFLIP protein acting as a negative regulator of caspase-8 and thereby inhibits Fas-mediated apoptosis in mucosal inflammation that is essential for wound healing and tissue repair [16,17]. Importantly, TGF-β is known to be one of the most potent cytokines in the regulation of mediators (TGF-α, EGF, IL-1, IL-2, IFN-γ) and plays an important role in the prevention of intestinal epithelial destruction [18,19]. TGF-β1 expression is increased parallel to the increase of pro-inflammatory cytokine secretion in patients with UC and Crohn's disease (CD) [20]. NF-κB mediates the IL-1β induction of TGF-β1 gene expression and NF-κB RelA antisense oligonucleotides suppress TGF-β1 mRNA expression [21]. There are also studies implying that successful treatment of UC-related mucosal injury results in decrease of TGF-β1 level in plasma and intestinal mucosa [22]. In this regard, the regulation of inflammatory response and IEC apoptosis may be a promising therapeutic modality for UC.

NF-κB signal pathway plays a pivotal role in regulating the production of pro-inflammatory cytokines and apoptosis of IEC in UC, which contribute to cytokine-mediated mucosal tissue damage, leading to a breakdown in the mucosal barrier [23,24]. Increased NF-κB activation has been detected in the mucosa of patients with IBD and in a murine colitis model, and inhibition of NF-κB with a specific p65 antisense oligonucleotide is effective in preventing experimental models of IBD and efficiently down-regulates cytokine production by intestinal macrophages from Crohn's disease (CD) patients [25,26]. NF-κB can be activated by diverse stimuli (e.g., pro-inflammatory cytokines, microbes and microbial products, and oxidative stress) that signal its activation through the catalytic IκB kinase β (IKKβ) [23,27]. IKKβ phosphorylates NF-κB-bound IκBs in the cytoplasm and targets their degradation, thereby leading to subsequent release of NF-κB dimmers, which then translocate from the cytoplasm to the nucleus and activate the transcription of multiple κB-dependent target genes [28], including pro-inflammatory cytokines (TNF-α, IL-1α, IL-6, IL-8, IL-12, MCP-1, interferon-γ), death and survival proteins (Bcl-2, Bcl-xl, Bcl-xs, Bax, p53, Myc, Fas), intercellular adhesion molecules (ICAM), COX-2 and iNOS [29,30]. Growing evidence reveals that the inhibition of NF-κB activity by either directed blockade of RelA (p65) or suppression of IκBα degradation or IKKβ activity may lead to alleviating the severity of intestinal inflammation [26,31]. Therefore, the modulation of NF-κB signaling pathway could be the main target for the treatment of IBD.

Folium syringae leaves have been used in herbal medicines to treat inflammatory intestinal disease such as acute enteritis and bacillary dysentery in China for a long time. Iridoid glycosides (IG) is the main active fraction extracted from *F. syringae* leaves, with high content of syringopicroside [32]. Although our previous studies indicate that IG exert conspicuous anti-inflammatory effects on UC *in vivo* by scavenging reactive oxygen species (ROS) and inhibiting relative pro-inflammatory cytokines [33]. The molecular mechanisms of IG involved in protection against UC are still not entirely clear. In the present study, we further explored whether its mechanism was associated with modulating NF-κB signaling pathway and IEC apoptosis. The protective effects of IG on dextran sulfate sodium (DSS)-induced colitis were assessed by macroscopic score and histological analysis as well as by determination of inflammation markers such as MPO activity and the mRNA expressions of pro-inflammatory cytokines such as TNF-α and IL-8. The activity of COX-2 and TGF-β1 were also evaluated. In order to elucidate the probable mechanisms of IG in ameliorating inflammatory injury in experimental colitis, the anti-inflammatory effects of IG on activation change of NF-κB signaling pathway and the relative expressions of serial genes involved in IEC apoptosis were evaluated by immunohistochemistry, western blotting and real-time quantitative PCR, respectively.

Materials and Methods

Animals and reagents

Male Sprague-Dawley rats weighing 200–220 g, were supplied by Slaccas Laboratory Animal Co. Ltd. (Shanghai, China). The rats were maintained in standard cages in a controlled room (temperature 24–25°C, humidity 70–75%, lighting regiment of 12L/12D) and fed with standard rodent diet. All animal experiments were approved under animal protocol number SCXK (Zhe) 2008-0033 by Zhejiang Medical Laboratory Animal Administration Committee. Experimental animals were treated according to Guideline of Laboratory Animal Care from Chinese Ministry of Science and Technology in 2006 (Available from: http://www.most.gov.cn/fggw/zfwj/zfwj2006/200609/t20060930_54389. htm).

F. syringae leaves were collected in Heilongjiang Province, China, in September 2008. Voucher specimens (No. 20080916) of this material was identified by Professor Jianming Wang, and deposited at Heilongjiang University of Chinese Medicine. The iridoid glycosides fraction was purified using D-141 macroporous adsorption resin column from *F. syringae* leaves based on previously described procedures [32]. The content of syringopicroside in the iridoid glycosides fraction reached 55.74%.

No specific permits were required for the described field studies. The field studies did not involve endangered or protected species.

Salicylazosulfapyridine (SASP) was purchased from Sine Pharmaceutical Co. Ltd. (Shanghai, China). DSS was provided by MP Biomedicals (M.W. = 36–50 kDa, USA). Apoptosis detection kit was supplied by Boster Bio-engineering limited company (Wuhan, China). Bax kit was purchased from Santa Cruz Biotechnologies (USA). The primers for real-time quantitative RT-PCR were synthesized from GeneCore Biotechnologies Co. Ltd. (Shanghai, China).

Induction of colitis and experimental design

Rats (n = 60) were adapted for 1 week and randomly assigned to 6 groups (n = 10). Drinking water containing 4% dextran sulfate sodium (DSS) was provided for 1 week to induce colitis [34]. Following 7 days of DSS administration, IG (80, 160 and 240 mg/kg) were suspended in 0.9% saline solution and administered twice daily by oral gavage for 14 days, respectively. Positive control group received SASP in a dose of 150 mg/kg twice daily. Normal and model groups received the vehicle in a comparable volume (10 ml/kg body weight), respectively.

Macroscopic assessment and histological study of colon damage

The rats were checked daily for body weight, behavior, stool consistency and the presence of gross blood in stool. At the end of the experimental period, rats were sacrificed using an overdose of anesthetic. The entire colon was excised from the cecum to the anus and opened longitudinally. Colon length as an indirect marker of inflammation was measured. Macroscopic damage was assessed using a validated scoring system with slight modifications [35,36]. The numerical rating score were as follows: 0, no inflammation; 1, local hyperemia without ulcers, and/or stool consistency; 2, ulceration without hyperemia; 3, ulceration and adhesions at one site; 4, two or more sites of inflammation and ulceration extending >1 cm; and 5, ulceration extending more than 2 cm.

Colonic tissues were fixed in 4% buffered paraformaldehyde, then dehydrated through graded concentrations of ethanol, subsequently embedded in paraffin, and finally sectioned in 4 μm thick sections. After dewaxing and rehydration, the sections were stained with hematoxylin-eosin (H&E) according to standard procedures for histological evaluation. The colonic pieces were collected from inflamed portions after samples were taken for histological examination and frozen in liquid nitrogen to quantify biochemical parameters.

Determination of myeloperoxidase (MPO) activity

Myeloperoxidase (MPO) activity was determined with the O-dianisidine method [37], using a MPO detection kit (Nanjing Jiancheng Bioengineering Institute). Colon tissues were washed in ice-cold physiological saline to remove fecal residues and weighed on analytical scale, then homogenized three times in 9 volumes of ice-cold physiological saline. The MPO activity was measured with a spectrophotometer (756pc Shanghai Spectrum Instrument Co. Ltd., China) by absorbance at 460 nm. MPO activity was defined as the quantity of enzyme degrading 1 μmol of peroxide per minute at 37°C and was expressed in units per gram weight of wet tissue.

Immunohistochemical analysis

Colon tissues were fixed in 4% buffered paraformaldehyde and 4 μm sections were prepared from paraffin-embedded tissues. After deparaffinization in xylene and rehydration in a series of graded alcohol, endogenous peroxidase was quenched with 3.0% hydrogen peroxide in methanol for 30 min. For the heat rehabilitation of antigen, slides were immersed in 10 mmol/L citrate buffer (pH 6.0) and performed by microwave for 10 minutes, then cooled for 20 minutes. Slides were incubated with polyclonal primary antibody of Bax (diluted to 1:100) overnight at 4°C. The sections were washed three times with phosphate-buffered saline (PBS) and incubated with polyclonal rabbit anti-mouse biotinylated secondary antibody (Dako, CA, USA) at room temperature for 30 min. After washing with PBS, the sections were incubated with 3, 3′-diaminobenzidine solution (Sigma, St Louis, MO, USA) until a brown reaction product could be visualized. Sections were washed with PBS and stained with haematoxylin. Then the sections were dehydrated with increasing concentration of ethanol, mounted with neutral gum, and observed under an Olympus BH-2 microscope.

Analysis of intestinal epithelial cell apoptosis

Apoptotic epithelial cells in colonic tissue were analyzed using the terminal deoxynucleotidyl transferase (TdT)-mediated dUTP-biotin nick end labeling (TUNEL) assay according to the manufacturer's instruction. TUNEL-positive nuclei were clearly identified as brown-stained nuclei, which indicated the presence of DNA fragmentation due to apoptosis. TUNEL-positive cells were determined by observing 1000 cells in randomly selected fields.

Western blot analysis

Colon tissues were pounded to pieces in liquid nitrogen, then disrupted by homogenization on ice in hypotonic lysis buffer containing: 20 mmol/L N-2-Hydroxyethylpiperazine-N′-2′-ethanesulfonic Acid (HEPES) pH 7.8, 1.5 mmol/L $MgCl_2$, 420 mmol/L NaCl, 1 mmol/L ethylenediamine tetraacetic acid (EDTA), 1 mmol/L ethylene glycol bis (2-aminoethyl ether)-N,N,N′N′-tetraacetic acid (EGTA), 1 mmol/L dithiothreitol (DTT), 0.5 mmol/L phenylmethyl sulfonylfluoride (PMSF), 15 μg/ml trypsin inhibitor, 3 μg/ml pepstatin, 2 μg/ml leupeptin, 40 μmol/L benzidamin, 1% Nonidet P-40 and 20% glycerol. Homogenates were centrifuged at 4°C (12,000 g, 15 min). The supernatants were collected as nuclear extracts in aliquots and stored at −80°C for western blotting analysis. Protein concentrations were determined by Bradford assay.

Equal amounts of protein (40 μg/lane) were separated on 10% sodium dodecylsulfate-polyacrylamide gel electrophoresis (SDS-PAGE) and transferred to a nitrocellulose membrane. Membranes were blocked in 5% skim milk dissolved in 10 mmol/L Tris-HCl, pH 7.5, 100 mmol/L NaCl and 0.1% Tween-20, and incubated with anti-NF-κBp65, anti-IκBα, anti-IKKβ, anti-β-actin (Santa Cruz Biotechnology) and anti-phosphserine IκBα polyclonal antibodies (Cell signaling, Beverly, USA) at dilution of 1:500, 1:500, 1:500, 1:1000 and 1:500, respectively. The membranes were washed three times for 15 min with Tween-20/Tris-buffered saline (TTBS) and incubated with horseradish peroxidase-conjugated secondary antibodies (diluted to 1:2000, Santa Cruz Biotechnology). Blots were again washed with TTBS, and then developed by enhanced chemiluminescence detection regents (ECL, Amersham). The protein bands were quantified by the average ratios of integral optic density (IOD) following normalization to the housekeeping gene.

Real-time quantitative RT-PCR

Total RNA was isolated from colonic tissue using Trizol reagent (Invitrogen, Carlsbad, CA, USA). For each sample, 1 μg of RNA was reverse-transcribed (RT) using AMV reverse transcriptase (Promega), 1 mmol/L deoxyribonucleotide triphosphate (dNTP) (GibcoBRL), and oligo (dT_{12-18}) 0.5 μg/μl (GibcoBRL). ABI TaqMan 2×PCR Master mix of primers (Applied Biosystems, Foster City, CA, USA) and TaqMan MGB probes (FAM dye-labeled) were used for the target genes and pre-developed 18S rRNA (VIC-dye-labeled probe). Real-time RT-PCR was performed using an ABI Prism 9700 sequence detection system (Applied Biosystems, Foster City, CA) with specific primers for rat NF-κBp65, IκBα, IKKβ, TNF-α, IL-8, TGF-β1, COX-2, Fas, FasL, Bcl-2, Caspase-3. β-actin was used as a housekeeping gene. All primers were designed by Primer Premier 5.0 software (Molecular Biology Insights, USA). The primer sequences used in PCR amplification are shown in Table 1. Thermal cycler parameters were as follows: one cycle of 50°C for 2 min, 95°C for 10 min, and 40 cycles of denaturation (95°C, 30 s) and combined annealing/extension (60°C, 30 s). Duplicate cycle threshold (CT) values were analyzed in Microsoft Excel using the comparative CT $(\Delta\Delta C_T)$ method as described by the manufacturer. The amount of target $(2^{-\Delta\Delta CT})$ was obtained by normalizing it to an endogenous reference (18S rRNA) and relative to a calibration curve.

Table 1. Sequences of the amplification primers used in the real-time RT-PCR.

mRNA Species		Oligonucleotides (5'→3')
NF-κBp65	forward	ACCTGGAGCAAGCCATTAGC
	reverse	CGGACCGCATTCAAGTCATA
IκBα	forward	TGGAGCCGACCTCAATAAACC
	reverse	TGCGACTGTGAACCACGATG
IKKβ	forward	AGCTCTGGAACCTCCTGAAGA
	reverse	AGCTCCAGTCTAGGGTCGTGA
TNF-α	forward	GCCAATGGCATGGATCTCAAAG
	reverse	CAGAGCAATGACTCCAAAGT
IL-8	forward	CTCCAGCCACACTCCAACAGA
	reverse	CACCCTAACACAAAACACGAT
TGF-β1	forward	CGCAACAACGCAATCTATG
	reverse	CCCTGTATTCCGTCTCCTT
COX-2	forward	ACTACGCCGAGATTCCTGACA
	reverse	ACTGATGAGTGAAGTGCTGGG
Fas	forward	AACTTCTATTGCAATGCTTCTCTCTGT
	reverse	CAAGGCTCAAGGATGTCTTCAA
FasL	forward	CACCAACCACAGCCTTAGAGTATCA
	reverse	ACTCCAGAGATCAAAGCAGTTCCA
Bcl-2	forward	TCAAACAGAGGTCGCATGCT
	reverse	CATCTGCACACCTGGATCCA
Caspase-3	forward	GAGGCCGACTTCCTGTATGC
	reverse	TGACCCGTCCCTTGAATTTC
β-actin	forward	TGGAATCCTGTGGCATCCATGAAAC
	reverse	TAAAACGCAGCTCAGTAACAGTCCG

Statistical analysis

The results were expressed as the mean ± SD. SPSS 16.0 statistical software was used for the analysis. Differences between groups were compared using one way analysis of variance and two-tailed Student's t test. $P<0.05$ was considered significant.

Results

Iridoid glycosides ameliorate DSS-induced colitis

The therapeutic efficacy of IG on experimental colitis was assessed by body weight change, colon length, disease activity index (DAI), histological analysis and MPO activity. Severe drug-induced colitis was observed from the 4th day after DSS administration, which was characterized by obvious hyperemia, edema, stool consistency and ulceration (Fig. 1C). The animals of normal group averagely increased (13.89±2.01)% in the body weight, whereas a dramatic body weight loss and shortened colon length accompanied with obvious diarrhea in DSS group was observed as a result of the colitis, and was maintained during the experimental period (Fig. 1A and B). Administration of SASP effectively suppressed body weight loss and colon shortening. However, treatment of IG (80–240 mg/kg) could significantly reverse the changes of two parameters induced by DSS in a dose-dependent manner. Histological studies showed that inflamed tissue had marked necrosis of colonic mucosa, hyperemia and adhesions to adjacent bowel wall. Additionally, MPO activity was significantly increased after DSS administration compared with

normal group. Administration with SASP could improve the acute inflammatory response. Nevertheless, treatment with IG dose-dependently inhibited these pathological symptoms and MPO activity with lower DAI (Fig. 1C, D, E and F). In particular, IG (240 mg/kg) had a better therapeutic effect than SASP. This result strongly suggested that the inhibition of neutrophil infiltration was a mechanism for the protective effects of IG in experimental colitis.

Effect of iridoid glycosides on key inflammatory cytokine expression

In order to test whether treatment with IG may modulate the inflammatory process through the regulation of the expressions of key NF-κB-dependent cytokines, the mRNA levels of TNF-α, IL-8, TGF-β1 and COX-2 in colonic tissue were examined by real-time quantitative RT-PCR. As shown in Fig. 2, the mRNA levels of TNF-α, IL-8, TGF-β1 and COX-2 in DSS model group showed a significantly high expression compared with normal control group ($P<0.01$). In contrast, administration of SASP obviously decreased the expressions of TNF-α, IL-8, TGF-β1 and COX-2 mRNA. Especially, IG treatment inhibited the expressions of the four inflammatory genes in a dose-dependent manner to some degree (Fig. 2 A, B, C and D). Maximum inhibition effect was observed with IG at a dose of 240 mg/kg.

Effect of iridoid glycosides on IEC apoptosis

To study whether experimental colitis is associated with IEC apoptosis and the effect of IG on IEC apoptosis, we measured TUNEL staining in colonic tissues. As shown in Fig. 3B, few apoptotic cells were observed in normal group, whereas colon tissues demonstrated a marked appearance of dark brown apoptotic cells and intercellular apoptotic fragments after treatment with DSS ($P<0.01$, Fig. 3C). In contrast, administration of SASP obviously decreased the number of apoptotic epithelial cells and apoptotic fragments (Fig. 3D). Treatment with IG remarkably reduced the percentages of TUNEL-positive cells in a dose-dependent manner ($P<0.01$, Fig. 3E, F and G). In particular, IG in a dose of 240 mg/kg was the most effective in suppressing IEC apoptosis.

Effect of iridoid glycosides on the expressions of serial genes involved in IEC apoptosis

As it could be informed from Fig. 4A, the mRNA levels of Fas and FasL in normal group were very low. Both of their expression levels in the colonic epithelia of DSS-induced model group were significantly higher than those of normal group ($p<0.01$). In contrast, administration of SASP effectively inhibited FasL mRNA expression ($p<0.05$), whereas the mRNA level of Fas had no significant difference compared with DSS group ($p>0.05$). Treatment with IG dose-dependently decreased the mRNA expressions of Fas and FasL. Especially, IG in a dose of 240 mg/kg was the most effective in down-regulating the mRNA levels of Fas and FasL.

Immunohistochemistry and real-time PCR results showed that the protein expression of Bax in DSS group was distinctly elevated compared with normal group ($p<0.01$, Fig. 5), whereas no significant difference of Bcl-2 mRNA level was found between DSS group and normal group ($p>0.05$, Fig. 4B). SASP obviously suppressed Bax protein expression level. But it had no effect on the mRNA expression of Bcl-2. Nevertheless, IG treatment significantly diminished the induced upregulation of Bax protein expressions in a dose-dependent manner. IG (240 mg/kg) was the most effective in reducing the protein expression of Bax

A

B

C

(a) Normal group   (b) DSS group

(c) SASP group   (d) IG 240 mg/kg group

D

(a)

(b)

(c)

(d)

E

F

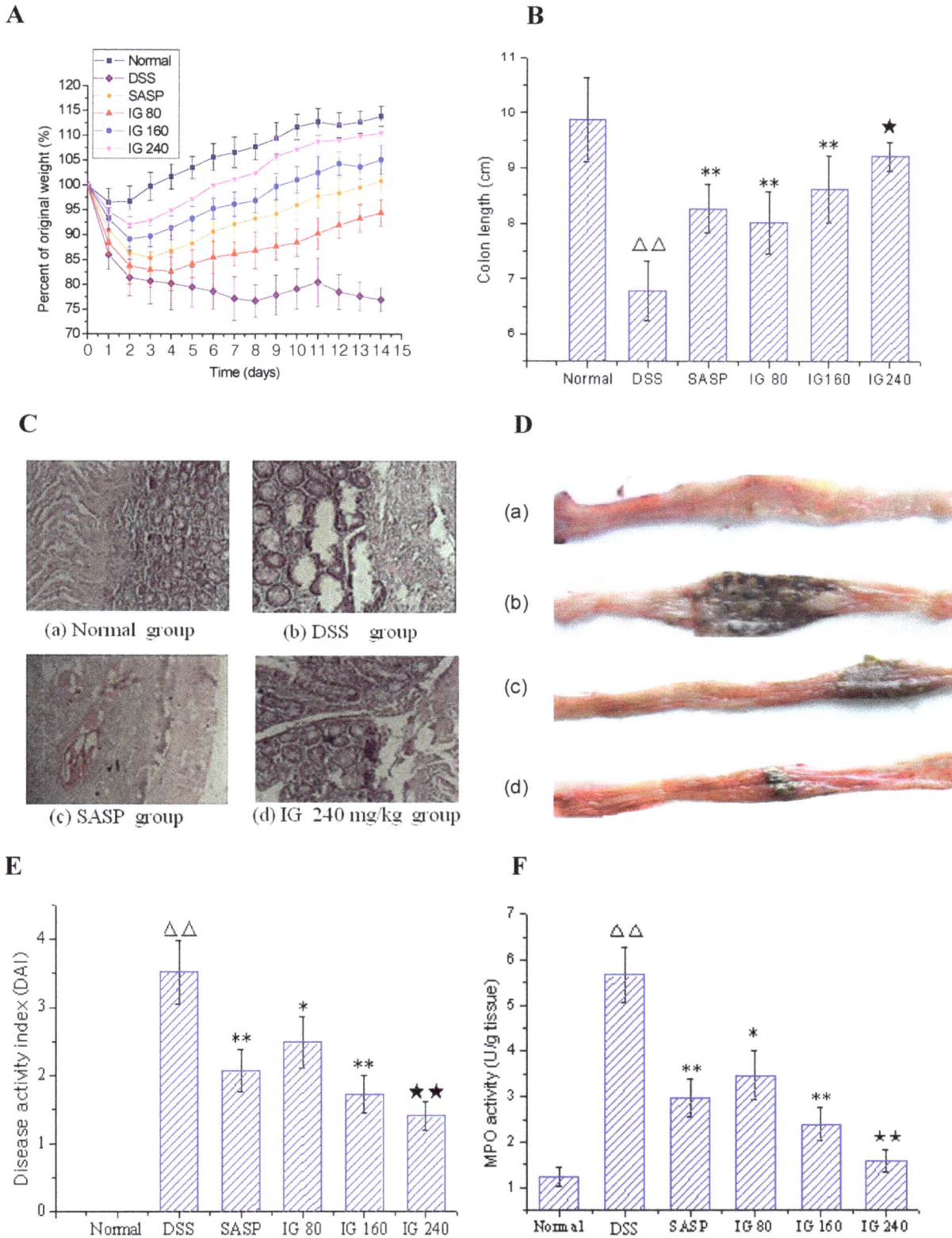

Figure 1. Iridoid glycosides (IG) ameliorate the clinical, macroscopic and histological features of acute colitis model. Colitis was induced by 4% DSS in drinking water. Rats were administrated p.o. at different dose of IG 80, 160 and 240 mg/kg twice daily for 14 days after administration of DSS. All rats were sacrificed on the 14 day after the first IG administration. The severity of colonic injury and the clinical evaluation were monitored by weight changes (A), colon length (cm) (B) histological analysis (C), macroscopic signs (D: a, normal group; b, DSS group; c, SASP group; d, high dose group of IG 240 mg/kg), disease activity index (E) and MPO activity (U/g tissue) (F). Representative macroscopic and histological analysis of rat colonic tissue in normal group, DSS group and high dose group of IG (240 mg/kg) (C and D) were shown in this figure. SASP (150 mg/kg p.o.) was used

as a positive control. IG administration dose-dependently diminished these parameters. The data are expressed as the mean ± standard deviation (Mean ± SD). ΔΔ p<0.01 versus normal group; * p<0.05, ** p<0.01 versus DSS group; ★ p<0.05, ★★ p<0.01 versus SASP group.

(P<0.01, Fig. 5). In addition, IG could dose-independently up-regulate the mRNA level of Bcl-2 (P<0.01, Fig. 4B).

As shown in Fig. 4C, the Caspase-3 mRNA expression of colonic epithelia cells in DSS group was markedly increased compared with normal group (p<0.01). Administration of SASP effectively inhibited Caspase-3 mRNA expression (p<0.01). The Caspase-3 mRNA level of colonic epithelia in IG group was significantly decreased in a dose-dependent manner compared to that in DSS group. Furthermore, the effect of IG in a dose of 240 mg/kg was prior to that of SASP (p<0.05).

Our study suggested that one mechanism underlying the protective effect of IG involved in the regulation of serial genes associated with IEC apoptosis in experimental colitis.

Effect of iridoid glycosides on NF-κB signal pathway

NF-κB activation can be regulated at several steps, including the nuclear translocation of its p65/RelA component and phosphorylation/degradation of IκBα [28]. In addition, IκBα phosphorylation is mediated by the activation of IKKβ unit of the IKK complex in numerous cell systems [23]. To further determine the impact of IG on cytokine-induced signal transduction in experimental colitis, we investigated the expression levels of representative upstream and downstream signal proteins involved in NF-κB activation using real-time PCR and Western blotting analysis. A significant increase in the mRNA and protein expressions of NF-κBp65 and IKKβ were observed in colonic epithelia cells of DSS-induced model group (p<0.01, Fig. 6A, C

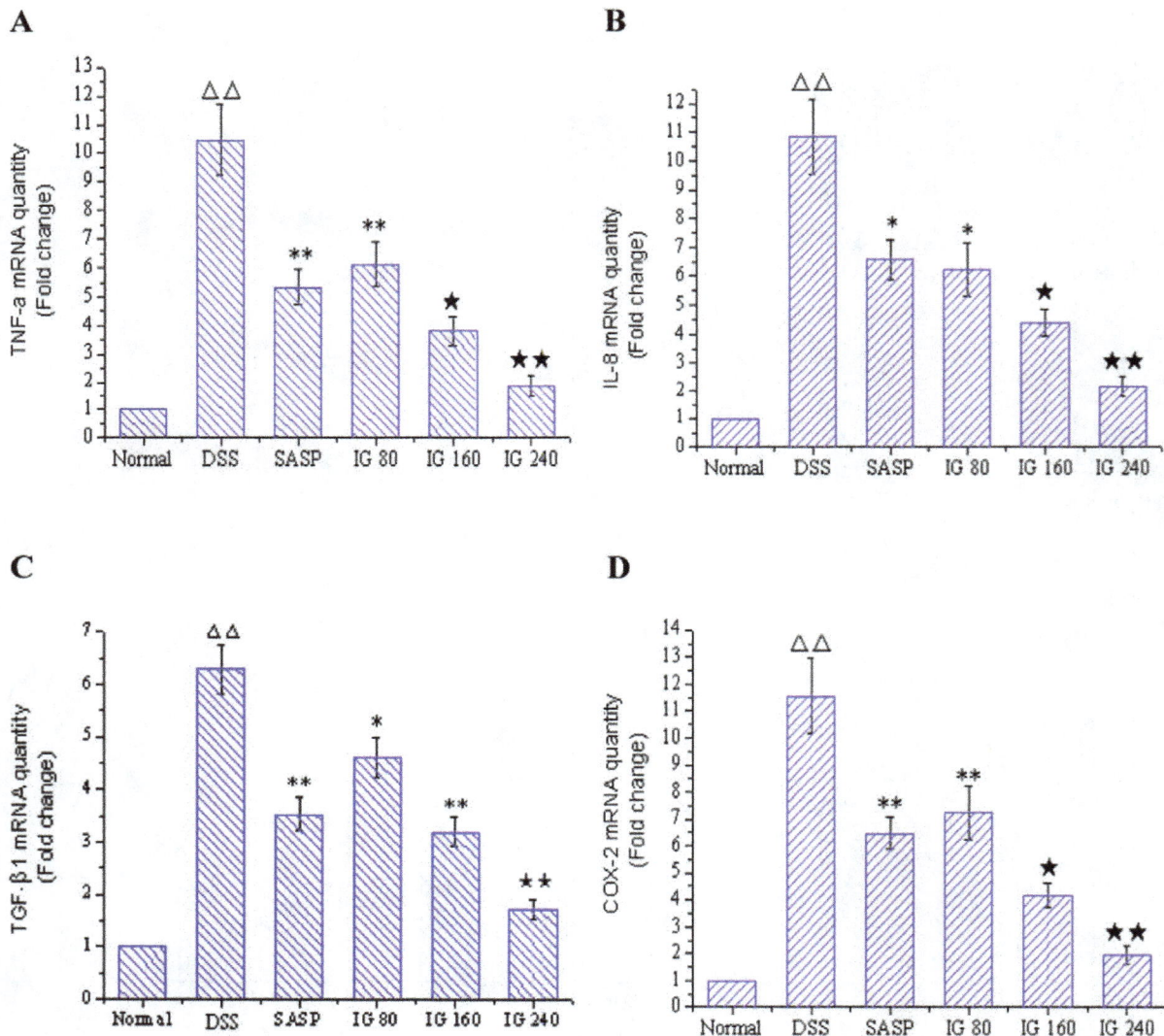

Figure 2. Effect of iridoid glycosides on the mRNA expressions of TNF-α, IL-8, TGF-β1 and COX-2 in DSS-induced colitis. Rats were administered with IG (80, 160, 240 mg/kg/day p.o.) for 14 days. SASP (150 mg/kg/day p.o.) was used as a positive control. The mRNA expressions of (A) TNF-α, (B) IL-8, (C) TGF-β1 and (D) COX-2 were determined using real-time quantitative PCR. The data are expressed as the mean ± standard deviation (Mean ± SD). ΔΔ p<0.01 vs normal group; * p<0.05, ** p<0.01 vs DSS group; ★ p<0.05, ★★ p<0.01 vs SASP group.

A

B C D

E F G

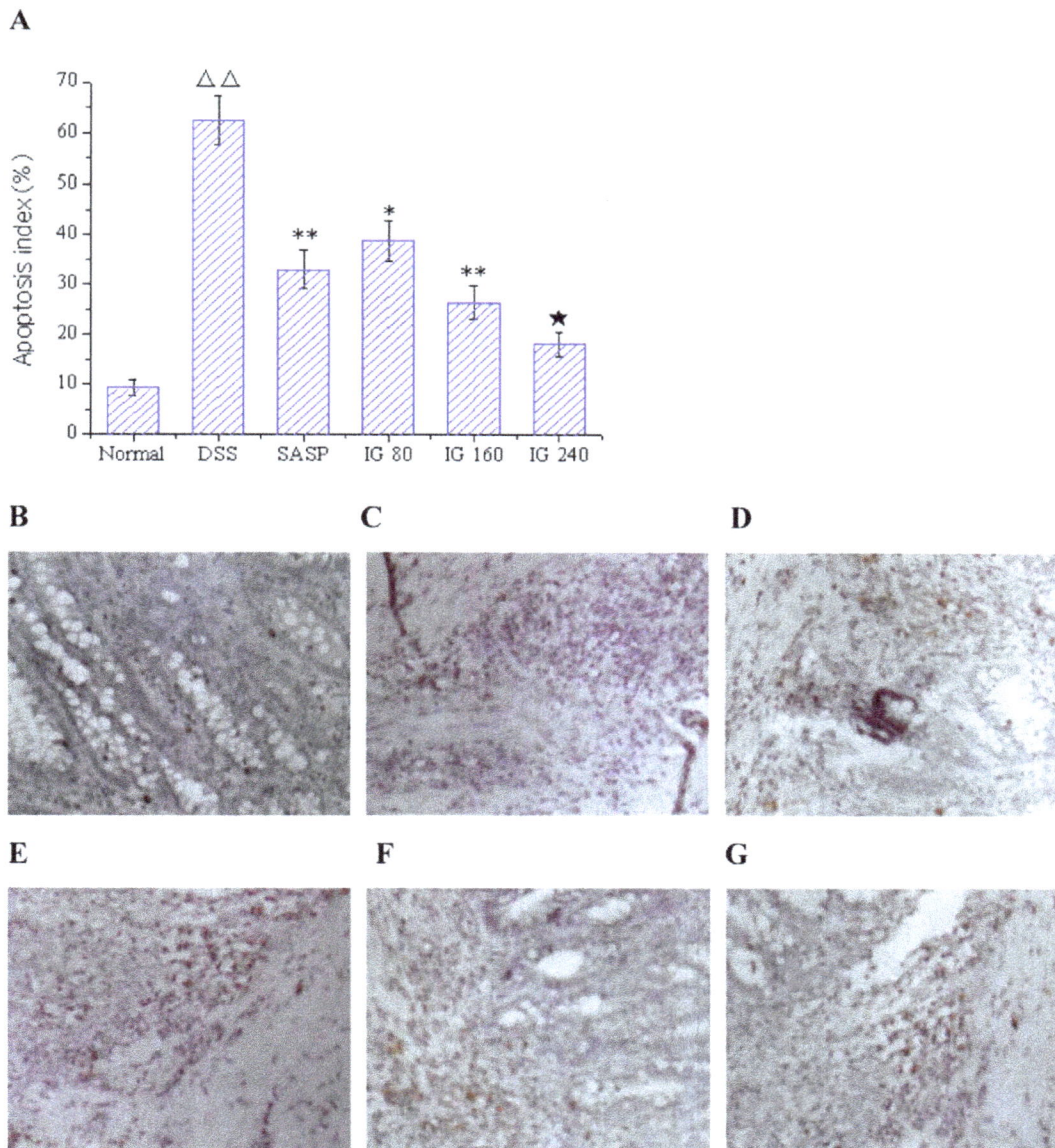

Figure 3. Effect of iridoid glycosides on intestinal epithelial cells apoptosis. Apoptotic cells in the colon tissues were detected using TUNEL assay. Cells with nuclei that stained dark brown were considered to be TUNEL-positive. (A) Apoptosis index (%); (B) Normal group, (C) DSS Model group; (D) SASP group; (E) IG 80 mg/kg, (F) IG 160 mg/kg and (G) IG 240 mg/kg (original magnification ×400). Apoptosis index indicated that the percentage of TUNEL-positive cells significantly decreased in a dose-dependent manner after treatment with IG compared with the DSS Model group. Data were expressed as mean ±SD (each group, n = 10). ΔΔ p<0.01 versus normal group; * p<0.05, ** p<0.01 versus DSS group; ★ p<0.05 versus SASP group.

and D). Furthermore, the degradation and phosphorylation of IκBα were distinctively induced in colonic epithelia cells of DSS-induced rats compared with normal group (p<0.01, Fig. 6B and D). In contrast, administration of SASP obviously reduced NF-κBp65 and IKKβ expressions in DSS-induced colitis, and the phosphorylation/degradation of IκBα were effectively suppressed, too. In accordance with the data presented in Fig. 6A and D, IG inhibited NF-κB nuclear translocation as indicated by dose-dependently decreasing p65/RelA expression and IκBα degradation in colonic epithelia cells compared with that in DSS group. However, IG (240 mg/kg) exerted the optimum effect in suppressing NF-κBp65 level and IκBα degradation. On the other hand, IG significantly blocked IκBα phosphorylation and IKKβ

activity in a dose-independent manner (p<0.05, Fig. 6C and D). IG (160 mg/kg) showed the maximum inhibition effect.

These results indicated that IG markedly blocked NF-κB signaling pathway in experimental colitis by inhibiting its binding to target DNA and suppressing IκBα phosphorylation/degradation and IKKβ activity in IEC.

Discussion

The present study was undertaken to investigate the potential anti-inflammatory and anti-apoptosis effects of IG on experimental colitis induced by DSS and the mechanisms involved. NF-κB signaling pathway regulates multiple κB-dependent genes involved

A

B

C

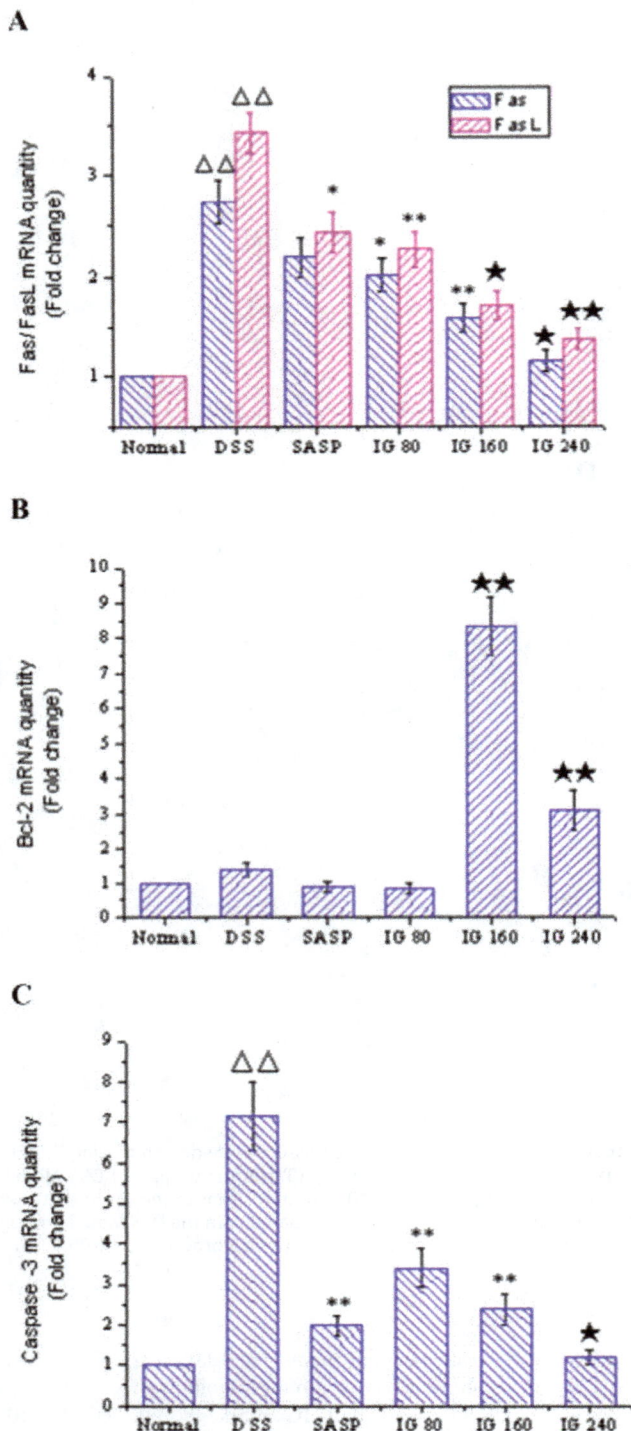

Figure 4. Effect of iridoid glycosides on the mRNA expressions of Fas/FasL, Bcl-2 and Caspase-3 in DSS-induced colitis. Rats were administered with IG (80, 160, 240 mg/kg/day p.o.) for 14 days. SASP (150 mg/kg/day p.o.) was used as a positive control. The mRNA expressions of (A) Fas/FasL, (B) Bcl-2 and (C) Caspase-3 were determined using real time quantitative PCR. The data are expressed as the mean ± standard deviation (Mean ± SD). ΔΔ p<0.01 vs normal group; * p<0.05, ** p<0.01 vs DSS group; ★ p<0.05, ★★ p<0.01 vs SASP group.

in the inflammatory response and cell apoptosis and represents an ideal target for the molecular therapy of UC [23,38]. Therefore, understanding the molecular mechanisms involved in this pathway is an essential step towards countering the damaging effects of pro-inflammatory mediators and cell apoptosis in IBD. In our previous study, IG, the main active fraction extracted from *F. syringae* leaves, has been known to possess strong anti-inflammatory activities and acts as an inhibitor for NF-κBp65 and oxidative-free radicals in experimental colitis [33]. However, the mechanism whereby IG inhibits NF-κB activity and IEC apoptosis has not been investigated. On the basis of the above, we hypothesized that IG might also modulate IκB/NF-κB pathway in DSS-induced colitis, through which it could inhibit intestinal inflammation and IEC apoptosis *in vivo*.

To confirm the validity of these hypotheses, first, we investigated the effect of IG on NF-κB-mediated inflammatory cytokine expression in DSS-induced colitis, which represents several characteristics resembling human UC. Recent studies have demonstrated increased production of pro-inflammatory cytokines including TNF-α, IL-1β, IL-6, IL-8, ICAM-1 and COX-2 in IBD that are known to play a key role in the modulation of intestinal immune system [29,33]. TNF-α released from macrophages in the early inflammatory response plays an important role in experimental colitis and it is likely the regulator key of the inflammatory cascade in IBD. IL-6 and IL-8 could stimulate neutrophil chemotaxis and relate to the presence of necrosis in the colon which led to tissue destruction. COX-2 is an important NF-κB-dependent mediator, in both of acute murine colitis and colitis-related cancer. The COX-2 level was increased in IBD and in colon cancer [39,40]. Therefore, blockade of these inflammatory mediators can offer an alternative therapy for UC. However, it is insufficient for achieving the optimal therapeutic effects only to block individual factors in a multifactorial inflammatory disease. Actually, individual factor such as cytokine or COX-2 only represents a downstream target, whereas NF-κB is just the final common pathway of the inducible expression of these pro-inflammatory genes or rate-limiting step in the inflammatory cascade of UC [33,38]. Increased NF-κB activation has been detected in the intestinal lamina propria of patients with IBD, and in a acute murine colitis model [26,29]. The cytokine-induced IκB/NF-κB signaling cascade is complex, involving the participation of multiple kinases and adapter proteins. The critical rate-limiting step in the activation of the NF-κB pathway is the catalytic IκB kinase (IKK) [41]. Cytokine (TNF-α and IL-1β) or bacterial product signaling converge on the IKK complex to trigger IκBα phosphorylation and ultimately NF-κB activity in numerous cell systems [4,42]. Activation of NF-κB then upregulates the expression of numerous κB-dependent pro-inflammatory genes involved in intestinal inflammation, including TNF-α, IL-6, IL-8, ICAM-1, iNOS, and COX-2 [29,43]. IKK is made up of two kinases, IKKα and IKKβ. Whereas IKKα is activated by an only limited set of stimuli, IKKβ activation occurs upon receptor-mediated stimulation by a broad set of microbial or host-derived ligands [44]. Gene depletion studies have demonstrated that IKKβ, but not IKKα, plays an essential role in NF-κB activation [41]. In order to achieve the optimal therapeutic effects, the application of a therapeutic strategy that interferes with NF-κB pathway (the upstream target) in the cascade of inflammation, namely, the blockade of simultaneously the expression of multiple pro-inflammatory genes, might be more effective than suppressing individual factor in treatment of UC. To demonstrate the effect of IG on NF-κB pathway, we utilized real-time quantitative PCR and Western blotting to determine NF-κBp65 level, IKKβ activity and IκBα phosphorylation/degradation in colonic tissue. The

A

B

C

D

E

F

G

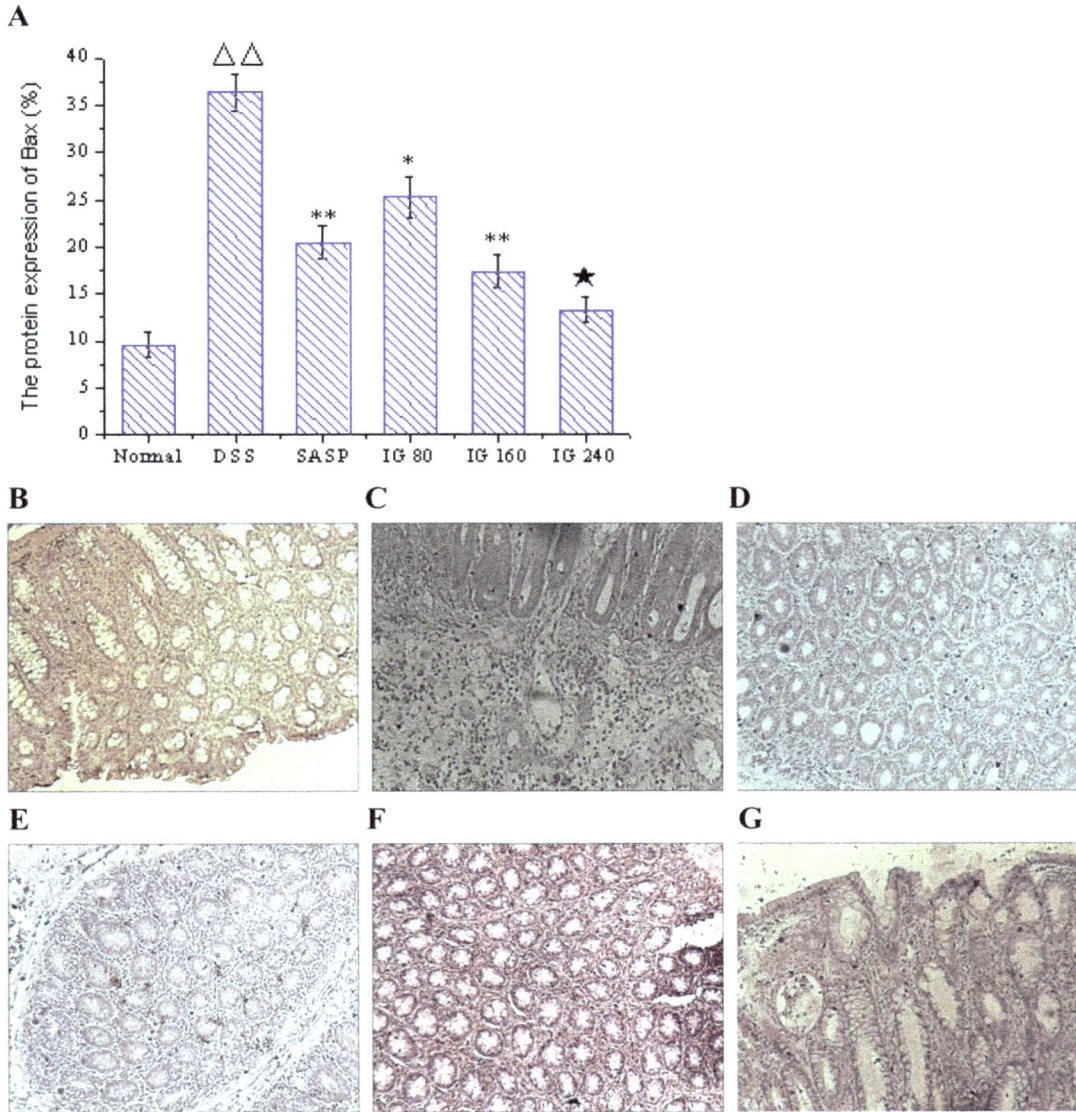

Figure 5. Immunohistochemical localization for Bax. There was few specific expression of Bax in normal tissue (B). Protein expression of Bax was significantly increased in the epithelial cell, intestine glands and in the inflammatory cells infiltrating in the tissue of model animals (C). Treatment of SASP (150 mg/kg), Bax protein expression was obviously reduced (D). Administration with IG (80 mg/kg, E; 160 mg/kg, F; 240 mg/kg, G), protein expression of Bax was effectively inhibited in both mucosa and submucosa in dose-dependent manner (A). Specific expression of Bax was very weak in the colonic tissue of high-dose group (G). Original magnification 400×.

results indicated that the protein and mRNA expressions of NF-κBp65 and IKKβ were significantly increased in DSS-treated rats. NF-κBp65 mRNA expression was dose-dependently inhibited and IKKβ decreased dose-independently after administration of IG for 2 weeks. Moreover, DSS strongly induced IκBα phosphorylation and triggered IκBα degradation in colonic tissue. IG also blocked IκBα phosphorylation/degradation in a dose-dependent manner. On the other hand, our study indicated that the levels of TNF-α, IL-8 and COX-2 in DSS group were increased more distinctly than normal group and reduced dose-dependently after treatment with IG in response to NF-κBp65 and IKKβ activity. In addition, the effect of IG at dose of 160 mg/kg and 240 mg/kg were all prior to SASP. Since the promoter regions of TNF-α, IL-8 and COX-2 had also been shown to contain consensus binding motifs for NF-κB. In the present study, we firstly infer that anti-

inflammatory effect of IG may be linked with inhibition of multiple pro-inflammatory genes through blockade of IκB/NF-κB pathway in experimental colitis.

Second, to clarify whether IG could modulate IEC apoptosis in UC *in vivo*, we investigated the effect of IG on the relative expression level of a series of apoptosis genes in DSS-induced colitis. Recent evidence suggests that NF-κB activates the transcription of many genes capable of regulating apoptosis, known as the "cell-death substrates" [45]. Fas/FasL is an important pathway of involved in the induction of epithelial cell apoptosis in UC [38]. When UC occurred, the expression of FasL is markedly upregulated on the surface of infiltrating cytotoxic lymphocytes in active UC and binds the Fas receptor on the basolateral epithelial membrane [46]. Fas associated death domain recruits molecules, including procaspase-8, to form the death-

A

B

C

D

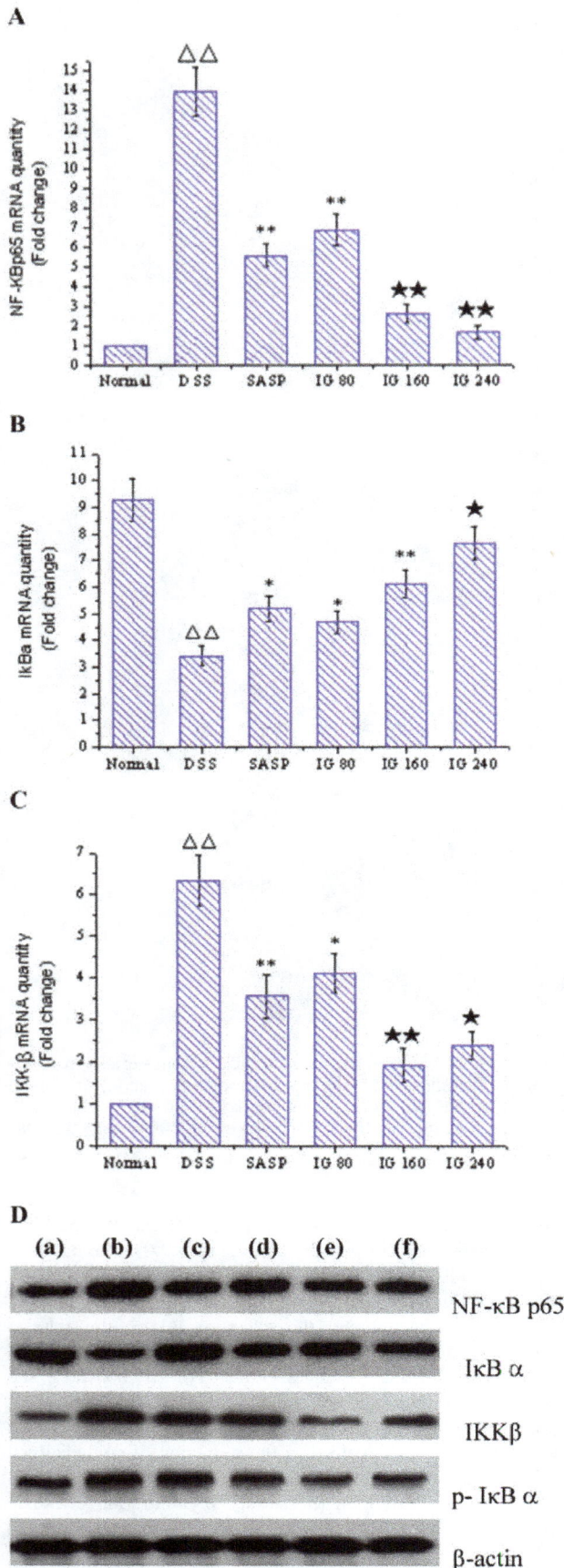

Figure 6. Iridoid glycosides blocks NF-κB activation by inhibiting NF-κB p65 mRNA expression, IκBα phosphorylation/degradation and IKKβ activity in rats with DSS-induced colitis. The mRNA levels of (A) NF-κB p65, (B) IκB α and (C) IKKβ in colonic tissues were determined using real time quantitative PCR. Total protein was extracted and examined for NF-κB p65, IκB α, phosphor-IκB α and IKKβ expression by Western blotting (D: a, normal group; b, DSS group; c, SASP group; d, low dose group of IG 80 mg/kg; e, middle dose group of IG 160 mg/kg; f, high dose group of IG 240 mg/kg). Densitometry was made to following normalization to the control (housekeeping gene). The results are representative of three experiments performed on different samples. Data are expressed as the mean $\pm$ standard deviation (Mean $\pm$ SD). $\triangle\triangle$ $p < 0.01$ vs normal group; * $p < 0.05$, ** $p < 0.01$ vs DSS group; ★ $p < 0.05$, ★★ $p < 0.01$ vs SASP group.

inducing signaling complex [47]. Procaspase-8 is then cleaved into its activated form, and the apoptotic cascade ensues, culminating in the activation of executioner caspase-3 [48]. These interactions accelerate migration and activity of neutrophils, induce generation of excessive ROS through NF-κB activation and expression of FasL, and inhibit immune response at the inflammatory site, resulting in progressive mucosal lesion of UC [38,46]. Anti-apoptotic NF-κB target genes include TGF-β1, inhibitors of apoptosis proteins (IAP), and prosurvial members of the Bcl-2 gene kindred and so on [19,21]. As Bcl-2 could prolong the life of cells, it has been generally accepted as an anti-apoptosis gene. The apoptosis promoting gene Bax is a new member of Bcl-2 gene kindred, it could form a dimer with Bcl-2 to inhibit its function [49]. The relative expression ratio of Bax/Bcl-2 determines whether apoptosis occurs in IEC or not. Excessive expression of Bax promotes apoptosis, and when the expression of Bcl-2 gained advantage, the cells would continue to exist [50]. Among the anti-apoptotic regulatory proteins, TGF-β1 plays especially important role in the pathogenesis of IBD [51]. TGF-β1 expression can be induced by pro-inflammatory cytokines, such as IL-1β and TNF-α [21]. The general opinion showed that TGF-β1 expression in plasma is increased parallel to the increase in cytokine secretion due to inflammation in patients with UC and Crohn's disease (CD), which can be used as a marker for differential diagnosis of the active phase of both diseases [52]. Additionally, plasma TGF-β1 levels are affected by anti-inflammatory drugs such as glucocorticoid, sulfasalazine and 5-aminosalicylic acid [52,53]. The present study confirmed that DSS-induced colitis leads to a substantial increase of IEC apoptosis. Meanwhile, the mRNA and protein expressions of Fas/FasL, Bax and caspase-3 in colonic epithelia were significantly increased. Activation of these apoptosis genes increased the number of apoptotic cells, which might be one of the important mechanisms of colonic pathological changes in UC. After treatment with IG, activation of Fas/FasL, Bax and caspase-3 in colonic epithelia were markedly downregulated compared with DSS group, and the number of apoptosis cells was also decreased. In addition, our results showed persistent inflammation resulted in a significant upregulation of TGF-β1 expression and reduction of Bcl-2 expression. IG treatment dose-dependently reduced TGF-β1 level and increased the mRNA and protein expression of Bcl-2. These findings demonstrate, for the first time, the novel protective effects of IG against inflammation in colon, suggesting a potential clinical value in the treatment of IBD. Considering that the common effector pathway for regulating expression of these pro-inflammatory cytokines and apoptosis genes is IκB/NF-κB transduction system, IG could ameliorate experimental colitis through the blockade of NF-κB signaling.

Although IG had anti-inflammatory functions through acting on the IκB/NF-κB pathway, and these effects most probably contributed to its therapy of UC. Many upstream signaling proteins and downstream cytokines of NF-κB in which treatment of IG were also involved have not been completely demonstrated. The pro-inflammatory gene transcriptional program mediated by IκB/NF-κB pathway was induced by toll-like receptor (TLR) activation and subsequent recruitment of MyD88, followed by p38-dependent transcriptional activity of the NF-κB complex leading to induction of target genes, such as TNF-a, IL-27, IL-15, MMP-9, and VCAM-1 [43,54]. Therefore, our future studies will investigate these upstream targets and other downstream cytokines, in order to elucidate underlying molecular mechanisms responsible for the therapeutic effects of IG. Despite we demonstrated the protective effects of IG on preventing acute colitis in DSS-induced murine model, which has proven useful for examining the underlying pathophysiology of IBD. It should be further validate that whether IG would modulate the inflammation in different colitis models such as the IL-10 knock-out model and therapeutic trails for established colitis [43]. In addition, NF-κB activation has emerged as a hallmark for many human hematologic malignancies and solid tumors, most commonly because of persistent activation of the IKK complex [55], and IKK could be related to the development of colitis-associated cancer [56]. Intriguingly, a recent study demonstrated that 5-aminosalicylic acids (5-ASAs) are the most commonly prescribed anti-inflammatory drugs for IBD. Regular 5-ASA intake may reduce the risk of colorectal cancer in patients with IBD through anti-NF-κB action by direct inhibition of IKK [57]. In our study,

IG ameliorates experimental colitis through inhibiting NF-κB pathway by blockade of IKK activity. In view of this, the effect of IG on colitis-associated cancer should be further clarified by *in vitro* and *in vivo* studies to support this hypothesis.

In conclusion, the present results demonstrated that IG dose-dependently ameliorated the severity of DSS-induced colitis. The possible mechanisms in the protective effect of UC were concluded that IG could inhibit multiple pro-inflammatory molecules and modulate serial genes involved in IEC apoptosis through blocking NF-κB signal pathway. Additionally, numerous studies from clinical trial as well as animal studies have shown that few toxic effects or side effects are found with treatment of IG [58]. Recently, antisense oligonucleotide against NF-κB has been applied in the treatment of UC. However, its price was expensive and the safety need to be further identified. Therefore, IG, as natural inhibitor of NF-κB signaling pathway, could be a promising remedy for the treatment of IBD.

Acknowledgments

We thank Qiu Ming Li for helpful expertise in histology.

Author Contributions

Conceived and designed the experiments: XL. Performed the experiments: XL. Analyzed the data: XL JMW. Contributed reagents/materials/analysis tools: JMW. Wrote the paper: XL.

References

1. Eckmann L, Nebelsiek T, Fingerle AA, Dann SM, Mages J, et al. (2008) Opposing functions of IKKβ during acute and chronic intestinal inflammation. Proc Natl Acad Sci USA 105: 15058–15063.
2. Shanahan F, Bernstein CN (2009) The evolving epidemiology of inflammatory bowel disease. Curr Opin in Gastroenterol 25: 301–305.
3. Jun CD, Kim Y, Choi EY, Kim M, Park B, et al. (2006) Gliotoxin reduces the severity of trinitrobenzene sulfonic acid-induced colitis in mice: evidence of the connection between heme oxygenase-1 and the nuclear factor-κB pathway *in vitro* and *in vivo*. Inflamm Bowel Dis 12: 619–629.
4. Cheon JH, Kim JS, Kim JM, Kim N, Jung HC, et al. (2006) Plant sterol guggulsterone inhibits nuclear factor-kappaB signaling in intestinal epithelial cells by blocking IkappaB kinase and ameliorates acute murine colitis. Inflamm Bowel Dis 12: 1152–1161.
5. Kozuch PL, Hanauer SB (2008) Treatment of inflammatory bowel disease: a review of medical therapy. World J Gastroenterol 14: 354–377.
6. Seidelin JB, Nielsen OH (2008) Attenuated Apoptosis Response to Fas-ligand in Active Ulcerative Colitis. Inflamm Bowel Dis 14: 1623–1629.
7. Martin AR, Villegas I, Sanchez-Hidalgo M, de la Lastra CA (2006) The effects of resveratrol, a phytoalexin derived from red wines, on chronic inflammation induced in an experimentally induced colitis model. Brit J Pharmacol 147: 873–885.
8. Da Silva MS, Sánchez-Fidalgo S, Talero E, Cárdeno A, da Silva MA, et al. (2010) Anti-inflammatory intestinal activity of Abarema cochliacarpos (Gomes) Barneby & Grimes in TNBS colitis model. J Ethnopharmacol 128: 467–475.
9. O'Shea J, Ma A, Lipsky P (2002) Cytokines and autoimmunity. Nat Rev 2: 37–45.
10. Lammers KM, Vergopoulos A, Babel N, Rizzello F, Morselli C, et al. (2005) Probiotic therapy in the prevention of pouchitis onset: decreased interleukin-1β, interleukin-8 and interferon-γ gene expression. Inflamm Bowel Dis 11: 447–454.
11. Yao J, Wang JY, Liu L, Li YX, Xun AY, et al. (2010) Anti-oxidant effects of resveratrol on mice with DSS-induced ulcerative colitis. Arch Med Res 41: 288–294.
12. Talero E, Sanchez-Fidalgo S, Alarcon de la Lastra C, Illanes M, Calvo JR, et al. (2008) Acute and chronic responses associated with adrenomedullin administration in experimental colitis. Peptides 29: 2001–2012.
13. Seidelin JB, Nielsen OH (2003) Apoptosis in chronic inflammatory bowel disease. The importance for pathogenesis and treatment. Ugeskr Laeger 165: 790–792.
14. Strater J, Wellisch I, Riedl S, Walczak H, Koretz K, et al. (1997) CD95 (APO-1/Fas)-mediated apoptosis in colon epithelial cells: a possible role in ulcerative colitis. Gastroenterology 113: 160–167.
15. Nagata S (1997) Apoptosis by death factor. Cell 88: 355–365.
16. Clavel T, Haller D (2007) Bacteria- and host-derived mechanisms to control intestinal epithelial cell homeostasis: implications for chronic inflammation. Inflamm Bowel Dis 13: 1153–1164.
17. Irmler M, Thome M, Hahne M, Schneider P, Hofmann K, et al. (1997) Inhibition of death receptor signals by cellular FLIP. Nature 388: 190–195.
18. Beck PL, Rosenberg IM, Xavier RJ, Koh T, Wong JF, et al. (2003) Transforming growth factor-β mediates intestinal healing and susceptibility to injury in vitro and in vivo through epithelial cells. Am J Pathol 162: 597–608.
19. Sakuraba H, Ishiguro Y, Yamagata K, Munakata A, Nakane A (2007) Blockade of TGF-β accelerates mucosal destruction through epithelial cell apoptosis. Biochem Biophys Res Commun 359: 406–412.
20. Kilic ZM, Ayaz S, Özin Y, Nadir I, Cakal B, et al. (2009) Plasma transforming factor-β1 level in inflammatory bowel disease. Turk J Gastroenterol 20: 165–170.
21. Lee KY, Ito K, Hayashi R, Jazrawi EP, Barnes PJ, et al. (2006) NF-κB and Activator Protein 1 Response Elements and the Role of Histone Modifications in IL-β1-Induced TGF-β1 Gene Transcription. J Immunol 176: 603–615.
22. Wiercińska-Drapalo A, Flisiak R, Prokopowicz D (2003) Effect of ulcerative colitis treatment on transforming growth factor β1 in plasma and rectal mucosa. Regul Peptides 113: 57–61.
23. Chae S, Eckmann L, Miyamoto Y, Pothoulakis C, Karin M, et al. (2006) Epithelial cell IκB-Kinase β has an important protective role in *clostridium difficile* toxin A-induced mucosal injury. J Immunol 177: 1214–1220.
24. Zhang DK, He FQ, Li TK, Pang XH, Cui de J, et al. (2010) Glial-derived neurotrophic factor regulates intestinal epithelial barrier function and inflammation and is therapeutic for murine colitis. J Pathol 222: 213–222.
25. Fiocchi C (1998) Inflammatory bowel disease: etiology and pathogenesis. Gastroenterology 115: 182–205.
26. Neurath MF, Pettersson S, Meyer zum Büschenfelde KH, Strober W (1996) Local administration of antisense phosphorothioate oligonucleotides to the p65 subunit of NF-kappa B abrogates established experimental colitis in mice. Nat Med 9: 998–1004.
27. Ghosh S, Karin M (2002) Missing pieces in the NF-κB puzzle. Cell 109: 81–96.
28. Hayden MS, Ghosh S (2008) Shared Principles in NF-κB Signaling. Cell 132: 344–362.
29. Lee JY, Kim JS, Kim JM, Kim N, Jung HC, et al. (2007) Simvastatin inhibits NF-κB signaling in intestinal epithelial cells and ameliorates acute murine colitis. Int Immunopharmacol 7: 241–248.
30. Malek R, Borowicz KK, Jargiello M, Czuczwar SJ (2007) Role of NF-κB in the central nervous system. Pharmacol Rep 59: 25–33.
31. Atreya I, Atreya R, Neurath MF (2008) NF-κB in inflammatory bowel disease. J Intern Med 263: 591–596.
32. Liu X, Wang J, Zhou C, Gan L (2010) Preparative separation and enrichment of syringopicroside from *Folium syringae* leaves with macroporous resins. J Biomed Biotechnol;accepted 28 November 2010, Article ID 572570, doi:10.1155/2010/572570.
33. Liu X, Wang JM (2011) Anti-inflammatory effects of iridoid glycosides fraction of *Folium syringae* leaves on TNBS-induced colitis in rats. J Ethnopharmacol 133: 780–787.

34. Cooper HS, Murthy SN, Shah RS, Sedergran DJ (1993) Clinicopathlolgic study of dextran sulfate sodium experimental murine colitis. Lab Invest 69: 238–249.

35. Wallace JL, Keenan CM, Gale D, Shoupe TS (1992) Exacerbation of experimental colitis by non-steroidal antinflammatory drugs is not related to elevate leukotriene B4 synthesis. Gastroenterology 102: 18–27.

36. Bobin-Dubigeon C, Collin X, Grimaud N, Robert JM, Le Baut G, et al. (2001) Effects of tumor necrosis factor-α synthesis inhibitors on rat trinitrobenzene sulphonic acid-induced chronic colitis. Eur J Pharmacol 421: 103–110.

37. Krawisz JE, Sharon P, Stenson WF (1984) Quantitative assay for acute intestinal inflammation based on myeloperoxidase activity. Assessment of inflammation in rat and hamster models. Gastroenterology 87: 1344–1350.

38. Mazzon E, Esposito E, Crisafulli C, Riccardi L, Muià C, et al. (2006) Melatonin modulates signal transduction pathways and apoptosis in experimental colitis. J Pineal Res 41: 363–373.

39. Nam SY, Kim JS, Kim JM, Lee JY, Kim N, et al. (2008) DA-6034, a derivative of flavonoid, prevents and ameliorates dextran sulfate sodium-induced colitis and inhibits colon carcinogenesis. Exp Biol Med (Maywood) 233: 180–191.

40. Singer II, Kawka DW, Schloemann S, Tessner T, Riehl T, et al. (1998) Cyclooxygenase 2 is induced in colonic epithelial cells in inflammatory bowel disease. Gastroenterology 115: 297–306.

41. Yang F, Tang E, Guan K, Wang CY (2003) IKKbeta plays an essential role in the phosphorylation of RelA/p65 on serine 536 induced by lipopolysaccharide. J Immunol 170: 5630–5635.

42. Malinin NL, Boldin MP, Kovalenko AV, Wallach D (1997) MAP3K-related kinase involved in NF-κB induction by TNF, CD95 and IL-1. Nature 385: 540–544.

43. Jobin C, Bradham CA, Russo MP, Juma B, Narula AS, et al. (1999) Curcumin blocks cytokine-mediated NF-κB activation and proinflammatory gene expression by inhibiting inhibitory factor I-κB kinase activity. J Immunol 163: 3474–3483.

44. Hayden MS, Ghosh S (2004) Signaling to NF-κB. Genes Dev 18: 2195–2224.

45. Kucharczak J, Simmons MJ, Fan Y, Gélinas C (2003) To be, or not to be: NF-κB is the answer-role of Rel/NF-κB in the regulation of apoptosis. Oncogene 22: 8961–8982.

46. Ueyama H, Kiyohara T, Sawada N, Isozaki K, Kitamura S, et al. (1998) High Fas ligand expression on lymphocytes in lesions of ulcerative colitis. Gut 43: 48–55.

47. Sayani FA, Keenan CM, Van Sickle MD, Amundson KR, Parr EJ, et al. (2004) The expression and role of Fas ligand in intestinal inflammation. Neurogastroenterol Motil 16: 61–74.

48. Barnhart BC, Pietras EM, Geciras-Schimnich A, Salmena L, Sayama K, et al. (2005) CD95 apoptosis resistance in certain cells can be overcome by noncanonical activation of caspase-8. Cell Death Differ 12: 25–37.

49. Scorrano L, Korsmeyer SJ (2003) Mechanisms of cytochrome C release by proapoptotic Bcl-2 family members. Biochem Biophys Res Commun 304: 437–444.

50. Ina K, Itoh J, Fukushima K, Kusugami K, Yamaguchi T, et al. (1999) Resistance of Crohn's disease T cells to multiple apoptotic signals is associated with a Bcl-2/Bax mucosal imbalance. J Immunol 63: 1081–1090.

51. Stadnicki A, Machnik G, Klimacka-Nawrot E, Wolanska-Karut A, Labuzek K (2009) Transforming growth factor-β1 and its receptors in patients with ulcerative colitis. Int Immunopharmacol 9: 761–766.

52. Kilic ZMY, Ayaz S, Özin Y, Nadir I, Cakal B, et al. (2009) Plasma transforming growth factor-β1 level in inflammatory bowel disease. Turk J Gastroenterol 20: 165–170.

53. Koelink PJ, Hawinkels LJ, Wiercinska E, Sier CF, ten Dijke P, et al. (2010) 5-Aminosalicylic acid inhibits TGF-β1 signalling in colorectal cancer cells. Cancer Lett 287: 82–90.

54. Gorina R, Font-Nieves M, Márquez-Kisinousky L, Santalucia T, Planas AM (2011) Astrocyte TLR4 activation induces a proinflammatory environment through the interplay between MyD88-dependent NFκB signaling, MAPK, and Jak1/Stat1 pathways. Glia 59: 242–255.

55. Luo JL, Kamata H, Karin M (2005) IKK/NF-κB signaling: balancing life and death-a new approach to cancer therapy. J Clin Invest 115: 2625–2632.

56. Greten FR, Eckmann L, Greten TF, Park JM, Li ZW, et al. (2004) IKKβ links inflammation and tumorigenesis in a mouse model of colitis-associated cancer. Cell 118: 285–296.

57. Weber CK, Liptay S, Wirth T, Adler G, Schmid RM (2000) Suppression of NF-κB activity by sulfasalazine is mediated by direct inhibition of IκB kinases α and β. Gastroenterology 119: 1209–1218.

58. Zhang LX (2009) The research progress of *Folium syringae* leaves. Strait Pharmaceutical Journal 21: 20–23.

9

TRIM27 Negatively Regulates NOD2 by Ubiquitination and Proteasomal Degradation

Birte Zurek[1], Ida Schoultz[2¤a], Andreas Neerincx[1], Luisa M. Napolitano[3,4], Katharina Birkner[1¤b], Eveline Bennek[5], Gernot Sellge[5], Maria Lerm[2], Germana Meroni[3], Johan D. Söderholm[2], Thomas A. Kufer[1]*

1 Institute for Medical Microbiology, Immunology and Hygiene, University of Cologne, Cologne, Germany, 2 Department of Clinical and Experimental Medicine, Faculty of Health Sciences, Linköping University, Linköping, Sweden, and Department of Surgery, Linköping, Sweden, 3 Cluster in Biomedicine (CBM), AREA Science Park, Trieste, Italy, 4 Telethon Institute of Genetics and Medicine, Naples, Italy, 5 Department of Medicine III, University Hospital Aachen, Aachen, Germany

Abstract

NOD2, the nucleotide-binding domain and leucine-rich repeat containing gene family (NLR) member 2 is involved in mediating antimicrobial responses. Dysfunctional NOD2 activity can lead to severe inflammatory disorders, but the regulation of NOD2 is still poorly understood. Recently, proteins of the tripartite motif (TRIM) protein family have emerged as regulators of innate immune responses by acting as E3 ubiquitin ligases. We identified TRIM27 as a new specific binding partner for NOD2. We show that NOD2 physically interacts with TRIM27 via the nucleotide-binding domain, and that NOD2 activation enhances this interaction. Dependent on functional TRIM27, ectopically expressed NOD2 is ubiquitinated with K48-linked ubiquitin chains followed by proteasomal degradation. Accordingly, TRIM27 affects NOD2-mediated pro-inflammatory responses. NOD2 mutations are linked to susceptibility to Crohn's disease. We found that TRIM27 expression is increased in Crohn's disease patients, underscoring a physiological role of TRIM27 in regulating NOD2 signaling. In HeLa cells, TRIM27 is partially localized in the nucleus. We revealed that ectopically expressed NOD2 can shuttle to the nucleus in a Walker A dependent manner, suggesting that NOD2 and TRIM27 might functionally cooperate in the nucleus. We conclude that TRIM27 negatively regulates NOD2-mediated signaling by degradation of NOD2 and suggest that TRIM27 could be a new target for therapeutic intervention in NOD2-associated diseases.

Editor: Edward Harhaj, Johns Hopkins School of Medicine, United States of America

Funding: This work was supported by grants from the German Research Foundation (DFG),grant SFB670-NG01 to TAK and grants from the Swedish Society of Medicine, the Regional Research Council of South-East Sweden (FORSS) and the Swedish Research Council division of Medicine and Gustav V 90th anniversary foundation to ML and JDS. GM is partly funded by the Italian Telethon Foundation. EB and GS acknowledge funding from the DFG, grant SE 1122/2-1. The funders had no role in study design, data collection and analysis, decision to publish, or preparation of the manuscript.

Competing Interests: The authors have declared that no competing interests exist.

* E-mail: thomas.kufer@uk-koeln.de

¤a Current address: School of Health and Medical sciences, Faculty of Medicine, Örebro University, Örebro, Sweden
¤b Current address: Institute of Cell Biology, ETH Zürich, Zürich, Switzerland

Introduction

Innate immune responses are characterized by recognition of invariant structural signatures of pathogens, so called pathogen-associated molecular patterns (PAMPs) as well as the recognition of danger-associated molecular patterns (DAMPs), which generally are compartmentalized host molecules that delocalize upon cell damage. Different types of pattern-recognition receptors (PRRs) show distinct subcellular localizations to recognize extracellular, vesicular or cytosolic PAMPs and DAMPs. NOD2 is a member of the nucleotide-binding domain and leucine-rich repeat containing protein family (NLR), many of which are important cytosolic PRRs [1–3]. NOD2 is composed of two N-terminal CARD domains recruiting the downstream signaling adaptor RIP2, a central nucleotide-binding domain (NBD) thought to mediate homooligomerization and a C-terminal leucine-rich repeat domain likely involved in pattern recognition. It is localized to the cytoplasm but is also partially found at the plasma membrane [4–7]. NOD2 induces signaling cascades in response to muramyl dipeptide (MDP), a bacterial peptidoglycan fragment, which activates NF-κB and MAP kinases and finally results in the transcription of proinflammatory cytokines, chemokines and antimicrobial peptides [8–10].

NOD2 gain-of-function mutations leading to uncontrolled NF-κB activation are found in severe autoinflammatory disorders like early-onset sarcoidosis (EOS) and Blau syndrome (BS) [11], underscoring the need to tightly regulate NOD2 activation. Other mutations in NOD2, predominantly fs1007, are linked with the development of Crohn's disease (CD), a multifactorial inflammatory bowel disease [11]. These mutations are located in the LRR-domain and result in a loss-of-function for MDP sensing. Several proteins like the cell polarity protein Erbin [4,12], the GTPase-activating protein Centaurin-β1 (CENTB1) [13], and the angio-associated migratory cell protein (AAMP) [14] have been shown to bind NOD2 and negatively regulate NOD2-mediated NF-κB activation. However, the contribution of NOD2 protein turn-over on signaling has not been elucidated.

Tripartite motif-containing (TRIM) proteins are present in all metazoans and over 60 TRIM proteins are encoded in the human genome [15]. They are involved in a broad range of biological processes including cell proliferation, differentiation, development, morphogenesis, and apoptosis and many TRIM proteins are expressed in response to interferons (IFNs) [16,17]. Members of the TRIM protein superfamily possess a RBCC motif at the N-terminus, which consists of a RING domain and one or two B-Box domains followed by a coiled-coil region. They differ from each other by their C-terminal domain. Most TRIM family members are, however, characterized by a PRY-SPRY (also called B30.2) domain which is suggested to serve as target binding site [18,19]. RING domains mediate the conjugation of proteins with ubiquitin, SUMO or ISG15 [20,21] and E3 ubiquitin ligase activity has been observed for several TRIM proteins. Recently, members of the TRIM family have been implicated in regulating antiviral and antimicrobial immune responses. The importance of TRIM proteins in regulating immune homeostasis is highlighted by inherited disorders that are associated with some of these genes: TRIM20 (pyrin) is mutated in the inflammatory disease familial Mediterranean fever (FMF) [22,23] and TRIM21 (Ro52) is one of the autoantigens detected in Sjögren's syndrome (SS) and systemic lupus erythematosus (SLE), two severe autoimmune disorders [24,25]. The most prominent example for antiviral activities of TRIM proteins is provided by TRIM5-α which is necessary to restrict retroviral infection in mammals, and in particular in higher primates [26].

TRIM27 (alternatively named RET finger protein (RFP)) is a member of the TRIM superfamily and exhibits the classical PRY-SPRY domain C-terminal of the RBCC motif. TRIM27 was initially identified as a part of the *rfp/ret* transforming gene generated by DNA rearrangements, in which the RING finger is essential for the oncogenic potential [27]. In accordance with the presence of a RING finger, TRIM27 has been shown to confer E3 ubiquitin ligase activity with the enzymes UBE2D1 and D3 [28] and to possess SUMO E3 ligase activity [29]. TRIM27 is highly expressed in mouse spleen and thymus [30] and in cells of the hematopoietic compartment [16]. In contrast to many other TRIM proteins, TRIM27 expression is not altered by type I and II IFNs [16,17]. TRIM27 exhibits either nuclear or cytosolic localization depending on the cell type [30,31]. Like other TRIM proteins, TRIM27 can form homooligomers mediated by the coiled-coil domain [31]. Heterooligomerization has been observed between TRIM27 and TRIM19 with the recruitment of the former to promyelocytic leukaemia nuclear bodies (PMLs) [32]. Furthermore, interaction with members of the protein inhibitors of activated STAT (PIAS) family results in targeting of TRIM27 to subnuclear compartments by TRIM27 SUMOylation [33]. A role for TRIM27 in transcriptional repression [34,35], the negative regulation of NF-κB and IFN-signaling pathways [36], apoptosis [37], and in cell cycle regulation [38] has been reported, suggesting that TRIM27 is involved in the control of multiple cellular processes.

Here we show that TRIM27 regulates innate immune responses by physical interaction with NOD2. We find that TRIM27 mediates K48-linked ubiquitination and subsequent proteasomal degradation of NOD2. Functionally, TRIM27 negatively influenced NOD2-mediated NF-κB activation. TRIM27 expression was enhanced in Crohn's patients, indicating a physiological role of TRIM27 in controlling NOD2 activity. Of note, ectopically expressed NOD2 colocalized with TRIM27 to the nucleus of HeLa cells, suggesting a new role for NOD2 in nuclear processes.

Results

TRIM27 is a new interaction partner of NOD2

Members of the TRIM protein family are emerging as important new regulators of innate immune responses. We were interested in whether TRIM proteins also contribute to NOD2 signaling. To search for TRIM proteins that physically interact with human NOD2, we conducted a yeast two-hybrid screen with a panel of human TRIM proteins as bait and NOD2 as prey. This identified interactions of NOD2 with TRIM8, TRIM27, and TRIM50 (Figure S1A). Of note, we observed homointeractions for all TRIM proteins indicating a correct folding [39]. Furthermore, TRIM27 formed heterointeractions with TRIM8 and TRIM18 (Figure S1A). Next, we verified interactions of NOD2 with TRIM8, TRIM27, and TRIM50. To this end, co-immunoprecipitations in human embryonic kidney (HEK293T) cells expressing Flag-NOD2 and myc-tagged TRIM proteins were performed. We observed interaction of NOD2 with TRIM27 (Figure 1A), but no robust interaction with the other TRIM proteins tested could be detected (data not shown). Importantly, NOD2 had a much higher binding affinity for TRIM27 than NOD1 (Figure 1A, 1B), which was confirmed by reciprocal co-immunoprecipitations (Figure 1B), suggesting specificity of the interaction.

To establish this interaction for endogenous TRIM27, we transfected HEK293T cells, which strongly express TRIM27 (Figure S2A), with Flag-NOD2 and immunoprecipitated NOD2. This revealed that also endogenous TRIM27 co-precipitated with NOD2 but not with the matrix alone (Figure 1C). Moreover, endogenous TRIM27 also bound endogenous NOD2 precipitated with the NOD2 specific antibody 6F6 (Figure S1B) from the colon cell line SW480 (Figure 1D). NOD2 is activated by MDP, a bacterial peptidoglycan fragment. To explore whether activation of NOD2 has an influence on NOD2-TRIM27 complex formation, we treated Nod2-expressing HEK293T cells with MDP prior to lysis. This revealed that NOD2 activation slightly increased its interaction with TRIM27 (Figure 1D).

To obtain additional *in vitro* evidence for the NOD2-TRIM27 interaction and to elucidate the necessary TRIM27 domain for interaction, we next performed protein-protein interaction assays. To this end, *in vitro*-transcribed and -translated NOD2 was incubated with recombinantly expressed, GST-tagged TRIM27 protein bound to glutathione-Sepharose. NOD2 strongly bound to TRIM27 WT and TRIM27 ΔRING and to a weaker extent to TRIM27 ΔRING+B-Box. Virtually no binding was observed to GST alone, which was used as control (Figure 1E). As reticulocyte lysates only contain a limited repertoire of endogenous proteins, this finding strongly suggest that the NOD2-TRIM27 interaction is direct. Collectively, these findings established that TRIM27 physically interacts with NOD2 in human cells.

TRIM27 PRY-SPRY and NOD2 NBD domains are sufficient for interaction

In order to elucidate the protein domains that mediate NOD2-TRIM27 interaction in more detail, we performed a series of co-immunoprecipitation experiments with NOD2 deletion mutants lacking the two CARD domains (ΔCARDs) or the LRRs (ΔLRR), or comprising only the CARD (CARDs) or NBD (NBD) domains (depicted in Figure 2A, upper panel). We found that NOD2 binding to TRIM27 was independent of the CARD domains and the LRRs. Instead, NOD2 NBD was sufficient to mediate the interaction (Figure 2A, lower panel). Of note, TRIM27 binding to NOD2 ΔLRR appeared to be stronger than to NOD2 WT. Next, we determined which domains in TRIM27 are needed for NOD2 binding. In agreement with our in vitro data (Figure 1E), deletion of the RING or both RING and B-Box domains did not abolish the interaction with NOD2. In contrast, we did not observe NOD2 binding to TRIM27 lacking the PRY-SPRY domain (TRIM27 ΔPRY-SPRY) (Figure 2B, lower panel). However, the expression of this construct was weak and we failed to obtain a

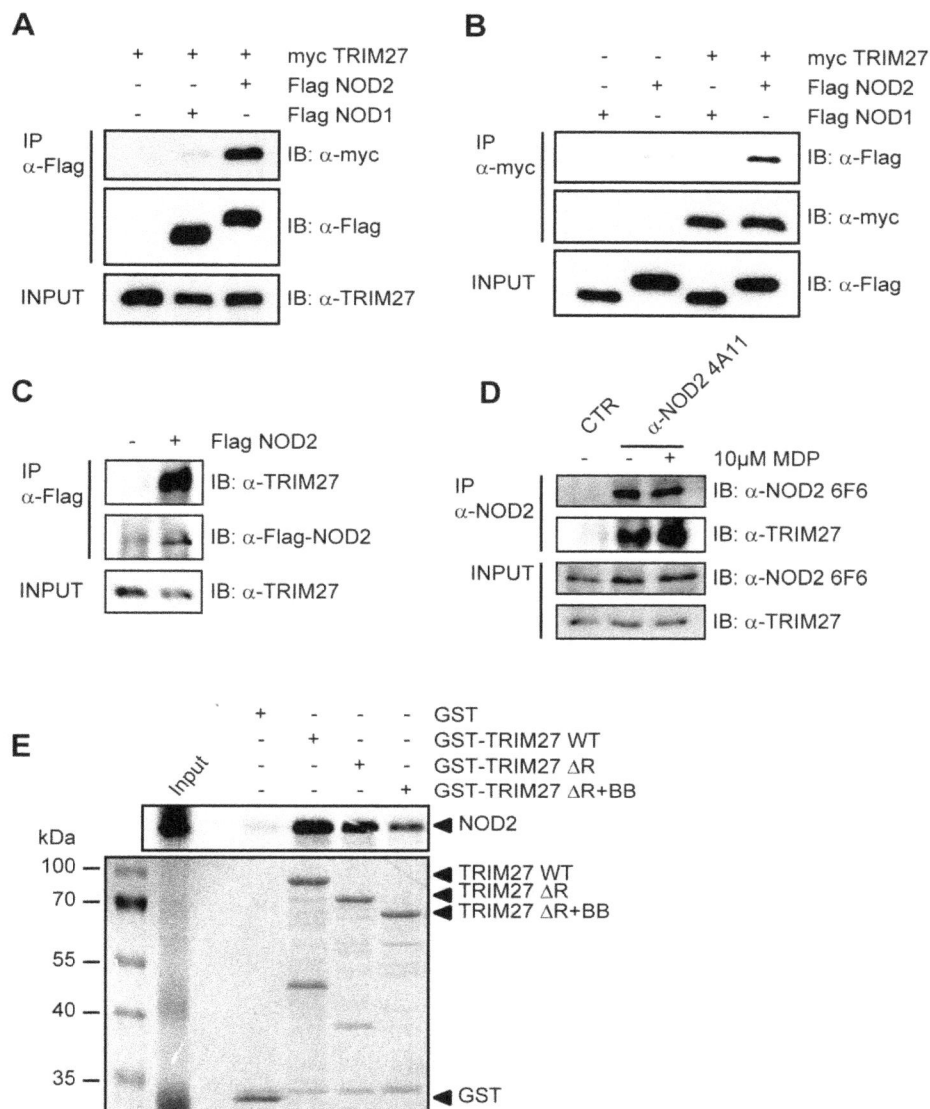

Figure 1. NOD2 physically interacts with TRIM27 via the NBD domain. A–C) Lysates of HEK293T cells expressing the indicated proteins were subjected to immunoprecipitation using anti-Flag (A and C) or anti-myc beads (B). Immunoblots of immunoprecipitates (IP) and total lysates (Input) were performed using the indicated antibodies. D) Immunoprecipitation of endogenous NOD2 from SW480 cells using the NOD2- specific monoclonal antibody 6F6. Cells were treated with 10 μM MDP for 3 h as indicated. Immunoblots of immunoprecipitates (IP) and total lysates (Input) were performed using the indicated antibodies. E) Protein-protein binding assays using *in vitro* transcribed and translated [35S]-methionine-labeled NOD2 and recombinant GST or GST-TRIM27 (WT, ΔRING or ΔRING+B-Box) bound to glutathione-Sepharose beads. The coomassie-stained gel (bottom) and the autoradiograph (top) of co-precipitated NOD2 are shown.

construct of this domain that expressed well in human cells. We thus cannot formally exclude that NOD2 weakly binds to this domain. However, we observed strong interaction of NOD2 with the TRIM27 PRY-SPRY domain alone (Figure 2B, lower panel), showing that the PRY-SPRY domain is sufficient for NOD2 binding.

TRIM27 contributes to NOD2 ubiquitination

To investigate if TRIM27 might be involved in ubiquitination of NOD2, we first determined basal NOD2 ubiquitination status in human cells. During expression in HEK293T cells, NOD2 but not NOD1 was poly-ubiquitinated at steady-state conditions as revealed by detection of conjugated HA-ubiquitin in immunopre-

cipitations of denatured lysates (Figure 3A). Using linkage-specific anti-ubiquitin antibodies we showed that the NOD2 ubiquitin chains reacted with an anti-K48-antibody (Figure 3B). Important-ly, RIP2, a known NOD2-interacting protein that is ubiquitinated upon NOD2 activation, did not significantly contribute to the ubiquitin signal detected in the NOD2 precipitate, as shown by siRNA-mediated depletion of RIP2 (Figure 3C). Recently, TRIM27 was shown to interact with a subset of E2 enzymes and to possess E3 ubiquitin ligase activity *in vitro* [28]. To investigate if TRIM27 contributes to the ubiquitination of NOD2, HEK293T cells were co-transfected with Flag-NOD2, myc-TRIM27 WT and HA-ubiquitin. The ubiquitin signal in NOD2 precipitates, detected either by anti-HA or the K48-linkage-specific antibody, was increased upon TRIM27 overexpression

(Figure 3D). In contrast, overexpression of a TRIM27 E3 ligase-deficient mutant (called 'TRIM27 E3' here), in which the two conserved catalytic cysteine residues within the TRIM27 RING domain (C16 and C31) were mutated to alanine, significantly reduced NOD2 ubiquitination compared to TRIM27 WT (Figure 3D). Of note, TRIM27 E3 still bound NOD2 to the same extent as TRIM27 WT, showing that this mutation did not affect binding affinity (Figure 3D).

Since NOD2 activation by MDP seemed to increase the binding affinity of the endogenous protein for TRIM27 (Figure 1D) we went on to explore in more detail how activation of NOD2 influences NOD2-TRIM27 complex formation and NOD2 ubiquitination. To this end, we performed co-immunoprecipitations in HEK293T cells expressing Flag-NOD2 and myc-TRIM27 following stimulation with 10 μM MDP at different time points. MDP induced NOD2 activation as monitored by IκBα degradation (Figure 3E). Moreover, binding of TRIM27 to NOD2 was enhanced over two-fold at 3 h after MDP stimulation compared to untreated controls and accordingly we observed a stronger ubiquitination of NOD2 after MDP treatment (Figure 3E).

Taken together, these data showed that NOD2 but not NOD1 is ubiquitinated and revealed a role for TRIM27 in this process, which was dependent on activation of NOD2.

TRIM27 contributes to proteasomal degradation of NOD2

K48-linked ubiquitination of proteins usually targets them for degradation by the 26S proteasome [40]. To investigate if NOD2 is subjected to proteasomal degradation, HEK293T cells expressing small amounts of Flag-NOD2 were treated with cycloheximide (CHX) to block protein neosynthesis and changes in NOD2 protein levels were followed by immunoblot analysis. This showed that NOD2 was readily degraded in a time-dependent manner (Figure 4A, upper panel), whereas NOD1 was not subjected to rapid protein turn-over (Figure S3A). TRIM27 WT overexpression only very slightly influenced the kinetic of NOD2 degradation (Figures 4A, upper panel, and S3B). However, overexpression of TRIM27 E3 strongly inhibited NOD2 degradation. This indicates that TRIM27 E3 acts as dominant negative over TRIM27 WT and endogenous TRIM27, which is expressed in these cells. To determine whether NOD2 degradation occurred via the 26S proteasome, we used the proteasome inhibitor bortezomib (MG-341). NOD2 degradation was inhibited in HEK293T cells expressing Flag-NOD2 treated with 100 nM bortezomib and poly-ubiquitinated NOD2 was strongly accumulated as early as 3 h after bortezomib treatment (Figure 4B).

To elucidate the contribution of endogenous TRIM27 on NOD2 degradation, TRIM27 expression was silenced in HEK293T using two different TRIM27-specific siRNA duplexes. Both siRNA duplexes reduced TRIM27 levels nearly to the detection limit as shown by immunoblot (Figure 4C). In cells transfected with non-targeting control siRNA NOD2 was readily degraded after CHX treatment as observed before (Figure 4C). In contrast, in cells treated with either of the two TRIM27-specific siRNA duplexes, NOD2 degradation was effectively inhibited.

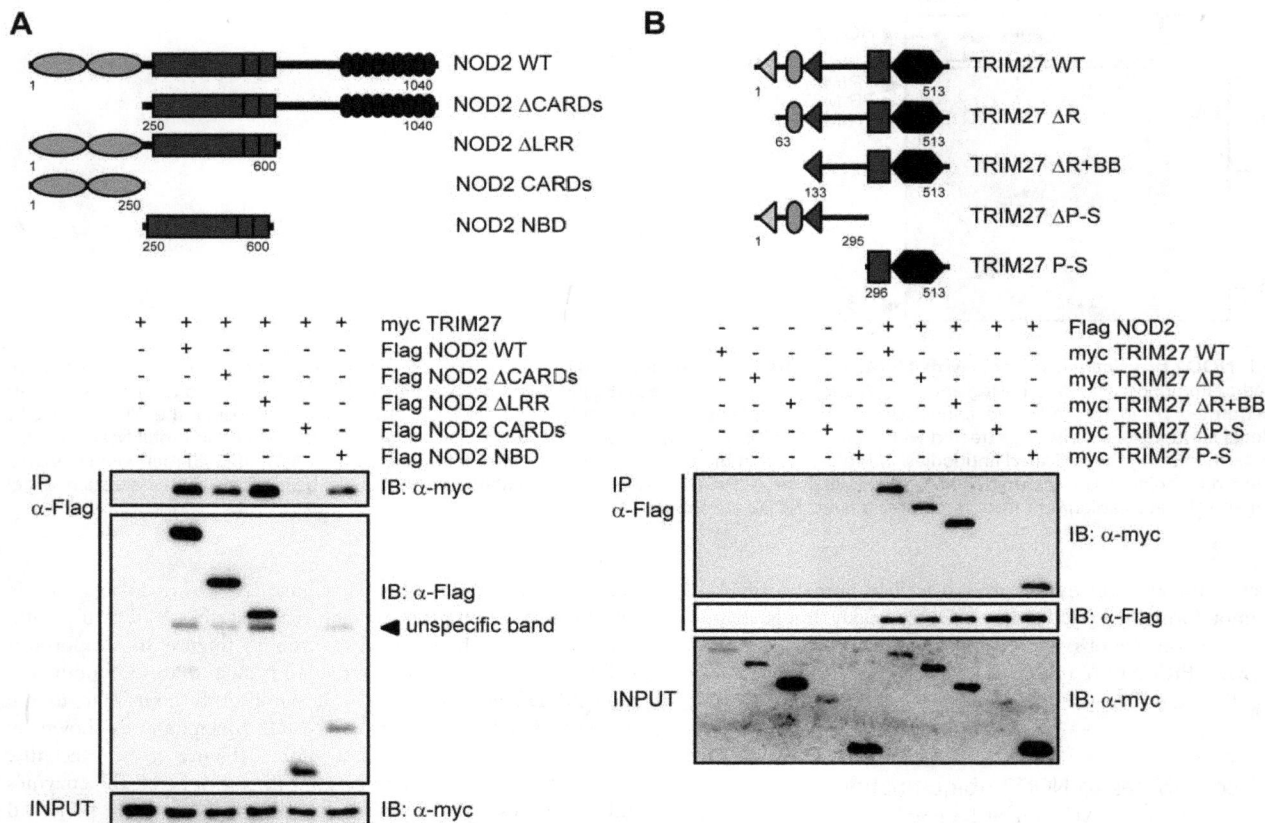

Figure 2. Mapping of the interaction domains in NOD2 and TRIM27. The depicted NOD2 (A) or TRIM27 (B) deletion constructs (upper panels) were used for the domain mapping. Lysates were subjected to immunoprecipitation using anti-Flag beads and immunoblotted with the indicated antibodies.

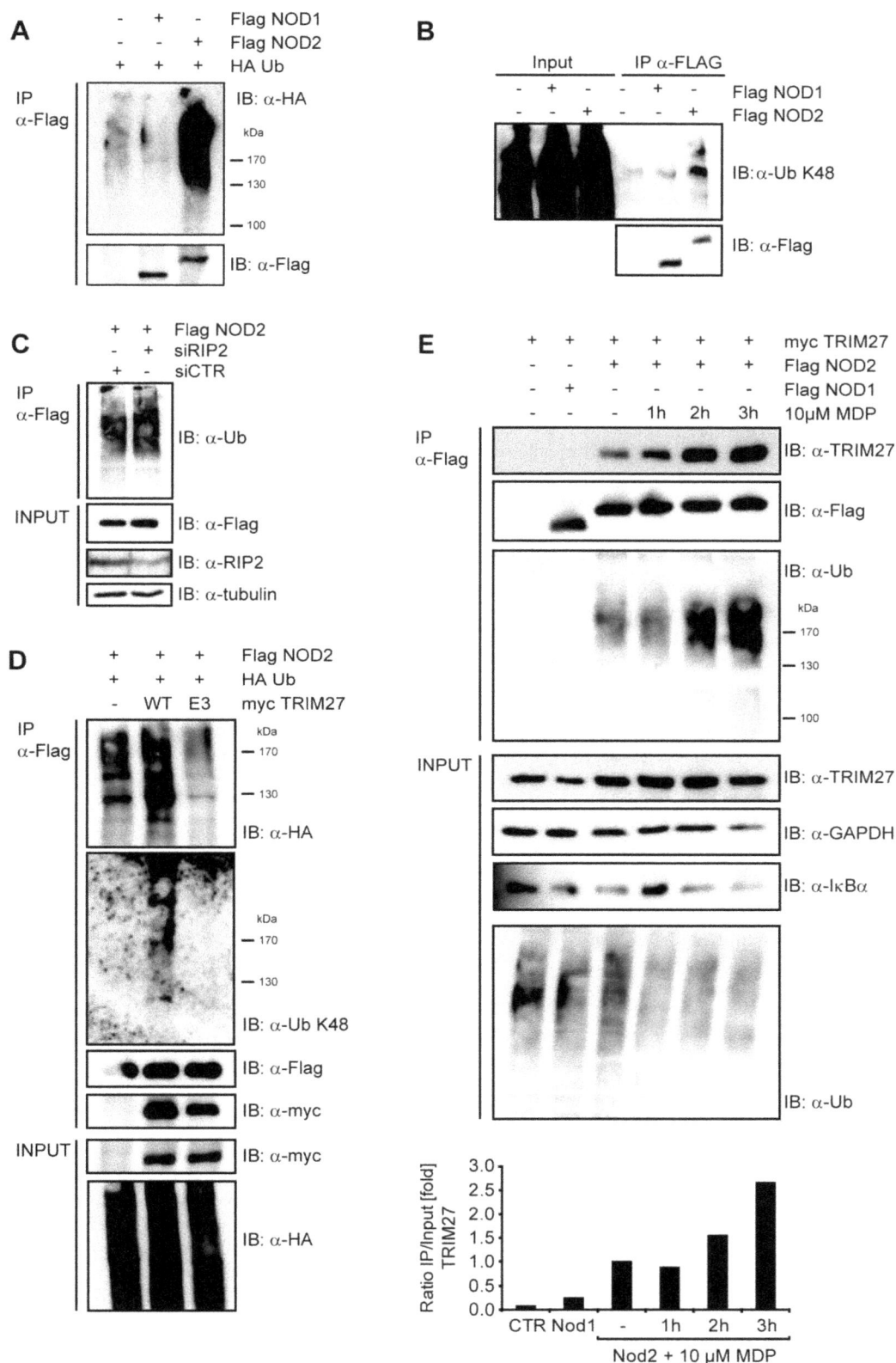

Figure 3. NOD2 is ubiquitinated. A) To determine NOD1 and NOD2 ubiquitination, denatured lysates of HEK293T cells expressing the indicated proteins were subjected to immunoprecipitation. Immunoprecipitates were immunoblotted using the indicated antibodies B) To determine the type of ubiquitin-linkage, lysates of HEK293T cells expressing the NOD1 or NOD2 were subjected to immunoprecipitation. Endogenous ubiquitin was revealed using a K48-link specific antibody. C) HEK293T cells were transfected for 72 h with siCTR, siTRIM27-1 or -3 after expression of Flag-NOD2 and HA-Ubiquitin. Immunoblots of immunoprecipitates (IP) and total lysates (Input) were performed using the indicated antibodies. D) TRIM27 and a E3

mutant of TRIM27 were expressed together with NOD2 and HA-ubiquitin in HEK293T cells. Immunoprecipitates were probed with the indicated antibodies. E) HEK293T cells expressing the indicated proteins were stimulated with 10 μM MDP for the indicated time. Lysates were subjected to immunoprecipitation as described in (C). Densitometric analysis of the TRIM27 signal in the immunoprecipitation normalized to the input signal is shown (bottom). Representative data of at least three independent experiments are shown.

Taken together, these data revealed that K48-linked ubiquitination occurred on NOD2 and that this targeted NOD2 for 26S proteasomal degradation in a TRIM27-dependent manner.

TRIM27 co-localized with ectopically expressed NOD2 in the nucleus

In HeLa cells, TRIM27 has been shown to localize to the nucleus [31], whereas in HEK293T cells TRIM27 is also found at distinct sub-cellular structures (Figure S2B, S2C). NOD2 has been shown to be a cytoplasmic protein that partially localizes to the plasma membrane [4–6], whereas other NLR proteins such as NLRC5 and CIITA also show nuclear localization [41–45]. We asked if NOD2 might also be able to shuttle to the nucleus and co-localize in this compartment with TRIM27 as previous experiments indicated that transiently overexpressed NOD2 is sometimes found in the nucleus [4]. To investigate this in more detail, we performed indirect immunofluorescence analysis in HeLa cells transfected with myc-NOD2 WT and blocked nuclear export using the specific nuclear export inhibitor leptomycin B (LMB). In the untreated samples, NOD2 WT mainly localized to the cytosol and was only partially found in the nucleus in less than 5% of the cells (Figure 5A, 5B). After LMB treatment, however, NOD2 WT was found in the nucleus in about 30% of the cells (Figure 5A, 5B). In contrast, NOD1 and a NOD2 Walker A mutant (K305R), which is unable to induce NF-κB activation [8], did not localize to the nucleus at all, even after LMB treatment (Figure 5A and Figure S2D). To substantiate these results, we prepared cytosolic and nuclear fractions from HEK293T cells expressing either Flag-NOD1, -NOD2 or -NOD2 K305R. Immunoprecipitation of the Flag-tagged proteins from the cytosolic and nuclear fractions revealed that a small portion of NOD2 was present in the nucleus without LMB treatment (Figure 5C). NOD2 nuclear localization was enhanced by about three-fold upon LMB treatment, as determined by normalized densitometric analysis (Figure 5C), which is in line with the data obtained in the cell-biological analysis. In contrast, NOD1 and NOD2 K305R were again found exclusively in the cytoplasm even after LMB treatment (Figure 5C). Importantly, also untagged NOD2 showed a nuclear enrichment after LMB treatment (Figure 5D), showing that nuclear localization of NOD2 is not an artifact of the epitope tag used above. Of note, the ability of NOD2 to trigger NF-κB activation upon MDP stimulation was unaffected when NOD2 was targeted to the nucleus by fusing it to a SV40 nuclear localization signal, showing that nuclear localization of NOD2 is not detrimental to its established function in bacterial sensing (data not shown).

Conclusively, our data show that at least ectopically expressed NOD2 is able to shuttle to the nucleus in a Walker A-dependent manner, which is reminiscent of the behavior of other NLRs, such as NLRC5 and CIITA [41–45].

TRIM27 negatively influences NOD2 signaling

Finally, we wanted to determine the influence of TRIM27 on NOD2-mediated signaling. In HEK293T cells, overexpression of TRIM27 significantly reduced MDP-induced NOD2-mediated NF-κB activation in a dose-dependent manner (Figure 6A). This effect of TRIM27 on NOD2-mediated signaling cannot be explained by inhibition of RIP2-NOD2 complex formation as NOD2 was still able to bind RIP2 in the presence of TRIM27

(Figure S4A). Importantly, TRIM27 overexpression had no significant influence on TNF-induced NF-κB activation (Figure 6B). Moreover, NF-κB activation induced by overexpression of IKK-β was also not significantly influenced by TRIM27 (Figure 6C), suggesting that TRIM27 acts upstream of the IKK-complex, likely at the level of NOD2.

Next, the effect of siRNA-mediated knock-down of endogenous TRIM27 on NOD2-mediated signaling was determined in THP1 cells that have a functional endogenous NOD2 signaling pathway [46] and express TRIM27 mRNA (Figure S2A). In line with a function of TRIM27 in regulating NOD2 signaling, although not significant, a tendency towards higher MDP-induced IL-8 secretion was observed with two different siRNAs tested (data not shown). This suggests that other described negative regulators of NOD2 can overcome missing regulation by TRIM27. Finally, to explore if TRIM27 expression might be linked to NOD2-associated diseases *in vivo*, we conducted immunohistological inspection of colon sections derived from healthy and active Crohn's disease (CD) patients. This showed that TRIM27 was well expressed in intestinal epithelial cells and to a lesser extent in cells of the lamina propria. In all these cells TRIM27 exhibited a primarily nuclear localization in these cells and appeared to be restricted to sub-nuclear compartments (Figure 6D). Of note, the TRIM27 signal appeared lower in healthy tissue compared to tissue derived from active Crohn's patients (Figure 6D). Analysis of TRIM27 mRNA expression in colon biopsy material of Crohn's disease patients confirmed a significant increase in TRIM27 expression in CD compared to healthy controls (Figure 6E).

Collectively, these data support a role for TRIM27 as a specific negative regulator of NOD2-mediated signaling and suggest a implication of TRIM27 in Crohn's disease.

Discussion

In this paper we report the identification of the E3 ubiquitin ligase TRIM27 as a new interaction partner for NOD2. Mapping studies indicated that NOD2 binds via its NBD domain to the TRIM27 B30.2/PRY-SPRY domain. The B30.2 domain is composed of the ~61 aa PRY and the ~140 aa SPRY domain and is most commonly found at the C-terminus of TRIM proteins [18]. The SPRY domain is evolutionarily more ancient as it is found in animals, plants and fungi, whereas the B30.2 domain is only found in vertebrates with an adaptive immune system [47]. In humans, B30.2/PRY-SPRY domains are only present at the C-terminus in TRIM proteins and in butyrophilin-related transmembrane glycoproteins (BTNs), which are receptors of the immunoglobulin superfamily [48]. Of note, the TRIM27 binding site for NOD2 correlates with the findings for other TRIM proteins: TRIM21 binds its interaction partners IRF3 and IRF8 via the B30.2/PRY-SPRY domain [49–51] and TRIM25 binds RIG-I via the C-terminal SPRY domain [52]. TRIM20 (also known as pyrin), regulates caspase-1 activation and IL-1β production by interacting with caspase-1 via its PRY-SPRY and with ASC via its PYD domain, respectively [53–55]. Mutations in the human TRIM20 PRY-SPRY domain are associated with inherited Familial Mediterranean Fever (FMF). TRIM20 knock-in mice expressing a TRIM20 with the mutant human PRY-SPRY domain reflect the inflammatory phenotype found in patients by

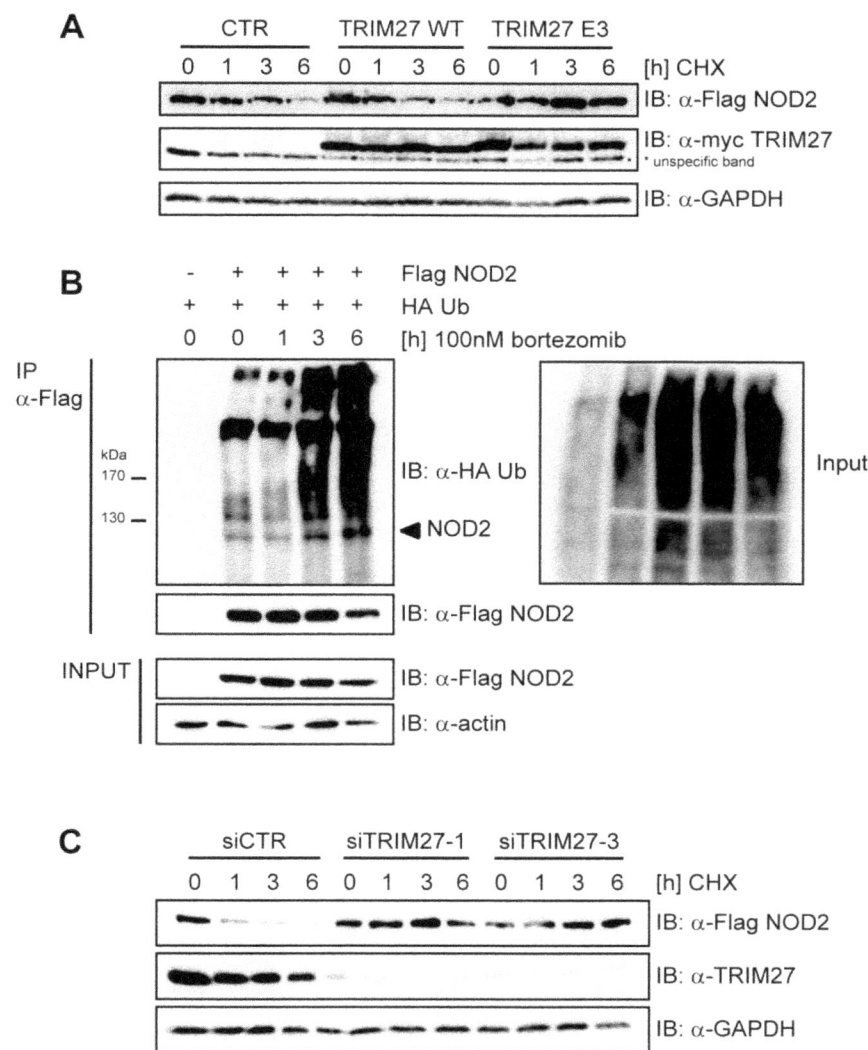

Figure 4. TRIM27 contributes to proteasomal degradation of NOD2. A) HEK293T cells transfected with low amounts of Flag-NOD2 and myc-TRIM27, E3 or CTR as indicated were treated with 30 µg/ml cyclohexímid (CHX) and immunoblots of total cell lysates (top) were performed using the indicated antibodies. GAPDH served as loading control. B) HEK293T cells expressing the indicated proteins were treated with 100 nM bortezomib. Lysates were subjected to immunoprecipitation as described in Figure 1A. Actin served as loading control. C) HEK293T cells transfected for 48 h with siCTR, siTRIM27-1 or -3 and subsequently with Flag-NOD2 were treated with 30 µg/ml CHX, as indicated. Immunoblots of total cell lysates were performed using the indicated antibodies. GAPDH served as loading control. Representative data of at least three independent experiments are shown (see also Fig. S3B).

forming spontaneous ASC-dependent, NLRP3-independent inflammasomes [56]. This clearly links the PRY-SPRY domain in TRIM20 to immune functions. Another intriguing example underscoring the involvement of PRY-SPRY domains in NLR regulation is present in zebrafish (*Danio rerio*). One class of NLR proteins in *D. rerio* comprises molecules harboring a PRY-SPRY domain fused to the canonical NLR sequence [57]. Of note, PRY-SPRY domains from *D. rerio* NLRs are closely related to zebrafish TRIMs, indicating domain shuffling during evolution [58]. This suggests that TRIM and NLR proteins have been tied together in evolution to function in innate immune responses.

TRIM proteins are involved in the regulation of PRR- and IFN-signaling pathways, typically by acting as ubiquitin ligases. TRIM-mediated ubiquitination events have been documented to both enhance immune response as shown i.e. for TRIM8, TRIM21, TRIM23, TRIM25 and TRIM56 [49,51,52,59–61] or inhibit

them as shown for TRIM21 and TRIM30-α [50,62,63]. We show here that also TRIM27 is involved in regulating PRR-signaling by negatively regulating NOD2. We observed that NOD2 is ubiquitinated by K48-linked ubiquitin chains and that this ubiquitination is enhanced by TRIM27 overexpression, whereas overexpression of an E3 ligase-deficient mutant of TRIM27 (TRIM27 E3) reduces NOD2 ubiquitination (Figure 4).

K48-linked ubiquitination usually targets proteins to degradation [40], which is partly mediated by TRIM proteins in PRR- and IFN-signaling pathways: Mouse TRIM30-α promotes ubiquitination and degradation – although not by proteasomal but rather by lysosomal degradation – of TAB2 and TAB3 thereby inhibiting TLR-induced NF-κB activation [63], whereas TRIM8 decreases SOCS-1 protein levels leading to an inhibition of IFN-γ-signaling repression by SOCS-1 [59]. Ubiquitinated NOD2 is also targeted to proteasomal degradation, as inhibition of the 26S proteasome

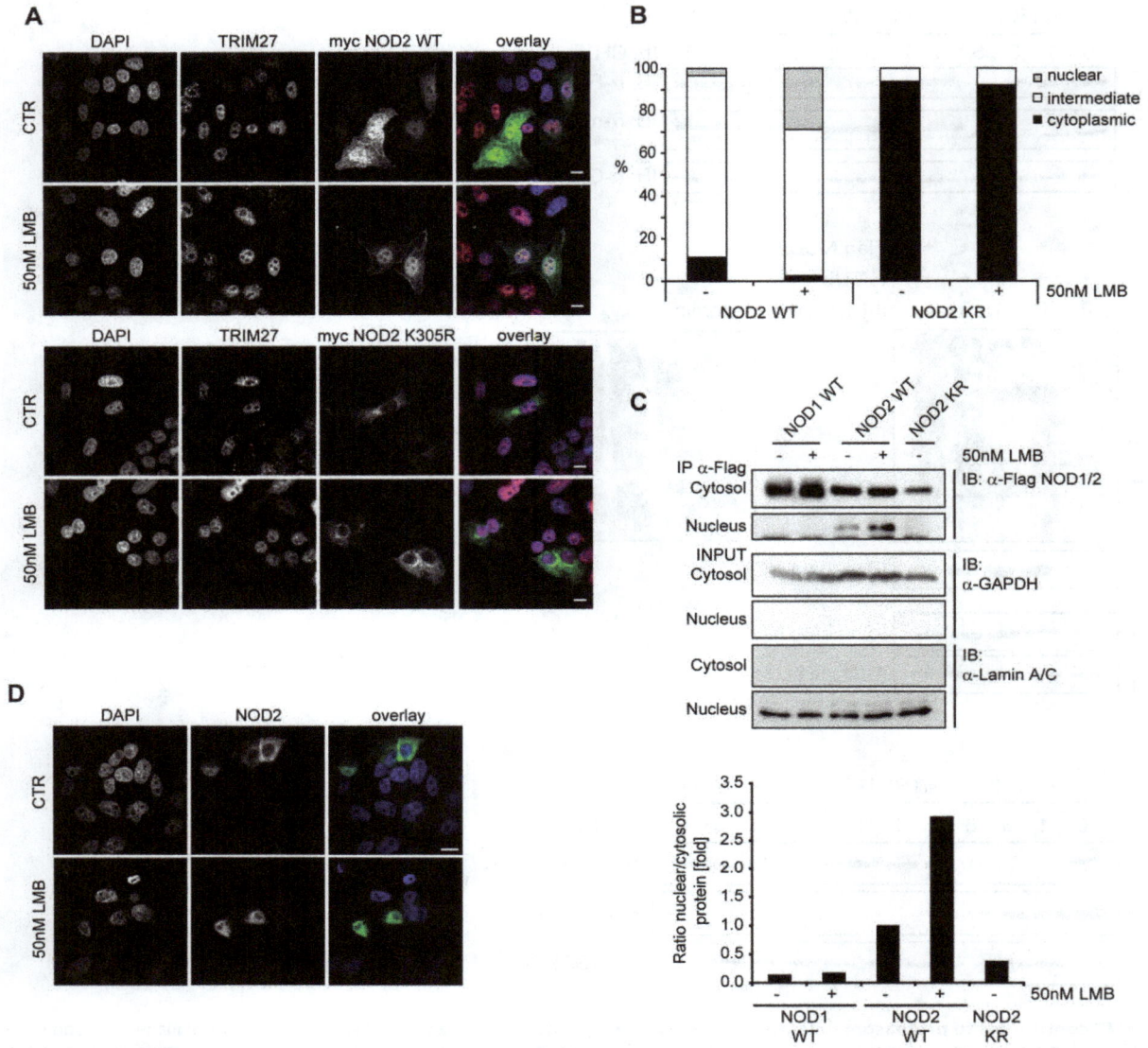

Figure 5. NOD2 WT localizes to the nucleus whereas NOD2 K305R or NOD1 do not. A) Indirect immunofluorescence micrographs of HeLa cells grown on coverslips and expressing myc-NOD2 WT (top) or myc-NOD2 K305R (bottom) were treated with 50 nM leptomycine B (LMB) for 4 h or left untreated. Images with signals for DAPI, TRIM27, myc-NOD2 and an overlay (blue: DAPI, red: TRIM27, green: NOD2) are shown. B) Quantification of NOD2 subcellular localization in HeLa cells expressing Flag-NOD2 WT or K305R, as indicated (n = 100). Data is representative of two independent experiments. C) Cellular fractions of HEK293T cells transfected with Flag-NOD1, -NOD2 WT or -NOD2 K305R, as indicated, and treated as described in A were generated. Immunoblots of precipitated protein and total lysates are shown. For densitometric analysis, cytosolic and nuclear signals were normalized to GAPDH and Lamin A/C, respectively. The ratio of nuclear to cytosolic protein is shown in fold. Representative data of at least three independent experiments are shown. D) Indirect immunofluorescence micrographs of HeLa cells expressing untagged-NOD2 WT treated with 50 nM leptomycine B (LMB) for 4 h or left untreated. Bars, 10 μm.

with bortezomib led to NOD2 protein stability and accumulation of ubiquitinated NOD2 (Figure 4B). Of note, NOD2 protein stability is effectively dependent on TRIM27. This is evidenced by the finding that knock-down of endogenous TRIM27 as well as overexpression of TRIM27 E3 inhibited NOD2 degradation (Figure 4A and 4C). The latter indicates that TRIM27 E3 acts as dominant negative over WT TRIM27 and endogenous TRIM27. We were surprised that overexpression of TRIM27 did not correlate with reduced NOD2 protein stability. Our interpretation is that this might be due to the activity of endogenous TRIM27 that might be sufficient to target even ectopically expressed NOD2 efficiently for degradation or that degradation at the proteasome is rate-limiting for overexpressed NOD2. TRIM27 has also been shown to confer SUMO E3 ligase activity [29]. However, we did not detect SUMOylated NOD2, suggesting that NOD2 might not be a substrate for TRIM27-mediated SUMOylation (data not shown). In most cases, proteins are ubiquitinated in the cytosol and are degraded in this compartment. However, also evidence for nuclear ubiquitination and protein degradation exists [64]. Based on our results showing that only a small fraction of NOD2 seems to shuttle to the nucleus (Figure 5) we suggest that NOD2 might be ubiquitinated in the cytoplasm.

Regulation of PRRs by ubiquitination and proteasomal degradation is a common theme for PRRs in animals and plants:

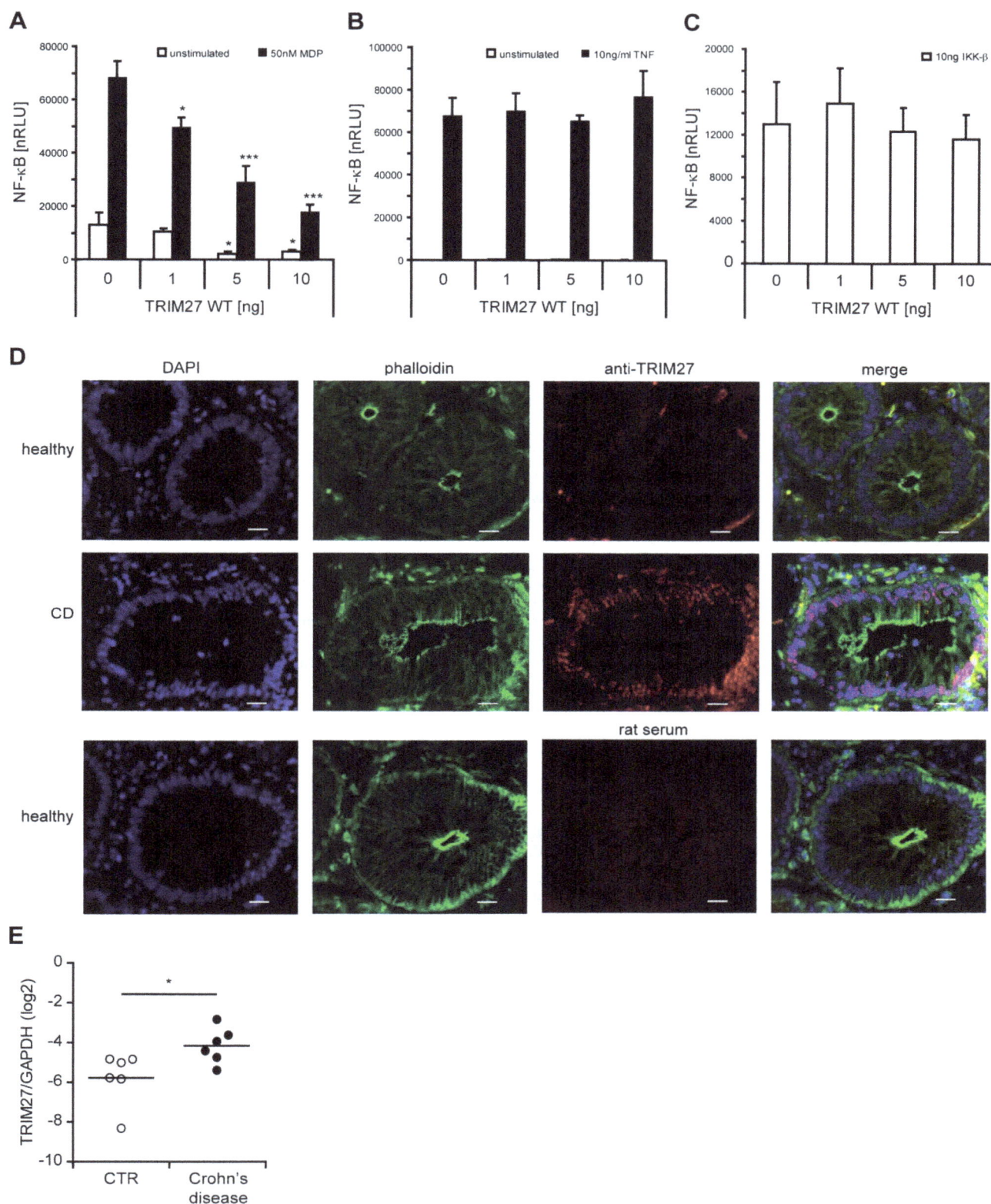

Figure 6. TRIM27 negatively regulates NOD2 signaling. A–C) NF-κB luciferase assays in HEK293T cells to determine the influence of TRIM27 overexpression on MDP-induced NOD2-mediated (A), TNF- (B), or IKK-β-induced (C) NF-κB activation. Normalized luciferase activity (nRLU) of unstimulated (white bars) and stimulated (black bars) samples is shown. Values are given as mean+SD (n = 3). *, P<0.05; ***, P<0.005. D. Sections from human colon derived from healthy and active Crohn's disease patients. Staining with DAPI (blue), phalloidin-FITC (green) and with α-TRIM27 antibody (red) is shown. Staining with a rat serum is shown as control in the lower panel (rat serum). Slides are representative for 3 control and 4 Crohn's disease patients. Scale bar = 20 μm. E. qRT-PCR of TRIM27 mRNA expression in colonic biopsies derived from patients with Crohn's disease

and controls (CTR) with no evidence of mucosal inflammation. Each symbol represents one patient. TRIM27 mRNA expression normalized to GAPDH is shown. *, P<0.05 (n = 6).

Triad3A is known to control TLR4 and TLR9 signaling [65] and plant FLS2 has been shown to be ubiquitinated and degraded in a negative feedback-loop by PUB12/13 [66]. Our data suggest that NOD2 signaling is regulated in a similar manner. Indeed, gene reporter assays in HEK293T cells showed that TRIM27 overexpression specifically reduces NOD2-mediated MDP-induced NF-κB activation in a dose-dependent manner, whereas TNF- and IKK-β-induced NF-κB activation is not affected. The negative regulating effects of TRIM27 on NOD2 signaling are not necessarily explained by NOD2 degradation but might also be due to circumvention of adaptor protein recruitment to the NOD2 complex. However, TRIM27 did not inhibit NOD2-RIP2 interaction (Figure S4A). In contrast to our findings, Zha et al. reported that TRIM27 interacts with IKK-α, IKK-β, IKK-ε and negatively regulates NF-κB, IFN-β and ISRE activation induced by these kinases in a RING-domain-independent manner [36]. The discrepancies between the two data sets remain unclear and need further independent investigation.

In contrast to most TRIM proteins, TRIM27 expression is not altered in response to IFNs [16,17]. Among the TRIM proteins induced by type I and II IFNs, many have been shown to confer antiviral activity, although IFN-inducibility is not a prerequisite for this [17,39]. Constitutively expressed TRIM proteins have also been shown to trigger antiviral immune responses. TRIM27 overexpression, however, did not influence Sendai virus-induced IFN-β activation (Figure S4B). We therefore assume that TRIM27 might predominantly function in other pathways including NOD2 signaling.

NOD2 has been reported to be localized in the cytosol and at the cell membrane at steady-state conditions. Unexpectedly, we found that ectopically expressed NOD2, in contrast to NOD1, can shuttle to the nucleus (Figure 5), dependently on a functional Walker A motif, i.e. ATPase activity. Although, a strong bipartite nuclear localization signal (NLS) in the NOD2 sequence could not be identified. Due to the low expression of endogenous NOD2, we were not able to establish the sub-cellular localization of endogenous NOD2. So although nuclear shuttling was verified for both NOD2 and epitope-tagged versions of NOD2 ectopically expressed in different cells by both cell biological and biochemical techniques, we cannot formally exclude that this is a particularity of ectopically expressed NOD2. Of note, also two other members of the human NLR family are known to shuttle to the nucleus. CIITA, one of the founding members of the NLR family, has long been recognized to regulate MHC class II gene expression by acting as a scaffold for DNA-binding transcription factor assembly in the nucleus [67,68]. Recently, also NLRC5 has been shown to localize to the nucleus and to regulate MHC class I expression [44,45,69]. Of note, nuclear translocation and functionality are also shown for several NLR-related plant R proteins. For tobacco N, barley MLA, arabidopsis RPS4 and potato RX R proteins nuclear localization is essential for defense activation [70–73]. For these it has been suggested that pathogen recognition takes place in the cytoplasm, whereas they act in the nucleus to induce transcriptional reprogramming to activate immune responses [74]. This is exemplified by the tobacco N protein, which confers resistance to Tobacco mosaic virus (TMV). Here MAP kinase activation in the cytosol is necessary for N-mediated resistance in addition to its nuclear functions [75,76]. In analogy, it is tempting to speculate if NOD2 might not only recognize pathogens and activate MAP kinases and NF-κB in the cytosol, but likely possess

additional nuclear functions to mediate and control immune responses. TRIM27 is known to be recruited to specific subnuclear compartments [33] and was suggested as a transcriptional repressor [34,35]. This raises the intriguing possibility that TRIM27, in addition to its role in NOD2 regulation, might be functionally involved in orchestrating NOD2 nuclear functions. Future research might help to address these open questions.

We and others recently demonstrated that some mutations in the NBD domain of NOD2 can result in enhanced NF-κB activation, whereas the corresponding mutations do not increase the activity of NOD1 [77]. This suggests that NOD2 is more prone for autoactivation compared to NOD1, requesting tighter control mechanisms to act on NOD2 to prevent unwanted auto-inflammatory responses. This is in line with the findings that I) more negative regulators are reported for NOD2 than for NOD1 [78,79], II) there are more disease-associated mutations found in NOD2 than in NOD1 [11], and III) NOD1 is expressed at basal levels in most tissues whereas NOD2 expression is more restricted and can be induced by pathogen stimuli [8,80–84]. Here, we add another difference between NOD1 and NOD2 regulation and show that NOD2, but not NOD1, is controlled by ubiquitination and subsequent proteasomal degradation dependent on TRIM27 E3 ligase activity. We identified TRIM27 as a negative regulator of NOD2-mediated inflammatory responses and detected enhanced TRIM27 expression in the colon of Crohn's disease patients. Clinically, this makes TRIM27 an interesting new target for NOD2-associated diseases. It is conceivable that targeting TRIM27 might be advantageous when NOD2 activity is altered, such as in Crohn's disease.

Materials and Methods

Plasmids

Plasmids encoding N-terminally Flag-tagged NOD1, NOD2 and deletion constructs of NOD2 (ΔCARD: aa250–1040; ΔLRR: aa1–600; CARD: aa1–250; NBD: aa250–600; LRR: aa600–1040) have been described [4,85]. Myc-NOD1 WT, myc-NOD2 WT and K305R were obtained by subcloning (BamHI-XhoI) into a modified pcDNA3.1 vector containing an N-terminal 3xmyc tag. Human TRIM27 cDNA was obtained from ImaGenes (Berlin, Germany) (GI 115387097). Full length TRIM27 and deletion constructs (ΔRING: aa63–513; ΔRING+BBox: aa133–513; ΔPRY-SPRY: aa1–295; PRY-SPRY: aa296–513) were generated by PCR and cloned into pGEX-II (kindly provided by I. Roux, Institute Pasteur, Paris) or a modified pcDNA3.1 vector (see above). Point mutations of myc-TRIM27 E3 ligase mutant (CC16/31AA) were generated by PCR mutagenesis according to the QuikChange Site-Directed Mutagenesis procedure (Stratagene). IFN-β luciferase reporter was a kind gift from M. Schröder (NUI Maynooth), IgK luciferase NF-κB-reporter and β-galactosidase expression plasmid were described previously [4]. VSV-tagged RIP2 was a kind gift from M. Thome (University Lausanne). The IKK-β plasmid was purchased from InvivoGen. pRK5-HA-ubiquitin (Addgene plasmid 17608) is described in [86]. All constructs were subjected to full-length DNA sequencing.

Two-hybrid analysis

Binary two-hybrid screening was performed as described by Gyuris et al. [87]. Briefly, the bait plasmids (pEG202) express the cDNA fused directionally to the first 202 residues of LexA under the control of the constitutive ADH promoter. Prey plasmids (pJG4-5) express the cDNA fused to the B42 activation domain, the SV40T nuclear localization signal and an HA-tag under the control of the inducible GAL1 promoter. EGY42/EGY48 diploid strain was generated by mating for every pairwise combination. Six LexA-operators lacZ in the pSH18-34 vector and a genome integrated 4 LexA-operators LEU2 are used as reporters. The expression of two reporters was used to establish the interaction, blue-turning colonies and growth in the absence of Leu.

Cell culture and siRNA

HEK293T cells were kindly provided by the Sansonetti lab (Institute Pasteur, Paris) [4], HeLa (ATCC #CCL-2) and SW480 (ATCC #CCL-228) cells were obtained from the ATCC. Cells were cultivated at 37°C in a 5% CO$_2$ atmosphere in Dulbecco's modified Eagle's medium (Biochrom AG) supplemented with 10% heat-inactivated fetal bovine serum (Biowest), penicillin and streptomycin (100 IU/ml and 100 mg/ml, respectively; Biochrom AG). Cells were continuously tested for absence of mycoplasma contamination by PCR.

All siRNA duplexes were obtained from Qiagen: siCTR (AllStars Negative Control, #1027281); siTRIM27-1 (target sequence AAGACTCAGTGTGCAGAAAAG); siTRIM27-3 (target sequence CAGAACCAGCTCGACCATTTA, Hs_RFP_6, SI03062794); siNOD2 (target sequence CTGCCACATGCAAGAAGTATA; Hs_CARD15_3, SI00133049); siRIP2 (target sequence ACGTATGATCTCTCTAATAGA).

Co-immunoprecipitation and immunoblotting

For co-immunoprecipitations, HEK293T cells were seeded in 6 cm dishes and were transiently transfected with 1 µg plasmid as indicated using Lipofectamin2000 (Invitrogen) or FuGene6 (Roche). Cells were lysed in NP40 buffer (150 mM NaCl, 50 mM Tris pH 7.4, 1% NP40) or RIPA buffer (150 mM NaCl, 50 mM Tris pH 7.4, 1% Triton X-100, 0.1% SDS, 0.5% deoxycholate) containing phosphatase inhibitors (20 µM β-glycerophosphate, 5 mM NaF, 100 µM Na$_3$VO$_4$) and protease inhibitors (Complete protease inhibitor cocktail with EDTA; Roche). Lysates were cleared for 20 min at 14,000× g at 4°C. Flag-tagged NOD2 was immunoprecipitated with anti-Flag beads (M2 agarose; Sigma), myc-tagged TRIM27 with anti-myc beads (c-myc AC, clone 9E10; Santa Cruz Biotechnology) for 3 h at 4°C. Beads were washed five times with lysis buffer before SDS loading buffer containing β-mercaptoethanol was added. Typically, 10-times more precipitate than input was loaded onto the gel. Proteins were separated by Laemmli sodium dodecylsulfate-polyacrylamide gel electrophoresis (SDS-PAGE) and subsequently transferred on nitrocellulose membrane (Bio-Rad) by semi-dry immunoblotting. Proteins were detected by incubation of the membrane successive with primary and secondary antibody and a final incubation with SuperSignal West Pico Chemiluminescent Substrate or Femto Maximum Sensitivity Substrate (Pierce). Signals were recorded on an electronic imaging system (LAS4000, Fujifilm). Primary antibodies were mouse anti-Flag M2 (1:2000; Stratagene), rabbit anti-myc (1:500; A-14, Santa Cruz Biotechnology), rabbit anti-TRIM27 (1:400; IBL), rabbit anti-HA (1:500; Y-11, Santa Cruz Biotechnology), mouse anti-ubiquitin (1:500; Santa Cruz Biotechnology), mouse anti-ubiquitin K48 (1:1000; Millipore), mouse anti-ubiquitin K63 (1:1000; Millipore), rat anti-NOD2 4A11 (1:100; [4]), rabbit anti-lamin A/C (1:500; Cell Signaling Technology), rabbit anti-GAPDH (1:1000; Santa Cruz Biotechnology) and rabbit anti-actin (1:1000; A2066, Sigma-Aldrich). Secondary antibodies were horseradish peroxidase (HRP)-conjugated goat anti-mouse IgG, light chain specific (1:4000; Jackson ImmunoR-

esearch Laboratories), HRP-conjugated goat anti-mouse IgG (1:4000; 170-6516, Bio-Rad), HRP-conjugated goat anti-rabbit IgG (1:4000; 170-6515, Bio-Rad) and HRP-conjugated goat anti-rat IgG (1:4000; Jackson ImmunoResearch Laboratories). All antibodies were diluted in 5% milk in PBS or TBS, according to the manufacturer's instructions.

Endogenous NOD2 was immunoprecipitated from SW480 cells lysed in NP40 buffer using the NOD2 specific monoclonal rat antibody 6F6 [6] bound to Protein-G Sepharose beads.

For testing for ubiquitination of NOD2, HEK293T cells were lysed in NP40 buffer containing 1% SDS and boiled for 10 min. Immunoprecipitations were conducted from these samples diluted 1:10 in NP40 buffer as described above.

Expression of recombinant GST-TRIM27

TRIM27 and its deletion constructs were expressed as N-terminal glutathione S-transferase (GST) fusion proteins in Rosetta2 (DE3) pLys E.coli cells (kindly provided by G. Praefcke) following overnight isopropyl 1-thio-β-d-galactopyranoside (IPTG, 100 µM; Sigma) induction at 20°C. Bacteria were lysed by a freeze-and-thaw cycle followed by addition of 1.5% sarkosyl (Sigma) and sonication. All GST fusion proteins were purified from bacterial extracts with glutathione-Sepharose (Amersham Biosciences), followed by extensive washing with buffer A (150 mM NaCl, 50 mM Tris pH 7.5, 2 mM DTT), buffer B (500 mM NaCl, 50 mM Tris pH 7.5, 2 mM DTT) and again buffer A. TRIM27 protein bound to glutathione-Sepharose was stored in buffer A at −80°C.

In vitro translation and GST-binding assay

In vitro transcription/translation (IVT) of NOD2 was performed from the Flag-NOD2 construct by T7 RNA polymerase (Promega) in the presence of L-[35S]-methionine (10 mCi/ml; Perkin Elmer) using the TnT coupled reticulocyte lysate system (Promega) according to the manufacturer's instructions. IVT preparation was diluted three times in PBS and incubated with recombinant TRIM27 protein bound to glutathione-Sepharose beads for 2 h at 4°C. Beads were precipitated and washed five times with RIPA buffer (150 mM NaCl, 50 mM Tris pH 7.4, 1% Triton, 0.1% SDS, 0.5% deoxycholate) before SDS loading buffer containing β-mercaptoethanol was added. Proteins were analyzed by Laemmli sodium dodecylsulfate-polyacrylamide gel electrophoresis (SDS-PAGE) followed by Coomassie brilliant blue staining. Autoradiographs were recorded using a PhosphorImager (Bio-Rad).

Indirect immunofluorescence microscopy

For indirect immunofluorescence microscopy, HeLa cells were seeded in 24-well plates on glass coverslips and transiently transfected with 0.8 µg of expression plasmids, as indicated using Lipofectamin2000 transfection reagent (Invitrogen) according to the manufacturer's instructions. After 24 h, cells were fixed with 3% paraformaldehyde (Roth) in PBS for 10 min and permeabilized with 0.5% Triton X-100 (Roth) in cold PBS for 5 min. Cells were blocked in 3% bovine serum albumin (BSA; Roth) in PBS for 20 min and incubated successively in primary and secondary antibodies. Primary antibodies: rabbit anti-TRIM27 (1:500; IBL) and mouse anti-myc (1:1000; 9E10, Sigma). Secondary antibody: goat anti-rabbit AlexaFluor 546 (1:250; Invitrogen Molecular Probes) and goat anti-mouse AlexaFluor 488 (1:250; Invitrogen Molecular Probes). DNA was stained with DAPI (5 µg/ml; Invitrogen Molecular Probes). Cells were mounted in ProLong Gold antifade reagent (Invitrogen Molecular Probes). Image acquisition of z-stacks was performed on an Olympus FV-1000 laser scanning microscope (objective: Olympus PlanApo, 60×/

1.40 oil, ∞/0.17) and images were processed using the ImageJ software [88].

Sub-cellular fractionation

For fractionation, HEK293T cells were seeded in 10 cm dishes and transiently transfected with 3 µg plasmid as indicated. After 24 h, cellular fractions were prepared using the Qproteome cell compartment kit (Qiagen). Flag-tagged proteins in the different fractions were precipitated using anti-Flag beads as described above.

Luciferase reporter assay

3×10^4 HEK293T cells per well were seeded in 96-well plates and transfected with 8.6 ng β-galactosidase, 13 ng luciferase NF-κB- or 10 ng IFN-β-reporter, different amounts of myc-TRIM27 and either with or without 0.1 ng NOD2 or 10 ng IKK-β expression plasmids as indicated, added up with pcDNA to 51 ng total DNA using FuGene6 (Roche). Cells were directly stimulated with 50 nM MDP, 10 ng/ml TNF (all obtained from InvivoGen) or 133 hemagglutination units (HAU)/ml Sendai virus (hen egg allantoid fluid; obtained from Charles River Laboratories) or left unstimulated, as indicated. After 16 h, cells were lysed in luciferase lysis buffer (25 mM Tris pH 8, 8 mM $MgCl_2$, 1% Triton, 15% glycerol, 1 mM DTT) and luciferase activity was measured using a standard plate luminometer. Standard deviation (SD) was calculated from triplets and luciferase activity was normalized as a ratio to β-galactosidase activity. All experiments were repeated independently at least three times.

RT-PCR

End point RT-PCR was performed using *Taq* polymerase (Fermentas) on cDNA obtained from isolated RNA of the indicated cell lines. RNA was isolated using the RNeasy kit (Qiagen) and 1 µg of total RNA was transcribed into cDNA using the First Strand cDNA synthesis kit (Fermentas) with an oligo (dT) primer (Fermentas). Primers for TRIM27 were obtained from Qiagen (QT00051954). For GAPDH, the following primer pair was used: GAPDH_fwd, GGTATCGTGGAAGGACTCAT-GAC; and GAPDH_rev, ATGCCAGTGAGCTTCCCGTT-CAG. The PCR products were separated by agarose gel electrophoresis and visualized using ethidium bromide.

qRT-PCR of TRIM27 from patient samples

Endoscopic biopsies were taken from the sigmoid colon of patients with mildly to moderately active Crohn's disease and controls. Only patients with no endoscopic or histological evidence of mucosal inflammation were included in the control group. Written informed consent was obtained from all patients before endoscopy. The study was approved by the local ethical committee of the University Hospital Aachen, Germany. Biopsies were immediately shock-frozen in liquid nitrogen and stored at −80°C. RNA from frozen tissue biopsies was isolated using PegGOLD RNAPure (PEQLAB Biotechnology) according to the manufacturer's instructions. 2 µg of RNA were treated with DNAseI (Invitrogen) before cDNA was generated by reverse transcription with 200 ng random hexamer primer (Invitrogen), 500 µM dNTPs (Invitrogen) and 4 U Omniscript Reverse Transcriptase (Quiagen) in 1× reverse transcriptase buffer for 1 h at 37°C. Real-time PCR was performed using Real Time PCR System 7300 (Applied Biosystems) and SYBRGreenER qPCR Super Mix (Invitrogen). TRIM27 expression levels were normalized to GAPDH. Primers for TRIM27 were obtained from Qiagen (QT00051954). For GAPDH, the following primer pair was used:

GAPDH_fwd,   CAGCCTCAAGATCATCAGCA;   and GAPDH_rev, CCTTCCACGATACCAAAGTTGTC.

Immunfluorescence microscopy of human specimens

Colon biopsies from Crohn's disease and control patients were obtained during colonoscopy surgeries and placed in Tissue-Tek® (Sakura Finetek Europe B.V, Netherlands). Frozen samples were cut in 7 µm-sections and fixed with 4% paraformaldehyde for 15 minutes at 4°C. Slides were blocked for 1 hour with 50% (v/v) fetal calf serum and 50% (v/v) PBS/BSA 1% at room temperature. To assess TRIM27 expression anti-RET Finger Protein (RFP) rabbit IgG affinity purified primary antibody (0.1 µg/ml, IBL, Japan) and secondary Alexa Fluor 594 goat anti-rabbit IgG (H+L) (1:200 dilution, Invitrogen, USA) were used. F-Actin-staining was performed by using Phalloidin FITC labeled mixed isomers (2 µg/ml in DMSO, Sigma-Aldrich). Slides were mounted with Vectashield/DAPI stain (Vector Laboratories H-1200) and stored at 4°C in darkness prior to immunfluorescence microscopy. Images were captured with Zeiss AxioVision LE Rel. 4.4 on a Zeiss Axio Imager Z1 (Carl Zeiss Inc.) with a 20× objective.

Statistical analysis

Data are presented as mean+SD. Significance was assessed with the two-sample Student's t-test (*, $P<0.05$; **, $P<0.01$; ***, $P<0.005$)

Supporting Information

Figure S1   Screening for TRIM proteins interacting with NOD2. *A.* Results obtained from the Y2H screen using human NOD2 full length (NOD2 fl) and several human TRIM proteins as bait and prey, as indicated. x, weak interaction; "XX", strong interaction. *B.* Characterization of the rat 6F6 anti-NOD2 antibody. Western blot probed with 6F6, loaded with different amounts of whole cell lysates from SW480 cells and SW480 cells treated with a NOD2 specific siRNA for 48 h is shown.

Figure S2   TRIM27 mRNA expression and cellular localization. *A.* End-point RT-PCR analysis of TRIM27 mRNA expression in different cell lines. Amplification of GAPDH served as control. *B.* Indirect immunofluorescence micrographs of HeLa and HEK cells grown on coverslips. Images with signals for DAPI, TRIM27 and an overlay (blue: DAPI, red: TRIM27) are shown. *C.* HeLa cells were stimulated with 10 µM MDP for 3 h or left unstimulated. Cellular fractions were prepared using the Qproteome cell compartment kit. Immunoblot analysis was performed using the indicated antibodies. *D.* Indirect immunofluorescence micrographs of HeLa cells grown on coverslips and expressing myc-NOD1 were treated with 50 nM LMB for 4 h or left untreated. Images with signals for DAPI, myc-NOD1 and an overlay (blue: DAPI, green: NOD1) are shown. Bars, 10 µm.

Figure S3   NOD2 but not NOD1 is degraded. *A.* HEK cells expressing Flag-NOD1 or –NOD2 were treated with 30 µg/ml CHX, as indicated. Immunoblots of total cell lysates (top) were performed using the indicated antibodies. GAPDH served as loading control. Densitometric analysis (bottom) of the NOD1 and NOD2 signals normalized to GAPDH is shown. *B.* HEK293T cells transfected with Flag-NOD2 and myc-TRIM27, E3 or CTR as indicated were treated with 30 µg/ml cycloheximid (CHX) and immunoblots of total cell lysates (top) were performed using the indicated antibodies. GAPDH served as loading control (related to Figure 4A).

Figure S4 Effect of TRIM27 on RIP2/Nod2 interaction and IFN signalling.

A. Lysates of HEK cells expressing the indicated proteins were subjected to immunoprecipitation using anti-Flag beads. Immunoblots of immunoprecipitates (IP) and total lysates (Input) were performed using the indicated antibodies. *B.* To determine the influence of TRIM27 on Sendai virus-induced IFN-β promoter activation, HEK293T cells were transfected with different amounts of TRIM27, as indicated, and an IFN-β promotor luciferase reporter system. Cells were then infected with 133 HAU/ml Sendai virus. Normalized luciferase activity (nRLU) is shown. Values are given as mean+SD.

Acknowledgments

We thank Peter Söderkvist (University of Linköping) for continuous support and helpful discussions. We are grateful to Gerrit Praefcke and Kirstin Keusekotten (University of Cologne) for advice in TRIM protein expression and purification and Maureen Menning for perfect technical assistance. Finally, we want to thank Martin Krönke (University of Cologne) for his continuous support.

Author Contributions

Conceived and designed the experiments: ML GM JDS TAK. Performed the experiments: BZ IS AN LMN KB EB. Analyzed the data: GS ML GM JDS TAK. Contributed reagents/materials/analysis tools: GM GS. Wrote the paper: BZ IS ML GM JDS TAK.

References

1. Ting JP, Duncan JA, Lei Y (2010) How the noninflammasome NLRs function in the innate immune system. Science 327: 286–290.
2. Chen G, Shaw MH, Kim YG, Nunez G (2009) NOD-like receptors: role in innate immunity and inflammatory disease. Annu Rev Pathol 4: 365–398.
3. Magalhaes JG, Sorbara MT, Girardin SE, Philpott DJ (2011) What is new with Nods? Curr Opin Immunol 23: 29–34.
4. Kufer TA, Kremmer E, Banks DJ, Philpott DJ (2006) Role for erbin in bacterial activation of Nod2. Infect Immun 74: 3115–3124.
5. Barnich N, Aguirre JE, Reinecker HC, Xavier R, Podolsky DK (2005) Membrane recruitment of NOD2 in intestinal epithelial cells is essential for nuclear factor-{kappa}B activation in muramyl dipeptide recognition. J Cell Biol 170: 21–26.
6. Legrand-Poels S, Kustermans G, Bex F, Kremmer E, Kufer TA, et al. (2007) Modulation of Nod2-dependent NF-kappaB signaling by the actin cytoskeleton. J Cell Sci 120: 1299–1310.
7. Philpott DJ, Girardin SE (2010) Nod-like receptors: sentinels at host membranes. Curr Opin Immunol 22: 428–434.
8. Ogura Y, Inohara N, Benito A, Chen FF, Yamaoka S, et al. (2001) Nod2, a Nod1/Apaf-1 family member that is restricted to monocytes and activates NF-kappaB. J Biol Chem 276: 4812–4818.
9. Kobayashi K, Inohara N, Hernandez LD, Galan JE, Nunez G, et al. (2002) RICK/Rip2/CARDIAK mediates signalling for receptors of the innate and adaptive immune systems. Nature 416: 194–199.
10. Kobayashi KS, Chamaillard M, Ogura Y, Henegariu O, Inohara N, et al. (2005) Nod2-dependent regulation of innate and adaptive immunity in the intestinal tract. Science 307: 731–734.
11. Borzutzky A, Fried A, Chou J, Bonilla FA, Kim S, et al. (2009) NOD2-associated diseases: Bridging innate immunity and autoinflammation. Clin Immunol.
12. McDonald C, Chen FF, Ollendorff V, Ogura Y, Marchetto S, et al. (2005) A role for Erbin in the regulation of Nod2-dependent NF-kappaB signaling. J Biol Chem 280: 40301–40309.
13. Yamamoto-Furusho JK, Barnich N, Xavier R, Hisamatsu T, Podolsky DK (2006) Centaurin beta1 down-regulates nucleotide-binding oligomerization domains 1- and 2-dependent NF-kappaB activation. J Biol Chem 281: 36060–36070.
14. Bielig H, Zurek B, Kutsch A, Menning M, Philpott DJ, et al. (2009) A function for AAMP in Nod2-mediated NF-kappaB activation. Mol Immunol. 46:2647–54.
15. Sardiello M, Cairo S, Fontanella B, Ballabio A, Meroni G (2008) Genomic analysis of the TRIM family reveals two groups of genes with distinct evolutionary properties. BMC Evol Biol 8: 225.
16. Rajsbaum R, Stoye JP, O'Garra A (2008) Type I interferon-dependent and -independent expression of tripartite motif proteins in immune cells. Eur J Immunol 38: 619–630.
17. Carthagena L, Bergamaschi A, Luna JM, David A, Uchil PD, et al. (2009) Human TRIM gene expression in response to interferons. PLoS One 4: e4894.
18. Ozato K, Shin DM, Chang TH, Morse HC III (2008) TRIM family proteins and their emerging roles in innate immunity. Nat Rev Immunol 8: 849–860.
19. McNab FW, Rajsbaum R, Stoye JP, O'Garra A (2011) Tripartite-motif proteins and innate immune regulation. Curr Opin Immunol. 23:46–56.
20. Bailly V, Lauder S, Prakash S, Prakash L (1997) Yeast DNA repair proteins Rad6 and Rad18 form a heterodimer that has ubiquitin conjugating, DNA binding, and ATP hydrolytic activities. J Biol Chem 272: 23360–23365.
21. Deshaies RJ, Joazeiro CA (2009) RING domain E3 ubiquitin ligases. Annu Rev Biochem 78: 399–434.
22. French FMF Consortium (1997) A candidate gene for familial Mediterranean fever. Nat Genet 17: 25–31.
23. International FMF Consortium (1997) Ancient missense mutations in a new member of the RoRet gene family are likely to cause familial Mediterranean fever. The International FMF Consortium. Cell 90: 797–807.
24. Harley JB, Alexander EL, Bias WB, Fox OF, Provost TT, et al. (1986) Anti-Ro (SS-A) and anti-La (SS-B) in patients with Sjogren's syndrome. Arthritis Rheum 29: 196–206.
25. Ishii T, Ohnuma K, Murakami A, Takasawa N, Yamochi T, et al. (2003) SS-A/Ro52, an autoantigen involved in CD28-mediated IL-2 production. J Immunol 170: 3653–3661.
26. Nakayama EE, Shioda T (2010) Anti-retroviral activity of TRIM5 alpha. Rev Med Virol 20: 77–92.
27. Hasegawa N, Iwashita T, Asai N, Murakami H, Iwata Y, et al. (1996) A RING finger motif regulates transforming activity of the rfp/ret fusion gene. Biochem Biophys Res Commun 225: 627–631.
28. Napolitano LM, Jaffray EG, Hay RT, Meroni G (2011) Functional interactions between ubiquitin E2 enzymes and TRIM proteins. Biochem J 434: 309–319.
29. Chu Y, Yang X (2011) SUMO E3 ligase activity of TRIM proteins. Oncogene 30: 1108–1116.
30. Tezel G, Nagasaka T, Iwahashi N, Asai N, Iwashita T, et al. (1999) Different nuclear/cytoplasmic distributions of RET finger protein in different cell types. Pathol Int 49: 881–886.
31. Cao T, Borden KL, Freemont PS, Etkin LD (1997) Involvement of the rfp tripartite motif in protein-protein interactions and subcellular distribution. J Cell Sci 110 (Pt 14): 1563–1571.
32. Cao T, Duprez E, Borden KL, Freemont PS, Etkin LD (1998) Ret finger protein is a normal component of PML nuclear bodies and interacts directly with PML. J Cell Sci 111 (Pt 10): 1319–1329.
33. Matsuura T, Shimono Y, Kawai K, Murakami H, Urano T, et al. (2005) PIAS proteins are involved in the SUMO-1 modification, intracellular translocation and transcriptional repressive activity of RET finger protein. Exp Cell Res 308: 65–77.
34. Shimono Y, Murakami H, Hasegawa Y, Takahashi M (2000) RET finger protein is a transcriptional repressor and interacts with enhancer of polycomb that has dual transcriptional functions. J Biol Chem 275: 39411–39419.
35. Bloor AJ, Kotsopoulou E, Hayward P, Champion BR, Green AR (2005) RFP represses transcriptional activation by bHLH transcription factors. Oncogene 24: 6729–6736.
36. Zha J, Han KJ, Xu LG, He W, Zhou Q, et al. (2006) The Ret finger protein inhibits signaling mediated by the noncanonical and canonical IkappaB kinase family members. J Immunol 176: 1072–1080.
37. Dho SH, Kwon KS (2003) The Ret finger protein induces apoptosis via its RING finger-B box-coiled-coil motif. J Biol Chem 278: 31902–31908.
38. Patel CA, Ghiselli G (2005) The RET finger protein interacts with the hinge region of SMC3. Biochem Biophys Res Commun 330: 333–340.
39. Reymond A, Meroni G, Fantozzi A, Merla G, Cairo S, et al. (2001) The tripartite motif family identifies cell compartments. Embo J 20: 2140–2151.
40. Hershko A, Ciechanover A (1998) The ubiquitin system. Annu Rev Biochem 67: 425–479.
41. Benko S, Magalhaes JG, Philpott DJ, Girardin SE (2010) NLRC5 limits the activation of inflammatory pathways. J Immunol 185: 1681–1691.
42. Cressman DE, Chin KC, Taxman DJ, Ting JP (1999) A defect in the nuclear translocation of CIITA causes a form of type II bare lymphocyte syndrome. Immunity 10: 163–171.
43. Harton JA, Cressman DE, Chin KC, Der CJ, Ting JP (1999) GTP binding by class II transactivator: role in nuclear import. Science 285: 1402–1405.
44. Meissner TB, Li A, Biswas A, Lee KH, Liu YJ, et al. (2010) NLR family member NLRC5 is a transcriptional regulator of MHC class I genes. Proc Natl Acad Sci U S A 107: 13794–13799.
45. Neerincx A, Rodriguez GM, Steimle V, Kufer TA (2012) NLRC5 Controls Basal MHC Class I Gene Expression in an MHC Enhanceosome-Dependent Manner. J Immunol 188: 4940–4950.
46. Uehara A, Yang S, Fujimoto Y, Fukase K, Kusumoto S, et al. (2005) Muramyldipeptide and diaminopimelic acid-containing desmuramylpeptides in

combination with chemically synthesized Toll-like receptor agonists synergistically induced production of interleukin-8 in a NOD2- and NOD1-dependent manner, respectively, in human monocytic cells in culture. Cell Microbiol 7: 53–61.

47. Rhodes DA, de Bono B, Trowsdale J (2005) Relationship between SPRY and B30.2 protein domains. Evolution of a component of immune defence? Immunology 116: 411–417.

48. Henry J, Ribouchon M, Depetris D, Mattei M, Offer C, et al. (1997) Cloning, structural analysis, and mapping of the B30 and B7 multigenic families to the major histocompatibility complex (MHC) and other chromosomal regions. Immunogenetics 46: 383–395.

49. Kong HJ, Anderson DE, Lee CH, Jang MK, Tamura T, et al. (2007) Cutting edge: autoantigen Ro52 is an interferon inducible E3 ligase that ubiquitinates IRF-8 and enhances cytokine expression in macrophages. J Immunol 179: 26–30.

50. Higgs R, Ni Gabhann J, Ben Larbi N, Breen EP, Fitzgerald KA, et al. (2008) The E3 ubiquitin ligase Ro52 negatively regulates IFN-beta production post-pathogen recognition by polyubiquitin-mediated degradation of IRF3. J Immunol 181: 1780–1786.

51. Yang K, Shi HX, Liu XY, Shan YF, Wei B, et al. (2009) TRIM21 is essential to sustain IFN regulatory factor 3 activation during antiviral response. J Immunol 182: 3782–3792.

52. Gack MU, Shin YC, Joo CH, Urano T, Liang C, et al. (2007) TRIM25 RING-finger E3 ubiquitin ligase is essential for RIG-I-mediated antiviral activity. Nature 446: 916–920.

53. Richards N, Schaner P, Diaz A, Stuckey J, Shelden E, et al. (2001) Interaction between pyrin and the apoptotic speck protein (ASC) modulates ASC-induced apoptosis. J Biol Chem 276: 39320–39329.

54. Chae JJ, Wood G, Masters SL, Richard K, Park G, et al. (2006) The B30.2 domain of pyrin, the familial Mediterranean fever protein, interacts directly with caspase-1 to modulate IL-1beta production. Proc Natl Acad Sci U S A 103: 9982–9987.

55. Chae JJ, Komarow HD, Cheng J, Wood G, Raben N, et al. (2003) Targeted disruption of pyrin, the FMF protein, causes heightened sensitivity to endotoxin and a defect in macrophage apoptosis. Mol Cell 11: 591–604.

56. Chae JJ, Cho YH, Lee GS, Cheng J, Liu PP, et al. (2011) Gain-of-Function Pyrin Mutations Induce NLRP3 Protein-Independent Interleukin-1beta Activation and Severe Autoinflammation in Mice. Immunity 34: 755–768.

57. Laing KJ, Purcell MK, Winton JR, Hansen JD (2008) A genomic view of the NOD-like receptor family in teleost fish: identification of a novel NLR subfamily in zebrafish. BMC Evol Biol 8: 42.

58. van der Aa LM, Levraud JP, Yahmi M, Lauret E, Briolat V, et al. (2009) A large new subset of TRIM genes highly diversified by duplication and positive selection in teleost fish. BMC Biol 7: 7.

59. Toniato E, Chen XP, Losman J, Flati V, Donahue L, et al. (2002) TRIM8/GERP RING finger protein interacts with SOCS-1. J Biol Chem 277: 37315–37322.

60. Arimoto K, Funami K, Saeki Y, Tanaka K, Okawa K, et al. (2010) Polyubiquitin conjugation to NEMO by triparite motif protein 23 (TRIM23) is critical in antiviral defense. Proc Natl Acad Sci U S A 107: 15856–15861.

61. Tsuchida T, Zou J, Saitoh T, Kumar H, Abe T, et al. (2010) The ubiquitin ligase TRIM56 regulates innate immune responses to intracellular double-stranded DNA. Immunity 33: 765–776.

62. Hu Y, Mao K, Zeng Y, Chen S, Tao Z, et al. (2010) Tripartite-motif protein 30 negatively regulates NLRP3 inflammasome activation by modulating reactive oxygen species production. J Immunol 185: 7699–7705.

63. Shi M, Deng W, Bi E, Mao K, Ji Y, et al. (2008) TRIM30 alpha negatively regulates TLR-mediated NF-kappa B activation by targeting TAB2 and TAB3 for degradation. Nat Immunol 9: 369–377.

64. von Mikecz A (2006) The nuclear ubiquitin-proteasome system. J Cell Sci 119: 1977–1984.

65. Chuang TH, Ulevitch RJ (2004) Triad3A, an E3 ubiquitin-protein ligase regulating Toll-like receptors. Nat Immunol 5: 495–502.

66. Lu D, Lin W, Gao X, Wu S, Cheng C, et al. (2011) Direct ubiquitination of pattern recognition receptor FLS2 attenuates plant innate immunity. Science 332: 1439–1442.

67. Steimle V, Otten LA, Zufferey M, Mach B (1993) Complementation cloning of an MHC class II transactivator mutated in hereditary MHC class II deficiency (or bare lymphocyte syndrome). Cell 75: 135–146.

68. Zika E, Ting JP (2005) Epigenetic control of MHC-II: interplay between CIITA and histone-modifying enzymes. Curr Opin Immunol 17: 58–64.

69. Staehli F, Ludigs K, Heinz LX, Seguin-Estevez Q, Ferrero I, et al. (2012) NLRC5 deficiency selectively impairs MHC class I- dependent lymphocyte killing by cytotoxic T cells. J Immunol 188: 3820–3828.

70. Tameling WI, Baulcombe DC (2007) Physical association of the NB-LRR resistance protein Rx with a Ran GTPase-activating protein is required for extreme resistance to Potato virus X. Plant Cell 19: 1682–1694.

71. Wirthmueller L, Zhang Y, Jones JD, Parker JE (2007) Nuclear accumulation of the Arabidopsis immune receptor RPS4 is necessary for triggering EDS1-dependent defense. Curr Biol 17: 2023–2029.

72. Burch-Smith TM, Schiff M, Caplan JL, Tsao J, Czymmek K, et al. (2007) A novel role for the TIR domain in association with pathogen-derived elicitors. PLoS Biol 5: e68.

73. Shen QH, Saijo Y, Mauch S, Biskup C, Bieri S, et al. (2007) Nuclear activity of MLA immune receptors links isolate-specific and basal disease-resistance responses. Science 315: 1098–1103.

74. Liu J, Coaker G (2008) Nuclear trafficking during plant innate immunity. Mol Plant 1: 411–422.

75. Liu Y, Jin H, Yang KY, Kim CY, Baker B, et al. (2003) Interaction between two mitogen-activated protein kinases during tobacco defense signaling. Plant J 34: 149–160.

76. Jin H, Liu Y, Yang KY, Kim CY, Baker B, et al. (2003) Function of a mitogen-activated protein kinase pathway in N gene-mediated resistance in tobacco. Plant J 33: 719–731.

77. Zurek B, Proell M, Wagner RN, Schwarzenbacher R, Kufer TA (2012) Mutational analysis of human NOD1 and NOD2 NACHT domains reveals different modes of activation. Innate Immun. 18:100–11.

78. Lecat A, Piette J, Legrand-Poels S (2010) The protein Nod2: an innate receptor more complex than previously assumed. Biochem Pharmacol 80: 2021–2031.

79. Kufer TA (2008) Signal transduction pathways used by NLR-type innate immune receptors. Mol Biosyst 4: 380–386.

80. Sabbah A, Chang TH, Harnack R, Frohlich V, Tominaga K, et al. (2009) Activation of innate immune antiviral responses by Nod2. Nat Immunol 10: 1073–1080.

81. Oh HM, Lee HJ, Seo GS, Choi EY, Kweon SH, et al. (2005) Induction and localization of NOD2 protein in human endothelial cells. Cell Immunol 237: 37–44.

82. Rosenstiel P, Fantini M, Brautigam K, Kuhbacher T, Waetzig GH, et al. (2003) TNF-alpha and IFN-gamma regulate the expression of the NOD2 (CARD15) gene in human intestinal epithelial cells. Gastroenterology 124: 1001–1009.

83. Gutierrez O, Pipaon C, Inohara N, Fontalba A, Ogura Y, et al. (2002) Induction of Nod2 in myelomonocytic and intestinal epithelial cells via nuclear factor-kappa B activation. J Biol Chem 277: 41701–41705.

84. Ogura Y, Lala S, Xin W, Smith E, Dowds TA, et al. (2003) Expression of NOD2 in Paneth cells: a possible link to Crohn's ileitis. Gut 52: 1591–1597.

85. Kufer TA, Kremmer E, Adam AC, Philpott DJ, Sansonetti PJ (2008) The pattern-recognition molecule Nod1 is localized at the plasma membrane at sites of bacterial interaction. Cell Microbiol 10: 477–486.

86. Lim KL, Chew KC, Tan JM, Wang C, Chung KK, et al. (2005) Parkin mediates nonclassical, proteasomal-independent ubiquitination of synphilin-1: implications for Lewy body formation. J Neurosci 25: 2002–2009.

87. Gyuris J, Golemis E, Chertkov H, Brent R (1993) Cdi1, a human G1 and S phase protein phosphatase that associates with Cdk2. Cell 75: 791–803.

88. Rasband WS (2007) ImageJ. Bethesda, Maryland, USA: U.S. National Institutes of Health.

10

From SNPs to Genes: Disease Association at the Gene Level

Benjamin Lehne[1], Cathryn M. Lewis[1,2], Thomas Schlitt[1]*

1 Department of Medical and Molecular Genetics, King's College London, London, United Kingdom, **2** Social, Genetic and Developmental Psychiatry Centre, Institute of Psychiatry, King's College London, London, United Kingdom

Abstract

Interpreting Genome-Wide Association Studies (GWAS) at a gene level is an important step towards understanding the molecular processes that lead to disease. In order to incorporate prior biological knowledge such as pathways and protein interactions in the analysis of GWAS data it is necessary to derive one measure of association for each gene. We compare three different methods to obtain gene-wide test statistics from Single Nucleotide Polymorphism (SNP) based association data: choosing the test statistic from the most significant SNP; the mean test statistics of all SNPs; and the mean of the top quartile of all test statistics. We demonstrate that the gene-wide test statistics can be controlled for the number of SNPs within each gene and show that all three methods perform considerably better than expected by chance at identifying genes with confirmed associations. By applying each method to GWAS data for Crohn's Disease and Type 1 Diabetes we identified new potential disease genes.

Editor: Raya Khanin, Memorial Sloan Kettering Cancer Center, United States of America

Funding: This work was supported by King's College London (KCL) and the KCL Systems Biomedicine Graduate Program (SBGP). The funders had no role in study design, data collection and analysis, decision to publish, or preparation of the manuscript.

Competing Interests: The authors have declared that no competing interests exist.

* E-mail: thomas.schlitt@kcl.ac.uk

Introduction

Genome-Wide Association Studies (GWAS) link genetic variants to phenotypes. One common study design in human disease genetics is to compare a group of diseased individuals (cases) to a group of healthy individuals (controls) for a large number of Single Nucleotide Polymorphisms (SNPs). The frequency of each allele is compared between cases and controls using a χ^2 statistic, which can be transformed into a measure for the probability of the data arising under no association between disease and SNP (p-value). Currently, GWAS are carried out using microarray technology, genotyping up to one million SNPs in parallel. Because a statistical test is performed for each SNP, careful multiple hypothesis testing procedures are employed to ensure the identification of association signals with genome-wide significance, typically with a p-value $p < 5 \cdot 10^{-8}$ [1]. In most GWAS only a few SNPs pass this correction and although this approach has led to the discovery of several novel disease-linked variants, it ignores thousands of SNPs with "suggestive" p-values that fail to reach the stringent threshold for genome-wide significance, but may reflect evidence for association. Several approaches try to make use of these "suggestive" p-values through the incorporation of prior biological knowledge [2,3,4,5,6,7,8,9,10,11,12]. The best known is Gene Set Enrichment Analysis (GSEA) [3,13], which assesses whether predefined sets of genes are overrepresented within a sample. Genes that are members of the same gene-set are typically involved in a common biological process as defined by e.g. the Gene Ontology [14] or biological pathways as defined by databases such as KEGG [15]. In a similar way, protein networks have been consulted [10,11] with the objective of identifying subnetworks of interacting proteins. Individually none of the proteins within such a subnetwork might be significantly associated, but overall a subnetwork might show statistically significant association with a disease.

All of these studies face very similar methodological problems: GWAS report association for individual SNPs, whereas functional information typically exists for proteins or genes. Therefore SNPs have to be assigned to genes and their individual association signals combined. This can be done in different ways and one must take into consideration that the number of SNPs per gene can vary to a great extent. The most widely used approach is to take the most significant p-value per gene [2,3,4,5,6,7,8]; however this can introduce a substantial bias in the downstream analysis if the number of SNPs per gene is not controlled for [9]. In this work we systematically compare three methods to analyse GWAS data at the gene level. We also propose a way to control for differences in the number of SNPs per gene based on permutations of the disease status and demonstrate its effectiveness. Based on GWAS data for Crohn's disease (CD) and Type 1 Diabetes (T1D) genotyped by the Wellcome Trust Case Control Consortium [16], we evaluate the performance of the different methods using sets of disease genes that were identified and replicated by the most recent meta-analyses [17,18].

Methods

Quality Control and Association Testing

GWAS of seven diseases have been performed by the WTCCC [16]. Approximately 3,000 shared controls and 2,000 cases were genotyped for seven diseases, including Crohn's Disease (CD) and Type 1 Diabetes (T1D), on the Affymetrix GeneChip 500K Mapping Array Set. We re-analyzed the WTCCC I data using PLINK v1.06 [19]. In addition to SNPs and individuals in the exclusion lists provided with the genotyping data, we applied more stringent quality control criteria than the original study, because our analysis includes moderate associations which are more susceptible to study biases. Based on the pooled case/control dataset we excluded SNPs with Hardy-Weinberg equilibrium p<0.001, a minor allele frequency of less than 0.01 or genotyping call-rates of less than 0.97. Association testing was performed using the Cochran Armitage trend test (1df). We manually checked the most strongly associated SNPs for every disease to ensure consistency with the original WTCCC I results. To take into account inflated test statistics caused by population stratification we corrected test statistics using the genomic control metric λ_{median} [20]. The estimated λ_{median} (for simplicity denominated as λ) for CD ($\lambda = 1.12$) and T1D ($\lambda = 1.06$) are in good agreement with the original values reported by the WTCCC ($\lambda = 1.11$ and $\lambda = 1.05$ for CD and T1D, respectively). For both diseases, 500,000 permutations of the disease status were performed using the PLINK max(T) permutation method and association p-values were calculated. Table 1 summarises the GWAS data analysis for CD and T1D.

To further assess the effect of population stratification on our analyses we performed principal component analysis (PCA) of the CD and T1D data using EIGENSTRAT [21]. We then performed association testing using logistic regression to incorporate the first two principal components as covariates. For both diseases, 1,000 permutations of the disease status were performed using logistic regression and the PLINK max(T) permutation method.

Gene to SNP assignment

A tab-delimited text-file (seq_gene.md) containing genomic coordinates for all genes was downloaded from the NCBI ftp-server [22] in November 2009. Only entries for the human reference sequence (NCBI assembly GRCh37) and protein-coding genes were retained. Genes mapping to sex-chromosomes, the mitochondrial chromosome, unassembled contigs or alternative haplotypes were discarded. SNPs on the GeneChip 500K Mapping Array Set were assigned to the remaining genes. Because this genotyping platform is based on the previous assembly of the human genome (NCBI 36) all SNP positions were converted to the latest assembly using the "Lift-Over" tool on the GALAXY

website [23]. SNPs were assigned to a gene if they are located within its primary transcript or 40 kilobases (kb) upstream or downstream. These boundaries are chosen based on the distribution of association signal with respect to protein-coding genes [24]. When a SNP could be assigned to multiple genes because of overlapping flanking windows, the closest gene was chosen.

The WTCCC study found the strongest association signal for Type 1 Diabetes (T1D) within the Major Histocompatibility Complex (MHC) region on chromosome 6. The MHC region has high levels of linkage disequilibrium (LD) and harbours many genes. This causes the association signal to be spread over many genes, thereby artificially inflating the number of genes with associated SNPs. We therefore excluded the MHC region (chromosome 6, position 25,930,839 to position 33,495,825, NCBI assembly GRCh37) in all analyses of the T1D dataset, which removed 1,473 SNPs and 185 genes. In total, approximately 290,000 SNPs were assigned to 17,000 protein coding genes. Table 1 summarises the SNP to gene assignment for CD and T1D.

Assessment of LD on SNP to gene assignment

In order to assess the effect of LD we repeat our analyses, but take into account LD to extend the assignment of SNPs to genes. We use PLINK v1.06 [19] to obtain a list of SNP pairs in LD ($r^2>0.8$) based on the GWAS data for CD and T1D [16]. SNPs are added to the initial assignment if they are in LD ($r^2>0.8$) with a SNP in a gene or its 40 kb flanking windows, including SNPs that have already been assigned to other genes. Taking into account LD adds approximately 6,000 (2%) additional SNPs to the analyses.

Deriving a gene-wide test statistic for each gene

Each gene has n SNPs assigned to it with $n \in N_0$. Let the test statistics in the gene be T_i, $i = 1, \dots n$. Under the null hypothesis of no association, T_i has a χ_1^2 distribution (χ^2 distribution with one degree of freedom); high values of T_i indicate evidence for association. To obtain a gene-wide test statistic, we use three summary statistics for T_i:

1. **maxT:** the maximum value of T_i (maximum χ_1^2 value) for each gene is chosen;
2. **meanT:** the arithmetic mean test statistic (mean χ_1^2 value) for each gene is calculated;
3. **topQ:** the highest quartile of all test statistics T_i (highest quartile of all χ_1^2 values) in a gene are selected and their mean is calculated. If n is not a multiple of 4 the number of SNPs considered for topQ is rounded up to the next integer (e.g. if a gene has 5 SNPs the mean of the largest two test statistics is calculated).

Deriving an empirical p-value (p_{emp}) for each gene

We derive test statistics for each gene in the observed dataset and in 500,000 randomised datasets derived from permutations of the disease status. For each gene we tabulate the number of permuted data sets in which we observe a higher gene-wide test statistic than in the observed data set, thus deriving an empirical p-value p_{emp}.

Because we compare observed and permuted test statistics for every gene, a significantly associated gene requires a p_{emp} value that is also controlled for the number of genes tested. Assuming there are approximately 20,000 protein-coding genes in the human genome, a Bonferroni correction requires a p-value threshold of $p_{emp} = 0.05 \times 1/20,000 = 2.5 \times 10^{-6}$. In order to be able to obtain

Table 1. Overview statistics of the analysed GWAS datasets and the gene to SNP assignment for Crohn's Disease (CD) and Type 1 Diabetes (T1D).

	CD	T1D
Number of cases before QC	2,009	2,000
Number of cases after QC	1,752	1,964
Number of controls before QC	3,004	3,004
Number of controls after QC	2,938	2,938
Genomic Control metric λ	1.12	1.06
Protein-coding genes on chromosome 1–22	20,919	20,919
Protein-coding genes after SNP to gene assignment	17,006	17,006
Protein-coding genes after QC	16,326	16,146
SNPs on the Affymetrix GeneChip 500K Mapping Array Set	500,568	500,568
SNPs assigned to genes (chromosome 1–22)	290,571	289,098
SNPs assigned to genes after QC	227,418	225,973

p-values of that magnitude we perform 500,000 permutations of the disease status. Empirical p-values are derived for each gene for all three methods to derive gene-wide test statistics.

Uncontrolled vs. empirical p-value

To compare the different methods we rank genes for each gene-wide test statistic method. This is done before and after deriving p_{emp} values (i.e. controlling for the number of variants per gene and LD) resulting in six different sets of ranks. When p_{emp} values are identical for two or more genes we use the gene-wide test statistics to resolve ties. Based on the ranks we calculate pairwise Spearman rank correlation coefficients between all six sets for the top 500 genes: For each gene, we sum the ranks across all six gene sets, and select the 500 genes with the highest summed ranks.

To analyse the effect of deriving p_{emp} values for individual genes we convert the gene-wide test statistics to p-values assuming test statistics have a χ_1^2 distribution. For each gene the uncontrolled p-value is plotted against the p_{emp} value for all three methods.

Table 2. Replicated Disease Genes for Crohn's Disease from [17] and their ranks for each method.

| hgnc | Number of SNPs per gene n | Rank of gene for | | |
		rank maxT	rank meanT	rank topQ
NOD2	13	1	3	2
ATG16L1	11	2	1	1
IL23R	21	3	4	3
NKX2-3	26	5	5	5
PTPN2	20	7	11	10
IRGM	5	8	2	6
ZNF365	91	18	149	67
GCKR	6	31	81	76
CREM	12	34	59	46
C13orf31	6	43	136	78
IL12B	14	55	45	94
SP140	18	64	110	56
CDKAL1	127	83	486	248
C11orf30	22	336	164	180
VAMP3	1	357	356	348
CCR6	14	602	291	319
DNMT3A	9	612	667	399
MTMR3	23	827	788	715
FADS1	3	980	921	1002
NDFIP1	19	1020	754	506
TAGAP	4	1169	3445	1203
IKZF3	8	1192	4281	995
DENND1B	22	1337	3818	1855
THADA	59	1500	1157	1206
JAK2	17	2074	3065	3038
PTGER4	4	2620	4084	2622
PTPN22	4	3457	2465	3498
SMAD3	42	4071	11565	9918
CPEB4	21	4108	4080	3842
ICOSLG	5	6041	8465	6570
PRDM1	18	6151	4859	5241
IL2RA	20	6698	8568	5229
BACH2	49	8022	3687	2962
MAP3K7IP1	6	8040	6149	6685
PLCL1	56	8317	3347	3754
ICAM3	2	9345	9596	9415
UBE2D1	4	10217	12176	10212
TNFSF11	21	11858	9547	9927
ZMIZ1	72	14061	5704	9596

Performance

To assess the performance of the three methods for deriving p_{emp} values we calculate Receiver Operating Characteristic (ROC) curves, which estimate the accuracy of a prediction by comparing the True Positive Rate (TPR = True Positives/Positives) with the False Positive Rate (FPR = False Positives/Negatives) [25]. In this analysis we used as positives a list of successfully replicated disease genes from meta-analyses of T1D [18] and CD [17]. We only chose loci that either contain a single gene or a for which a unique candidate gene has been proposed [17,18]. This results in 39 and 27 true positive genes for CD and T1D, respectively (Tables 2, S1 and S2). We assume that all other genes are negatives. We rank all genes within both lists (positives and negatives) by their p_{emp} values, and used their gene-wide test statistics to resolve ties when p_{emp} values are identical for two or more genes. For each gene the relative rank within the positives is plotted against the relative rank within the negatives to derive the ROC curve, and the areas under the curve (AUC) were calculated.

All scripts written for the analyses presented are available from authors upon request.

Results

Number of SNPs per gene

The Affymetrix 500K GeneChip includes approximately 500,000 SNPs distributed over the whole genome. We assign these SNPs to their closest protein-coding gene if a SNP is located less than 40 kb from a gene. Approximately 290,000 SNPs were assigned to genes, of which 227,000 were left after QC for specific disease data sets (Table 1). Genes vary substantially in size, which leads to different numbers of SNPs assigned to each gene (Figure 1). Of 20,919 protein-coding genes 17,006 have at least one SNP assigned; most of these genes (~77% or 13,083 genes) have fewer than 10 SNPs; 6.5% (1,097 genes) have more than 50 SNPs. The

largest number of SNPs assigned to a single gene is 1,008 (*CSMD1*, gene length: 818 kb).

We performed analyses of GWAS data for both Crohn's Disease (CD) and Type 1 Diabetes (T1D). In the following section we present results for CD. Results for T1D are comparable and presented in supplementary material.

Deriving a gene-wide test statistic for each gene

To measure association of a SNP with the disease we compare genotype frequencies between cases and controls and calculate a genomic control-corrected test statistic based on an Armitage trend test for every SNP. To obtain a gene-wide measure of association we first derive three summary statistics: **maxT** (the maximum test statistic for each gene), **meanT** (the mean test statistic for each gene), and **topQ** (the mean of the highest quartile

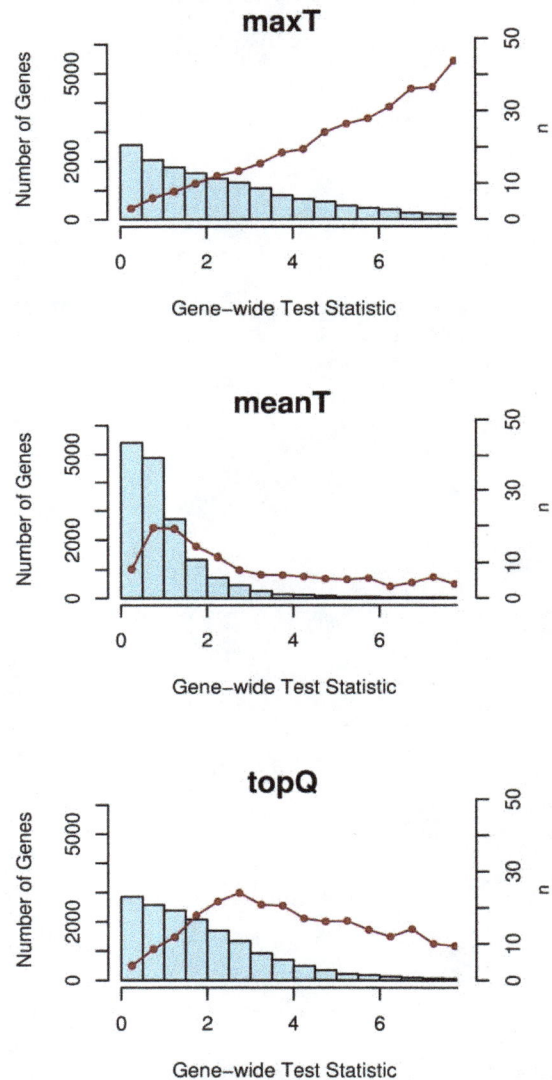

Figure 2. Confounding effect of the number of SNPs per gene (Crohn's Disease). Multiple test statistics are combined for each gene using three different methods (maxT, meanT, topQ). For each method, the gene-wide test statistic is correlated with the number of SNPs per gene. For these histograms, genes are binned according to their gene-wide test statistic (left axis). The red dots show the mean number of SNPs per gene for every bin (right axis).

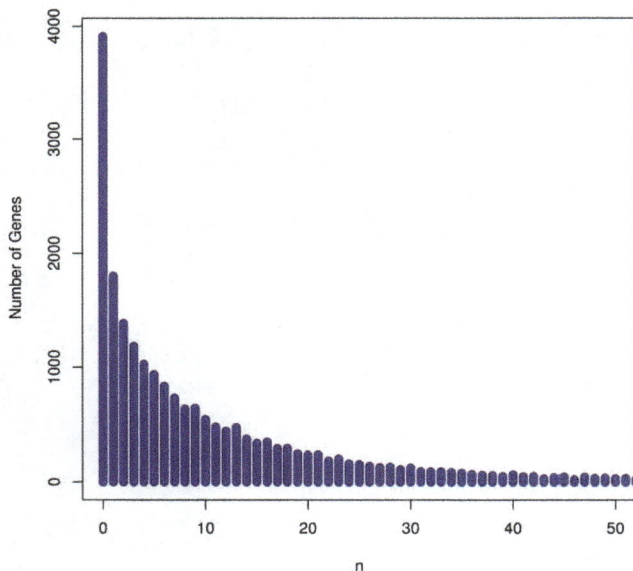

Figure 1. Distribution of the number of SNPs assigned to genes. We assigned SNPs on the Affymetrix 500K genotyping array to protein-coding genes. SNPs were assigned to a gene if they are located within the transcribed region or within a 40 kilobase flanking window around the transcribed region. Where flanking windows overlapped SNPs were assigned to their closest gene only.

of all test statistics in a gene). Here we illustrate how each summary statistic is subject to confounding factors that have to be controlled for. The gene-wide test statistic is correlated with the number of SNPs per gene, n (Figures 2 and S1), as follows.

- For **maxT** the test statistic increases approximately linearly with n (Pearson correlation coefficient r = 0.36). Even if there is no association, genes with many SNPs assigned are more likely to have a SNP with a high test statistic, by chance.

- A different effect occurs for **meanT**, whereby genes with many SNPs tend to have gene-wide test statistics close to one, whereas genes with few SNPs tend to be at the extremes of the distribution, i.e. to have either very low or very high gene-wide test statistics. Under the null hypothesis of no association, the test statistic has a χ_1^2 distribution, with a mean of 1. When calculating meanT, genes with more SNPs are therefore likely to have gene-wide test statistics close to 1, whereas genes with few SNPs are more affected by individual SNPs with extreme test statistic.

- An effect similar to meanT is observed for **topQ**: Genes with fewer SNPs tend to have extreme gene-wide test statistics whereas genes with many SNPs tend to have a gene-wide test statistic close to $\chi^2 \approx 3$. This value is higher than for the meanT method since only the top 25% of SNPs per gene are selected.

Deriving an empirical p-value for each gene

The distribution of the summary statistics for each gene is not known and impossible to derive analytically, since it depends on the pattern of LD within each gene. We therefore derive an empirical p-value p_{emp} for each gene from permuted datasets (see Methods). By comparing the observed to the permuted test statistics we maintain LD structure and account for differences in the number of SNPs per gene. The observed p_{emp} values are appropriately controlled for the number of SNPs per gene; we observe no correlation between the number of SNPs per gene and the p_{emp} value (Figures 3 and S2). For each of the three methods to combine test statistics, the p_{emp} values are approximately uniformly distributed. The high proportions of very low p_{emp} values (Figures 3 and S2) are likely due to true association signal.

Uncontrolled vs. empirical p-value

Although different methods yield different levels of association for a given gene, the results are correlated. Between the three methods to derive p_{emp} values, we observe an average Spearman rank correlation coefficient of 0.74 when considering the top 500 genes (Tables S1 and S2). The average Spearman rank correlation coefficient between the three methods before deriving p_{emp} values (i.e. controlling for the number of variants per gene and LD) is only 0.30, which reflects the different biases introduced by the methods to derive gene-wide test statistics

The p_{emp} values are controlled for the number of SNPs per gene and the correlation structure, but how does the control affect individual genes? To address this question, we convert the combined test statistics to p-values assuming test statistics have a χ_1^2 distribution. These uncontrolled p-values are plotted against the p_{emp} values for all three methods (Figures 4 and S3):

- For the **maxT** method, genes with many SNPs (large n) are more likely to have a high test statistic and therefore a low uncontrolled p-value. When deriving p_{emp} values we control for n. The control has very little impact on genes with $n = 1$ and in that case the empirical and the uncontrolled p-values are very similar (lying along the diagonal in Figures 4 and S3). For

genes with higher n the control is stronger and p_{emp} values are higher than the uncontrolled p-values.

- For **meanT** we observe a sigmoid-like distribution. That is explained by the effect of varying n: We compare permuted to observed test statistics. If there is no association the expected test statistic is 1. Therefore the expected meanT values for the permuted datasets are 1, i.e. with increasing n the permuted meanT is more likely to be 1. For genes with large n this leads to extreme p_{emp} values when we compare observed to the permuted meanT. As a result the distribution for genes with large n shows a stronger curvature than for genes with small n. When the observed meanT value is 1 (uncontrolled p-value

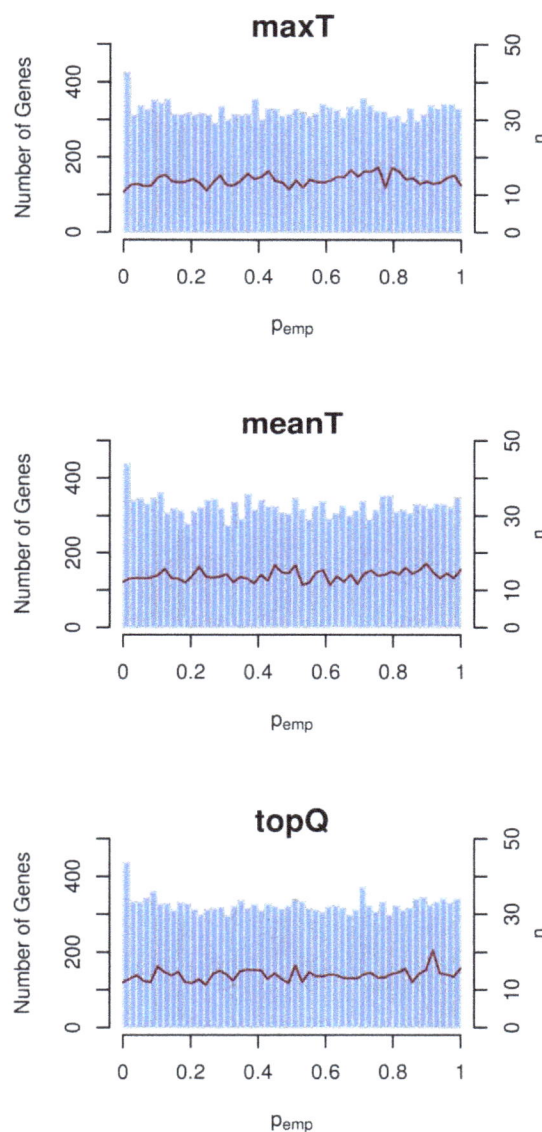

Figure 3. Distribution of empirical p-value (p_{emp}) for Crohn's Disease from 500,000 permutations of the disease labels. Genes were assigned to 50 bins according to their p_{emp}. Histogram shows the number of genes with p_{emp} values (left axis). The red line shows the mean number of SNPs per gene for every bin (right axis). In contrast to the gene-wide test statistics we observe no correlation of the number of SNPs per gene with p_{emp} for any method. We observe an increase of genes with very low p_{emp} values caused by the actual association signal.

maxT

meanT

topQ

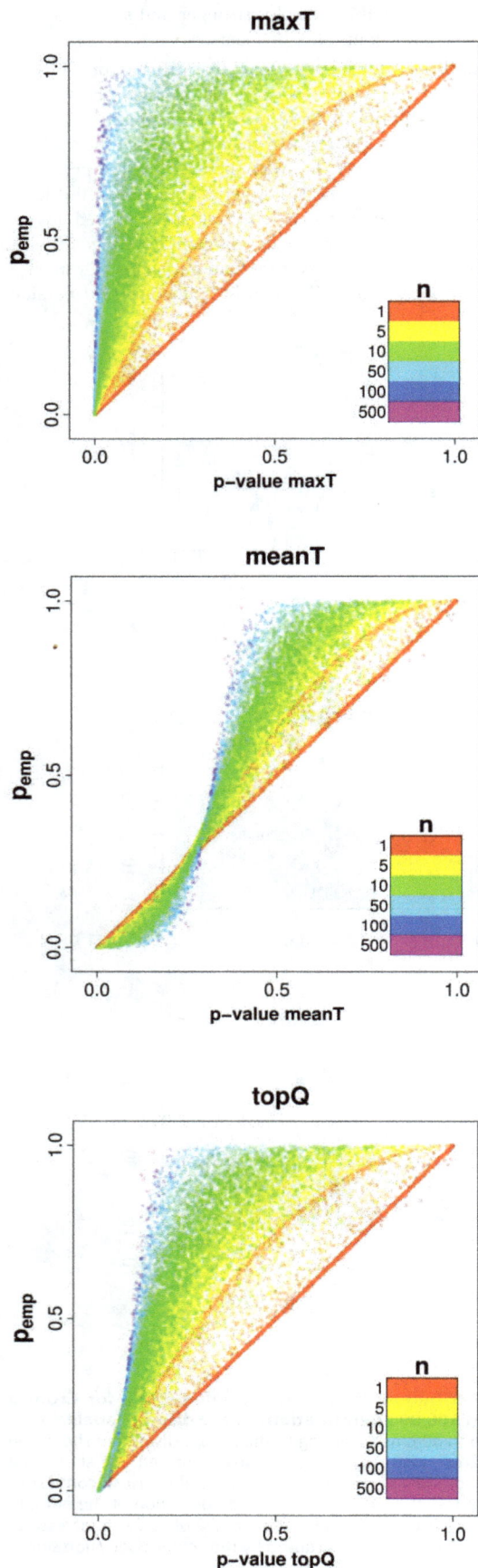

Figure 4. Empirical p-values vs. uncontrolled p-values (Crohn's Disease). For each gene the p_{emp} is plotted against the uncontrolled p-value (based on the gene-wide test statistic). Each point represents a gene and is coloured according to the number of SNPs assigned to a gene (n). Genes with few SNPs have p_{emp} values similar to the uncontrolled p-value and therefore cluster along the diagonal. For genes with higher number of SNPs the distribution depends on the method to combine test statistics.

= 0.317) the control is (on average) not affected by n. Therefore the points representing genes with different n overlap at meanT = 1.

- The distribution for **topQ** is similar to maxT, but the gradient for genes with many SNPs is less steep.

Performance

To assess the performance of the different methods of combining test statistics we plot Receiver Operating Characteristic (ROC) curves for CD and T1D (Figure 5) using two sets of confirmed disease genes [17,18] under the assumption that all other genes are not associated (see Methods). The known disease genes are based on meta-analyses CD [17] and T1D [18]. Based on genomic loci that successfully replicated the authors selected the most likely candidate gene considering known involvement in the immune system, association with other auto-immune disorders and location of the most strongly associated SNP. Although the resulting gene list may contain genes which are not associated with the trait, it is the best currently available dataset to assess the performance of our methods for measuring genetic association at the gene-level.

All three p_{emp} methods give considerably better results than expected by chance. For both diseases the topQ method performs slightly better than maxT and meanT, although all three methods perform similarly with differences in the areas under the curve (AUC) of less than 2%. The performance of the different methods for the two diseases might depend on the number of SNPs assigned to the known disease genes. For genes with many SNPs the association signal can get diluted, as it is the case for the CD disease gene *ZNF365*, which has 91 SNPs (Table 2). Its maxT is 23.74 which corresponds to $p_{emp} = 0.0001$, but the meanT and the topQ for this gene are 2.46 ($p_{emp} = 0.0041$) and 8.32 ($p_{emp} = 0.0010$), respectively. Consequently the performances measured here by the AUCs depend on the properties of the known disease genes and we can only assume that they are characteristic for disease genes that have not been identified yet.

Several known disease genes were consistently ranked very low by all three methods (Table 2). For some of these genes the associated SNPs are over 40 kb from the gene (e.g. *PTPN22*), or the associated SNP is located in the adjacent gene (e.g. *ORMDL3*). Other confirmed disease genes were ranked low because the associated SNP has not been genotyped by the WTCCC (e.g. *JAK2*) or did not show any association (e.g. *PLCL1*).

Linkage Disequilibrium

Our analysis is influenced by linkage disequilibrium (LD) and some of the top ranked genes (Table 3) are part of the same LD region, reflecting the fact that a true association signal could extend over a large region of the genome if it falls into a large LD block. Most of the SNPs in such a region would appear to be associated with the phenotype which can result in several genes with significant empirical p-values. For example, *CYLD* and *SNX20* have p_{emp} values smaller than 5.4×10^{-5}; they are located upstream and downstream of *NOD2* and are located in the same

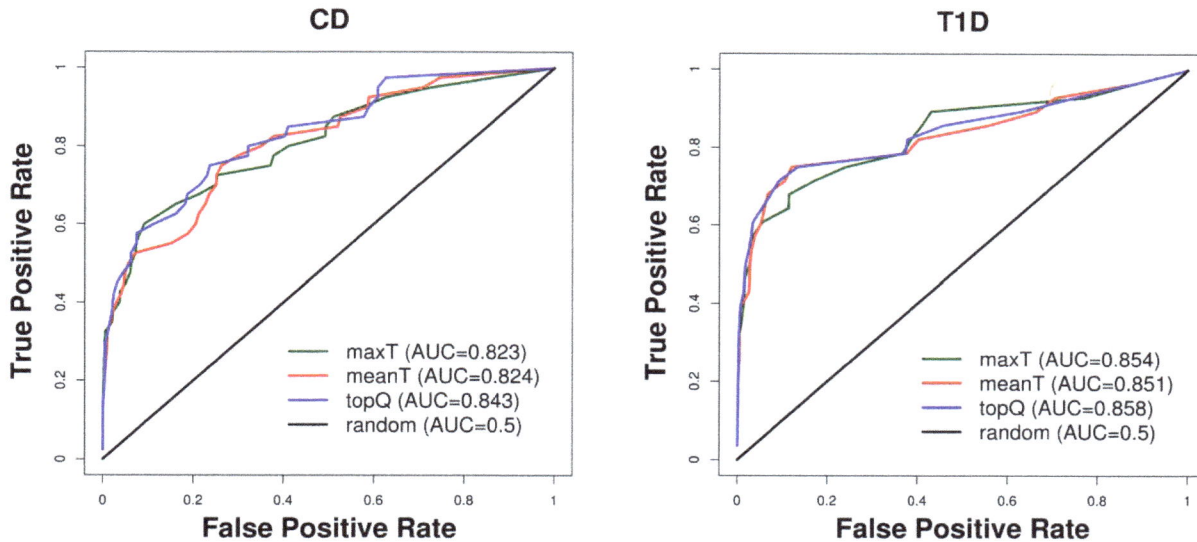

Figure 5. Receiver Operating Characteristic (ROC) curves for Crohn's Disease (CD) and Type 1 Diabetes (T1D). To assess the performance of different methods to combine test statistics we plot the proportion of confirmed disease genes (True Positive Rate) against their rank within the whole set of genes (False Positive Rate).

LD block as *NOD2*. Their association is most probably an artefact of the confirmed association of the *NOD2* gene [26,27,28]. To further assess the impact of LD on our analyses we extended the initial gene to SNP assignment. In addition to SNPs located within the gene or a 40 kb flanking window we include SNPs in LD ($r^2 > 0.8$) with any SNP in this region. This increases the average number of SNPs per gene to 15.5 (from 13.9) and the total number of SNPs assigned to genes to over 296,000 (from 290,000) (Figure S4). Including LD in the gene to SNP assignment has only a moderate effect: Although AUC values show a small increase for each method (<1.3%), only a small minority of genes is affected (Figure S5). Gene ranks obtained with and without taking into account LD are highly correlated (Spearman rank correlation r = 0.98 for each method and disease). Only 3 genes out of the top 100 have a rank above 100 when including LD (maxT for CD) and all genes discussed here and shown in the tables only marginally change their rank or p-value.

Population Stratification

Our primary analysis method is testing for association with the Cochran Armitage Trend Test, with genomic control correction for population ancestry, as this makes performing large numbers of permutations computationally tractable. To assess the effect of population stratification on our analysis in more detail we performed Principal Component Analysis [21] for both datasets. We repeated association testing using logistic regression and adjusting for the first two principal components (PC-correction). This reduced the genomic control measure for CD from $\lambda = 1.12$ to $\lambda = 1.08$, with no reduction observed for T1D ($\lambda = 1.06$). Adjusting for up to 10 PCs did not reduce λ any further. The correlation between gene ranks of our primary analysis and after correction for population stratification was high (CD-maxT R = 0.932, CD-meanT R = 0.942, CD-topQ R = 0.940, T1D-maxT R = 0.997, T1D-meanT R = 0.998, T1D-topQ R = 0.998). Gene ranks for CD are more affected than for T1D: out of the top 100 genes of our primary analysis, 78 are within the top 100 genes after PC-correction, and all 100 are within the top 204 genes (maxT, Figure S6). For T1D, 86 out of the top 100 genes of our primary analysis are within the top 100 after PC-correction and all 100 are within the top 143 genes

(maxT, Figure S6). Correcting for two principal components only marginally affects the performance of our methods: AUC values increased by <0.6% for both CD and T1D.

Associated Genes

All genes discussed here only marginally change their rank or p-value after correcting for two principal components or when considering LD for the SNP to gene assignment. For CD we find 7 out of 39 known disease genes (true positives) within the top 30 genes when we rank all genes based on p_{emp} values (derived from maxT). We use their gene-wide test statistics to resolve ties when p_{emp} values are identical for two or more genes (Table 3). The genes *STAT3* (maxT rank 27) and *SBNO2* (maxT rank 26) are located within known disease loci, but are not part of the true positive list because the association signal extends over several genes [17]. Both loci did not reach genome-wide significance in the original WTCCC study and their association was only confirmed in a more recent large-scale meta-analyses. *STAT3* and *SBNO2* can be linked to the *IL10/STAT3* anti-inflammatory pathway [29], which has been implicated with CD [2,17,30].

Another promising candidate for CD might be *DAG1* (dystroglycan 1), ranked 23rd for maxT. It is located within a large LD block whose association has been replicated and that encompasses about 35 genes [17]. *DAG1* is a cell surface receptor which is used by several known pathogens [31,32] and there has been speculation about a role for *DAG1* in the uptake of *Mycobacterium avium* ssp. *paratuberculosis* and the aetiology of Crohn's Disease [33].

For T1D five out of 27 known disease genes are within the top 30 (based on maxT, Tables S3 and S4). Of the top 30 genes, 14 fall into a large LD region on chromosome 12 (position 111,348,628 to position 112,947,717), which contains 15 genes. According to Todd *et al.* [34] the most probable causal gene for this region is *SH2B3*. The authors detected a highly associated non-synonymous SNP in exon 3 of *SH2B3*, which had not been genotyped in the WTCCC study [16]. Two SNPs that were genotyped in the WTCCC are assigned to *SH2B3* and show moderate association ($p = 3 \times 10^{-5}$ and $p = 7 \times 10^{-4}$). Since 40 other SNPs in the region show stronger association, *SH2B3* is only ranked 26 (by maxT).

Table 3. The top 30 ranked genes for Crohn's Disease (CD) using the maxT method.

HGNC symbol	Chr location	Region (Mb)	n	p-value maxT	p-value meanT	p-value topQ	rank maxT	rank meanT	rank topQ
C1orf141	1p31	67.56-67.59	26	2.0E-06	8.7E-04	6.0E-06	9	60	9
IL23R	1p31	67.63-67.73	21	>2.0E-06	>2.0E-06	>2.0E-06	3	4	3
IL12RB2	1p31	67.77-67.86	17	6.0E-06	1.4E-03	6.8E-04	10	76	54
ATG16L1	2q37	234.16-234.20	11	>2.0E-06	>2.0E-06	>2.0E-06	2	1	1
USP4	3p21	49.31-49.38	5	2.1E-04	1.0E-04	1.1E-04	28	22	23
TCTA	3p21	49.45-49.45	2	1.1E-04	2.0E-06	1.1E-04	21	8	22
AMT	3p21	49.45-49.46	3	7.1E-05	2.0E-06	7.1E-05	19	7	17
DAG1	3p21	49.51-49.57	4	1.2E-04	2.4E-05	1.2E-04	23	14	24
BSN	3p21	49.59-49.71	13	1.6E-04	2.9E-04	1.6E-05	13	32	13
APEH	3p21	49.71-49.72	1	7.3E-05	7.3E-05	7.3E-05	20	19	18
IP6K1	3p21	49.76-49.82	1	2.2E-04	2.2E-04	2.2E-04	29	27	31
SLC22A5	5q31	131.71-131.73	9	1.4E-05	3.3E-05	1.4E-05	12	35	12
C5orf56	5q31	131.75-131.80	13	2.0E-05	4.0E-06	6.0E-06	15	10	8
IRGM	5q33	150.23-150.23	5	>2.0E-06	>2.0E-06	>2.0E-06	8	2	6
ZNF300	5q33	150.27-150.28	10	>2.0E-06	2.0E-06	>2.0E-06	6	9	7
TRIM10	6p21	30.12-30.13	2	1.9E-04	6.6E-04	1.9E-04	25	51	26
HLA-DQB1	6p21	32.63-32.63	11	2.8E-05	3.8E-04	2.1E-04	16	39	29
HLA-DQA2	6p21	32.71-32.72	29	1.1E-04	1.2E-05	1.6E-05	22	12	15
C7orf33	7q36	148.29-148.31	13	2.4E-04	4.6E-04	1.0E-04	30	42	21
LOC100130652	10p15	3.87-3.87	24	1.4E-04	8.8E-02	4.1E-02	24	1,600	809
ZNF365	10q21	64.13-64.43	91	5.8E-05	4.1E-03	9.6E-04	18	149	67
NKX2-3	10q24	101.29-101.30	26	>2.0E-06	>2.0E-06	>2.0E-06	5	5	5
SNX20	16q12	50.70-50.72	3	1.2E-05	5.4E-05	1.2E-05	11	17	11
NOD2	16q12	50.73-50.77	13	>2.0E-06	>2.0E-06	>2.0E-06	1	3	2
CYLD	16q12	50.78-50.84	16	>2.0E-06	>2.0E-06	>2.0E-06	4	6	4
STAT3	17q21	40.47-40.54	13	2.1E-04	2.0E-04	8.5E-05	27	26	19
PTPN2	18p11	12.79-12.88	20	>2.0E-06	7.9E-06	6.0E-06	7	11	10
SBNO2	19p13	1.11-1.17	3	2.0E-04	1.9E-04	2.0E-04	26	24	27
RSHL1	19q13	46.30-46.32	1	1.6E-05	1.6E-05	1.6E-05	14	13	14
ZGPAT	20q13	62.34-62.37	1	3.4E-05	3.4E-05	3.4E-05	17	15	16

Genes are ordered by chromosome and genomic position; n denominates the number of SNPs per gene. The last three columns show the corresponding ranks for the three methods. *italics*: genes that are within the true positive list.

Discussion

Based on GWAS data for two common diseases we present three different methods to combine individual test statistics at a gene level. For all methods the gene-wide test statistic is correlated with the number of SNPs per gene. Based on permutations of the disease status we derive an empirical p-value for each gene and show that it is controlled for the number of SNPs within the gene. To assess the performances of the p_{emp} methods we derive ROC curves based on two sets of disease genes that were replicated in the most recent meta-analyses [17,18]. The p_{emp} methods distinguish different genetic architectures underlying a disease: for maxT a single mutation within a gene contributes to the disease (i.e. one SNP within a gene shows association); for meanT mutations spread all over the gene contribute to the disease (i.e. all or many SNPs within a gene show association): in the case of topQ only a few mutations within a gene contribute to the disease (i.e. a subset of the SNPs within a gene show association). All three methods performed substantially better than expected by chance at identifying these genes, thus justifying our approach. The performances of the three methods were similar, demonstrating the robustness of the permutation approach. This is also reflected by the correlations between empirical p-values for each method for the top 500 genes. For some genes however, results can vary across the methods, as illustrated by *ZNF365* (Table 2). To identify all potentially associated genes, results from all methods should be considered. As the methods are correlated, integration results in a moderate increase in the number of genes. For example, the union of the top 500 genes for all three methods consists of 678 genes.

In this work we perform gene-wide analyses on two independent GWAS datasets. We observe the same overall properties for gene-wide test statistics and p_{emp}-values. Furthermore for both datasets our methods successfully reproduced known disease associations showing the robustness of our approach. In addition to the methods presented here other methods have been proposed, including multi-marker association tests [35,36,37,38] and variations [39,40,41] of Fisher's method to combine p-values [42]. Recently, two studies proposed approaches to control for confounding factors (e.g. number of SNPs per gene) which do not require genotyping data [12,43]. Further studies will be required to determine how these methods compare.

An open problem that still has to be addressed is the effect of LD. Correlation between the SNPs of a gene can impact the combined test statistic for meanT and topQ method. Because multiple associations can be caused by a single causal SNP a high meanT or topQ might not reflect several independent associations. Correlation between the SNPs of a gene can therefore change the nature of the method to combine test statistics. Furthermore LD makes it difficult to allocate association signal to the correct gene. A number of groups have proposed computational approaches to prioritize genes within LD blocks [6,44,45]. They have been shown to give reasonably good results and could be combined with our approach.

Another approach is to use imputed genotypes, which will increase the density of SNPs and therefore the proportion of genes that are captured. Hong et al. [9] were able to include over 800 additional genes (5%) in their gene-wide analysis of GWAS data, but levels of statistical significance for most other genes remain unchanged compared to using genotyped SNPs only. Assigning SNPs to genes is not straight forward as regulatory elements such as enhancers can be many kilobases away from the transcribed region. In addition some disease-associated variants are located in so-called gene deserts that cannot be linked to protein-coding genes or any other functional elements. Ultimately functional studies are necessary to determine which gene is implicated in a disease process. The methodology demonstrated here is instrumental in automatically identifying the relevant genes that might be implicated in inherited disorders and provides an unbiased ranked list of genes for experimental validation.

Currently GWAS are moving from microarray based technology towards next-generation sequencing (NGS). NGS, in principle, allows for the identification of all genetic variants. As the number of genetic variants in a given individual is far higher [46] than the number of SNPs genotyped using microarray technology, the number of tests is going to increase dramatically. There is a need for new analytical methods that combine association signals over several genetic variants or all variants within a gene, particularly for rare variants which may individually lack power to show significant association. Testing for combined association of all rare variants within a gene overcomes this problem, as demonstrated for simulated data and sequence data of previously known disease genes [47,48,49].

With the emergence of next-generation sequencing, GWAS will increasingly be analysed on gene level. Gene-level association measurements allow the application of gene-set enrichment analysis and related methods, which will ultimately improve the understanding of the underlying molecular mechanism. The methods proposed here provide an accurate and powerful approach to summarise evidence for association within genes and could be used to design functional follow-up studies.

Supporting Information

Figure S1   Confounding effect of the number of SNPs per gene (Type 1 Diabetes). Multiple test statistics are combined for each gene using three different methods (maxT, meanT, topQ). For each method, the gene-wide test statistic is correlated with the number of SNPs per gene. For these histograms, genes are binned according to their gene-wide test statistic (left axis). The red dots show the mean number of SNPs per gene for every bin (right axis).

Figure S2   Distribution of empirical p-value (p_{emp}) for Type 1 Diabetes from 500,000 permutations of the disease labels. Genes were assigned to 50 bins according to their p_{emp}. Histogram shows the number of genes with p_{emp} values (left axis). The red line shows the mean number of SNPs per gene for every bin (right axis). In contrast to the gene-wide test statistics we observe no correlation of the number of SNPs per gene with p_{emp} for any method. We observe an increase of genes with very low p_{emp} values caused by the actual association signal.

Figure S3   Empirical p-values vs. uncontrolled p-values (Type 1 Diabetes). For each gene the p_{emp} is plotted against the uncontrolled p-value (based on the gene-wide test statistic). Each point represents a gene and is coloured according to the number of SNPs assigned to a gene (n). Genes with few SNPs have p_{emp} values similar to the uncontrolled p-value and therefore cluster along the diagonal. For genes with higher number of SNPs the distribution depends on the method to combine test statistics.

Figure S4   Distribution of the number of SNPs assigned to genes. We assigned SNPs on the Affymetrix 500K genotyping array to protein-coding genes. SNPs were assigned to a gene if they are located within the transcribed region or within a 40 kilobase flanking window around the transcribed region. In addition SNPs in linkage disequilibrium (LD, r2>0.8) with these SNPs were included.

Figure S5   Effect of Linkage Disequilibrium (LD). Gene ranks after assigning SNPs to genes based on genomic distance only are plotted against gene ranks after assigning SNPs to genes based on genomic distance and linkage disequilibrium (LD, r2> 0.8). The top 500 ranks are compared for CD and T1D and all three methods to derive pemp-values.

Figure S6   Effect of Population Stratification. Gene ranks based on an armitage trend test are plotted against gene ranks based on logistic regression and adjusting for two principal components. The top 500 ranks are compared for CD and T1D and all three methods to derive pemp-values.

Table S1   Pairwise Spearman rank correlation for the different methods to combine test statistics before and after controlling for multiple hypothesis testing for Crohn's Disease. For the correlation the top 500 genes were considered.

Table S2   Pairwise Spearman rank correlation for the different methods to combine test statistics before and after controlling for multiple hypothesis testing for Type 1 Diabetes. For the correlation the top 500 genes were considered.

Table S3   Replicated Disease Genes for Type 1 Diabetes (T1D) and their ranks for each method.

Table S4   The top 30 genes for Type 1 Diabetes (T1D) ranked using the maxT method. Genes are ordered by chromosome and genomic position; n denominates the number of SNPs per gene. The last three columns show the corresponding ranks for the three methods. *italics:* genes that are within the true positive list.

Acknowledgments

We thank Daniel Crouch, Natalie Prescott, Roli Roberts, Mike Weale, Jo Knight and everyone in the Statistical Genetics Unit for comments and discussion.

We would like to thank the National Institutes of Health Research comprehensive Biomedical Research Centre at Guy's and St Thomas' NHS Foundation Trust in partnership with King's College London (cBRC) for providing access to their high-performance computing cluster.

This study makes use of data generated by the Wellcome Trust Case-Control Consortium. A full list of the investigators who contributed to the generation of the data is available from www.wtccc.org.uk. Funding for the Wellcome Trust Case-Control Consortium was provided by the Wellcome Trust under award 076113 and 085475.

Author Contributions

Conceived and designed the experiments: BL CML TS. Performed the experiments: BL. Analyzed the data: BL. Contributed reagents/materials/analysis tools: BL CML TS. Wrote the paper: BL CML TS. Obtained permission to use GWAS data: TS.

References

1. Dudbridge F, Gusnanto A (2008) Estimation of significance thresholds for genomewide association scans. Genet Epidemiol 32: 227–234.

2. Wang K, Zhang H, Kugathasan S, Annese V, Bradfield JP, et al. (2009) Diverse genome-wide association studies associate the IL12/IL23 pathway with Crohn Disease. Am J Hum Genet 84: 399–405.

3. Wang K, Li M, Bucan M (2007) Pathway-Based Approaches for Analysis of Genomewide Association Studies. Am J Hum Genet 81.

4. Holden M, Deng S, Wojnowski L, Kulle B (2008) GSEA-SNP: applying gene set enrichment analysis to SNP data from genome-wide association studies. Bioinformatics 24: 2784–2785.

5. Torkamani A, Topol EJ, Schork NJ (2008) Pathway analysis of seven common diseases assessed by genome-wide association. Genomics 92: 265–272.

6. Elbers CC, van Eijk KR, Franke L, Mulder F, van der Schouw YT, et al. (2009) Using genome-wide pathway analysis to unravel the etiology of complex diseases. Genet Epidemiol 33: 419–431.

7. Holmans P, Green EK, Pahwa JS, Ferreira MA, Purcell SM, et al. (2009) Gene ontology analysis of GWA study data sets provides insights into the biology of bipolar disorder. Am J Hum Genet 85: 13–24.

8. Perry JRB, McCarthy MI, Hattersley AT, Zeggini E, Weedon MN, et al. (2009) Interrogating Type 2 Diabetes Genome-Wide Association Data Using a Biological Pathway-Based Approach. Diabetes 58: 1463–1467.

9. Hong MG, Pawitan Y, Magnusson PK, Prince JA (2009) Strategies and issues in the detection of pathway enrichment in genome-wide association studies. Hum Genet 126: 289–301.

10. Baranzini SE, Galwey NW, Wang J, Khankhanian P, Lindberg R, et al. (2009) Pathway and network-based analysis of genome-wide association studies in multiple sclerosis. Hum Mol Genet 18: 2078–2090.

11. Brorsson C, Hansen NT, Lage K, Bergholdt R, Brunak S, et al. (2009) Identification of T1D susceptibility genes within the MHC region by combining protein interaction networks and SNP genotyping data. Diabetes, Obesity and Metabolism 11: 60–66.

12. Segre AV, Groop L, Mootha VK, Daly MJ, Altshuler D (2010) Common inherited variation in mitochondrial genes is not enriched for associations with type 2 diabetes or related glycemic traits. PLoS Genet 6.

13. Mootha VK, Lindgren CM, Eriksson KF, Subramanian A, Sihag S, et al. (2003) PGC-1alpha-responsive genes involved in oxidative phosphorylation are coordinately downregulated in human diabetes. Nat Genet 34: 267–273.

14. Ashburner M, Ball CA, Blake JA, Botstein D, Butler H, et al. (2000) Gene Ontology: tool for the unification of biology. Nat Genet 25: 25–29.

15. Kanehisa M, Goto S (2000) KEGG: Kyoto Encyclopedia of Genes and Genomes. Nucleic Acids Res 28: 27–30.

16. Wellcome Trust Case Control Consortium T (2007) Genome-wide association study of 14,000 cases of seven common diseases and 3,000 shared controls. Nature 447: 661–678.

17. Franke A, McGovern DP, Barrett JC, Wang K, Radford-Smith GL, et al. (2010) Genome-wide meta-analysis increases to 71 the number of confirmed Crohn's disease susceptibility loci. Nat Genet 42(12): 1118–25.

18. Barrett JC, Clayton DG, Concannon P, Akolkar B, Cooper JD, et al. (2009) Genome-wide association study and meta-analysis find that over 40 loci affect risk of type 1 diabetes. Nat Genet 41(6): 703–7.

19. Purcell S, Neale B, Todd-Brown K, Thomas L, Ferreira MAR, et al. (2007) PLINK: A Tool Set for Whole-Genome Association and Population-Based Linkage Analyses. Am J Hum Genet 81: 559–575.

20. Devlin B, Roeder K (1999) Genomic control for association studies. Biometrics 55: 997–1004.

21. Price AL, Patterson NJ, Plenge RM, Weinblatt ME, Shadick NA, et al. (2006) Principal components analysis corrects for stratification in genome-wide association studies. Nat Genet 38: 904–909.

22. National Center for Biotechnology Information (NCBI). Available: ftp://ftp.ncbi.nih.gov Accessed 2009 Nov 3.

23. Galaxy. Available: http://galaxy.psu.edu/. Accessed 2009 Nov 5.

24. Lehne B, Lewis CM, Schlitt T (2011) Exome localization of complex disease association signals. BMC Genomics 12: 92.

25. Lasko TA, Bhagwat JG, Zou KH, Ohno-Machado L (2005) The use of receiver operating characteristic curves in biomedical informatics. Journal of Biomedical Informatics 38: 404–415.

26. Ogura Y, Bonen DK, Inohara N, Nicolae DL, Chen FF, et al. (2001) A frameshift mutation in NOD2 associated with susceptibility to Crohn's disease. Nature 411: 603–606.

27. Hampe J, Cuthbert A, Croucher PJ, Mirza MM, Mascheretti S, et al. (2001) Association between insertion mutation in NOD2 gene and Crohn's disease in German and British populations. Lancet 357: 1925–1928.

28. Hugot JP, Chamaillard M, Zouali H, Lesage S, Cezard JP, et al. (2001) Association of NOD2 leucine-rich repeat variants with susceptibility to Crohn's disease. Nature 411: 599–603.

29. El Kasmi KC, Smith AM, Williams L, Neale G, Panopoulos AD, et al. (2007) Cutting edge: A transcriptional repressor and corepressor induced by the STAT3-regulated anti-inflammatory signaling pathway. J Immunol 179: 7215–7219.

30. Wang K, Li M, Hakonarson H (2010) Analysing biological pathways in genome-wide association studies. Nat Rev Genet 11: 843–854.

31. Cao W, Henry MD, Borrow P, Yamada H, Elder JH, et al. (1998) Identification of -Dystroglycan as a Receptor for Lymphocytic Choriomeningitis Virus and Lassa Fever Virus. Science 282: 2079–2081.

32. Rambukkana A, Yamada H, Zanazzi G, Mathus T, Salzer JL, et al. (1998) Role of -Dystroglycan as a Schwann Cell Receptor for Mycobacterium leprae. Science 282: 2076–2079.

33. Warth A (2008) Is [alpha]-dystroglycan the missing link in the mechanism of enterocyte uptake and translocation of Mycobacterium avium paratuberculosis. Medical Hypotheses 70: 369–374.

34. Todd JA, Walker NM, Cooper JD, Smyth DJ, Downes K, et al. (2007) Robust associations of four new chromosome regions from genome-wide analyses of type 1 diabetes. Nat Genet 39: 857–864.

35. Ballard DH, Aporntewan C, Lee JY, Lee JS, Wu Z, et al. (2009) A pathway analysis applied to Genetic Analysis Workshop 16 genome-wide rheumatoid arthritis data. BMC Proc 3(Suppl 7): S91.

36. Chapman J, Whittaker J (2008) Analysis of multiple SNPs in a candidate gene or region. Genet Epidemiol 32: 560–566.

37. Buil A, Martinez-Perez A, Perera-Lluna A, Rib L, Caminal P, et al. (2009) A new gene-based association test for genome-wide association studies. BMC Proc 3(Suppl 7): S130.

38. Cui Y, Kang G, Sun K, Qian M, Romero R, et al. (2008) Gene-centric genomewide association study via entropy. Genetics 179: 637–650.

39. Moskvina V, Craddock N, Holmans P, Nikolov I, Pahwa JS, et al. (2008) Gene-wide analyses of genome-wide association data sets: evidence for multiple common risk alleles for schizophrenia and bipolar disorder and for overlap in genetic risk. Mol Psychiatry.

40. Yu K, Li Q, Bergen AW, Pfeiffer RM, Rosenberg PS, et al. (2009) Pathway analysis by adaptive combination of P-values. Genet Epidemiol 33: 700–709.

41. De la Cruz O, Wen X, Ke B, Song M, Nicolae DL (2010) Gene, region and pathway level analyses in whole-genome studies. Genet Epidemiol 34: 222–231.

42. Fisher RA (1932) Statistical Methods for Research Workers. London: Oliver & Boyd.

43. Li MX, Gui HS, Kwan JS, Sham PC (2011) GATES: A Rapid and Powerful Gene-Based Association Test Using Extended Simes Procedure. Am J Hum Genet 88: 283–293.

44. Raychaudhuri S, Plenge RM, Rossin EJ, Ng ACY, Purcell SM, et al. (2009) Identifying Relationships among Genomic Disease Regions: Predicting Genes at Pathogenic SNP Associations and Rare Deletions. PLoS Genet 5: e1000534.

45. Franke L, van Bakel H, Fokkens L, de Jong ED, Egmont-Petersen M, et al. (2006) Reconstruction of a functional human gene network, with an application for prioritizing positional candidate genes. Am J Hum Genet 78: 1011–1025.

46. Frazer KA, Ballinger DG, Cox DR, Hinds DA, Stuve LL, et al. (2007) A second generation human haplotype map of over 3.1 million SNPs. Nature 449: 851–861.

47. Price AL, Kryukov GV, de Bakker PI, Purcell SM, Staples J, et al. (2010) Pooled association tests for rare variants in exon-resequencing studies. Am J Hum Genet 86: 832–838.

48. Li B, Leal SM (2008) Methods for detecting associations with rare variants for common diseases: application to analysis of sequence data. Am J Hum Genet 83: 311–321.

49. Madsen BE, Browning SR (2009) A groupwise association test for rare mutations using a weighted sum statistic. PLoS Genet 5: e1000384.

11

The Cannabinoid 1 Receptor (*CNR1*) 1359 G/A Polymorphism Modulates Susceptibility to Ulcerative Colitis and the Phenotype in Crohn's Disease

Martin Storr[1]*, **Dominik Emmerdinger**[2], **Julia Diegelmann**[2], **Simone Pfennig**[2], **Thomas Ochsenkühn**[2], **Burkhard Göke**[2], **Peter Lohse**[3], **Stephan Brand**[2]

1 Division of Gastroenterology, Department of Medicine, University of Calgary, Calgary, Alberta, Canada, 2 Department of Medicine II – Grosshadern, Ludwig-Maximilians-University Munich, Munich, Germany, 3 Department of Clinical Chemistry – Grosshadern, Ludwig-Maximilians-University Munich, Munich, Germany

Abstract

Background: Recent evidence suggests a crucial role of the endocannabinoid system, including the cannabinoid 1 receptor (CNR1), in intestinal inflammation. We therefore investigated the influence of the *CNR1* 1359 G/A (p.Thr453Thr; rs1049353) single nucleotide polymorphism (SNP) on disease susceptibility and phenotype in patients with ulcerative colitis (UC) and Crohn's disease (CD).

Methods: Genomic DNA from 579 phenotypically well-characterized individuals was analyzed for the *CNR1* 1359 G/A SNP. Amongst these were 166 patients with UC, 216 patients with CD, and 197 healthy controls.

Results: Compared to healthy controls, subjects A/A homozygous for the *CNR1* 1359 G/A SNP had a reduced risk to develop UC (p = 0.01, OR 0.30, 95% CI 0.12–0.78). The polymorphism did not modulate CD susceptibility, but carriers of the minor A allele had a lower body mass index than G/G wildtype carriers (p = 0.0005). In addition, homozygous carriers of the G allele were more likely to develop CD before 40 years of age (p = 5.9×10^{-7}) than carriers of the A allele.

Conclusion: The CNR1 p.Thr453Thr polymorphism appears to modulate UC susceptibility and the CD phenotype. The endocannabinoid system may influence the manifestation of inflammatory bowel diseases, suggesting endocannabinoids as potential target for future therapies.

Editor: Syed A. Aziz, Health Canada, Canada

Funding: M. Storr is supported by grants from the Deutsche Forschungsgemeinschaft (DFG STO645/2-2), the Crohn's and Colitis Foundation of Canada (CCFC), and a grant from the University of Calgary (URGC-1011592). J. Diegelmann received a grant from the University of Munich (Promotionsstipendium). S. Brand is supported by grants from the DFG (BR 1912/5-1), the Else Kraner-Fresenius-Stiftung (Else Kraner Fresenius Memorial Stipendium 2005; P50/05/EKMS05/62), by the Ludwig-Demling Grant 2007 from DCCV e.V., and grants from the Ludwig-Maximilians University Munich (Excellence Initiative - Investment Fund 2008 and FaFoLe program). The funders had no role in study design, data collection and analysis, decision to publish, or preparation of the manuscript.

Competing Interests: The authors have declared that no competing interests exist.

* E-mail: mstorr@ucalgary.ca

Introduction

Anecdotal reports suggest that marijuana- or tetrahydrocannabinol-containing products may be effective in alleviating symptoms in patients with ulcerative colitis (UC) and Crohn's disease (CD). [1,2] This is supported by recent studies of our group and others suggesting that pharmacological activation of the cannabinoid 1 (CB$_1$) receptor with selective receptor agonists decreases the inflammatory response in various murine models of colonic inflammation including dinitrobenzene sulphonic acid (DNBS)-, trinitrobenzene sulphonic acid (TNBS)- and dextran sodium sulfate (DSS)-induced colitis. [3–7] Interestingly, pharmacological blockade of CB$_1$ receptors or genetic ablation of CB$_1$ receptors (*CNR1*$^{-/-}$ mice) aggravates intestinal inflammation in these models, [3,7] emphasizing the physiological relevance of the CB$_1$ receptor in the protection against intestinal inflammation. Increased mucosal levels of the endocannabinoid anandamide during intestinal inflammation in humans further stress the role of the CB$_1$ receptor and the endocannabinoid system in

intestinal inflammation. [4] Thus, present knowledge suggests up-regulation of endocannabinoids as an important protective mechanism in intestinal inflammation.

The endocannabinoid system and the CB$_1$ and CB$_2$ receptors seem to be crucially involved in the regulation of multiple physiological functions, e.g. in the heart, where they relax coronary arteries and decrease cardiac work, [8] in organ perfusion, [9] in metabolic homeostasis, [10,11] and in the regulation of bone mass by osteoclasts, [12] as well as in the protection against stress responses, inflammation, and associated repair mechanisms. [13,14] Although recent evidence suggests that the endocannabinoid system is involved in many physiological and pathophysiological functions of the gastrointestinal tract such as intestinal motility, secretion, and intestinal inflammation [3,15–20], the exact mechanisms underlying these findings are not yet known. It was recently suggested that CB$_1$ signaling may be up-regulated during colitis, [3] but it is unknown whether this is a specific feature of the colitis model or a general response to intestinal inflammation.

Moreover, the role of the CB$_1$ receptor in human inflammatory bowel disease (IBD) has not been clarified. Increased anandamide levels were found in mucosal biopsies from UC patients, suggesting a role of the endocannabinoid system in UC. [4] In contrast, the colonic expression of the endocannabinoid 2-acyl-glycerol (2-AG) is not increased in UC. [4] So far, however, no other studies analyzing the endocannabinoid system or the pharmacological effects of cannabinoids in human IBD have been published.

Gastrointestinal inflammation is likely the result of multiple factors, e.g., increased pro-inflammatory stimuli and reduced protective capability. The overall balance between pro- and anti-inflammatory mechanisms may determine the progression and severity of intestinal inflammation. [21,22] Given the results of recent genome-wide association studies, [23] genetic susceptibility is an important factor contributing to IBD development. Moreover, knowledge of genetic susceptibility factors could provide important pathophysiologic insights for the generation of novel IBD therapeutics.

Considering our previous work on the endocannabinoid system in murine intestinal inflammation, [3,6,7,24] we hypothesized that genetic variants in the CNR1 gene, which may modulate CB$_1$ receptor function, could be associated with an increased susceptibility to IBD. To test our hypothesis, we genotyped a cohort of more than 550 individuals including 382 IBD patients and analyzed whether the 1359 G/A (p.Thr453Thr; rs1049353) single nucleotide polymorphism (SNP) within the CNR1 gene encoding the CB$_1$ receptor modulates the susceptibility to CD and UC or results in a certain IBD phenotype. The selection of the CNR1 1359 G/A SNP was based on previous studies reporting that this polymorphism is associated with other disorders modulated by the endocannabinoid system such as alcohol dependence and hebephrenic schizophrenia. [25,26]

Methods

Ethics Statement

The study was approved by the Ethics Committee of the Medical Faculty of the University of Munich. All participating subjects gave their written, informed consent prior to the genetic analysis.

Human Study Population

The study population comprised 579 individuals, including 216 patients with CD, 166 with UC, and 197 healthy, unrelated controls. Patients and controls were recruited at the IBD center of the Ludwig-Maximilians-University Munich, Campus Grosshadern, from September 2002 to December 2006. The diagnoses of CD and UC were established following clinical guidelines, using endoscopic, radiological, and histopathologic criteria. Table 1 shows the baseline characteristics of the study population. All 197 controls were unrelated, healthy individuals of Caucasian origin and sex-matched (by frequency) to the CD group. Controls were healthy blood donors without a history or family history of IBD. Demographics and routine clinical data (including location and behavior of IBD, disease-related complications, and prescription data of immunosuppressive and immunomodulatory therapy e.g., azathioprine, 6-mercaptopurine, methotrexate, infliximab) were recorded by retrospective analysis of the clinical charts by two independent investigators and an interview including a questionnaire at the time of enrollment. All data were collected blind to the CNR1 genotype. Patients with CD or UC were grouped according to age at diagnosis, disease localization, and behavior status of the Vienna classification, [27] and the recent modifications suggested by the Montreal classification. [28]

DNA Extraction and Genotyping of the CNR1 Polymorphism

Recently, a guanosine-to-adenine substitution at nucleotide position 1359 has been identified in the CNR1 gene (rs1049353) [25,29]. Thus, three genotypes (GG, GA, AA) are possible. Genomic DNA was isolated from peripheral blood leukocytes by standard procedures using the DNA blood mini kit from Qiagen (Hilden, Germany). Genotyping was done as previously described [7,30]. Briefly, a single 20-µl PCR was performed to genotype this

Table 1. Demographic characteristics of the study population.

	(1) CD (n=216)	(2) UC (n=166)	(3) Controls (n=197)	(1) vs (2) p value	(1) vs (3) p value	(2) vs (3) p value
Gender						
Male (%)	105 (48.6%)	83 (50.0%)	114 (58.0%)	p=0.84	p=0.06	p=0.14
Female (%)	111 (51.4%)	83 (50.0%)	83 (42.0%)			
Age (yr)						
Mean ± SD	41.4±11.8	43.3±14.4	43.9±21.6	p=0.17	p=0.19	p=0.75
Range	17–71	19–85	0–80			
Body mass index						
Mean ± SD	23.1±3.9	24.2±4.2		p=0.02		
Range	16–34	16–41				
Age at diagnosis (yr)						
Mean ± SD	28.1±11.4	31.8±13.7		p=0.006		
Range	7–67	9–81				
Disease duration (yr)						
Mean ± SD	13.5±8.5	11.5±7.6		p=0.016		
Range	2–44	1–40				
Positive family history of IBD (%)	30 (13.9%)	21 (12.7%)		p=0.76		

site using approximately 200 ng of genomic DNA and 20 pmol each of the following primers 5′-GAAAGCTGCATCAA-GAGCCC-3′ (forward) and 5′-TTTTCCTGTGCTGCCA-GGG-3′ (reverse). Other conditions were as follows: 1.5 mM $MgCl_2$, 400 μM of each dNTP, 1.25 U Taq polymerase, and 1× reaction buffer (Life Technologies, Rockville, MD). DNA amplification was performed with 40 cycles of 94°C, 60°C, and 72°C for 30 seconds each, preceded by a single cycle of 95°C for 15 minutes and followed by a single cycle of 72°C for 5 minutes. Five μl of the resulting 111 bp PCR product were then digested overnight with 10 U of MspI (New England Biolabs, Beverly, MA) at 37°C. This resulted in fragments of 92 and 19 bp, when a G was present at nucleotide position 385, while the fragment remained uncut, when an A was present. Restriction digests were analyzed by electrophoresis of the digestion mixture in a 2% agarose gel stained with ethidium bromide. The assay was verified by sequencing the PCR product and the digested PCR fragments of all possible genotypes.

Statistics

Fisher's exact test was used for comparison between categorical variables. All tests were two-tailed. P values <0.05 were considered as significant. Analyses were performed using SPSS 14.0.1 software for Windows.

Results

The CNR1 1359 G/A (p.Thr453Thr) Polymorphism Modulates UC but Not CD Susceptibility

Given the above reported increased CB_1 receptor expression in several models of intestinal inflammation and previous studies implicating the *CNR1* 1359 G/A (p.Thr453Thr) SNP in endocannabinoid-mediated diseases, [25,31] we investigated whether this polymorphism modulates susceptibility and phenotype of CD and UC. The demographic characteristics of the IBD and control population analyzed are given in Table 1. The CD patients were classified with regard to their disease phenotype, considering disease location, the age at diagnosis, and disease behaviour by using the Montreal classification. [27,28] The majority of patients had an onset of the disease in their mid20s (mean age at first diagnosis of CD: 28.1±11.4 years). The mean age at first diagnosis of UC was 31.8±13.7 years. 13.9% of the CD patients and 12.7% of the UC patients had a positive family history of IBD.

The results of the CNR1 p.Thr453Thr genotyping analysis in 216 CD patients, 166 UC patients, and 197 controls are shown in Table 2. The frequencies of heterozygous and homozygous carriers of this polymorphism did not differ significantly from the expected ratio according to the Hardy-Weinberg law. Patients with UC were less likely to be 1359 A/A homozygous (p = 0.01, OR 0.30, 95% CI 0.12–0.78). In contrast, this polymorphism did not influence susceptibility to CD (Table 2).

The CNR1 1359 G/A (p.Thr453Thr) Polymorphism Modulates Disease Onset and Body Mass Index in CD

In Table 3, we provide a detailed genotype-phenotype analysis of the *CNR1* 1359 G/A polymorphism in CD patients. Carriers of the 1359 A/A genotype were likely to have a lower body weight (p = 0.0005). In addition, homozygous carriers of the major G allele were more likely to develop CD before 40 years of age (p = 5.9×10^{-7}) than carriers of the minor A allele. There was no association between the CNR1 p.Thr453Thr polymorphism and disease location, use of immunosuppressive drugs, family history of IBD, CD-related surgery, stenoses, and abscesses (Table 3). In

Table 2. Genotype frequencies of *CNR1* 1359 G/A (p.Thr453Thr) polymorphism in patients with Crohn's disease (CD) and ulcerative colitis (UC) as well as in controls.

	(1) GG	(2) GA	(3) AA	(1) vs. (2)	(1) vs. (3)
CD	115 (53.3%)	86 (39.8%)	15 (6.9%)	**CD vs. Controls**	
(n = 216)				p = 0.83	p = 0.28
Controls	103 (52.3%)	73 (37.0%)	21 (10.7%)	**UC vs. Controls**	
(n = 197)					
				p = 0.74	**p = 0.01 OR 0.30 CI 0.12–0.78**
UC	97 (58.4%)	63 (38.0%)	6 (3.6%)	**CD vs. UC**	
(n = 166)				p = 0.52	p = 0.17

addition, the CNR1 p.Thr453Thr polymorphism did not influence the UC phenotype (Table 4).

Discussion

We analyzed the effect of the CNR1 p.Thr453Thr polymorphism on IBD susceptibility and disease phenotype. This study was based on our previous results which suggested that CB_1 receptor signaling is involved in defense mechanisms in response to acute intestinal inflammation in animal models. [3,7] Based on this knowledge, we hypothesized that differential CB_1 receptor expression, e.g., modulated by genetic factors, may contribute to IBD susceptibility. In the present study, we focused on the 1359 G/A polymorphism within the *CNR1* gene encoding the CB_1 receptor, given the importance of this nucleotide substitution in other endocannabinoid-mediated disorders such as alcohol dependence [25] and schizophrenia [32]. Although the CNR1 1359 G/A (p.Thr453Thr) SNP is a silent mutation, which does not result in an amino acid exchange, it might be associated with alterations e.g. in RNA splicing. [33]

Our study demonstrated an association with UC susceptibility but not with CD susceptibility. The prevalence of 1359 A/A homozygous carriers was 10.7% in the control population, 6.9% in CD patients, and only 3.6% in UC patients. The genotype frequencies found for our control population were within the values expected from Hardy-Weinberg equilibrium and were similar to a previous German control cohort. [29] However, given the limited size of the study population and the low prevalence of 1359 A/A homozygous carriers among UC patients, this finding has to be confirmed in larger replication cohorts. Furthermore, given that the study was primarily designed to detect differences in the frequency of IBD risk alleles, the control population was selected only regarding absence of IBD and other chronic diseases as well as being negative for a family history of IBD. Therefore a selection bias resulting in differences e.g. in BMI can not be excluded though it is intriguing that a lower BMI was found with CD and not with UC.

The human *CNR1* gene is localized on chromosome 6q14–q15. [34] Interestingly, an earlier genome-wide family-based linkage study found an association of this region with celiac disease [35]. We recently demonstrated that celiac disease and UC (but not CD) share another common susceptibility locus on chromosome 4q27. [36] Although none of the recent genome-wide association studies demonstrated the *CNR1* gene as a major IBD susceptibility gene, a previous genome scan in 260 IBD-affected relative pairs found

Table 3. Association between the *CNR1* 1359 G/A (p.Thr453Thr) genotype and CD characteristics.

	(1) GG (n = 114)	(2) GA (n = 86)	(3) AA (n = 15)	(1) vs (2) P value	(1) vs (3) P value	(1) vs (2)+(3) P value
Male sex	56 (49.1%)	41 (47.7%)	8 (53.3%)	p = 0.89	p = 0.79	p = 1.00
Body mass index (kg/m^2)						
Mean ± SD	23.9±4.0	22.1±3.5	22.0±3.6	**p = 0.001**	**p = 0.05**	**p = 0.0005**
Range	16–34	16–32	18–31			
Age at diagnosis (yr)						
Mean ± SD	26.9±10.6	29.7±12.0	27.2±14.1	p = 0.09	p = 0.78	p = 0.11
Range	7–57	13–67	16–52			
Disease duration (yr)						
Mean ± SD	13.1±8.4	14.4±8.9	10.8±7.6	p = 0.31	p = 0.31	p = 0.52
Range	2–44	3–35	3–26			
Age (yr)						
Mean ± SD	39.9±11.5	44.0±11.7	37.2±12.1	**p = 0.01**	p = 0.46	**p = 0.05**
Range	17–70	23–71	19–56			
Age at diagnosis						
<17 years (A1)	0 (0.0%)	0 (0.0%)	0 (0.0%)	**p = 8.6×10^{-8}**	p = 0.33	**p = 5.9×10^{-7}**
17–40 years (A2)	89 (78.1%)	35 (40.7%)	10 (66.7%)			
>40 years (A3)	25 (21.9%)	51 (59.3%)	5 (33.3%)			
Location						
Terminal ileum (L1)	12 (10.5%)	8 (9.3%)	2 (13.3%)	p = 1.00	p = 0.67	p = 1.00
Colon (L2)	19 (16.7%)	18 (20.9%)	4 (26.7%)	p = 0.47	p = 0.47	p = 0.39
Ileocolon (L3)	60 (52.6%)	43 (50.0%)	7 (46.7%)	p = 0.78	p = 0.79	p = 0.68
Upper GI (L4)	23 (20.2%)	17 (19.8%)	2 (13.3%)	p = 1.00	p = 0.73	p = 0.86
Ileal involvement (L1 + L3)	72 (63.2%)	51 (59.3%)	9 (60.0%)	p = 0.66	p = 0.78	p = 0.18
Behaviour						
Non-sticturing, Non penetrating (B1)	22 (19.3%)	17 (19.8%)	4 (26.7%)	p = 1.00	p = 0.50	p = 0.86
Stricturing (B2)	33 (28.9%)	18 (20.9%)	3 (20.0%)	p = 0.25	p = 0.56	p = 0.21
Penetrating (B3)	59 (51.8%)	51 (59.3%)	8 (53.7%)	p = 0.32	p = 1.00	p = 0.34
Use of immunosuppressive agents	90 (78.9%)	64 (74.4%)	11 (73.3%)	p = 0.50	p = 0.74	p = 0.42
Extraintestinal manifestations	80 (70.2%)	55 (64.0%)	11 (73.3%)	p = 0.36	p = 1.00	p = 0.47
Positive family history of IBD	29 (25.4%)	13 (15.1%)	3 (20.0%)	p = 0.08	p = 0.76	p = 0.09
Surgery because of CD	65 (57.0%)	54 (62.8%)	8 (53.3%)	p = 0.47	p = 0.79	p = 0.58
Fistulas	59 (51.8%)	51 (59.3%)	8 (53.3%)	p = 0.32	p = 1.00	p = 0.34
Stenosis	78 (68.4%)	58 (67.4%)	9 (60.0%)	p = 0.88	p = 0.56	p = 0.77
Abscesses	41 (36.0%)	32 (37.2%)	4 (26.7%)	p = 0.88	p = 0.57	p = 1.00

[1]Disease behavior was defined according to the Montreal classification [28]. A stricturing disease phenotype was defined as presence of stenosis without penetrating disease. The diagnosis of stenosis was made surgically, endoscopically, or radiologically (using MRI enteroclysis).
[2]Immunosuppressive agents included azathioprine, 6-mercaptopurine, 6-thioguanin, methotrexate, and/or infliximab.
[3]Extraintestinal manifestations were defined as one or more of the following IBD-related diseases: non-medication-induced arthropathies (e.g., ankylosing spondylitis, sacroileitis, peripheral arthritis), eye involvement (e.g., episcleritis and/or iritis/uveitis), skin involvement (e.g., erythema nodosum and pyoderma gangrenosum), non-medication-induced biliary disease (e.g., sclerosing cholangitis).
[4]Only surgery related to CD-specific problems (e.g., fistulectomy, colectomy, ileostomy) was included.

nominal evidence for linkage of IBD to loci on chromosome 6q (lod = 2.21 between D6S2436/D6S305). [37]

We recently confirmed a number of CD susceptibility genes found in genome-wide associations studies such as *NOD2*, [38,39] *IL23R*, [40] and *ATG16L1* [41], but we also demonstrated differences in the genetic susceptibility to CD [42], suggesting that there are differences in the genetic susceptibility to IBD even between different Caucasian populations. In addition, other genetic associations such as those of *TLR4* SNPs with CD susceptibility shown by our group [43] were not among the major

CD susceptibility genes in a recent meta-analysis of genome-wide scans, although this gene has been confirmed as a CD susceptibility gene. [44]

Currently, it is unknown if the *CNR1* 1359 G/A (p.Thr453Thr) SNP modulates CB_1 receptor expression or function. Particularly changes at amino acid positions 418–439 seem to be associated with a lack of receptor desensitization [45], and allelic variation in the *CNR1* gene was suggested to be associated with a lower rather than a higher receptor activity, [46] but detailed studies investigating receptor activity based on different *CNR1* genotypes

Table 4. Association between *CNR1* 1359 G/A (p.Thr453Thr) genotype and UC disease characteristics.

	(1) GG (n = 97)	(2) GA (n = 63)	(3) AA (n = 6)	(1) vs. (2) p value	(1) vs. (3) p value	(2) vs. (3) p value	(1) vs. (2)+(3) p value
Male sex	47 (48.5%)	32 (50.8%)	4 (66.7%)	p = 0.87	p = 0.44	p = 0.68	p = 0.75
Body mass index (kg/m^2)							
Mean ± SD	23.8±3.7	24.4±4.9	26.5±4.6	p = 0.46	p = 0.27	p = 0.39	p = 0.30
Range	16–32	18–41	20–32				
Age at diagnosis (yr)							
Mean ± SD	31.7±13.9	31.7±13.4	34.5±17.0	p = 0.99	p = 0.70	p = 0.70	p = 0.92
Range	9–73	14–81	13–57				
Disease duration (yr)							
Mean ± SD	11.9±6.5	12.3±8.7	14.2±11.1	p = 0.79	p = 0.64	p = 0.70	p = 0.68
Range	2–2 9	2–41	4–36				
Age (yr)							
Mean ± SD	43.7±14.2	43.9±15.1	48.7±11.9	p = 0.93	p = 0.37	p = 0.40	p = 0.79
Range	21–81	20–86	37–68				
Location							
Rectum	21 (21.7%)	7 (11.1%)	1 (16.7%)	p = 0.13	p = 1.00	p = 0.55	p = 0.10
Left-sided	28 (28.9%)	28 (44.4%)	2 (33.3%)	p = 0.06	p = 1.00	p = 0.69	p = 0.07
Pancolitis	48 (49.4%)	28 (44.4%)	3 (50.0%)	p = 0.63	p = 1.00	p = 1.00	p = 0.64
Use of immunosuppressive agents	67 (69.1%)	48 (76.2%)	4 (66.7%)	p = 0.37	p = 1.00	p = 0.63	p = 0.39
Use of infliximab	27 (27.8%)	11 (17.5%)	1 (16.7%)	p = 0.18	p = 1.00	p = 1.00	p = 0.14
Surgery due to UC	4 (4.1%)	0 (0.0%)	0 (0.0%)	p = 0.15	p = 1.00	p = 1.00	p = 0.14
Fistulas	4 (4.1%)	3 (4.8%)	0 (0.0%)	p = 1.00	p = 1.00	p = 1.00	p = 1.00
Stenosis	15 (15.5%)	4 (6.3%)	1 (16.7%)	p = 0.13	p = 1.00	p = 0.37	p = 0.15
Abscesses	5 (5.2%)	4 (6.3%)	0 (0.0%)	p = 0.74	p = 1.00	p = 1.00	p = 1.00
Extraintestinal manifestations	14 (14.4%)	11 (17.5%)	0 (0.0%)	p = 0.66	p = 1.00	p = 0.58	p = 0.83
Positive family history	15 (15.5%)	6 (9.5%)	0 (0.0%)	p = 0.34	p = 0.59	p = 1.00	p = 0.24

[1]Immunosuppressive agents included azathioprine, 6-mercaptopurine, and/or infliximab.
[2]Only UC-related surgery (e.g., colectomy) was included.
[3]Extraintestinal manifestations were defined as one or more of the following IBD-related diseases: non-medication-induced arthropathies (e.g., ankylosing spondylitis, sacroileitis, peripheral arthritis), eye involvement (e.g., episcleritis and iritis/uveitis), skin involvement (e.g., erythema nodosum and pyoderma gangrenosum), non-medication-induced biliary disease (e.g., sclerosing cholangitis).

are lacking. The assumption that allelic variation is associated with reduced CB1 activity would also explain the low BMI found in the 1359 A/A homozygous CD patients. Consistent with these data, the 1359 G/G wildtype genotype has been shown to be associated with an increased BMI and overweight in an Italian study of a healthy population. [47] A low BMI in CD patients is also considered to be an indicator of high disease activity. Therefore, 1359 A/A homozygosity could contribute to a more severe disease phenotype. This would be consistent with our results in $CNR1^{-/-}$ mice, demonstrating that these knockout mice take a more fulminate course in DNBS and DSS colitis. [3] However, functional experiments have to analyze if CNR1 signaling is indeed decreased in 1359 A/A homozygous patients.

Our findings add evidence that targeting the CB$_1$ receptor system may modulate intestinal inflammation, suggesting this receptor as a potential target for future treatments. Similarly, animal models suggest that CB$_1$ receptor activation with exogenous CB$_1$ receptor agonists induces protection against intestinal inflammation. [3,5] Therefore, the increased CB$_1$ receptor expression seen in murine colitis models is likely an intrinsic protective mechanism to counter-regulate the deleterious effects of intestinal inflammation. The physiological importance of the CB$_1$ receptor and the endocannabinoid system becomes obvious when endocannabinoid levels are increased by blocking their degradation. Under these circumstances, intestinal inflammation is reduced and the CB$_1$ receptor is involved in this protection, emphasizing the important pathophysiological role of this system in intestinal inflammation. [7] Whether monitoring of CB$_1$ receptor function or genotyping can identify responders of future treatments targeting the CB$_1$ receptor remains speculative and has to be clarified in clinical trials.

In summary, we demonstrate that the *CNR1* 1359 G/A polymorphism modulates IBD susceptibility and phenotype. Specifically, we show that 1359 A/A homozygosity protects against UC and that CD patients carrying the minor A allele have a later disease onset and a lower BMI. These findings have to be confirmed in a larger replication study. Given the low prevalence of 1359 A/A homozygous carriers, this likely can be achieved only in a large multicenter trial. Nevertheless, our findings provide further evidence that endocannabinoids modulate intestinal inflammation, suggesting that this system could act as a target for future therapeutic interventions.

Author Contributions

Conceived and designed the experiments: MS JD TO BG PL SB. Performed the experiments: DE. Analyzed the data: MS DE JD SP PL SB.

Contributed reagents/materials/analysis tools: MS TO BG PL. Wrote the paper: MS SB.

References

1. Grinspoon L, Bakalar JB (1995) Marihuana as medicine. A plea for reconsideration. JAMA 273: 1875–1876.
2. Grinspoon L (1999) The future of medical marijuana. Forsch Komplementärmed 6 Suppl 3: 40–43.
3. Massa F, Marsicano G, Hermann H, Cannich A, Monory K, et al. (2004) The endogenous cannabinoid system protects against colonic inflammation. J Clin Invest 113: 1202–1209.
4. D'Argenio G, Valenti M, Scaglione G, Cosenza V, Sorrentini I, et al. (2006) Up-regulation of anandamide levels as an endogenous mechanism and a pharmacological strategy to limit colon inflammation. FASEB J 20: 568–570.
5. Kimball ES, Schneider CR, Wallace NH, Hornby PJ (2006) Agonists of cannabinoid receptor 1 and 2 inhibit experimental colitis induced by oil of mustard and by dextran sulfate sodium. Am J Physiol Gastrointest Liver Physiol 291: G364–G371.
6. Sibaev A, Massa F, Yuce B, Marsicano G, Lehr HA, et al. (2006) CB1 and TRPV1 receptors mediate protective effects on colonic electrophysiological properties in mice. J Mol Med 84: 513–520.
7. Storr M, Keenan CM, Emmerdinger D, Zhang H, Yuce B, et al. (2008) Targeting endocannabinoid degradation protects against experimental colitis in mice: involvement of CB_1 and CB_2 receptors. J Mol Med 86: 925–936.
8. Hiley CR (2009) Endocannabinoids and the Heart. J Cardiovasc Pharmacol.
9. Caraceni P, Pertosa A, Giannone F, Domenicali M, Grattagliano I, et al. (2009) Antagonism of the cannabinoid CB-1 receptor protects rat liver against ischemia-reperfusion injury complicated by endotoxemia. Gut 58: 1135–1143.
10. Sarzani R, Bordicchia M, Marcucci P, Bedetta S, Santini S, et al. (2009) Altered pattern of cannabinoid type 1 receptor expression in adipose tissue of dysmetabolic and overweight patients. Metabolism 58: 361–367.
11. Scheen AJ (2009) The endocannabinoid system: a promising target for the management of type 2 diabetes. Curr Protein Pept Sci 10: 56–74.
12. Idris AI, van 't Hof RJ, Greig IR, Ridge SA, Baker D, et al. (2005) Regulation of bone mass, bone loss and osteoclast activity by cannabinoid receptors. Nat Med 11: 774–779.
13. Maresz K, Pryce G, Ponomarev ED, Marsicano G, Croxford JL, et al. (2007) Direct suppression of CNS autoimmune inflammation via the cannabinoid receptor CB1 on neurons and CB2 on autoreactive T cells. Nat Med 13: 492–497.
14. Teixeira-Clerc F, Julien B, Grenard P, Tran Van NJ, Deveaux V, et al. (2006) CB1 cannabinoid receptor antagonism: a new strategy for the treatment of liver fibrosis. Nat Med 12: 671–676.
15. De Petrocellis L, Cascio MG, Di Marzo V (2004) The endocannabinoid system: a general view and latest additions. Br J Pharmacol 141: 765–774.
16. Storr M, Yuce B, Goeke B (2006) Perspectives of cannabinoids in gastroenterology. Z Gastroenterol 44: 185–191.
17. Storr M, Yuce B, Andrews C, Sharkey KA (2008) The role of the endocannabinoid system in the pathophysiology and treatment of irritable bowel syndrome. Neurogastroenterol Motil 20: 857–868.
18. Izzo AA, Camilleri M (2008) Emerging role of cannabinoids in gastrointestinal and liver diseases: basic and clinical aspects. Gut 57: 1140–1155.
19. Di Carlo G, Izzo AA (2003) Cannabinoids for gastrointestinal diseases: potential therapeutic applications. Expert Opin Investig Drugs 12: 39–49.
20. Izzo AA, Camilleri M (2008) Emerging Role of Cannabinoids in Gastrointestinal and Liver Diseases: Basic and Clinical Aspects. Gut 57: 1140–1155.
21. Mayer EA, Collins SM (2002) Evolving pathophysiologic models of functional gastrointestinal disorders. Gastroenterology 122: 2032–2048.
22. Barbara G, De Giorgio R, Stanghellini V, Cremon C, Corinaldesi R (2002) A role for inflammation in irritable bowel syndrome? Gut 51 Suppl 1: i41–i44.
23. Barrett JC, Hansoul S, Nicolae DL, Cho JH, Duerr RH, et al. (2008) Genome-wide association defines more than 30 distinct susceptibility loci for Crohn's disease. Nat Genet 40: 955–962.
24. Storr MA, Keenan CM, Zhang H, Patel KD, Makriyannis A, et al. (2009) Activation of the cannabinoid 2 receptor (CB(2)) protects against experimental colitis. Inflamm Bowel Dis 15: 1678–1685.
25. Schmidt LG, Samochowiec J, Finckh U, Fiszer-Piosik E, Horodnicki J, et al. (2002) Association of a CB1 cannabinoid receptor gene (CNR1) polymorphism with severe alcohol dependence. Drug Alcohol Depend 65: 221–224.
26. Ujike H, Takaki M, Nakata K, Tanaka Y, Takeda T, et al. (2002) CNR1, central cannabinoid receptor gene, associated with susceptibility to hebephrenic schizophrenia. Mol Psychiatry 7: 515–518.
27. Gasche C, Scholmerich J, Brynskov J, D'Haens G, Hanauer SB, et al. (2000) A simple classification of Crohn's disease: report of the Working Party for the World Congresses of Gastroenterology, Vienna 1998. Inflamm Bowel Dis 6: 8–15.
28. Silverberg MS, Satsangi J, Ahmad T, Arnott ID, Bernstein CN, et al. (2005) Toward an integrated clinical, molecular and serological classification of inflammatory bowel disease: Report of a Working Party of the 2005 Montreal World Congress of Gastroenterology. Can J Gastroenterol 19 Suppl A: 5–36.
29. Gadzicki D, Muller-Vahl K, Stuhrmann M (1999) A frequent polymorphism in the coding exon of the human cannabinoid receptor (CNR1) gene. Mol Cell Probes 13: 321–323.
30. Storr M, Emmerdinger D, Diegelmann J, Yuece B, Pfennig S, et al. (2008) The role of fatty acid hydrolase (FAAH) gene variants in inflammatory bowel disease. Aliment Pharmacol Ther 29: 542–551.
31. Horne AW, Phillips JA, III, Kane N, Lourenco PC, McDonald SE, et al. (2008) CB1 expression is attenuated in Fallopian tube and decidua of women with ectopic pregnancy. PLoS ONE 3: e3969.
32. Leroy S, Griffon N, Bourdel MC, Olie JP, Poirier MF, et al. (2001) Schizophrenia and the cannabinoid receptor type 1 (CB1): association study using a single-base polymorphism in coding exon 1. Am J Med Genet 105: 749–752.
33. Komar AA (2007) Silent SNPs: impact on gene function and phenotype. Pharmacogenomics 8: 1075–1080.
34. Hoehe MR, Caenazzo L, Martinez MM, Hsieh WT, Modi WS, et al. (1991) Genetic and physical mapping of the human cannabinoid receptor gene to chromosome 6q14–q15. New Biol 3: 880–885.
35. King AL, Yiannakou JY, Brett PM, Curtis D, Morris MA, et al. (2000) A genome-wide family-based linkage study of coeliac disease. Ann Hum Genet 64: 479–490.
36. Glas J, Stallhofer J, Ripke S, Wetzke M, Pfennig S, et al. (2009) Novel genetic risk markers for ulcerative colitis in the chromosome 4q27 region harboring IL2/IL21 region are in epistasis with IL23R and suggest a common genetic background for ulcerative colitis and celiac disease. Am J Gastroenterol 104: 1737–1744.
37. Barmada MM, Brant SR, Nicolae DL, Achkar JP, Panhuysen CI, et al. (2004) A genome scan in 260 inflammatory bowel disease-affected relative pairs. Inflamm Bowel Dis 10: 513–520.
38. Schnitzler F, Brand S, Staudinger T, Pfennig S, Hofbauer K, et al. (2006) Eight novel CARD15 variants detected by DNA sequence analysis of the CARD15 gene in 111 patients with inflammatory bowel disease. Immunogenetics 58: 99–106.
39. Seiderer J, Schnitzler F, Brand S, Staudinger T, Pfennig S, et al. (2006) Homozygosity for the CARD15 frameshift mutation 1007fs is predictive of early onset of Crohn's disease with ileal stenosis, entero-enteral fistulas, and frequent need for surgical intervention with high risk of re-stenosis. Scand J Gastroenterol 41: 1421–1432.
40. Glas J, Seiderer J, Wetzke M, Konrad A, Torok HP, et al. (2007) rs1004819 is the main disease-associated IL23R variant in German Crohn's disease patients: combined analysis of IL23R, CARD15, and OCTN1/2 variants. PLoS ONE 2: e819.
41. Glas J, Konrad A, Schmechel S, Dambacher J, Seiderer J, et al. (2007) The ATG16L1 gene variants rs2241879 and rs2241880 (T300A) are strongly associated with susceptibility to Crohn's disease in the German population. Am J Gastroenterol 103: 682–691.
42. Glas J, Seiderer J, Pasciuto G, Tillack C, Diegelmann J, et al. (2009) rs224136 on chromosome 10q21.1 and variants in PHOX2B, NCF4, and FAM92B are not major genetic risk factors for susceptibility to Crohn's disease in the German population. Am J Gastroenterol 104: 665–672.
43. Brand S, Staudinger T, Schnitzler F, Pfennig S, Hofbauer K, et al. (2005) The role of Toll-like receptor 4 Asp299Gly and Thr399Ile polymorphisms and CARD15/NOD2 mutations in the susceptibility and phenotype of Crohn's disease. Inflamm Bowel Dis 11: 645–652.
44. De Jager PL, Franchimont D, Waliszewska A, Bitton A, Cohen A, et al. (2007) The role of the Toll receptor pathway in susceptibility to inflammatory bowel diseases. Genes Immun 8: 387–397.
45. Jin W, Brown S, Roche JP, Hsieh C, Celver JP, et al. (1999) Distinct domains of the CB1 cannabinoid receptor mediate desensitization and internalization. J Neurosci 19: 3773–3780.
46. Siegfried Z, Kanyas K, Latzer Y, Karni O, Bloch M, et al. (2004) Association study of cannabinoid receptor gene (CNR1) alleles and anorexia nervosa: differences between restricting and binging/purging subtypes. Am J Med Genet B Neuropsychiatr Genet 125B: 126–130.
47. Gazzerro P, Caruso MG, Notarnicola M, Misciagna G, Guerra V, et al. (2007) Association between cannabinoid type-1 receptor polymorphism and body mass index in a southern Italian population. Int J Obes (Lond) 31: 908–912.

12

Inflammation Drives Dysbiosis and Bacterial Invasion in Murine Models of Ileal Crohn's Disease

Melanie Craven[1], Charlotte E. Egan[2], Scot E. Dowd[3], Sean P. McDonough[4], Belgin Dogan[1], Eric Y. Denkers[2], Dwight Bowman[2], Ellen J. Scherl[5], Kenneth W. Simpson[1]*

1 Department of Clinical Sciences, College of Veterinary Medicine, Cornell University, Ithaca, New York, United States of America, 2 Department of Microbiology and Immunology, College of Veterinary Medicine, Cornell University, Ithaca, New York, United States of America, 3 MR DNA (Molecular Research), Shallowater, Texas, United States of America, 4 Department of Pathology, College of Veterinary Medicine, Cornell University, Ithaca, New York, United States of America, 5 Division of Gastroenterology and Hepatology, Jill Roberts Inflammatory Bowel Disease Center, Weill Cornell Medical College, Cornell University, New York, New York, United States of America

Abstract

Background and Aims: Understanding the interplay between genetic susceptibility, the microbiome, the environment and the immune system in Crohn's Disease (CD) is essential for developing optimal therapeutic strategies. We sought to examine the dynamics of the relationship between inflammation, the ileal microbiome, and host genetics in murine models of ileitis.

Methods: We induced ileal inflammation of graded severity in C57BL6 mice by gavage with *Toxoplasma gondii*, *Giardia muris*, low dose indomethacin (LDI;0.1 mg/mouse), or high dose indomethacin (HDI;1 mg/mouse). The composition and spatial distribution of the mucosal microbiome was evaluated by 16S rDNA pyrosequencing and fluorescence in situ hybridization. Mucosal *E. coli* were enumerated by quantitative PCR, and characterized by phylogroup, genotype and pathotype.

Results: Moderate to severe ileitis induced by *T. gondii* (day 8) and HDI caused a consistent shift from >95% Gram + Firmicutes to >95% Gram - Proteobacteria. This was accompanied by reduced microbial diversity and mucosal invasion by adherent and invasive *E. coli*, mirroring the dysbiosis of ileal CD. In contrast, dysbiosis and bacterial invasion did not develop in mice with mild ileitis induced by *Giardia muris*. Superimposition of genetic susceptibility and *T. Gondii* infection revealed greatest dysbiosis and bacterial invasion in the CD-susceptible genotype, NOD2$^{-/-}$, and reduced dysbiosis in ileitis-resistant CCR2$^{-/-}$ mice. Abrogating inflammation with the CD therapeutic anti-TNF-α-mAb tempered dysbiosis and bacterial invasion.

Conclusions: Acute ileitis induces dysbiosis and proliferation of mucosally invasive *E. coli*, irrespective of trigger and genotype. The identification of CCR2 as a target for therapeutic intervention, and discovery that host genotype and therapeutic blockade of inflammation impact the threshold and extent of ileal dysbiosis are of high relevance to developing effective therapies for CD.

Editor: Markus M. Heimesaat, Charité, Campus Benjamin Franklin, Germany

Funding: This work was supported by grants from NY Presbyterian/Weill Cornell Medical College, the Jill Roberts Center for Inflammatory Bowel Disease and NIH (Eric Denkers: AI083526). The funders had no role in study design, data collection and analysis, decision to publish, or preparation of the manuscript.

Competing Interests: Dr. Scot Dowd is an employee of MR DNA (Molecular Research), Shallowater, TX, and performed the 16S pyrosequencing analysis. This does not represent a conflict of interest. The pyrosequencing was performed in a blinded fashion. Dr. Dowd is an expert in the analysis of 16S data and helped to evaluate the consequences of intestinal inflammation on the intestinal microbiome.

* E-mail: kws5@cornell.edu

Introduction

Inflammatory bowel diseases (IBD) encompass a complex of inflammatory intestinal disorders that are increasing in global prevalence and typified by recurrent flares of acute on chronic inflammation. [1,2] Traditionally, IBD comprises two distinct entities, Crohn's Disease (CD) and ulcerative colitis (UC), [1,2,3] both widely accepted to arise from the convergence of genetic susceptibility, enteric bacteria, the immune response, and environmental factors such as smoking, stress and diet. [3–10].

The best-characterized genetic susceptibility locus in CD has been mapped to NOD2, with polymorphisms reported in 20–30% of CD patients. [11] The NOD2 gene encodes an intracellular pathogen recognition receptor that, on sensing the bacterial muramyl dipeptide, evokes a pro-inflammatory response mediated by NF-B. [12,13] The effect of NOD2 polymorphisms in CD are incompletely understood, but appear to culminate in impaired bactericidal defenses and unchecked intestinal inflammation. [14,15] More recently, genome-wide studies have shown CD-associated polymorphisms in autophagy-related 16-like protein 1

(ATG16L1) and immunity-related GTPase family, M, (IRGM), genes involved in killing intracellular microbes. [6,16,17] Clearly, the emerging theme in CD genetics involves the abnormal interfacing of innate immunity with intestinal microbes.

Bacteria play a pivotal role in CD pathogenesis, purportedly via loss of immune tolerance to endogenous flora. [2,4,18,19] However more recent work shows global imbalances of the intestinal microbiome in CD, termed 'dysbiosis,' typified by a predominance of 'aggressive' species such as *Proteobacteria* relative to 'protective' species such as *Firmicutes*. A novel pathotype within *Proteobacteria*, Adherent and Invasive *E. coli* (AIEC), is increasingly associated with CD, and can invade and persist intracellularly within epithelial cells and macrophages. [20–23] A role for AIEC in CD is further supported by their ability to induce granulomas *in vitro* and to exploit host defects conferred by CD-associated polymorphisms in ATG16L, IRGM and NOD2. [24,25].

Here we examine the dynamics of the relationship between inflammation and the ileal microbiome in murine models of ileitis incorporating environmental triggers and pathomechanisms of relevance to CD: *Toxoplasma gondii*, *Giardia muris* and indomethacin. While *T. gondii* is not typically associated with CD, it induces granulomatous ileitis of Th1-type immunopathology in C57BL/6 mice that mimics ileal CD. [26,27] The development of inflammation in this model is also microbial dependent. [27,28] Giardia muris infection is associated with mild to moderate small intestinal inflammation characterized by intraepithelial cell infiltration, altered villus morphology, decreased disaccharidae activity and T cell dependence. [29,30] Indomethacin induces dose-dependant small intestinal damage in mice that involves the enteric flora, cytokines such as TNF-a, and TLR-4 mediated signaling. [31].

We show that moderate to severe ileitis is induced by *T. gondii* and indomethacin, and causes a consistent pattern of dysbiosis, characterized by reduced microbial diversity and a global shift in the ileal microbiome from >95% Gram +, to >95% Gram - species. Mucosal invasion by *E. coli* with an AIEC-pathotype accompanies severe ileitis and dysbiosis. In contrast, dysbiosis and bacterial invasion did not develop in mice with mild ileitis induced by *Giardia muris*. Next we show that dysbiosis induced by *T. gondii* is significantly muted and bacterial invasion prevented when we limit the inflammatory response via deletion of pro-inflammatory chemokine receptor, CCR2. In contrast, we observe heightened dysbiosis and *E. coli* invasion when we induce ileitis in the absence of NOD2. Lastly, abrogating inflammation with anti-TNF-α, a mainstay of CD management, limits the extent of dysbiosis and bacterial invasion. In summary, we establish that acute ileitis induces dysbiosis and proliferation of mucosally invasive *E. coli*, irrespective of trigger and genotype. We discover that therapeutic blockade of inflammation may indirectly control dysbiosis, and speculate that failure to completely resolve acute dysbiosis may set the scene for chronic microbial-driven inflammation in CD.

Materials and Methods

Mice

Eight to 12 week old female C57BL/6 and Swiss Webster mice were purchased from Jackson Laboratory and Taconic Farms. Breeding pairs of $CCR2^{-/-}$ and $Nod2^{-/-}$ mice were purchased from The Jackson Laboratory. Mice were established under specific pathogen-free conditions in the Transgenic Mouse Facility at Cornell University, which is American Association of Laboratory Animal Care accredited. Samples of ileum were obtained after rinsing the intestine of fecal contents with 10 ml sterile PBS introduced via a sterile gavage needle.

Toxoplasma Gondii Infections

Type II *T. gondii* cysts (ME49) were obtained from chronically infected Swiss Webster mice by homogenizing brains in sterile PBS. Groups of age-matched C57BL/6 wild type, $CCR2^{-/-}$ and $Nod2^{-/-}$ mice were infected with 100 cysts by gavage, and ileum harvested at 4 (n = 5/group, T4) and 8 (n = 5/group, T8) days post-infection. Five uninfected control mice were gavaged with sterile PBS and ileum harvested on day 8. Samples of ileum were obtained after rinsing the intestines of fecal contents with 10 ml sterile PBS introduced via a sterile gavage needle.

Indomethacin

Indomethacin solubilized in PBS was administered by gavage to C57BL/6 mice at a low dosage (LDI) of 0.1 mg/mouse/day (n = 5) for 5 days, and a high dosage (HDI) of 1 mg/mouse/day for 3 days (n = 5). Ileum was harvested on day 7 (LDI) and day 3 (HDI).

Giardia Muris Infections

2×10^5 *G. muris* trophozoites were administered to C57BL/6 mice by gavage. Ileum was harvested at 7 (n = 5, G7) and 14 days (n = 5, G14) post-infection. Five uninfected control mice received sterile PBS by gavage and ileum was harvested on day 14.

Anti-TNF-α mAb Treatment

Rat anti-mouse TNF-α (clone XT22.11) was purified from hybridoma supernatants by passage over a protein G sepharose column (Invitrogen). Mice were injected intraperitoneally with 3 mg anti-TNF-α or 3 mg of control rat IgG (Jackson ImmunoResearch) on days 3, 5 and 7 post- *T. gondii* infection of mice from Taconic Farms.

Histopathology

Hematoxylin and eosin stained ileal sections were examined by a blinded pathologist. An ileitis score (0 to 9) was calculated for each section by summing the degree of cellular infiltration (0 = normal, 1 = minimal, 2 = moderate, 3 = severe), extent of architectural abnormality (0 = normal, 1 = minimal, 2 = moderate, 3 = severe), and the presence or absence of ulcers, necrosis and neutrophils (0 or 1). Villus height and crypt depth were measured and a crypt:villus ratio calculated for each section.

Pyrosequencing

Pyrosequencing was performed using the bTEFAP method. [32,33,34] DNA was amplified using 27F-519R primers, labeled with linkers and tags, and pyrosequencing performed by Titanium chemistry FLX sequencing (Roche Applied Science, Indianapolis, IN). Data were curated and only high quality sequence reads (Phred20) used, with the final data annotated with BLASTn and analyzed as described previously. [32,33,34].

Fluorescence in situ Hybridization (FISH)

Formalin-fixed, paraffin-embedded sections of ileum mounted on Probe-On Plus slides (Fisher Scientific, Pittsburgh, PA, USA) were screened by FISH with probes targeting 16S rDNA for eubacteria, *E. coli* and Enterobacteriaceae (IDT, Coralville, IA, USA) as previously described. [20,35] Sections were examined with an Olympus BX51 epifluorescence microscope. Images were captured with a DP-70 camera and processed using DP Manager (Olympus America, Center Valley, PA, USA).

Quantitative PCR

Total bacteria and *E. coli* (uidA gene) were quantified as previously described. [20,35,36] A standard curve was generated using DNA from *E. coli* of known concentration. Bacterial DNA was normalized to biopsy size using murine 18S rRNA (Eurogentec, Seraing, Belgium). Bacterial number was expressed as colony-forming unit (CFU)/10^6 murine cells.

E. coli Characterization

E. coli strains were cultured from PBS-rinsed ileum as previously described. [35] Three to 5 *E. coli* colonies per biopsy were screened by RAPD-PCR and the major phylogenetic groups determined by triplex PCR. [20] Isolates differing in overall genotype were selected for subsequent analyses and stored at $-80°C$. Fresh non-passaged bacteria were used throughout. Isolates were serotyped and screened for heat-labile toxin, heat-stable toxins a and b, Shiga-like toxin types 1 and 2, cytotoxic necrotizing factors 1 and 2, and intimin-γ at the *E. coli* Reference Center, Penn State University. [37].

The presence of additional genes related to virulence in *E. coli* was determined by PCR (Table S6). [20,38,39,40].

The ability of *E. coli* isolates to invade Caco-2 cells, and replicate in J774 macrophages was determined as previously described. [20,35].

Statistical Analysis

For comparisons involving >2 groups, Kruskal-Wallis and Mann-Whitney post-test were applied (non-parametric data) or ANOVA with Tukey Kramer post hoc analysis (parametric data). Comparisons between 2 groups were performed using Mann-Whitney. Pyrosequencing data was analyzed as described in Supplementary Methods available online. Chi-square was used to create the association plots for microbial families as described in Supplementary Methods available online. For all evaluations, $p<0.05$ was considered significant.

Results

T. gondii and Indomethacin Trigger Acute Ileitis

Granulomatous ileitis is present in approximately 70% of CD patients, thus our first aim was to establish clinically relevant murine models of ileitis using enteric infections (*T. gondii*, *G. muris*) and NSAID ingestion (indomethacin). *T. gondii* is known to induce ileitis with CD-like immunopathology in C57BL/6 mice, i.e. $CD4^+$ T-cell mediated inflammation dominated by Th1 cytokines TNF-α and IFN-γ. [41,42] We show that peroral infection with *T. gondii* strain ME49 in C57BL/6 mice induces moderate to severe ileitis (ileitis score 4,range 3–6) within 8 days of infection (T8, Figure 1a). Histologic changes (summarized in Table S1) comprised granulomatous inflammation, villus atrophy, crypt hyperplasia, and Paneth cell and goblet cell depletion, comparable to CD. [2,42] In contrast, *G. muris* induced minimal to mild ileitis (ileitis score 1, range 1–1) and mucosal hyperplasia within 14 days of infection (G14, Figure 1a). Peroral indomethacin induced dose-dependent injury; low dosage (LDI) caused mild to moderate ileitis (ileitis score 2, range 1–4), whereas high dosage (HDI, Figure 1a) caused death in 2 mice, and ileal ulceration and necrosis of crypt cells in one and three of the survivors respectively (ileitis score 5, range 5–7). These results establish that we can induce ileitis of graded severity using environmental triggers of relevance to CD.

Acute Ileitis is Associated with Dysbiosis and E. coli Invasion

To capture the microbial response to induced inflammation, we analyzed the composition and spatial distribution of the ileal microbiome by pyrosequencing and FISH analysis. The ileum of healthy C57BL/6mice, was dominated by Gram+ bacteria, with 98% of sequences classed as phylum *Firmicutes*, (Figure 1b, Tables S2 and S3). Moderate to severe ileitis in the *T. gondii* (T8) and indomethacin (HDI) models induced a dramatic shift ($p<0.0001$) to >99% Gram- bacteria, as depicted in the pyrosequencing dendgram (Figure 1b) and the association plot (Figure 1c). In T8, 92% of sequences were classed as *Proteobacteria* and 7% *Bacteroides*. In HDI, 75% of sequences were classed as *Proteobacteria* and 24% *Bacteroidetes*. Ileitis was also associated with marked loss of microbial diversity, from 25 genera in controls (97% of maximum predicted genera), to 11 and 13 genera in T8 and HDI (100% of maximum predicted genera) respectively (Table S5 and Figure S1). These observations were confirmed and extended by FISH analysis, which revealed large numbers of mucosa-associated bacteria and invasive *E. coli* in all T8 and HDI mice (Figure 1d).

In contrast, dysbiosis and bacterial invasion did not develop in mice with minimal (G7, G14) or mild (T4, LDI) ileitis (Figure 1d). We conclude that moderate to severe ileitis induces dysbiosis and *E. coli* invasion in the absence of genetic susceptibility.

Severe Ileitis is Associated with E. coli Proliferation

We next quantified the numbers of total bacteria and *E. coli* in ileal tissue by real-time PCR. [20,36] In T8, the total bacterial load increased relative to controls ($p<0.01$), as did *E. coli* ($p<0.01$, Figure 2a, b). In addition, total bacterial load and *E. coli* were significantly greater in T8 versus T4 (total bacteria, T8 vs T4 $p<0.01$, and *E. coli*, T8 vs T4 $p<0.01$). In HDI there was a significant increase in *E. coli* ($p<0.05$). In contrast, in mice with minimal to mild ileal pathology (G14, T4), the median total bacterial counts were lower than controls ($p<0.01$) and *E. coli* did not increase. In summary, inflammation modulates the number of total bacteria and *E. coli*.

Ileitis-associated E. coli Strains are Clonal and Display an Adherent and Invasive Pathotype

E. coli was cultured from 2/5 T4 mice with mild ileitis, and 8/8 mice (T8 and HDI) with moderate to severe ileitis. All 32 *E. coli* isolates were phylogroup B1, and 29 had an identical RAPD banding pattern (Figure 2c). Representative strains from the dominant and minor RAPD groups were designated CUMT8 (serotype 08:H21) and CUMT4 (serotype 055:H8) respectively. CUMT4 was isolated from a single mouse (T4) co-colonized with CUMT8 (Figure 2b). Both CUMT8 and CUMT4 lacked the common virulence genes found in pathogenic *E. coli*, and carried genes associated with AIEC (hemolysin co-regulated protein, long polar fimbriae, and a Type II secretion system). [20,35] Phenotypically, CUMT8 and CUMT4 behaved like the CD-associated AIEC strain LF82, and were able to invade epithelial cells and persist within macrophages (Figure 2d). [21] These results demonstrate that ileitis of different etiologies induces proliferation of Adherent and Invasive *E. coli*.

Abrogating Ileitis by CCR2 Deletion Limits Dysbiosis and Prevents E. coli Invasion

To further explore the interdependence of dysbiosis and inflammation, we evaluated the ileal microbiome in the setting of a limited host immune response, utilizing the *T. gondii* trigger model and $CCR2^{-/-}$ mice. Polymorphisms in CCR2 are

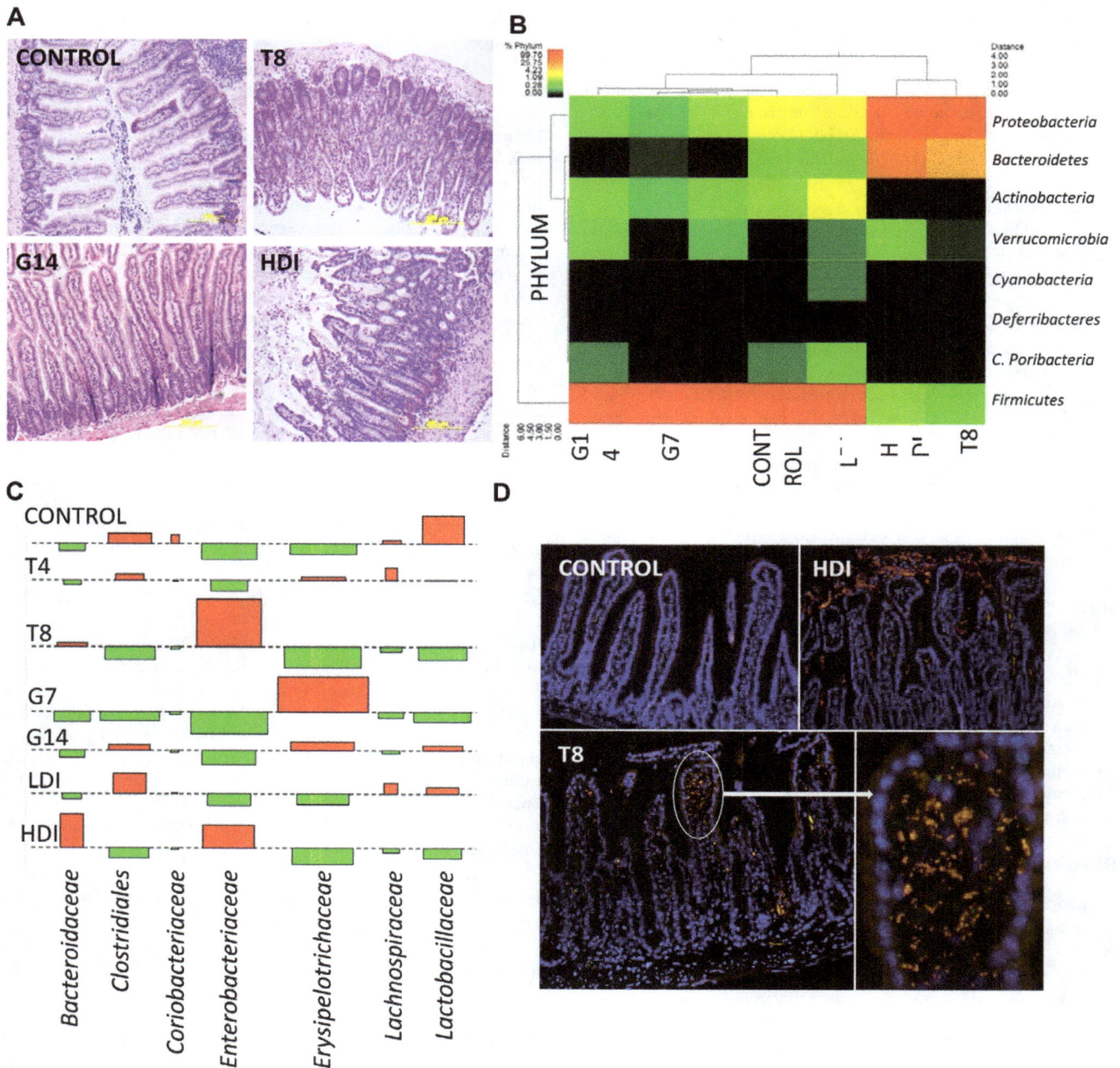

Figure 1. *T. gondii* infection and high dose indomethacin trigger severe ileitis, dysbiosis and mucosal *E. coli* invasion in C57BL/6 mice. (a) Histopathology. Normal ileal histology (inflammation score median =0, range 0–0) in control mice. Moderate to severe ileitis (4, 3–6) develops in *T. gondii* mice at 8 days post-infection (T8). *G. muris*-infected mice develop minimal inflammation (1, 1–1) and mucosal hyperplasia 14 days (G14). High dose indomethacin (HDI) induces severe ileitis (5, 5–7) (H&E 40x). (b) Pyrosequencing reveals a Gram− shift associated with ileitis. Gram+ bacteria predominate in control mice and mice with mild inflammation (G7, G14: Giardia 7 and 14 days p.i., T4: *T. gondii* 4 days p.i.; LDI: low-dose indomethacin). A shift to >95% Gram− bacteria dominated by the phyla *Proteobacteria* and *Bacteroidetes* (p<0.0001) is associated with moderate to severe ileitis in T8 and HDI mice. (c) Association plots of the number of sequences obtained by pyrosequencing corresponding to bacterial families. The area of each rectangle is proportional to the difference in observed and expected frequencies on chi square analysis. The observed frequency of a rectangle is indicated by position relative to baseline, increased (shaded red) or decreased (shaded green) highlighting the ileitis-associated shifts from *Firmicutes (Lactobacillaceae, Clostridiales)* to *Enterobacteriaceae* (T8, HDI) and *Erysipelotrichaceae* (G7, G14, T4). (d) Eubacterial FISH reveals scant luminal and mucosa-associated flora in control mice (EUB338-Cy3, non-EUB338-6FAM with DAPI counterstaining, 40x). Ileitis in T8 and HDI is associated with increased mucosal bacteria and invasive *E. coli* (*E. coli*-Cy3, EUB338-6FAM, 40x).

associated with CD, and mice lacking the pro-inflammatory chemokine receptor CCR2 are protected from *T. gondii*-induced intestinal damage. [41] Here, ileitis in CCR2$^{-/-}$ at day 8 post-

infection (CCR2$^{-/-}$8) was less severe (P<0.05) than T8 (Figure 3a, Table S1). Pyrosequencing in uninfected CCR2$^{-/-}$ (CCR2$^{-/-}$0) revealed 91% *Firmicutes*, and 8% *Bacteroidetes* (Figure 3d, Tables S3

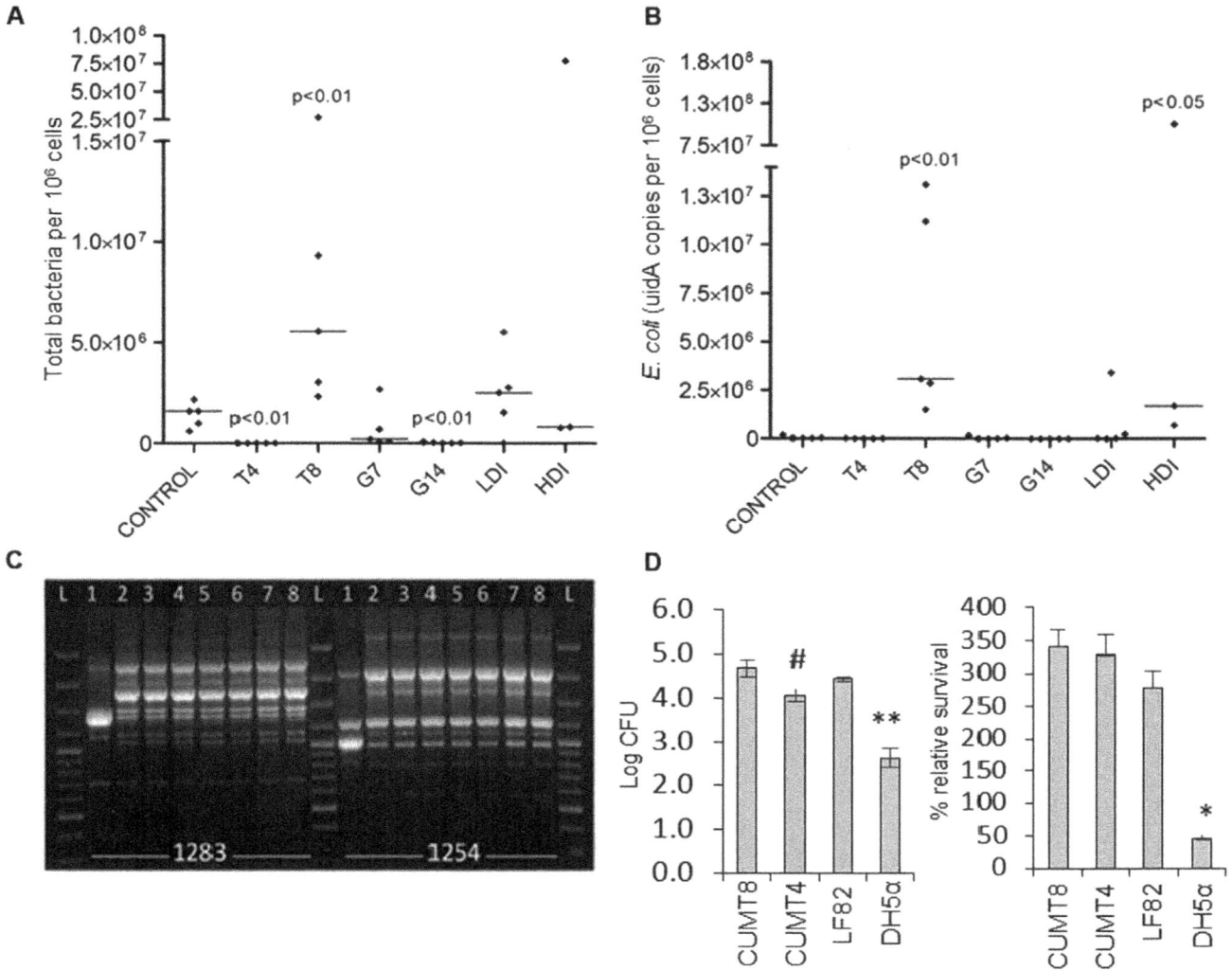

Figure 2. Ileitis-induced dysbiosis is associated with increased bacteria and clonal proliferation of adherent invasive E. coli (AIEC).
(a) Total bacteria quantified by real-time PCR, expressed as bacterial CFU per 10^6 murine cells. Moderate to severe ileitis in T8 is associated with increased bacteria relative to controls. Mild pathology (T4, G14) induces a decrease. (b) Moderate to severe ileitis (T8, HDI) induces E. coli proliferation (E. coli uidA quantification by real-time PCR). (c) Agarose gel electrophoresis showing the products of Random Amplification of Polymorphic DNA (RAPD-PCR) using primers 1283 and 1254. E. coli strains from: T4 (Lanes 1–3), T8 (4, 5) and HDI (6–8). Lane L, 100bp plus DNA ladder. E. coli isolates in lanes 2–8 are clonal, and a representative strain was designated CUMT8. E. coli in lane 1 was designated CUMT4. (d). Invasion and survival of E. coli CUMT8 and CUMT4 in cultured epithelial cells (Caco-2) and macrophages (J774). CUMT8 and CUMT4 invade, and persist intracellularly like CD-associated AIEC LF82, and better than commensal E. coli DH5α (* = P<0.01, ** = P<0.001 vs other strains). CUMT4 was less invasive than CUMT8 (# = P<0.01).

and S4). In CCR2$^{-/-}$8, 58% of sequences were G- *Proteobacteria*, 27% *Bacteroidetes* and 14% *Firmicutes*. Despite this marked shift from 95% Gram+ flora in CCR2$^{-/-}$0, to 84% Gram- flora in CCR2$^{-/-}$8 (p<0.0001), microbial diversity was actually increased in CCR2$^{-/-}$8, with 22 genera present (89% of maximum predicted genera) at day 8 versus 18 genera (90% of maximum predicted genera) at day 0 (Figure 3e). FISH revealed minimal mucosa-associated bacteria and no bacterial invasion in CCR2$^{-/-}$0 and CCR2$^{-/-}$8 (Figure 3a). Real-time PCR showed significantly (p<0.05) increased E. coli at day 8 (median: day 8 = 9.16×10^4, vs Day 0 = 8.8×10^3) but importantly this was much less (p<0.01) than in T8 (median 3.1×10^6) and HDI (1.68×10^6, Figure 2b). A single E. coli strain isolated from one CCR2$^{-/-}$8 mouse was clonal with CUMT8. We have shown that abrogating inflammation

limits dysbiosis by maintaining microbial diversity, controlling bacterial proliferation, and preventing E. coli invasion.

The CD-susceptible Genotype NOD2$^{-/-}$ Lowers the Threshold for Dysbiosis

To evaluate the impact of a CD-susceptible genotype on the inflammatory microbiome, we applied the *T. gondii* ileitis model to NOD2$^{-/-}$ mice. This resulted in development of ileitis at day 4 (ileitis score 2, range 1–4) and severe histiocytic and neutrophilic inflammation (ileitis score 5, range 5 to 7) by day 8 (NOD2$^{-/-}$8, Figure 3b). Pyrosequencing of uninfected mice showed a shift in the endogenous flora, with 53% *Firmicutes* and 46% *Bacteroidetes* in NOD2$^{-/-}$0, relative to 98% *Firmicutes* in uninfected wildtype mice (Figure 3d, 3e, Tables S3 and S4). By day 8 post-infection we observed a dramatic shift to 99.8% *Proteobacteria*. The diversity of

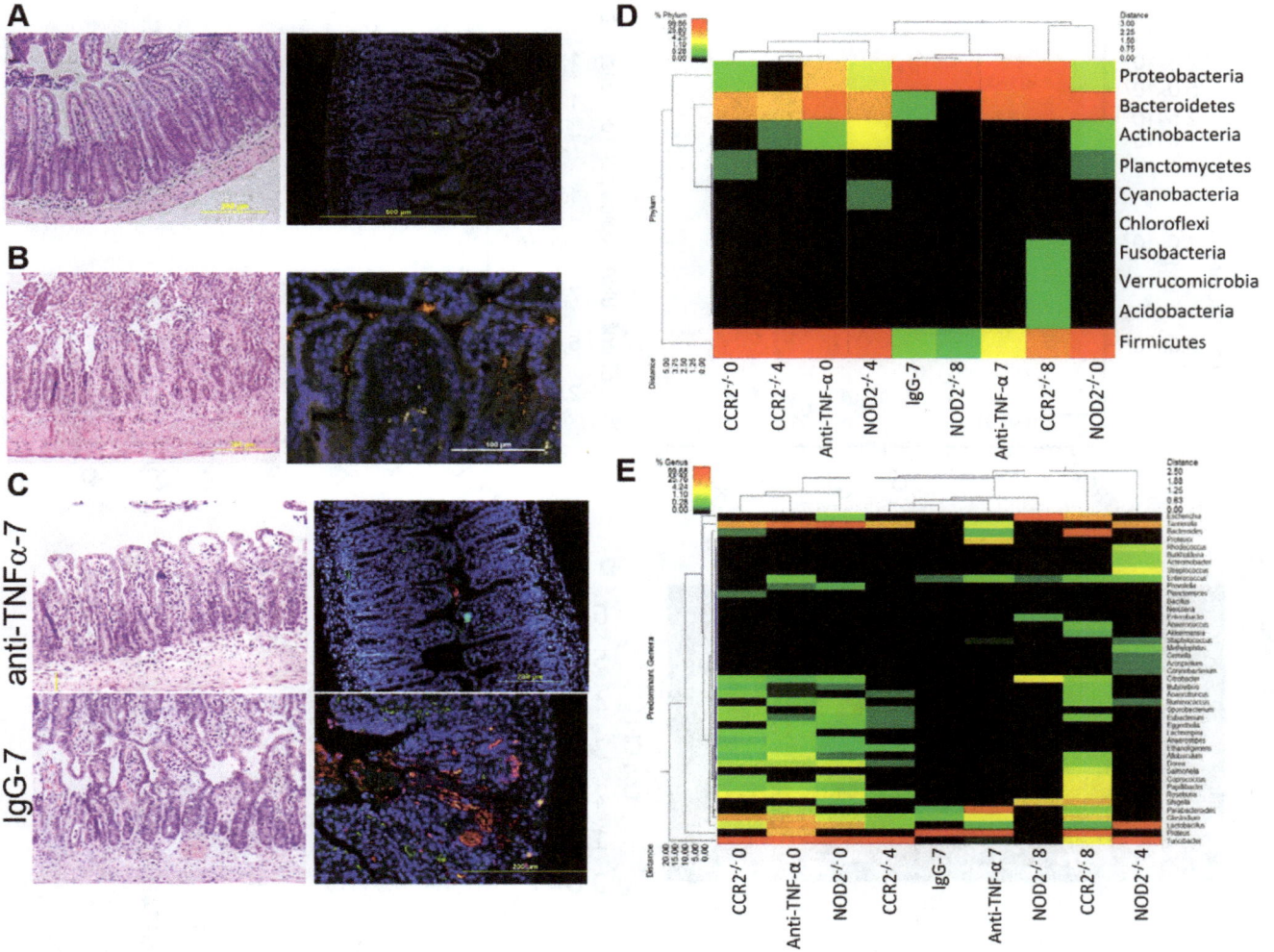

Figure 3. Dysbiosis and *E. coli* invasion are modulated by genetic susceptibility and pharmacotherapy. (a) CCR2$^{-/-}$8 (n = 5) are protected from *T. gondii*-induced ileitis (median inflammation score 3, range 2–3) and *E. coli* invasion. (b) NOD2$^{-/-}$8 (n = 5) develop severe ileitis (5, 5–7) and *E. coli* invasion. (c) anti-TNF-α mAb-7 (n = 5) reduces ileitis (4, 2–4 vs 4, 4–7) and decreases bacterial invasion relative to IgG-7 controls, n = 5). Histology, H&E 40x; FISH, CCR2$^{-/-}$8 and anti-TNF-α-7 = Cy3-EUB338/non-EUB338-6FAM; NOD2$^{-/-}$8 and IgG-7 = Cy3-*E. coli*/EUB338-6FAM, 40x. (d,e). Pyrosequencing reveals that *T. gondii*-induced dysbiosis is modulated by genetic susceptibility and pharmacotherapy. Abrogating ileitis maintains microbial diversity (CCR2$^{-/-}$8), whereas enhancing ileitis decreases diversity and increases *E. coli* (NOD2$^{-/-}$8). NOD2 deletion is associated with a baseline shift to *Bacteroidetes* (NOD2$^{-/-}$0). Anti-TNF-α mAb temper dysbiosis (anti-TNF-α-7 versus IgG-7).

the primary populations also decreased markedly, from 19 in NOD2$^{-/-}$0 (88% of maximum predicted genera), to only 6 genera in NOD2$^{-/-}$8 (100% of maximum predicted) as shown in Figure 3e. Large numbers of mucosa-associated bacteria and invasive *E. coli* were observed in all NOD2$^{-/-}$8 mice (Figure 3b), and *E. coli* increased from 1.13×10^3 uidA copies/10^6 cells in NOD2$^{-/-}$0, to 1.19×10^4 in NOD2$^{-/-}$8 (P<0.05). These results reveal that NOD2$^{-/-}$ perturbs the endogenous flora and enhances inflammation and dysbiosis in response to an injurious trigger.

Anti-TNF-α mAb Limits Dysbiosis and Reduces Bacterial Invasion

Biological agents targeting the pro-inflammatory cytokine tumor necrosis factor alpha (TNF-α), are increasingly used in the management of CD. [42] Thus, our final aim was to explore the impact of anti-TNF-α mAb on the inflammation-dysbiosis dynamic. Mice treated with anti-TNF-α mAb developed less

severe inflammation 7 days after *T. gondii* infection (ileitis score 4, range2–4)) than controls (ileitis score 4, range 4–7) receiving an irrelevant antibody (IgG-7, Figure 3c).

Pyrosequencing revealed a marked floral shift and loss of microbial diversity, from 71% *Firmicutes*, 21% *Bacteroidetes*, 6% *Proteobacteria* and 21 genera in uninfected controls (anti-TNF-α-0), to 99.7% *Proteobacteria* (99% *Proteus* spp.), and 4 genera in the IgG-7 group (Figure 3d, 3e, Tables S3 and S4). In anti-TNF-α-7, dysbiosis and loss of microbial diversity were tempered: 72% *Proteobacteria* (72% *Proteus spp.*), 21% *Bacteroidetes*, and 10 genera. We observed increased mucosa-associated and invasive bacteria in IgG-7 (5/5 mice with bacterial invasion) relative to anti-TNF-α-0 (0/5 mice), and anti-TNF-α-7 (low numbers of intramucosal bacteria in 3/5 mice) (Figure 3c). Interestingly, the vast majority of invasive bacteria in IgG-7 and anti-TNF-α-7 didn't hybridize with an *E. coli* probe. Based on pyrosequencing and bacterial culture, we suspect these invasive bacteria are *Proteus* spp. This contrasts with invasive *E. coli* in T8 and HDI, and likely reflects the relative abundance of *Proteus* in the endogenous flora of mice in this experiment that were purchased from Taconic Farms vs. Jackson Laboratories. These results show that anti-TNF-α treatment while not completely protective, decreases the inflammation-induced floral shift by maintaining greater microbial evenness and reducing bacterial invasion.

Discussion

The evidence is compelling that CD pathogenesis involves interplay between the intestinal microbiome, genetic susceptibility, the immune system, and environmental risk factors. Our limited understanding of these interrelationships has yet to reconcile the wide spectrum of CD phenotypes, but mapping their interactions is pivotal to understanding CD pathogenesis and identifying new therapeutic targets. Here we establish that acute ileitis induces a consistent shift in the microbiome from *Firmicutes* to *Proteobacteria*, accompanied by a reduction in microbial diversity and proliferation of AIEC. This 'inflammatory microbiome' recapitulates the dysbiosis of ileal CD. [20,43,44,45] When we superimposed a CD-susceptible genotype, NOD2$^{-/-}$, on *T. gondii*-induced ileitis, we enhanced inflammation and dysbiosis. Conversely, dysbiosis was tempered when we limited inflammation by CCR2 gene deletion, revealing a new potential therapeutic target in CD. Using anti-TNF-α mAb, a mainstay of CD therapy, we discover that dysbiosis can be reduced by pharmacologic manipulation of mucosal inflammation. We speculate that failure to resolve the inflamma-

tory microbiome after acute non-specific enteric injury may stimulate persistent microbial-drive inflammation in CD.

Many IBD susceptibility genes have been discovered, but similar advances in defining environmental risk factors have lagged. [8] Animal models of CD are usually chemically-induced, genetically engineered, or congenic rodent strains with limited relevance to the clinical setting and disease phenotype. [3,46] To specifically examine the interrelationship between the microbiome and inflammation in ileal CD, we utilized murine models of ileitis incorporating environmental triggers of relevance to CD. NSAID ingestion, infectious enteritis and stress are known IBD risks. [47,48] [10] While *T. gondii* is not typically associated with CD, it induces granulomatous ileitis of Th1-type immunopathology in C57BL/6 mice that mimics ileal CD. [26,27] The development of inflammation in this model is also microbial dependent. [27,28] Using these diverse stimuli we showed that the inflammatory microbiome is a common endpoint of ileitis, driven by severity of inflammation rather than the trigger. Our finding that mild ileitis (T4, G14) was associated with decreased bacterial load suggests an ability to limit dysbiosis until inflammation overwhelms. The mucosal hyperplasia in G14 mice raises the possibility that up-regulation of anti-microbial mucosal defenses may occur with mild injury. [49].

The question that naturally arises is whether the floral shift *per se* is in fact harmful, or a benign consequence of inflammation. However, consider that we show the degree of dysbiosis to directly relate to the severity of ileitis, and that invasive *E. coli* is always, and only, present in mice that develop a >95% G- shift. Further,

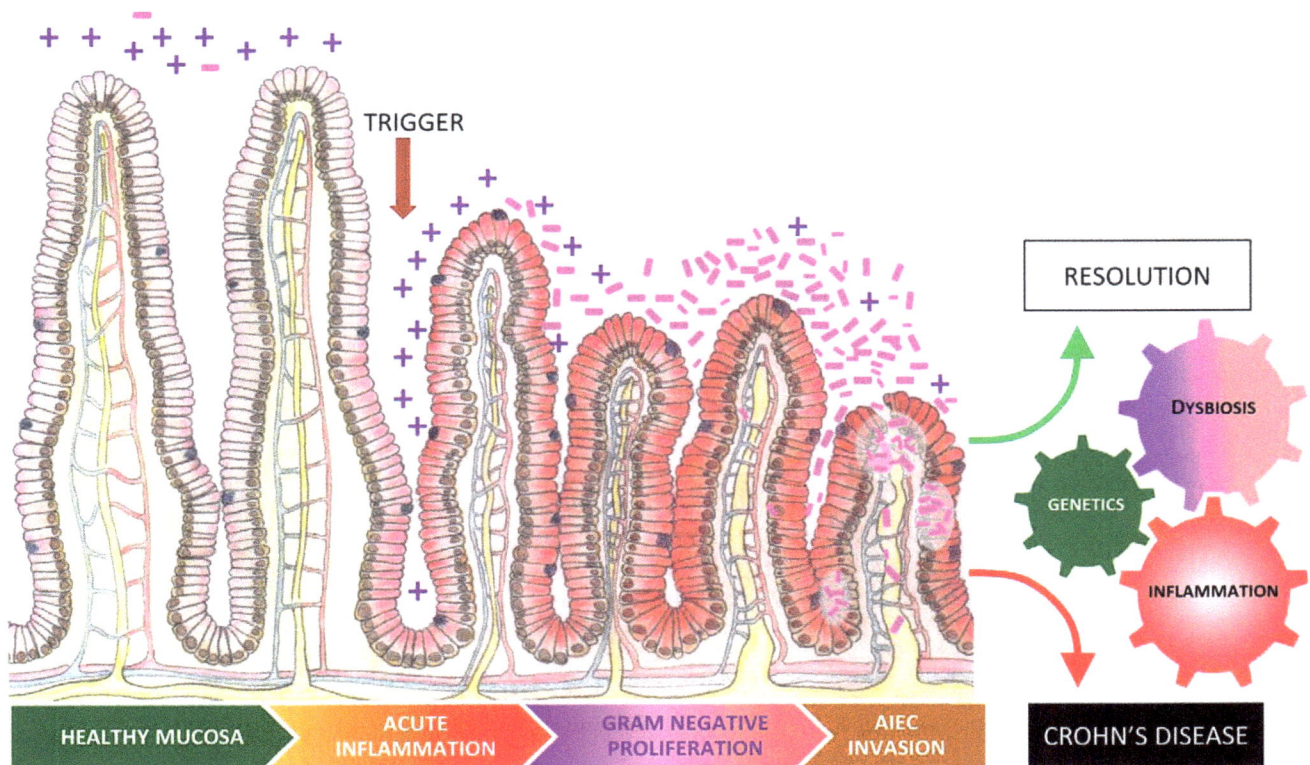

Figure 4. Inflammation drives dysbiosis, Gram negative proliferation and *E. coli* invasion. Independent of genotype, ileitis induces a progressive decrease in microbial diversity, a shift from *Firmicutes* (Gram+) to *Proteobacteria* (Gram−), and proliferation of AIEC. Superimposition of genetic susceptibility can lower (NOD2$^{-/-}$) or increase (CCR2$^{-/-}$) the threshold for dysbiosis in response to an external trigger. We speculate that genetic susceptibility may also influence the ability of an individual to resolve the self-perpetuating cycle of dysbiosis and inflammation generated by an acute insult.

the selection pressure exerted by inflammation is sufficiently strong to drive clonal proliferation of a single AIEC strain (CUMT8) in all mice with severe ileitis, independent of stimulus. Here we show for the first time that acute ileitis is closely linked to the proliferation of mucosally invasive *E. coli* with an AIEC pathotype. [20,21,35].

Increasingly implicated in CD in the US and Europe, AIEC have been isolated from the ileum of 36–38% of CD patients versus 6% of controls, and are associated with the severity of ileal CD. [20,50] Surprisingly little is known about the luminal microenvironment that promotes the proliferation of *E. coli* and disappearance of *Firmicutes* such as *Fecalibacterium prauznitzii*. A plethora of inflammation-associated factors could favor, or fail to regulate bacterial proliferation and virulence. [20,23,24,50] Specific mechanisms implicated in the adhesion and invasion of AIEC include bacterial factors such as flagellin [23] and Type I pili,[51] as well as host factors such as cell adhesion molecule CEACAM6[52] and the stress response protein Gp96. [53] Up-regulation of CEACAM6 and interaction with type 1 pili to promote adhesion and invasion is a potential pathomechanism for AIEC, but cannot account for our findings since mice do not express CEACAM6. [52] Notably, the highest *E. coli* counts were observed in mice with the most severe inflammation and dysbiosis, suggesting that quantification of mucosal *E. coli* may be a useful adjunct for monitoring CD activity. [20].

When we superimposed the effect of genotype on the inflammation-dysbiosis dynamic, we saw the most severe ileitis, dysbiosis, and *E. coli* invasion, in $NOD2^{-/-}$ mice. We postulate that this is attributable to altered sensing and reduced killing of luminal and intracellular *E. coli*. [11] Our observation of more *Bacteroidetes* sequences in uninfected $NOD2^{-/-}$ than other control groups suggests a pre-existing baseline floral shift. [54] Our findings indicate that NOD2 mutation confers greater vulnerability to inflammation and dysbiosis but importantly, absence of NOD2 was not a prerequisite for dysbiosis and invasion. This echoes the scenario in CD, where 60%–70% of CD patients show no NOD2 mutations. [11,55] Moreover, studies of identical twins elegantly show that microbial composition is determined by presence or absence of CD rather than genetic make-up alone. [45,56].

The interdependence of inflammation and dysbiosis is further supported by our findings in inflammation resistant $CCR2^{-/-}$ mice. CCR2 is a chemokine receptor for monocyte chemoattractant proteins (MCP1–4) and we have shown previously that mice lacking CCR2 are protected from *T. gondii*-induced ileal pathology. [41] The $CCR2^{-/-}$ model is relevant to CD pathogenesis because CCR2+ lamina propria lymphocytes are a specific feature of ileal CD [57] and polymorphisms in CCR2 have been associated with CD in several studies. [58,59] On this basis we suggest that pharmacologic blockade of this receptor, which has been demonstrated in mice, [60] may provide a novel pathway for therapeutic intervention in CD. In a similar vein, by controlling inflammation using anti-TNF-α mAb, we reduced dysbiosis, unmasking an effect of this therapy not previously appreciated. It has recently been shown that TNF-α can stimulate the replication of AIEC in infected macrophages hence the anti-TNF-α mAb may also have directly impacted the growth and proliferation of AIEC in the *T. gondii* infection model. [61].

In summary, this study has explored the dynamics of the relationship between ileal inflammation and alterations in the intestinal microbiome termed dysbiosis. On the basis of our observations we propose a model where the composition and spatial distribution of the ileal microbiome is regulated by inflammation independent of the injurious trigger (Figure 4).

Inflammation drives a progressive decrease in the microbial diversity or at the least a decrease in the evenness of the microbial population, a shift from Gram+ to Gram−, and the proliferation of mucosally invasive bacteria such as AIEC. The specific factors related to inflammation that induce dysbiosis remain to be elucidated. We speculate that inflammation related perturbations in the microenvironment such as increased availability of subtrates for growth of Gram −ve bacteria (e.g. iron and serum, dead or dying cells) and loss of niche and substrates for Gram +ve flora (e.g. mucus, goblet cells) underly this phenomenon. While the common end-point of inflammation is the inflammatory microbiome, genetic susceptibility can impact the threshold for dysbiosis in response to an external trigger. It seems plausible that genetic susceptibility may also influence the ability of an individual to resolve the self-perpetuating cycle of dysbiosis and inflammation generated by an acute insult.

Supporting Information

Figure S1 16S rDNA sequencing by genera. Moderate to severe ileitis in T8 and HDI induces a Gram negative shift dominated by >99% *Proteobacteria* and loss of microbial diversity, from 25 genera in controls, to 11 and 13 genera in T8 and HDI respectively.

Table S1 Histopathological evaluation of ileal inflammation and mucosal morphology.

Table S2 16S rDNA pyrosequencing sequence classification (% of total sequence number, n) by genus for ileitis trigger experiments (5 mice per group): Control - uninfected/untreated mice; T4, T8 - 4 and 8 days after *T. gondii* infection; G7, G14 - 7 and 14 days after *G. muris* infection. LDI, HDI: low dose (0.1 mg/mouse) and high dose (1 mg/mouse) indomethacin treatment.

Table S3 16S rDNA pyrosequencing data for all mouse groups, showing Shannon-Weaver bacterial diversity index, observed operative taxonomical units (OTU), the predicted maximum number of OTUs, rarefaction, and species richness estimators (ACE and Chao 1) at strain (1% dissimilarity), species (3%), and genus (5%) level.

Table S4 16S rDNA pyrosequencing data (% of total sequence number, n) by genus for control, CCR2, NOD2 and anti-TNF-α mAb experiments (5 mice per group).

Table S5 Maximum Predicted Operational Taxonomic units at >10,000 sequences and calculated percent of maximum observed by rarefaction for each sample.

Table S6 PCR primers for *E. coli* genotypic characterization.

Author Contributions

Conceived and designed the experiments: KS ED ES MC. Performed the experiments: MC CE ED DB BD SD. Analyzed the data: KS MC ED CE DB BD SM SD. Contributed reagents/materials/analysis tools: CE ED BD DB SD. Wrote the paper: KS MC ES ED.

References

1. Abraham C, Cho JH. (2009) Inflammatory bowel disease. N Engl J Med 361(21): 2066–2078.
2. Hanauer SB. (2006) Inflammatory bowel disease: Epidemiology, pathogenesis, and therapeutic opportunities. Inflamm Bowel Dis 12 Suppl 1: S3–9.
3. Xavier RJ, Podolsky DK. (2007) Unravelling the pathogenesis of inflammatory bowel disease. Nature 448(7152): 427–434.
4. Sartor RB. (2008) Microbial influences in inflammatory bowel diseases. Gastroenterology 134(2): 577–594.
5. Singh S, Graff LA, Bernstein CN. (2009) Do NSAIDs, antibiotics, infections, or stress trigger flares in IBD? Am J Gastroenterol 104(5): 1298–313; quiz 1314.
6. Van Limbergen J, Wilson DC, Satsangi J. (2009) The genetics of crohn's disease. Annu Rev Genomics Hum Genet 10: 89–116.
7. Packey CD, Sartor RB. (2009) Commensal bacteria, traditional and opportunistic pathogens, dysbiosis and bacterial killing in inflammatory bowel diseases. Curr Opin Infect Dis 22(3): 292–301.
8. Molodecky NA, Kaplan GG. (2010) Environmental risk factors for inflammatory bowel disease. Gastroenterol Hepatol (N Y) 6(5): 339–346.
9. Bernstein CN, Singh S, Graff LA, Walker JR, Miller N, et al. (2010) A prospective population-based study of triggers of symptomatic flares in IBD. Am J Gastroenterol 105(9): 1994–2002.
10. Mann EA, Saeed SA. (2011) Gastrointestinal infection as a trigger for inflammatory bowel disease. Curr Opin Gastroenterol.
11. Economou M, Trikalinos TA, Loizou KT, Tsianos EV, Ioannidis JP. (2004) Differential effects of NOD2 variants on crohn's disease risk and phenotype in diverse populations: A metaanalysis. Am J Gastroenterol 99(12): 2393–2404.
12. Inohara N, Ogura Y, Fontalba A, Gutierrez O, Pons F, et al. (2003) Host recognition of bacterial muramyl dipeptide mediated through NOD2. implications for crohn's disease. J Biol Chem 278(8): 5509–5512.
13. Maeda S, Hsu LC, Liu H, Bankston LA, Iimura M, et al. (2005) Nod2 mutation in crohn's disease potentiates NF-kappaB activity and IL-1beta processing. Science 307(5710): 734–738.
14. Eckmann L, Karin M. (2005) NOD2 and crohn's disease: Loss or gain of function? Immunity 22(6): 661–667.
15. Perez LH, Butler M, Creasey T, Dzink-Fox J, Gounarides J, et al. (2010) Direct bacterial killing in vitro by recombinant Nod2 is compromised by crohn's disease-associated mutations. PLoS One 5(6): e10915.
16. Massey DC, Parkes M. (2007) Genome-wide association scanning highlights two autophagy genes, ATG16L1 and IRGM, as being significantly associated with crohn's disease. Autophagy 3(6): 649–651.
17. Okazaki T, Wang MH, Rawsthorne P, Sargent M, Datta LW, et al. (2008) Contributions of IBD5, IL23R, ATG16L1, and NOD2 to crohn's disease risk in a population-based case-control study: Evidence of gene-gene interactions. Inflamm Bowel Dis 14(11): 1528–1541.
18. Swidsinski A, Ladhoff A, Pernthaler A, Swidsinski S, Loening-Baucke V, et al. (2002) Mucosal flora in inflammatory bowel disease. Gastroenterology 122(1): 44–54.
19. Rutgeerts P, Goboes K, Peeters M, Hiele M, Penninckx F, et al. (1991) Effect of faecal stream diversion on recurrence of crohn's disease in the neoterminal ileum. Lancet 338(8770): 771–774.
20. Baumgart M, Dogan B, Rishniw M, Weitzman G, Bosworth B, et al. (2007) Culture independent analysis of ileal mucosa reveals a selective increase in invasive escherichia coli of novel phylogeny relative to depletion of clostridiales in crohn's disease involving the ileum. ISME J 1(5): 403–418.
21. Darfeuille-Michaud A, Neut C, Barnich N, Lederman E, Di Martino P, et al. (1998) Presence of adherent escherichia coli strains in ileal mucosa of patients with crohn's disease. Gastroenterology 115(6): 1405–1413.
22. Martinez-Medina M, Aldeguer X, Lopez-Siles M, Gonzalez-Huix F, Lopez-Oliu C, et al. (2009) Molecular diversity of escherichia coli in the human gut: New ecological evidence supporting the role of adherent-invasive E. coli (AIEC) in crohn's disease. Inflamm Bowel Dis 15(6): 872–882.
23. Barnich N, Darfeuille-Michaud A. (2007) Adherent-invasive escherichia coli and crohn's disease. Curr Opin Gastroenterol 23(1): 16–20.
24. Lapaquette P, Glasser AL, Huett A, Xavier RJ, Darfeuille-Michaud A. (2010) Crohn's disease-associated adherent-invasive E. coli are selectively favoured by impaired autophagy to replicate intracellularly. Cell Microbiol 12(1): 99–113.
25. Meconi S, Vercellone A, Levillain F, Payre B, Al Saati T, et al. (2007) Adherent-invasive escherichia coli isolated from crohn's disease patients induce granulomas in vitro. Cell Microbiol 9(5): 1252–1261.
26. Liesenfeld O. (2002) Oral infection of C57BL/6 mice with toxoplasma gondii: A new model of inflammatory bowel disease? J Infect Dis 185 Suppl 1: S96–101.
27. Heimesaat MM, Fischer A, Jahn HK, Niebergall J, Freudenberg M, et al. (2007) Exacerbation of murine ileitis by toll-like receptor 4 mediated sensing of lipopolysaccharide from commensal escherichia coli. Gut 56(7): 941–948.
28. Heimesaat MM, Bereswill S, Fischer A, Fuchs D, Struck D, et al. (2006) Gram-negative bacteria aggravate murine small intestinal Th1-type immunopathology following oral infection with toxoplasma gondii. J Immunol 177(12): 8785–8795.
29. Gillon J, Thamery D AL, Ferguson A. (1982) Features of small intestinal pathology (epithelial cell kinetics, intraepithelial lymphocytes, disaccharidases) in a primary Giardia muris infection. Gut 23(6): 498–506.
30. Scott KG, Yu LC, Buret AG.Role of CD8+ and CD4+ T lymphocytes in jejunal mucosal injury during murine giardiasis (2004). Infect Immun 72(6): 3536–42.
31. Watanabe T, Higuchi K, Kobata A, Nishio H, Tanigawa T, et al. (2008) Nonsteroidal anti-inflammatory drug-induced small intestinal damage is Toll-like receptor 4 dependent. Gut. 57(2): 181–7.
32. Finegold SM, Dowd SE, Gontcharova V, Liu C, Henley KE, et al. (2010) Pyrosequencing study of fecal microflora of autistic and control children. Anaerobe 16(4): 444–453.
33. Gontcharova V, Youn E, Sun Y, Wolcott RD, Dowd SE. (2010) A comparison of bacterial composition in diabetic ulcers and contralateral intact skin. Open Microbiol J 4: 8–19.
34. Suchodolski JS, Dowd SE, Westermarck E, Steiner JM, Wolcott RD, et al. (2009) The effect of the macrolide antibiotic tylosin on microbial diversity in the canine small intestine as demonstrated by massive parallel 16S rRNA gene sequencing. BMC Microbiol 9: 210.
35. Simpson KW, Dogan B, Rishniw M, Goldstein RE, Klaessig S, et al. (2006) Adherent and invasive escherichia coli is associated with granulomatous colitis in boxer dogs. Infect Immun 74(8): 4778–4792.
36. Ott SJ, Musfeldt M, Ullmann U, Hampe J, Schreiber S. (2004) Quantification of intestinal bacterial populations by real-time PCR with a universal primer set and minor groove binder probes: A global approach to the enteric flora. J Clin Microbiol 42(6): 2566–2572.
37. DebRoy C, Maddox CW. (2001) Identification of virulence attributes of gastrointestinal escherichia coli isolates of veterinary significance. Anim Health Res Rev 2(2): 129–140.
38. Bach S, de Almeida A, Carniel E. (2000) The yersinia high-pathogenicity island is present in different members of the family enterobacteriaceae. FEMS Microbiol Lett 183(2): 289–294.
39. Germon P, Chen YH, He L, Blanco JE, Bree A, et al. (2005) ibeA, a virulence factor of avian pathogenic escherichia coli. Microbiology 151(Pt 4): 1179–1186.
40. Johnson JR, Stell AL. (2000) Extended virulence genotypes of escherichia coli strains from patients with urosepsis in relation to phylogeny and host compromise. J Infect Dis 181(1): 261–272.
41. Egan CE, Craven MD, Leng J, Mack M, Simpson KW, et al. (2009) CCR2-dependent intraepithelial lymphocytes mediate inflammatory gut pathology during toxoplasma gondii infection. Mucosal Immunol 2(6): 527–535.
42. Jones J, Panaccione R. (2008) Biologic therapy in crohn's disease: State of the art. Curr Opin Gastroenterol 24(4): 475–481.
43. Frank DN, St Amand AL, Feldman RA, Boedeker EC, Harpaz N, et al. (2007) Molecular-phylogenetic characterization of microbial community imbalances in human inflammatory bowel diseases. Proc Natl Acad Sci U S A 104(34): 13780–13785.
44. Swidsinski A, Loening-Baucke V, Lochs H, Hale LP. (2005) Spatial organization of bacterial flora in normal and inflamed intestine: A fluorescence in situ hybridization study in mice. World J Gastroenterol 11(8): 1131–1140.
45. Willing B, Halfvarson J, Dicksved J, Rosenquist M, Jarnerot G, et al. (2009) Twin studies reveal specific imbalances in the mucosa-associated microbiota of patients with ileal crohn's disease. Inflamm Bowel Dis 15(5): 653–660.
46. Mizoguchi A, Mizoguchi E. (2010) Animal models of IBD: Linkage to human disease. Curr Opin Pharmacol 10(5): 578–587.
47. Takeuchi K, Smale S, Premchand P, Maiden L, Sherwood R, et al. (2006) Prevalence and mechanism of nonsteroidal anti-inflammatory drug-induced clinical relapse in patients with inflammatory bowel disease. Clin Gastroenterol Hepatol 4(2): 196–202.
48. Felder JB, Korelitz BI, Rajapakse R, Schwarz S, Horatagis AP, et al. (2000) Effects of nonsteroidal antiinflammatory drugs on inflammatory bowel disease: A case-control study. Am J Gastroenterol 95(8): 1949–1954.
49. Ramasundara M, Leach ST, Lemberg DA, Day AS. (2009) Defensins and inflammation: The role of defensins in inflammatory bowel disease. J Gastroenterol Hepatol 24(2): 202–208.
50. Darfeuille-Michaud A, Boudeau J, Bulois P, Neut C, Glasser AL, et al. (2004) High prevalence of adherent-invasive escherichia coli associated with ileal mucosa in crohn's disease. Gastroenterology 127(2): 412–421.
51. Bringer MA, Rolhion N, Glasser AL, Darfeuille-Michaud A. (2007) The oxidoreductase DsbA plays a key role in the ability of the crohn's disease-associated adherent-invasive escherichia coli strain LF82 to resist macrophage killing. J Bacteriol 189(13): 4860–4871.
52. Barnich N, Carvalho FA, Glasser AL, Darcha C, Jantscheff P, et al. (2007) CEACAM6 acts as a receptor for adherent-invasive E. coli, supporting ileal mucosa colonization in crohn disease. J Clin Invest 117(6): 1566–1574.
53. Rolhion N, Barnich N, Bringer MA, Glasser AL, Ranc J, et al. (2010) Abnormally expressed ER stress response chaperone Gp96 in CD favours adherent-invasive escherichia coli invasion. Gut 59(10): 1355–1362.
54. Petnicki-Ocwieja T, Hrncir T, Liu YJ, Biswas A, Hudcovic T, et al. (2009) Nod2 is required for the regulation of commensal microbiota in the intestine. Proc Natl Acad Sci U S A 106(37): 15813–15818.
55. Ahmad T, Armuzzi A, Bunce M, Mulcahy-Hawes K, Marshall SE, et al. (2002) The molecular classification of the clinical manifestations of crohn's disease. Gastroenterology 122(4): 854–866.
56. Dicksved J, Halfvarson J, Rosenquist M, Jarnerot G, Tysk C, et al. (2008) Molecular analysis of the gut microbiota of identical twins with crohn's disease. ISME J 2(7): 716–727.

57. Connor SJ, Paraskevopoulos N, Newman R, Cuan N, Hampartzoumian T, et al. (2004) CCR2 expressing CD4+ T lymphocytes are preferentially recruited to the ileum in crohn's disease. Gut 53(9): 1287–1294.

58. Barrett JC, Hansoul S, Nicolae DL, Cho JH, Duerr RH, et al. (2008) Genome-wide association defines more than 30 distinct susceptibility loci for crohn's disease. Nat Genet 40(8): 955–962.

59. Palmieri O, Latiano A, Salvatori E, Valvano MR, Bossa F, et al. (2010) The -A2518G polymorphism of monocyte chemoattractant protein-1 is associated with crohn's disease. Am J Gastroenterol 105(7): 1586–1594.

60. Weisberg SP, Hunter D, Huber R, Lemieux J, Slaymaker S, et al. (2006) CCR2 modulates inflammatory and metabolic effects of high-fat feeding. J Clin Invest 116(1): 115–124.

61. Bringer MA, Billard E, Glasser AL, Colombel JF. Replication of Crohn's disease-associated AIEC within macrophages is dependent on TNF-α secretion. (2012) Lab Invest. 92(3): 411–9.

13

Characterization of Chromosomal Instability in Murine Colitis-Associated Colorectal Cancer

Marco Gerling[1]*, Rainer Glauben[1], Jens K. Habermann[2], Anja A. Kühl[3], Christoph Loddenkemper[3], Hans-Anton Lehr[4], Martin Zeitz[1], Britta Siegmund[1]

1 Medical Clinic I, Charité – Universitätsmedizin Berlin, Campus Benjamin Franklin, Berlin, Germany, 2 Laboratory for Surgical Research, Department of Surgery, University of Lübeck, Lübeck, Germany, 3 Institute of Pathology / RCIS, Charité – Universitätsmedizin Berlin, Campus Benjamin Franklin, Berlin, Germany, 4 Centre Hospitalier Universitaire Vaudois (CHUV), Institut Universitaire de Pathologie, Lausanne, Switzerland

Abstract

Background: Patients suffering from ulcerative colitis (UC) bear an increased risk for colorectal cancer. Due to the sparsity of colitis-associated cancer (CAC) and the long duration between UC initiation and overt carcinoma, elucidating mechanisms of inflammation-associated carcinogenesis in the gut is particularly challenging. Adequate murine models are thus highly desirable. For human CACs a high frequency of chromosomal instability (CIN) reflected by aneuploidy could be shown, exceeding that of sporadic carcinomas. The aim of this study was to analyze mouse models of CAC with regard to CIN. Additionally, protein expression of p53, beta-catenin and Ki67 was measured to further characterize murine tumor development in comparison to UC-associated carcinogenesis in men.

Methods: The AOM/DSS model (n = 23) and IL-10$^{-/-}$ mice (n = 8) were applied to monitor malignancy development via endoscopy and to analyze premalignant and malignant stages of CACs. CIN was assessed using DNA-image cytometry. Protein expression of p53, beta-catenin and Ki67 was evaluated by immunohistochemistry. The degree of inflammation was analyzed by histology and paralleled to local interferon-γ release.

Results: CIN was detected in 81.25% of all murine CACs induced by AOM/DSS, while all carcinomas that arose in IL-10$^{-/-}$ mice were chromosomally stable. Beta-catenin expression was strongly membranous in IL-10$^{-/-}$ mice, while 87.50% of AOM/DSS-induced tumors showed cytoplasmatic and/or nuclear translocation of beta-catenin. p53 expression was high in both models and Ki67 staining revealed higher proliferation of IL-10$^{-/-}$-induced CACs.

Conclusions: AOM/DSS-colitis, but not IL-10$^{-/-}$ mice, could provide a powerful murine model to mechanistically investigate CIN in colitis-associated carcinogenesis.

Editor: Reiner Albert Veitia, Institut Jacques Monod, France

Funding: Studies were in part founded by the German Research Foundation (Deutsche Forschungsgemeinschaft) under No. DFG Si-749/5-3 and SFB633, www.dfg.de. The funders had no role in study design, data collection and analysis, decision to publish, or preparation of the manuscript. No additional external funding was received for this study.

Competing Interests: The authors have declared that no competing interests exist.

* E-mail: marco.gerling@charite.de

Introduction

Patients suffering from ulcerative colitis (UC) face an increased lifetime risk of developing colorectal cancer (CRC) [1]. Such inflammation-associated malignancies of the colorectum show distinct differences to sporadic carcinomas: they develop in younger patients, more often in males, and synchronous carcinomas are more frequently found [2]. On the genomic level, it has been hypothesized that chronic inflammation leads to increased chromosomal instability (CIN) by reactive oxygen and nitrogen species (RONS), hypermethylation of pericentromeric DNA regions, telomere attrition, and other less well defined mechanisms [3,4,5]. CIN is observed in chronic inflammatory conditions such as Barrett's esophagus, chronic hepatitis, and UC to a high extent [6,7,8]. In UC, aneuploidy as the measurable sequela of CIN can be applied as a predictive marker for malignant transformation and is detectable up to a decade prior to diagnosis of carcinoma [8,9]. Recently, it could be shown that CIN characterizes colitis-associated carcinomas (CACs) with a frequency reaching 100% in a set of 31 CACs analyzed, while contrarily only 75% of sporadic CRCs were found aneuploid [10,11]. Taken together, mounting evidence suggests a causal relationship between inflammation and CIN, with presence of CIN being a predictive marker for both, malignancy development and inferior prognosis once malignant transformation has occurred.

Elucidating causes and effects of CIN on a mechanistic level could therefore substantially aid the development of strategies to prevent and treat cancer with novel, targeted approaches. Thus, suitable animal models are highly desirable to accelerate research progress. Preferably, such models should show characteristics similar to their human counterparts, which in case of colitis-associated carcinogenesis indispensably comprise aneuploidy.

In addition to CIN, previous studies have demonstrated further differences between sporadic and colitis-associated carcinogenesis with regard to canonical pathways of malignant transformation:

It has long been known that p53-point mutations occur early in UC-associated neoplastic progression and correlate directly with aneuploidy [12,13,14,15].

In CRC and other tumors, activation of Wnt-signaling promotes cell survival and inhibits cell death. Subsequent to activation of the Wnt-signaling pathway, accumulation and translocation of beta-catenin from the cell membrane to the cytoplasm and nucleus can be observed, resulting in activation of a variety of target genes [16]. Only limited data exist on beta-catenin-expression in CAC. One study focusing on genetic alterations adjacent to the beta-catenin locus on chromosome 3p22-p21.3 could not find a difference between the frequency of loss of heterozygosity among UC-associated and sporadic carcinomas [17]. Contrarily, a recent study on Wnt-signaling activation in CAC concluded that the pathway is activated in an early phase of malignant transformation in colitis, and found nuclear beta-catenin staining helpful in detecting neoplasia in CAC [18].

A diversity of animal models of UC is commonly used. In one canonical model colitis is induced with dextran sulphate sodium (DSS) [19]. Interestingly, long term DSS administration alone can cause malignant transformation in rodents [20,21], while this effect is aggravated by additional application of azoxymethane (AOM), a mutagenic agent that by itself causes the development of colorectal tumors in mice [22]. Tumors induced with AOM alone do not show CIN [23]. A dose-dependent promoting effect of DSS for AOM-induced tumors has been reported, while CIN has not been studied in the AOM/DSS-model [24].

A complementary murine model of UC is the interleukin $10^{-/-}$ (IL-$10^{-/-}$)-mouse [25]. In this model, inflammatory changes commence in the distal colon at about three weeks of age and progress proximally without additional administration of external pathogens [26]. Colonic lesions are characterized by inflammatory infiltrates in the mucosa and submucosa as well as crypt abscesses [26]. It has been described that at six months of age, 60% of IL-$10^{-/-}$-mice develop adenocarcinomas [26]. We have previously shown that lumen filling tumors arise in IL-$10^{-/-}$ mice, which closely resemble human adenocarcinomas histologically [27]. Furthermore, it has been reported that neoplastic transformation in these mice can be aggravated by administration of celecoxib [25,27].

The aim of this project was to characterize murine inflammation-associated CRCs with regard to CIN and other known characteristics of their human counterpart. The extent of CIN in premalignant and malignant stages of two mouse models for colitis-mediated carcinogenesis was assessed. Furthermore, the protein expression of p53 and beta-catenin was evaluated in murine tumors, as well as in an exemplary set of human CACs. Ki67 staining served to determine the growth fraction of the tumors. Finally, inflammatory activity was confirmed via endoscopy, histology, as well as a local increase of the pro-inflammatory cytokine interferon-γ (IFNγ)

Materials and Methods

Ethical Considerations

Animal protocols were approved by the regional animal study committee of Berlin (LAGeSo, approval ID G0297/03) for both models used in this study.

Mice

All animals were purchased from Harlan Winkelmann (Borchen, Germany). Altogether, 23 mice treated with AOM and DSS as described below were used for this study. Complementarily, eight IL-$10^{-/-}$ mice were investigated.

AOM/DSS-induced tumor development

DSS and AOM were administered to C57BL/6J mice at six weeks of age as described previously [27]. Briefly, mice received a single intraperitoneal injection of the mutagenic agent AOM (12.5 mg/kg body weight). Starting at day five after the AOM application, 3.5% DSS was dissolved in the drinking water for three cycles of five days each with intermittent 14-day intervals of regular drinking water, thereby inducing a chronic DSS colitis. Endoscopic surveillance was performed as described below on a weekly basis and mice were sacrificed on day 50, at that point exhibiting either adenocarcinomas or colitis without overt neoplasms (see results, **table 1**).

In total, ten healthy, untreated C57BL/6J-mice were used as normal controls (**figure 1**).

IL-$10^{-/-}$-mice

At twelve weeks of age, the cyclooxygenase 2 inhibitor celecoxib (500 mg/mouse/day) was administered orally to IL-$10^{-/-}$ mice (C57BL/6J −background, n = 8) for five days as described previously [25]. Mice were observed for an additional four weeks and underwent weekly lower endoscopy, before being sacrificed with or without signs of malignant growth (**table 1**).

Endoscopic surveillance and post-mortem examination

Tumor development was monitored macroscopically using a high resolution mouse endoscope system (Karl Storz GmbH, Tuttlingen, Germany) as described previously [28]. Endoscopies were performed weekly starting one week after AOM-treatment and celecoxib-treatment, respectively. Based on observed tumor development, days 50 and 28 after beginning of each treatment were chosen as endpoint for the AOM/DSS and IL-$10^{-/-}$ group, respectively. Endoscopic procedures surveyed on a color monitor were recorded digitally (DSR-20MD, Sony, Cologne, Germany).

In addition to preparation of colonic tissue as described below, post-mortem autopsy was performed macroscopically. Particularly, to screen for distant metastases, fresh lung and liver tissue was cut into 5 mm sections, which were investigated for macroscopical signs of neoplasms.

DNA-image cytometry

Nuclear DNA ploidy assessments were performed by means of DNA-image cytometry using Feulgen-stained histological sections of 8 μm thickness. Staining procedures, cell selection criteria, and internal standardization were based on methods described previously [29]. An average number of 110 enterocyte nuclei (range 100 to 120, SD = 3.4) were measured per specimen after interactive selection using a digital imaging system (Ahrens ACAS, Hamburg, Germany). All DNA values were expressed in relation to internal staining controls (lymphocytes), which were given the value 2c. DNA profiles were classified according to Auer [29]. Histograms characterized by a single peak in the diploid or near-diploid region (1.5 c–2.5 c) were classified as type I. Type II histograms showed a single peak in the tetraploid region (3.5 c–4.5 c) or peaks in both the diploid and tetraploid regions (>90% of the total cell population). The number of cells with DNA values between the diploid and tetraploid region and those exceeding the tetraploid region (>4.5 c) was <10%. Type III histograms represented highly proliferating near-diploid cell populations and were comprised of DNA values ranging between the diploid and the tetraploid region. Only a small number of cells (<5%) showed more than 4.5 c. The DNA histograms of types I, II and III thus characterize euploid cell populations. Type IV histograms showed increased (>5%) and/or distinctly scattered DNA values exceeding the tetraploid region

Table 1. Ploidy assessment according to Auer's classification, p53-, beta-catenin-, and Ki67-immunohistochemistry for murine tissue analyzed.

No.	Auer	Aneuploid	p53	b-catenin	Ki67 / %
AOM-CA1	4	1	2	4	30
AOM-CA2	4	1	1	4	20
AOM-CA3	4	1	1	4	25
AOM-CA4	4	1	2	1	10
AOM-CA5	4	1	1	4	30
AOM-CA6	4	1	1	4	25
AOM-CA7	4	1	1	1	10
AOM-CA8	4	1	1	2	10
AOM-CA9	4	1	2	3	20
AOM-CA10	4	1	2	2	35
AOM-CA11	4	1	3	2	10
AOM-CA12	3	0	3	3	15
AOM-CA13	3	0	1	4	20
AOM-CA14	4	1	1	5	5
AOM-CA15	3	0	2	4	40
AOM-CA16	4	1	3	4	40
IL10-CA1	3	0	3	1	40
IL10-CA2	3	0	3	1	40
IL10-CA3	3	0	3	1	35
IL10-CA4	3	0	3	1	40
AOM-CNTRL1	3	0	1	2	20
AOM-CNTRL2	1	0	0	1	5
AOM-CNTRL3	1	0	1	1	5
AOM-CNTRL4	3	0	1	1	10
AOM-CNTRL5	3	0	2	1	15
AOM-CNTRL6	1	0	1	2	5
AOM-CNTRL7	3	0	2	2	15
IL10-CNTRL1	3	0	3	1	35
IL10-CNTRL2	3	0	2	1	35
IL10-CNTRL3	3	0	2	1	30
IL10-CNTRL4	3	0	2	1	25

AOM-CA$_n$: carcinomas of AOM/DSS-colitis. IL10CA$_n$: carcinomas of IL10$^{-/-}$-mice. CNTRL$_n$: premalignant tissue.
DNA-ploidy was assessed according to Auer (please refer to the text). p53 was assessed semiquantitatively, 0: no expression, 1 1–20% positive mucosa cells, 2: 21–50%, 3>50%
Beta-catenin: 1: membranous, 2: membranous-cytoplasmatic, 3: cytoplasmatic, 4: cytoplasmatic-nulcear, to 5, nuclear.

(>4.5 c). These histograms were suggested to reflect aneuploid populations of enterocyte nuclei.

Colon organ culture and cytokine measurements

Murine colons were cut open longitudinally and washed in PBS. Strips of 1 cm² were placed in 48 flat-bottom well culture plates containing 0.5 ml of serum-free RPMI 1640 with penicillin (100 U/ml) and streptomycin (100 µg/ml), and were incubated at 37°C for 24 h. Culture supernatants were harvested, assayed for IFNγ, and total protein content was quantified using the Bio-Rad protein assay (Bio-Rad Laboratories, Munich, Germany). Murine IFNγ was determined by specific ELISA according to the

manufacturer's protocols (BD Biosciences, Heidelberg, Germany) with a quantification range from 20 pg/ml to 10 ng/ml.

Histopathology and Immunohistochemistry

All tumors and mucosa specimens were subjected to *Hematoxylin & Eosin* (H&E) staining for histopathology assessment by an experienced pathologist (H.-A. L). From AOM/DSS-treated mice or IL-10$^{-/-}$ mice, complete colons were fixed. Paraffin sections were stained with H&E. Histological signs of inflammation were evaluated as a combined score of inflammatory cell infiltration (0–3) and tissue damage (0–3), resulting in a score ranging from 0 to 6 as described previously [30]. Tumor size was scored as follows: 0, no adenoma; 1, focal; 2, expanded and/or confluent; 3, expanded and raised; and 4, lumen filling. Antibodies for p53, beta-catenin, and Ki67 were purchased from DAKO (Hamburg, Germany; anti-Ki67 antibody; clone TEC3; rat IgG2a), New England Biolabs (Frankfurt, Germany; anti-beta-catenin antibody; clone 6B3, rabbit IgG), and Cell Signaling (Danvers, MA, USA; anti-p53 antibody, Ser15; polyclonal rabbit). Staining procedures were performed according to the manufacturers' protocols. At least ten high power fields were used to semiquantitatively assess protein expression. For immunohistochemistry scoring please refer to **table 1**.

Statistical Analyzes

Statistical data analyzes were performed using Microsoft Excel 2003, DigDB v7.1.3.3 (Sunnyvale, CA, USA), and XLStat Pro v7.5 (Addinsoft, New York, NY, USA). Data are expressed in means (using standard error of means, SEM). For inductive inference, nonparameteric rank-sum tests were used to compare location parameters of data distributions. Two independent samples, e.g. of different ploidy status, were compared using Wilcoxon's test. Corresponding frequencies were analyzed by means of Fisher's exact test. The type 1 error rate was set to 5%.

Results

Administration of AOM/DSS and IL-10 deficiency result in colitis-mediated carcinomas

In total, 16 out of 23 mice treated with AOM and DSS developed colorectal neoplasms after an average age of seven weeks post AOM administration. Tumor development could be followed endoscopically and tumors closely resembled human adenocarcinomas histologically. In mice that developed neoplasms (n = 16), tumor number ranged from two to 19 per animal with a median of nine tumors per mouse (**figure 1a**). From each individual, one representative tumor was chosen for further analyses on the basis of tumor size. However, in only one out of 16 cases, invasion through the colonic wall was observed, while all other carcinomas were characterized by obstructing intraluminar growth without infiltration beyond the lamina propria mucosae. Neoplasms were seen exclusively in the colon.

In IL-10$^{-/-}$ mice, at an average age of 15 weeks upcoming dysplasias progressed to infiltrating adenocarcinomas in a total of four animals (out of eight animals observed as described in "methods"). Tumor number ranged from seven to 24 tumors per animal, with a median of 16 neoplasms per mouse. One tumor of each animal was chosen for downstream analyses as described above. Neoplastic transformation was constrained to the colorectum.

Macroscopic distant metastases were seen neither after AOM/DSS-treatment nor in IL-10$^{-/-}$ mice.

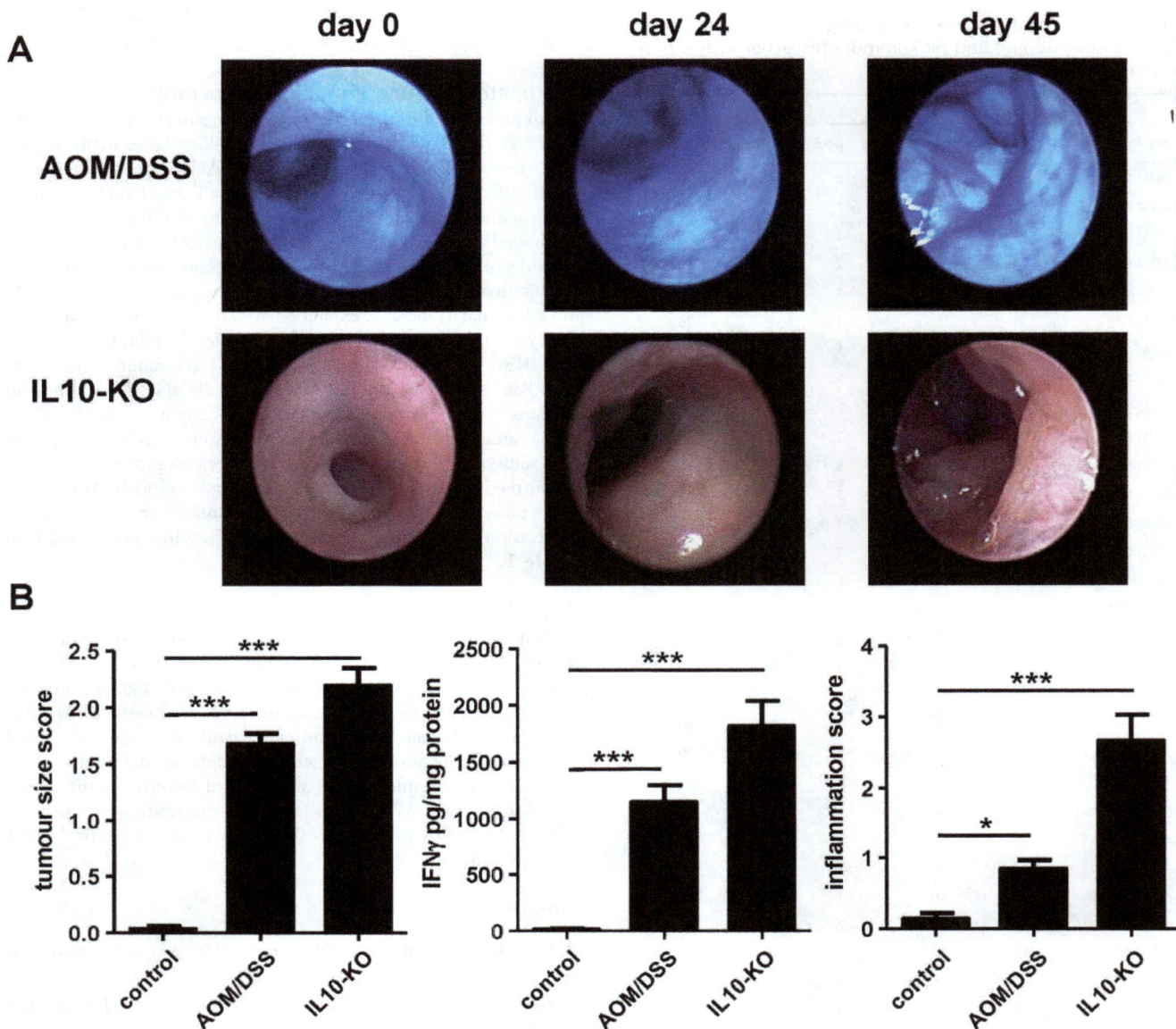

Figure 1. Murine models of inflammation-driven carcinogenesis. (A) Endoscopic images of inflamed mucosa and tumor of AOM/DSS-colitis as well as the IL10$^{-/-}$ model. Tumorigenesis was assessed by high resolution endoscopy *in vivo*. Methylene blue was used to enhance dysplasia detection as shown exemplarily for AOM/DSS colitis (B) Tumor size as rated by the tumor size score described in the methods section, IFNγ -levels, and inflammation score as assessed in H.E. staining for untreated controls, AOM/DSS-mice, and IL10$^{-/-}$ mice. Bars represent means, whishkers represent standard error of the mean (SEM). Colonic mucosa samples of 10 healthy untreated C57BL/6J-mice were applied to assess histologic parameters and IFNγ -expression.

Chronic intestinal inflammation in both models as prerequisite for tumorigenesis

Chronic inflammation at the site of tumorigenesis was characterized by a significant increase of the histological inflammation score in parallel to elevated IFNγ levels in the colon culture supernatants of both models when compared to healthy controls (**figure 1b**).

IL-10$^{-/-}$ colitis results in chromosomally stable tumors

A total of four IL-10$^{-/-}$ mice developed invasive colorectal carcinomas devoid of CIN. **Figure 2a** shows a DNA-histogram of inflamed mucosa and an example of an invasive carcinoma in IL-10$^{-/-}$ mice, both depicting a diploid-proliferative pattern. Histograms indicate a proliferating tumor without gross instability of the genome. In total, all four carcinomas of IL-10$^{-/-}$ mice presented diploid patterns. Likewise, all non-neoplastic mucosa samples showed diploid histograms. All non-neoplastic mucosa samples that were applied for DNA-cytometry and IHC presented with signs of chronic inflammation (average inflammation score of 2.1), while absence of neoplasia was ensured histologically (tumor score = 0).

AOM induced tumors that arise in mice treated with DSS show signs of gross CIN

Non-malignant mucosa after administration of AOM and DSS revealed a diploid pattern in DNA-cytometry (n = 7/7). Chronic inflammation was present in all non-neoplastic biopsies with an average inflammation score of 0.5, tumor score = 0.

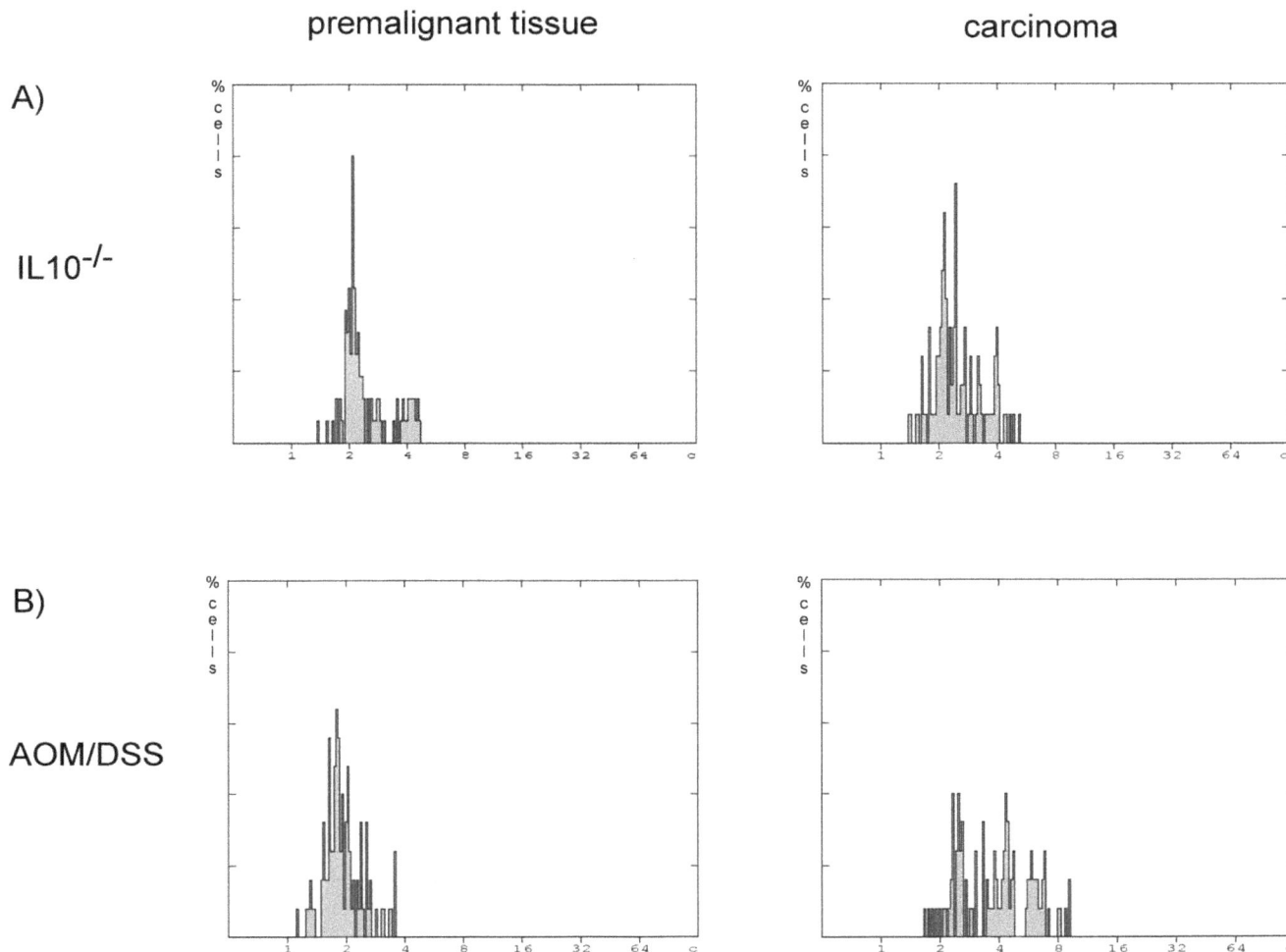

Figure 2. DNA-histograms. (A) Representative DNA histograms on logarithmic scale of premalignant and malignant tissue of IL-10$^{-/-}$ mice. Both histograms depict diploid proliferative patterns. (B) Mice treated with AOM/DSS showed diploid-proliferative patterns in premalignant stages. In the here presented example of CAC, 23% of all cells measured exceeded the threshold of 4.5 c, representing an aneuploid cell population.

Overt colorectal neoplasms on the basis of AOM/DSS-colitis presented aneuploidy with a significant amount of cells exceeding 4 c (**figure 2b**). In total, 13 out of 16 carcinomas arising in AOM/DSS-colitis showed aneuploidy reflecting CIN. The frequency of aneuploidy differed significantly between AOM/DSS-induced tumors and IL-10$^{-/-}$-induced tumors (p = 0.007).

Protein expression of CRC-associated gene products differs between both tumor types

In all IL-10$^{-/-}$ carcinomas (n = 4), membranous beta-catenin localization was found, while this was the case for two out of 16 AOM/DSS-induced tumors. In nine out of 16 AOM/DSS-induced carcinomas, nuclear or nuclear and cytoplasmatic beta-catenin expression was observed (**table 1**). The distribution of beta-catenin expression differed significantly between both groups (p = 0.020). In four out of seven non-malignant controls of AOM/DSS-colitis, membranous localization was observed, while the remaining three mucosa samples were characterized by membranous and cytoplasmatic expression, none showed nuclear expression. All four non-malignant controls of IL-10$^{-/-}$ colitis presented membranous expression of beta-catenin.

In IL-10$^{-/-}$ colitis as well as in IL-10$^{-/-}$-induced tumors, very high levels of p53-protein expression were detected. In contrast, while p53 expression was still elevated in AOM/DSS-colitis, it was significantly below that observed in IL-10$^{-/-}$ tumors (p = 0.010, **table 1**). In addition, premalignant mucosa of AOM/DSS-colitis revealed significantly lower p53-expression than AOM/DSS-induced CRCs (p = 0.015).

Within the group of AOM/DSS-induced tumors, there was neither a significant correlation between the presence of aneuploidy and beta-catenin expression (p = 0.580) nor between aneuploidy and p53 expression (p = 0.730). The growth fraction of the tumor was generally higher in IL-10$^{-/-}$-induced than in AOM/DSS-colitis-induced carcinomas (**table 1**). Thus, high expression of Ki67 was observed for premalignant mucosa of IL-10$^{-/-}$ animals, while it was low in premalignant stages of AOM/DSS-induced colitis (**table 1, figure 3**).

Discussion

Previously, a significantly higher frequency of aneuploidy reflecting chromosomal instability in human colitis-associated carcinomas as compared to the sporadic counterpart has been

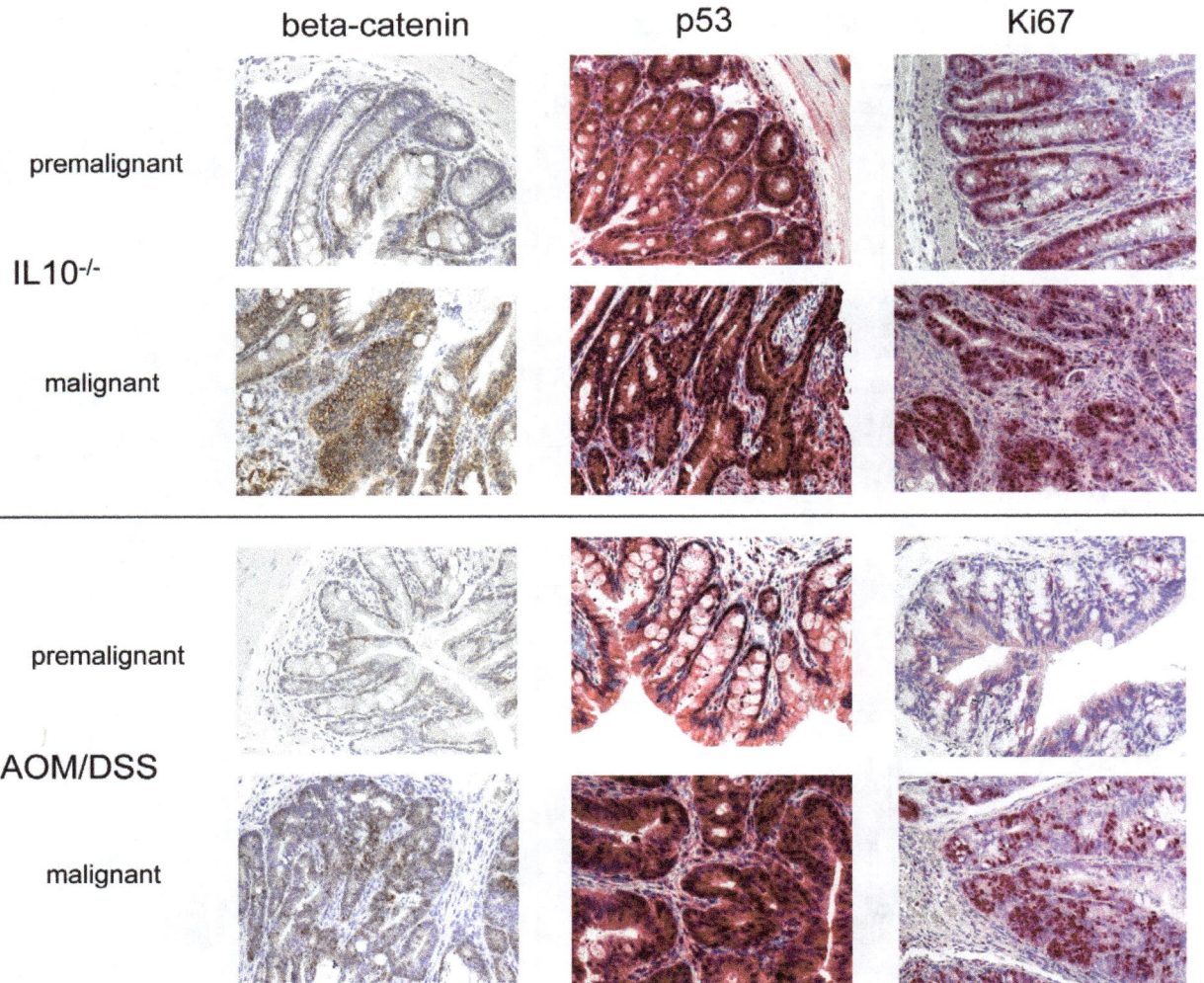

Figure 3. Immunohistochemistry for beta-catenin, p53 and Ki67 of murine premalignant tissue and CACs, details of 100x magnification.

described [10]. To assess whether canonical mouse models of colitis-associated carcinogenesis exist that equally exhibit signs of CIN, we investigated ploidy patterns in murine colitis-associated neoplasms of two murine models of CAC.

In IL-10$^{-/-}$ mice, neoplasms develop that resemble human adenocarcinomas, which has been described previously [26,31,32]. Severity of inflammation can be aggravated and malignant transformation accelerated by additional administration of celecoxib [25]. Carcinomas of the IL-10$^{-/-}$/celecoxib model did not exhibit signs of genomic instability in our study. Contrarily, tumors arising in the AOM/DSS-model presented with gross aneuploidy in the vast majority of cases. Although the number of specimens investigated differed between both groups with a considerably smaller number in the IL-10$^{-/-}$-group, differences in the frequency of aneuploidy reached the level of significance. The presence of biological differences between CACs in both models is furthermore suggested by differential expression of beta-catenin.

In IL-10$^{-/-}$ mice no extrinsic carcinogen is required to induce tumorigenesis. However, the complete absence of a critical cytokine for intestinal homeostasis represents an unphysiological state, even though altered IL-10 expression has previously been associated with human UC [33,34]. Our data provide evidence that chronic inflammation due to IL-10 deficiency does not induce CIN, despite the presence of severe colonic inflammation. Moreover, further characterization of the tumors indicates that beta-catenin expression in premalignant stages and in carcinomas is confined to the cell membrane. This seems to stand in contrast to human CACs, in which APC mutations are thought to inhibit beta-catenin degradation and thereby promote nuclear transloca-tion, although detailed data in humans is missing [18], whereas the high expression of phosphorylated p53 observed in these tumors is congruent with results in human UC-associated carcinomas [13].

In AOM/DSS colitis, an extrinsic carcinogen is needed to induce malignant transformation. Administration of DSS – and thereby initiation of chronic colitis – accelerates malignancy development, rendering the model particularly interesting for the study of colitis-associated carcinogenesis [22,35]. Here, we could show that a high percentage of CACs that arise after AOM/DSS treatment exhibit CIN (81.25%). This finding is particularly remarkable since it has previously been demonstrated that CRCs induced by administration of AOM alone, which therefore arise devoid of chronic inflammation, are genetically stable [23]. Thus, it can be hypothesized that similar to human colitis, murine colonic inflammation induces or significantly contributes to CIN. AOM/DSS colitis might therefore provide a powerful model to study the development of inflammation-induced CIN *in vivo*. Furthermore, in AOM/DSS induced tumors, cytoplasmatic and/or nuclear translocation of beta-catenin was observed, indicating activation of the Wnt-signaling pathway [18,36].

Expression of phosphorylated p53 was increased in AOM/DSS induced tumors, alongside with an increase in growth fraction as compared to premalignant stages. No association between the presence of aneuploidy and expression of p53 or beta-catenin could be shown, which might be due to insufficient numbers (n = 3 for the diploid group). Larger studies would be necessary to elucidate differential expression of tumor-associated proteins in relation to CIN in this murine model.

In neither of both models investigated in this study, macroscopic distant metastases could be observed. This is in line with previous findings [26,37], but stands in contrast to CRCs in humans, in which liver metastases occur in up to 50% of patients during the course of the disease [38]. In this context, inevitable limitations to translate biological findings from mice into the human system have to be appreciated. For CIN in inflammation-associated carcinogenesis specifically, telomere shortening could be associated with increased genomic instability [39]. As differences exist between murine and human telomere biology with mice bearing longer telomeres and constitutive telomerase activity [40], it might be questionable to address telomere attrition in the AOM/DSS model. However, e. g. in murine epithelial cancers, telomere and telomerase dysfunction have been shown to be pivotal for tumor development, exemplifying a possible role for telomere biology in

murine carcinogenesis [41]. Furthermore, other mechanisms such as chromatid cohesion defects have been associated with CIN in CRC, which involve proteins highly similar in man and mice and studied in both organisms [42,43].

In summary, IL-10-deficient mice do not represent a suitable animal model for the study of the CIN pathway of carcinogenesis. In addition, tumor development in this model does not depend on beta-catenin translocation.

Contrarily, with presence of aneuploidy and beta-catenin activation, the model of AOM/DSS-colitis might provide a valuable tool to gain a more detailed insight into the molecular architecture of inflammation-associated carcinogenesis and mechanistically investigate colitis-associated carcinogenesis with special regard to CIN.

Acknowledgments

The authors wish to express their gratitude to Katja Grollich for performing immunohistochemistry and Gisela Grosser-Pape for excellent assistance in preparation of slides for DNA-cytometry. Grants from the Werner and Clara Kreitz Foundation and the German Cancer Aid (DKH #108446: the *North German Tumorbank of Colorectal Cancer*) are gratefully acknowledged.

Author Contributions

Conceived and designed the experiments: MG JKH MZ BS. Performed the experiments: MG RG AAK. Analyzed the data: MG RG JKH BS. Contributed reagents/materials/analysis tools: H-AL CL. Wrote the paper: MG BS.

References

1. Bernstein CN, Blanchard JF, Kliewer E, Wajda A (2001) Cancer risk in patients with inflammatory bowel disease: a population-based study. Cancer 91: 854–862.
2. Pohl C, Hombach A, Kruis W (2000) Chronic inflammatory bowel disease and cancer. Hepatogastroenterology 47: 57–70.
3. Kanai Y (2010) Genome-wide DNA methylation profiles in precancerous conditions and cancers. Cancer Sci 101: 36–45.
4. Yan B, Peng Y, Li CY (2009) Molecular analysis of genetic instability caused by chronic inflammation. Methods Mol Biol 512: 15–28.
5. Risques RA, Lai LA, Brentnall TA, Li L, Feng Z, et al. (2008) Ulcerative colitis is a disease of accelerated colon aging: evidence from telomere attrition and DNA damage. Gastroenterology 135: 410–418.
6. Paulson TG, Maley CC, Li X, Li H, Sanchez CA, et al. (2009) Chromosomal instability and copy number alterations in Barrett's esophagus and esophageal adenocarcinoma. Clin Cancer Res 15: 3305–3314.
7. Goldberg-Bittman L, Kitay-Cohen Y, Hadari R, Yukla M, Fejgin MD, et al. (2008) Random aneuploidy in chronic hepatitis C patients. Cancer Genet Cytogenet 180: 20–23.
8. Habermann J, Lenander C, Roblick UJ, Kruger S, Ludwig D, et al. (2001) Ulcerative colitis and colorectal carcinoma: DNA-profile, laminin-5 gamma2 chain and cyclin A expression as early markers for risk assessment. Scand J Gastroenterol 36: 751–758.
9. Befrits R, Hammarberg C, Rubio C, Jaramillo E, Tribukait B (1994) DNA aneuploidy and histologic dysplasia in long-standing ulcerative colitis. A 10-year follow-up study. Dis Colon Rectum 37: 313–319; discussion 319–320.
10. Gerling M, Meyer KF, Fuchs K, Igl BW, Fritzsche B, et al. (2010) High Frequency of Aneuploidy Defines Ulcerative Colitis-Associated Carcinomas: A Comparative Prognostic Study to Sporadic Colorectal Carcinomas. Ann Surg 252(1): 84–89.
11. Araujo SE, Bernardo WM, Habr-Gama A, Kiss DR, Cecconello I (2007) DNA ploidy status and prognosis in colorectal cancer: a meta-analysis of published data. Dis Colon Rectum 50: 1800–1810.
12. Yin J, Harpaz N, Tong Y, Huang Y, Laurin J, et al. (1993) p53 point mutations in dysplastic and cancerous ulcerative colitis lesions. Gastroenterology 104: 1633–1639.
13. Brentnall TA, Crispin DA, Rabinovitch PS, Haggitt RC, Rubin CE, et al. (1994) Mutations in the p53 gene: an early marker of neoplastic progression in ulcerative colitis. Gastroenterology 107: 369–378.
14. Chaubert P, Benhattar J, Saraga E, Costa J (1994) K-ras mutations and p53 alterations in neoplastic and nonneoplastic lesions associated with longstanding ulcerative colitis. Am J Pathol 144: 767–775.
15. Harpaz N, Peck AL, Yin J, Fiel I, Hontanosas M, et al. (1994) p53 protein expression in ulcerative colitis-associated colorectal dysplasia and carcinoma. Hum Pathol 25: 1069–1074.
16. Su LK, Vogelstein B, Kinzler KW (1993) Association of the APC tumor suppressor protein with catenins. Science 262: 1734–1737.
17. Tomlinson I, Ilyas M, Johnson V, Davies A, Clark G, et al. (1998) A comparison of the genetic pathways involved in the pathogenesis of three types of colorectal cancer. J Pathol 184: 148–152.
18. Claessen MM, Schipper ME, Oldenburg B, Siersema PD, Offerhaus GJ, et al. WNT-pathway activation in IBD-associated colorectal carcinogenesis: potential biomarkers for colonic surveillance. Cell Oncol 32: 303–310.
19. Okayasu I, Hatakeyama S, Yamada M, Ohkusa T, Inagaki Y, et al. (1990) A novel method in the induction of reliable experimental acute and chronic ulcerative colitis in mice. Gastroenterology 98: 694–702.
20. Ishioka T, Kuwabara N, Oohashi Y, Wakabayashi K (1987) Induction of colorectal tumors in rats by sulfated polysaccharides. Crit Rev Toxicol 17: 215–244.
21. Yamada M, Ohkusa T, Okayasu I (1992) Occurrence of dysplasia and adenocarcinoma after experimental chronic ulcerative colitis in hamsters induced by dextran sulphate sodium. Gut 33: 1521–1527.
22. Tanaka T, Kohno H, Suzuki R, Yamada Y, Sugie S, et al. (2003) A novel inflammation-related mouse colon carcinogenesis model induced by azoxymethane and dextran sodium sulfate. Cancer Sci 94: 965–973.
23. Guda K, Upender MB, Belinsky G, Flynn C, Nakanishi M, et al. (2004) Carcinogen-induced colon tumors in mice are chromosomally stable and are characterized by low-level microsatellite instability. Oncogene 23: 3813–3821.
24. Suzuki R, Kohno H, Sugie S, Tanaka T (2005) Dose-dependent promoting effect of dextran sodium sulfate on mouse colon carcinogenesis initiated with azoxymethane. Histol Histopathol 20: 483–492.
25. Hegazi RA, Mady HH, Melhem MF, Sepulveda AR, Mohi M, et al. (2003) Celecoxib and rofecoxib potentiate chronic colitis and premalignant changes in interleukin 10 knockout mice. Inflamm Bowel Dis 9: 230–236.
26. Berg DJ, Davidson N, Kuhn R, Muller W, Menon S, et al. (1996) Enterocolitis and colon cancer in interleukin-10-deficient mice are associated with aberrant cytokine production and CD4(+) TH1-like responses. J Clin Invest 98: 1010–1020.
27. Glauben R, Sonnenberg E, Zeitz M, Siegmund B (2009) HDAC inhibitors in models of inflammation-related tumorigenesis. Cancer Lett 280: 154–159.
28. Becker C, Fantini MC, Wirtz S, Nikolaev A, Kiesslich R, et al. (2005) In vivo imaging of colitis and colon cancer development in mice using high resolution chromoendoscopy. Gut 54: 950–954.

29. Auer GU, Caspersson TO, Gustafsson SA, Humla SA, Ljung BM, et al. (1980) Relationship between nuclear DNA distribution and estrogen receptors in human mammary carcinomas. Anal Quant Cytol 2: 280–284.

30. Siegmund B, Lehr HA, Fantuzzi G (2002) Leptin: a pivotal mediator of intestinal inflammation in mice. Gastroenterology 122: 2011–2025.

31. Beatty PL, Plevy SE, Sepulveda AR, Finn OJ (2007) Cutting edge: transgenic expression of human MUC1 in IL-10$^{-/-}$ mice accelerates inflammatory bowel disease and progression to colon cancer. J Immunol 179: 735–739.

32. Chichlowski M, Sharp JM, Vanderford DA, Myles MH, Hale LP (2008) Helicobacter typhlonius and Helicobacter rodentium differentially affect the severity of colon inflammation and inflammation-associated neoplasia in IL10-deficient mice. Comp Med 58: 534–541.

33. Castro-Santos P, Suarez A, Lopez-Rivas L, Mozo L, Gutierrez C (2006) TNFalpha and IL-10 gene polymorphisms in inflammatory bowel disease. Association of -1082 AA low producer IL-10 genotype with steroid dependency. Am J Gastroenterol 101: 1039–1047.

34. Franke A, Balschun T, Karlsen TH, Sventoraityte J, Nikolaus S, et al. (2008) Sequence variants in IL10, ARPC2 and multiple other loci contribute to ulcerative colitis susceptibility. Nat Genet 40: 1319–1323.

35. Clapper ML, Cooper HS, Chang WC (2007) Dextran sulfate sodium-induced colitis-associated neoplasia: a promising model for the development of chemopreventive interventions. Acta Pharmacol Sin 28: 1450–1459.

36. Clevers H (2006) Wnt/beta-catenin signaling in development and disease. Cell 127: 469–480.

37. Rosenberg DW, Giardina C, Tanaka T (2009) Mouse models for the study of colon carcinogenesis. Carcinogenesis 30: 183–196.

38. Benson AB, 3rd (2007) Epidemiology, disease progression, and economic burden of colorectal cancer. J Manag Care Pharm 13: S5–18.

39. O'Sullivan JN, Bronner MP, Brentnall TA, Finley JC, Shen WT, et al. (2002) Chromosomal instability in ulcerative colitis is related to telomere shortening. Nat Genet 32: 280–284.

40. Wright WE, Shay JW (2000) Telomere dynamics in cancer progression and prevention: fundamental differences in human and mouse telomere biology. Nat Med 6: 849–851.

41. Artandi SE, Chang S, Lee SL, Alson S, Gottlieb GJ, et al. (2000) Telomere dysfunction promotes non-reciprocal translocations and epithelial cancers in mice. Nature 406: 641–645.

42. Kurze A, Michie KA, Dixon SE, Mishra A, Itoh T, et al. (2010) A positively charged channel within the Smc1/Smc3 hinge required for sister chromatid cohesion. Embo J 30: 364–378.

43. Barber TD, McManus K, Yuen KW, Reis M, Parmigiani G, et al. (2008) Chromatid cohesion defects may underlie chromosome instability in human colorectal cancers. Proc Natl Acad Sci U S A 105: 3443–3448.

14

Direct Bacterial Killing *In Vitro* by Recombinant Nod2 is Compromised by Crohn's Disease-Associated Mutations

Laurent-Herve Perez[1,9], Matt Butler[1,9], Tammy Creasey[1], JoAnn Dzink-Fox[3], John Gounarides[2], Stephanie Petit[1], Anna Ropenga[1], Neil Ryder[3], Kathryn Smith[1], Philip Smith[1], Scott J. Parkinson[1]*

1 Gastrointestinal Disease Area, Novartis Institutes for Biomedical Research, Horsham, United Kingdom, 2 Analytical Sciences, Novartis Institutes for Biomedical Research, Cambridge, Massachusetts, United States of America, 3 Infectious Disease Area, Novartis Institutes for Biomedical Research, Cambridge, Massachusetts, United States of America

Abstract

Background: A homeostatic relationship with the intestinal microflora is increasingly appreciated as essential for human health and wellbeing. Mutations in the leucine-rich repeat (LRR) domain of Nod2, a bacterial recognition protein, are associated with development of the inflammatory bowel disorder, Crohn's disease. We investigated the molecular mechanisms underlying disruption of intestinal symbiosis in patients carrying Nod2 mutations.

Methodology/Principal Findings: In this study, using purified recombinant LRR domains, we demonstrate that Nod2 is a direct antimicrobial agent and this activity is generally deficient in proteins carrying Crohn's-associated mutations. Wild-type, but not Crohn's-associated, Nod2 LRR domains directly interacted with bacteria *in vitro*, altered their metabolism and disrupted the integrity of the plasma membrane. Antibiotic activity was also expressed by the LRR domains of Nod1 and other pattern recognition receptors suggesting that the LRR domain is a conserved anti-microbial motif supporting innate cellular immunity.

Conclusions/Significance: The lack of anti-bacterial activity demonstrated with Crohn's-associated Nod2 mutations *in vitro*, supports the hypothesis that a deficiency in direct bacterial killing contributes to the association of Nod2 polymorphisms with the disease.

Editor: Niyaz Ahmed, University of Hyderabad, India

Funding: The study was funded by the Novartis Institutes for Biomedical Research which employs all of the authors and supports their research activities. Outside of this influence, the funders had no role in study design, data collection and analysis, decision to publish, or preparation of the manuscript.

Competing Interests: All of the authors are employees of the Novartis Institutes for Biomedical Research (NIBR). Novartis are assignees of a patent submitted for applications related to this work.

* E-mail: Scott.Parkinson@novartis.com

9 These authors contributed equally to this work.

Introduction

Crohn's disease is a chronic relapsing inflammatory bowel disorder characterised by transmural and discontinuous lesions of the intestinal tract [1],[2]. It is generally accepted that the characteristic gut inflammation of Crohn's (as well as ulcerative colitis) is the result of a robust immune response against commensal bacteria in the gastrointestinal tract. Currently, it is not clear what underlies this loss of tolerance, however patients demonstrate increased levels of attaching/effacing and intracellular bacteria consistent with an initiating role for bacteria in the pathogenesis of the disease [3]. Environmental factors (such as smoking) as well as genetic factors also play a role in disease pathogenesis [4]. Genome-wide linkage studies of Crohn's disease families initially identified a susceptibility locus on chromosome 16 [5]. This linkage was subsequently confirmed as being a result of mutations in the intracellular pattern recognition receptor (PRR) Nod2 [6]. Three distinct Nod2 single nucleotide polymorphisms (SNPs) have been associated with increased risk of developing Crohn's disease. All three are coding mutations contained within (G908R, 3020insC), or adjacent to (R702W), the LRR domain at the C-terminus of the protein. LRR domains are common to many PRRs and are believed to confer sensitivity to pathogen-associated molecular patterns (PAMPs).

Results

Unlike *H. pylori's* part in the pathogenesis of stomach ulcers, a single pathogen associated with development of Crohn's disease has not been demonstrated although several have been proposed [7]. Due to their constant exposure to the microbiota of the gastrointestinal tract, epithelial cells are the primary point of contact with the commensal flora. In order to investigate the mechanism by which Nod2 protects the gastrointestinal tract, polyclonal antibodies were raised against recombinant human Nod2 LRR domains and used to examine the localisation of endogenous Nod2 in an intestinal epithelial cell line incubated with a non-pathogenic *Escherichia coli* strain (Figure 1a). In the absence of bacteria, Nod2 was expressed at low levels and distributed throughout the cytosol (Figure S1). Following incuba-

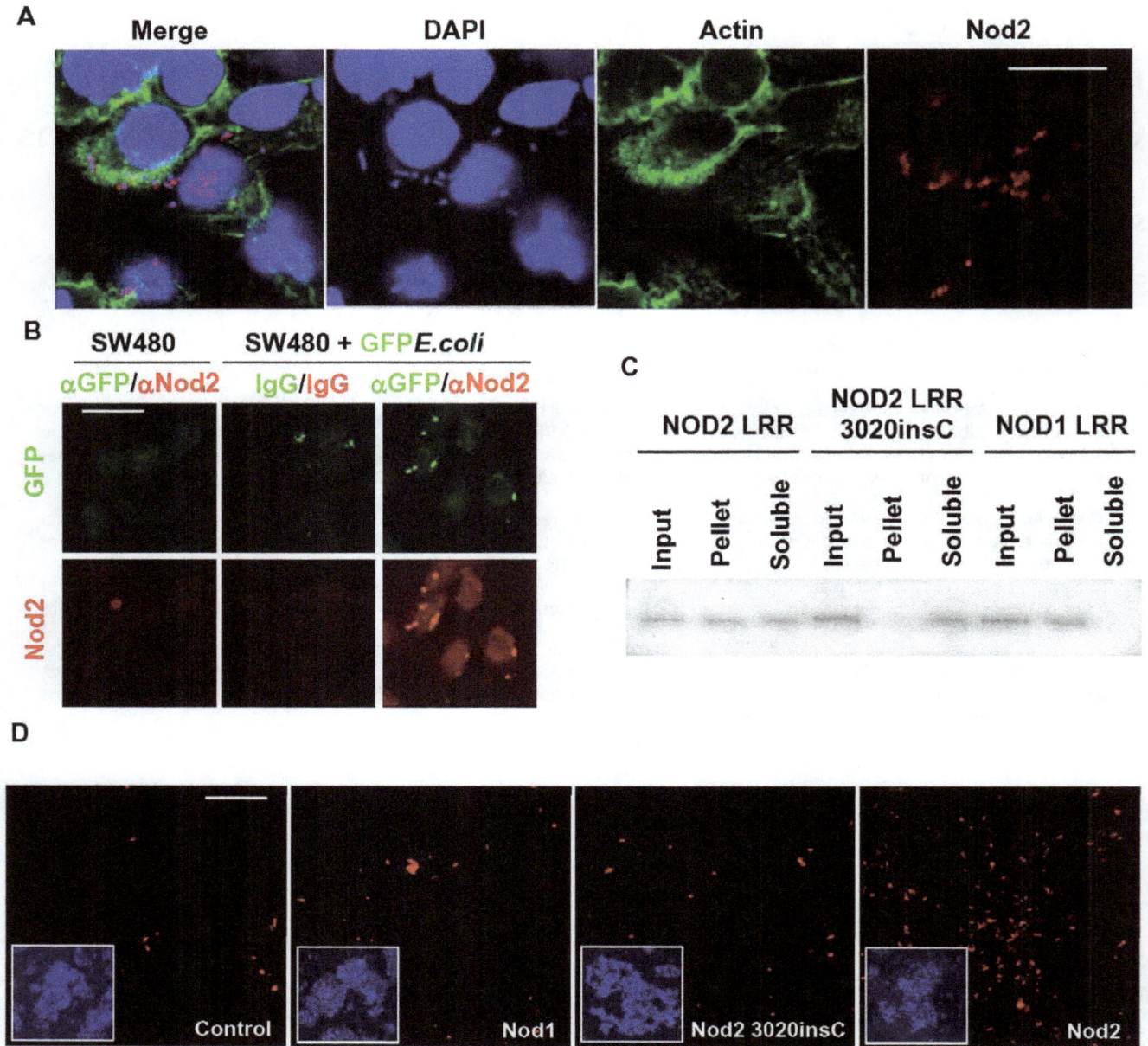

Figure 1. Nod2, but not the Crohn's-associated 3020insC mutation, directly associates with bacteria. A, SW480 intestinal epithelial cells were used to investigate the distribution of endogenous Nod2 protein following inoculation of the cells with *E.coli* (ATCC 25922) at an MOI of 1000:1. Cells were processed for immunofluorescence using a polyclonal antibody raised against the LRR domain of Nod2, immunopurified on the antigen and further processed on an *E.coli* lysate column to remove contaminating anti-bacterial antibodies. Controls are shown in Figure S1 demonstrating specificity of the Nod2 antibody. Bar = 15 μm. **B**, *E.coli* expressing GFP were generated by transformation of ATCC 25922 with a cDNA encoding GFP in pUC19. SW480 cells were treated as described in Figure 1a. An antibody against GFP was used to enhance the GFP signal although the fluorescent protein was generally visible (centre top panel). Isotype antibody control for GFP (chicken IgY) and rabbit IgG processed on an *E.coli* lysate column were used as controls (centre panels). Bar = 30 μm. **C**, Association of His-tagged recombinant protein derived from cDNAs encoding Nod2 LRR, Nod2 3020insC LRR and Nod1 LRR domains with *E.coli*. 10 ng of each protein was added to approximately 10^6 bacteria in 100 μl of LB media, incubated for 30 minutes at room temperature, and the samples centrifuged at low speed to collect the bacteria and associated proteins. The bacterial pellet and supernatants were reconstituted in equal volumes and loaded on an SDS-PAGE gel. Following transfer to nitrocellulose, the samples were analysed by Western blot using an anti-His antibody (Sigma). **D**, Direct binding of Nod2, but not Nod2 3020insC, to *E.coli* in vitro. Recombinant Nod2, Nod2 3020insC or Nod1 LRR domains (35 μg/ml) were added to *E.coli* at 37°C overnight. Bacteria were collected by centrifugation, washed and the association of LRR domains determined by immunofluorescent labelling of the bacteria with anti-Nod2 antibody (described in Figure 1a) and goat anti-rabbit 2° antibody. A sample of the labelled bacteria were placed on a sealed coverslip and analysed by fluorescent microscopy. Insets demonstrate the presence of comparable numbers of bacteria in each of the images as demonstrated by DAPI staining. Bar = 10 μm.

tion with *E.coli* for 2 hours, Nod2 aggregated within the cytoplasm of the cells (Figure 1a, Figure S1). The observed Nod2-positive structures were consistent with the size and characteristic shape of *E.coli* and were co-stained with DAPI. The presence of these bacteria inside the exposed cells was surprising considering the strain used (FDA strain Seattle 1946 [DSM 1103, NCIB 12210, ATCC25922]) is a biosafety level 1 bacterium that, to our knowledge, has not demonstrated any previous evidence of pathogenic potential. We next generated GFP-expressing *E.coli* and repeated the experiment to confirm that Nod2 was recruited to bacteria-containing structures within the cell (Figure 1b). Nod2 is generally believed to be a sensor of muramyl dipeptide (MDP), a component of the bacterial proteoglycan coat. Until now, a direct interaction between Nod2 and bacteria has not been demonstrated. We tested this possibility *in vitro* and confirmed that recombinant Nod2 LRR domains associated directly with *E.coli* using two different assays for direct bacterial binding. Recombinant Nod2, Nod2 3020insC and Nod1 LRR domains were incubated with *E.coli*, collected by centrifugation, and the distribution of the Nod2 and Nod1-derived proteins in the bacterial pellet and/or supernatant determined by Western blot (Figure 1c). This assay demonstrated a significant accumulation of Nod2 LRR domains with the bacterial pellet. This association was not observed using the 3020insC LRR domain. Nod1 LRR also distributed with the bacterial pellet demonstrating that it too can directly recognise bacteria. In addition, purified LRR domains of Nod2 were associated with *E. coli* as demonstrated by staining of the bacteria with an antibody raised against the LRR domain of Nod2 (Figure 1d). Incubation of bacteria with Nod1 LRR domains did not give significant staining above background (Control) despite Nod1 LRR domain association with *E.coli* (Figure 1c) demonstrating the specificity of the antibody for Nod2. The LRR domains containing the 3020insC polymorphism could not be detected on the bacteria above background levels suggesting this Crohn's-associated polymorphism confers an inherent defect in bacterial recognition. Direct interaction of the Nod2 LRR domain with the gram-positive bacteria *E. faecalis* was also demonstrated (Figure S2).

We next investigated the consequences of the observed LRR interaction with bacteria. Following overnight treatment of various bacterial strains with Nod2 LRR domains, a pellet could be observed in the bottom of the treated, but not control tubes (not shown). Examination of the pellet by microscopy revealed aggregation of LRR-treated bacteria suggesting Nod2 LRR domains were directly influencing the phenotype of a broad range of bacteria (Figure S3). Therefore, we sought to identify and quantitate the impact of the Nod2 LRR domains on exposed bacteria. *E.coli* was cultured in LB media in the presence of the Nod2 LRR domains for 6 hours and the metabolic profile of the bacteria assessed. Metabolomic analysis revealed that Nod2 LRR domains induced significant and specific perturbations to cellular metabolism (Figure 2, Table S1). These included a 3-fold increase in γ-aminobutyrate, a 40–50% decrease in glutamate, aspartate and glutathione and a 2-fold increase in trimethylamine oxide (TMAO). The loss of glutathione would be expected to be detrimental to cell survival as glutathione is central to the regulation of intracellular K^+ and detoxification of methylglyoxal in *E.coli* [8]. The loss of cellular glutamate and aspartate coupled with an increase in γ-aminobutyrate suggests the induction of amino acid decarboxylases consistent with cytoplasmic acidification [9]. LRR domains carrying the 3020insC did not induce similar perturbations to the cellular metabolite profile suggesting proteins with Crohn's-associated mutations cannot target bacterial metabolism due to their lack of direct binding to the bacteria (Figure 1).

Previous reports have shown that Nod2 can protect cultured cells from bacterial infection and this activity is deficient in cells expressing the 3020insC polymorphism [10]. In addition, mice deficient in Nod2 (as well as mice carrying the equivalent mutation to the human 3020insC polymorphism) are more susceptible to infection by various bacteria [11]–[13]. Based on these reports and our own observations, we hypothesized that Nod2, directly binds to bacteria and kills them via the LRR domain. *E.coli* were incubated with increasing doses of the recombinant LRR domains of either Nod2 or Nod2 3020insC and the integrity of the bacterial membrane evaluated using a flow cytometric assay previously used to study the activity of anti-bacterial defensins [14]. Incubation with wild-type Nod2 LRR domain resulted in membrane depolarisation indicative of anti-bacterial activity (Figure 3a). This activity could not be observed with the Nod2 3020insC LRR domains. While *E.coli* were only partially susceptible to Nod2-induced membrane depolarisation, gram positive *B. subtilis* were completely depolarised by less than 10 μg/ml Nod2 (Figure 3b). Again, this activity was deficient when the 3020insC LRR domain was used. Since LRR domains of Nod1 could also directly bind to bacteria (Figure 1c), we hypothesised that the observed anti-bacterial activity for Nod2 might be a common property of LRR domains derived from pattern-recognition receptors. LRR domains from Nod1, Naip, Nalp3, CIITA and TLR2 were generated and their activity against *B.subtilis* assessed in the membrane depolarisation assay (Figure 3c). Nod1 demonstrated comparable efficacy against the bacteria as Nod2. Naip, Nalp3 and TLR2 LRR domains all demonstrated significant activity in this assay – although this was not as robust as with Nod2 and Nod1 against *B.subtilis*.

We further extended our analysis of Nod2 anti-bacterial activity using a variety of established anti-bacterial assays to confirm our initial observations. In an agar-diffusion assay anti-bacterial activity of Nod2 could be observed with a clear zone of growth exclusion of *B.subtilis* and *S. aureus* surrounding a well containing purified LRR domains (Figure 3c). We did not observe any evidence of anti-bacterial activity using LRR proteins carrying the 3020insC mutation while Nod1 LRR domains also demonstrated a clear efficacy in this assay. Anti-bacterial activity was also tested using an *in vitro* assay based on the correlation of ATP levels with bacterial number (Table S2). Comparing Nod2 and Nod1 anti-bacterial activity in this assay demonstrated clear differences in bacterial specificity. For example, Nod2 effectively targeted *E. faecalis* while Nod1 was selective over Nod2 for *K. pneumoniae*. Not all bacteria were insensitive to the 3020insC LRR domain. Indeed, the activity of Nod2 and Nod2 3020insC was comparable against *L. monocytogenes*. This assay was also used to investigate the anti-bacterial activity of the Crohn's-associated G908R Nod2 polymorphism. *L. monocytogenes* continued to proliferate in the presence of the G908R LRR domain but was sensitive to the 3020insC domains. However, the anti-bacterial activity was not completely deficient in the G908R protein since it targeted *B. subtilis* with comparable efficacy to the 3020insC LRR (although this activity was deficient compared to the wild-type LRR domains).

The most pronounced observation was the clear sensitivity of the aerobic gram-positive bacteria tested in this assay to the Nod2 LRR domain. This was not observed when anaerobic bacteria were tested for LRR sensitivity in a standard minimal inhibitory concentration (MIC) assay. This assay assesses the potency of antibiotics by determining the minimal concentration at which no visible bacterial growth can be observed. The sensitivity of 9 anaerobic bacterial strains to Nod2 and Nod1 LRR domains using this assessment are presented in Table 1. All bacteria were insensitive to the presence of LRR domains containing the

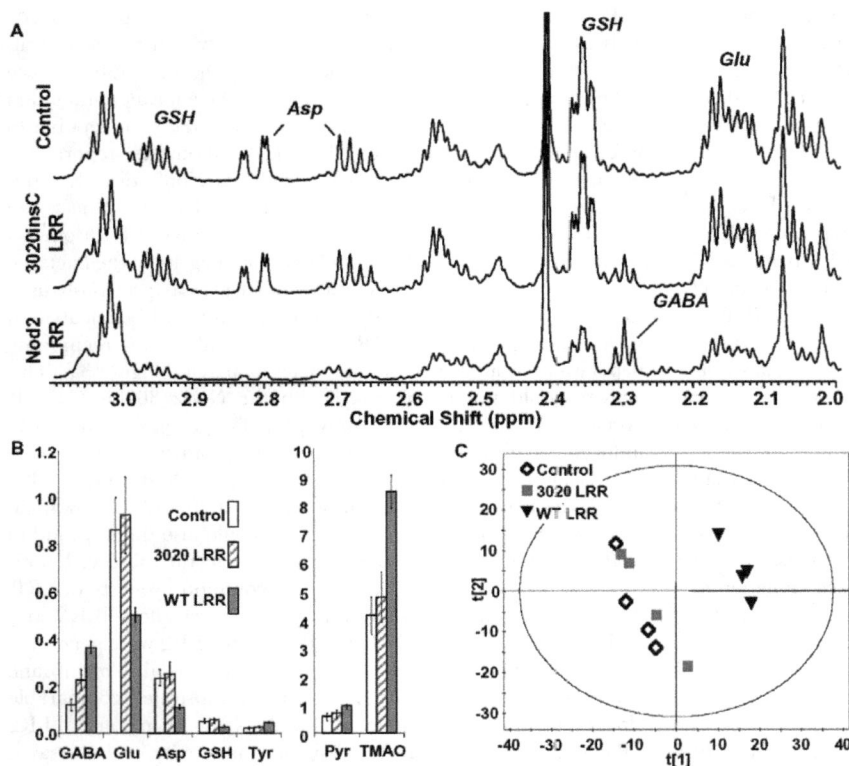

Figure 2. Nod2 LRR domains impact bacterial metabolism. A, Expansion of ^{1}H-NMR spectrum ($\delta{}^1$H 3.1 to 2.0 ppm) of cell extracts from Control (BSA treated), Nod2 LRR and Nod2 3020insC LRR domains as indicated. **B**, Metabolic perturbation induced by Nod2 LRR and Nod2 3020incC LRR treatment in *E. Coli*. GABA; γ-aminobutyrate, Glu; glutamate, Asp; aspartate, GSH; glutathione, Tyr; tyrosine, Pyr; pyruvate, TMAO; trimethylamine oxide. All metabolite changes indicated with Nod2 LRR were statistically significant versus control *E.coli* ($p < 0.05$, Student's T-test). The data are summarised in Table S1. **C**, Principle component analysis (PCA) score plot of *E.coli* metabolism treated as indicated with LRR domains from Nod2, Nod2 3020insC or BSA. PCA of the NMR data was performed using SIMCA-P v.10 (Umetrics AB, Umeå, Sweden). This data reduction method allows the visualization of the effect of treatment on the cellular metabolism, the clustering of groups of data is based solely on the similarity of the input spectral data. Each symbol represents the ^{1}H-NMR spectrum of an individual cell extract. The axis, principal component 1 (t[1]) and 2 (t[2]), represent the top two most abundant correlated variation within the data set. The separation of the WT LRR from the Control and 3020incC LRR cells is due to specific perturbations in cellular metabolism.

3020insC mutation. On a weight basis, Nod1 and Nod2 efficacy was comparable with a standard broad-range antibiotic (Ciprofloxacin). On a molar basis, Nod1 and Nod2 were potent against the majority of anaerobic bacteria tested with Nod2 LRR MICs ranging from approximately 30 nM (*P. anaerobius*) to 4 μM (*B. thetaiotamicron*). This establishes the Nod proteins as among the most potent endogenous anti-microbial peptides yet identified [15].

Discussion

These results have major implications for the pathogenesis of Crohn's disease. The compromised anti-bacterial activity demonstrated by the Crohn's-associated LRR domains should be considered alongside the signalling properties of the protein in any model of the molecular mechanisms associated with Nod2's role in Crohn's disease. Normal physiological events such as stress are associated with the onset of relapse in IBD patients and have been demonstrated to increase epithelial barrier permeability resulting in elevated levels of intracellular bacteria in normal animals [16],[17]. Breech of the epithelial barrier by bacteria would necessitate a response by the host to the invading microbe and Nod2 has a recognised role in coordinating innate immune responses to intracellular bacteria. In the context of Nod2 SNPs,

the data presented would support the hypothesis that initial recognition and potential lysis of the intracellular bacteria by Nod2 is deficient in genetically defined patient populations. It is conceivable that this could lead to persistent infection of the host by the bacteria. A robust immune response would then be initiated by redundant bacterial-sensing pathways in the host to contain and deal with the infection. This could account for the relapsing, remitting and focal character of the inflammation observed in Crohn's disease patients. Inflammatory responses are essential to maintaining a barrier between the host and its environment. The direct recognition of bacteria by Nod2 likely triggers a cellular inflammatory response to breech of host defences by potential pathogens. While polymorphisms in the Nod2 LRR domains confer sensitivity to developing Crohn's disease, mutations in the Nod2 NACHT domain are associated with other inflammatory disorders, such as Early-Onset Sarcoidosis and Blau syndromes [18],[19]. This leads us to speculate that the Nod2 Nacht domain mutations may mimic in part an association of the protein with bacteria resulting in an elevated basal cellular anti-bacterial signaling response (in the absence of a bacterial infection). The Nod2 Nacht domain mutations are associated with eye, joint and skin, but not intestinal inflammation whereas the Crohn's-associated LRR domain polymorphisms are generally associated with intestinal, but not with extraintestinal, manifestations. Our

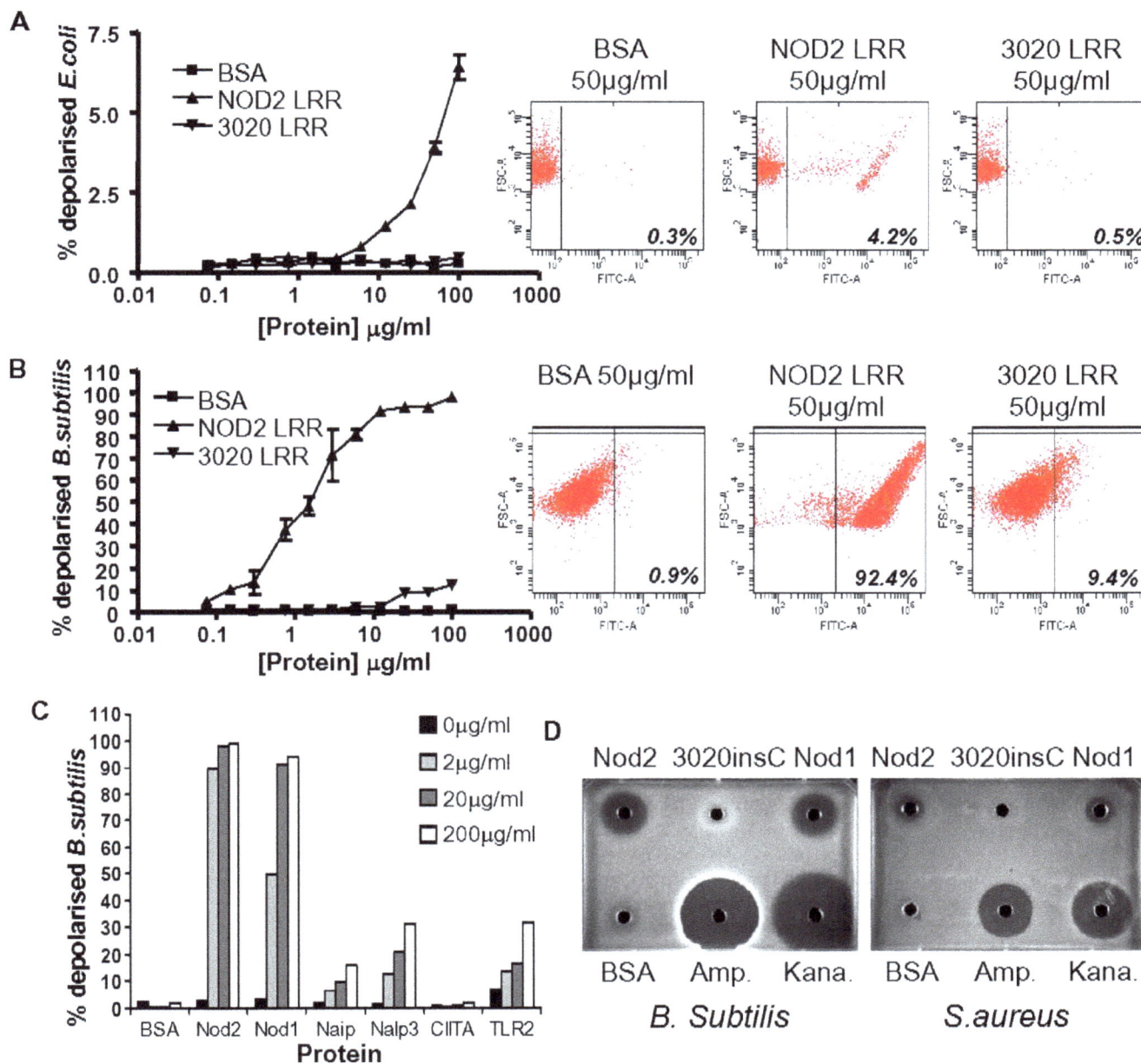

Figure 3. Bacterial killing by purified Nod2 LRR domains is deficient in the Crohn's-associated Nod2 3020insC mutant. Results shown are all representative of several experiments. **A,B**, Nod2 LRR domains influence the membrane polarity of *E.coli* and *B.subtilis*. Proteins were added at the concentration indicated to 5×10^5 bacteria in 100 µL growth medium and incubated for 2 hours at 37°C. 15 minutes prior to the end of the time course, 50 µl of 10 µg/ml DiBAC4 solution was added to each well. Plates were washed twice with 750 µl ice cold PBS/well. The percentage of depolarised bacteria taking up the dye was determined by flow cytometry. **C**, Anti-bacterial activity of Nod1 and Nod2 but not Nod2 3020insC LRR domains demonstrated by agar diffusion assay. Agar plates were inoculated with a lawn of the indicated bacteria. Approximately 0.5 cm diameter holes were punched into the agar with a sterile glass pipette and the indicated protein (BSA protein control or indicated LRR domain) or antibiotic (ampicillin or kanamycin) added to each well at a concentration of 0.5 mg/ml in sterile PBS. **D**, *B. subtilis* membrane polarity is influenced by the LRR domains from a range of pattern-recognition receptors. Bacteria were treated with the indicated LRR domains as described for Figure 3a and their effect on the membrane polarity of the bacteria evaluated.

data suggest that this may be due to a functional anti-bacterial LRR domain in the Nacht domain mutants suppressing any initiating bacterial infection in the gut that might lead to a Crohn's-like phenotype.

The discovery of a direct anti-microbial activity for Nod2 and Nod1 offers an explanation for the protection against bacterial infection conferred by expression of these proteins in cell lines and

is consistent with the increased sensitivity of Nod2 knockout mice to *Mycobacteria*, *Listeria* and *Salmonella* infection [10]–[13], [20]. These data also have implications for infectious diseases associated with other LRR domain-containing proteins. Using *B. subtilis* as a model organism, we observed anti-bacterial activity using LRR domains derived from Nalp3, NAIP and TLR2 indicating that the LRR domain is a common anti-bacterial motif. Significant effects

Table 1. LRR domain anti-bacterial activity against anaerobes.

	Nod1 LRR	Nod2 LRR	3020insC LRR	Ciprofloxacin
B.fragilis	16-32 (4)	4-32 (5)	>128 (3)	8 (2)
B.thetaiotamicron	64-128 (3)	32-128 (4)	>128 (3)	64 (1)
F.nucleatum	16-64 (2)	8->128 (3)	>128 (2)	2 (1)
P.intermedia	8 (1)	4-8 (2)	>128 (1)	1 (1)
E.lentum	16 (1)	8-16 (2)	>128 (1)	2 (1)
C.perfringens	16-32 (3)	4-32 (4)	>128 (3)	2 (2)
C.difficile*	16-32 (3)	4-32 (5)	128->128 (3)	8 (3)
P.anaerobius	2 (1)	´-2 (2)	>128 (1)	1 (1)
P.acnes	8 (1)	4-8 (2)	>128 (1)	1 (1)

Minimal Inhibitory Concentrations µg/ml [lowest – highest (n)],
*data is composite of testing against three different strains.

on *Listeria monocytogenes* were also observed with Nalp3 and TLR2 LRR domains using an ATP-based assay supporting this conclusion (Figure S4). Distinct categories of bacteria demonstrated sensitivity to different LRR domains suggesting that the LRR domains of individual PRRs have evolved to provide resistance to potential infection by specific pathogens. While many bacteria may be targeted directly by the LRR domains of the proteins that were tested, obvious candidates for future investigation are *Mycobacteria* for Nod2, *Legionella pneumophila* for NAIP and *Mycobacterium leprae* for TLR2 due to the evidence associating these proteins with susceptibility to infection in cells, animal models and their genetic links with patient populations [13],[21]–[26]. Nod2 deficiency in mice is associated with susceptibility to *Mycobacterial* infection [13]; a genus we did not consider in our study but one that has been debated as a candidate pathogen for Crohn's disease [27]–[29]. Nod2 SNPs associated with *Mycobacterial* infections are in general distinct from those observed in Crohn's disease or the Crohn's disease SNPs confer protection against *Mycobacterial*-dependent diseases [23],[24]. In addition, the Nod2-activating muramyl dipeptide motif in the bacterial proteoglycan coat is absent in *Mycobacteria*, although this does not preclude interaction of Nod2 with other PAMPs present on *Mycobacteria* [25]. Other SNPs identified in the leprosy, tuberculosis and Crohn's-susceptibility studies have identified common genes including IRGM, LRRK2 and TNFSF15 suggesting that a theme of host microbial defence underlies the pathogenesis of these diseases [23],[24],[30],[31].

Leucine-rich repeats are a conserved domain used in PRRs in most organisms and direct anti-bacterial activity may also play a significant role in innate defence against pathogens in plants via the R proteins [32]. Furthermore, agnathan fish possess an adaptive immune system based entirely on clonal rearrangement of LRRs rather than immunoglobulins and the resulting LRR domains demonstrate specificity for individual strains of bacteria [33]–[36]. Our data would predict that at least some of these LRR domains confer resistance to bacterial (and other microorganisms) infection by direct interaction and termination of the pathogen. This potential may underlie the conserved evolutionary development of the LRR domain as a PRR-associated motif.

In conclusion, our study has revealed a previously unappreciated anti-microbial activity for the LRR domains in a range of PRRs. Indeed, the clear association of Nod2 polymorphisms with defective bacterial killing suggests this function could significantly underlie the contribution of commensal flora to the pathogenesis

of Crohn's disease. In addition, the direct anti-microbial effects demonstrated with other LRR domains suggest that direct recognition and termination of pathogens underlies the association of PRRs with susceptibility to infectious diseases and offers a rationale for PRR links with the development of autoimmune diseases. Efforts are now required to understand the role of Nod2 anti-microbial activity *in vivo* and reconcile this with known inflammatory signalling pathways.

Materials and Methods

DNA cloning

The LRR domains of Nod1, Nod2 and Nod2 3020insC, Nalp3, NAIP, CIITA and TLR2 were generated by PCR using primers flanking the LRR domain. The PCR fragments encompassed nucleotides 2275 to 3124 of Nod2 (NM_022162), nt2165 to nt3286 of Nod1 (NM_006092), nt2856 to nt3857 of Nalp3 (NM_004895), nt3692 to nt4930 of NAIP (NM_004536), nt2204 to nt3526 of CIITA (NM_000246) and nt58 to nt1983 of TLR2 (NM_003264). The integrity of all inserted fragments were confirmed by DNA sequencing.

Protein purification

The LRR domains of Nod1, Nod2 and Nod2 3020insC, Nalp3, NAIP, CIITA and TLR2 were cloned in pDEST17 (Invitrogen) expressed in *Escherichia coli* Rossetta (DE3) cells (Novagen) and purified from inclusion bodies. The bacteria pellet were solubilized using Guanidine-HCl 6M and affinity purified by chromatography on a Ni–NTA column. Protein refolding was performed by a fast 10 fold dilution in PBS. A final purification step was performed using a HiLoad 16/60 Superdex 200 size-exclusion column. Purified proteins were visualized by Coomassie blue staining. The LRR domains were generally unstable, aggregated and demonstrated significant degradation upon storage. Nevertheless, comparable antibacterial activity was consistently demonstrated with over 20 individual protein preps.

Antibodies

Anti-Nod2 rabbit antisera recognising recombinant human LRR domains purified from bacteria were generated by Eurogentec. Antibodies recognising the antigen were purified from the serum using a Nod2 LRR domain protein column and passed through a bacterial affinity column (Pierce) to remove contaminating anti-bacterial antibodies.

In vitro anti-microbial assays

Bacterial viability was evaluated by standard MIC assay protocol in accordance with NCCLS standards [37]. The BacTiter-Glo microbial assay (Promega) was performed following the manufacturers instruction. Bacterial membrane depolarisation was assessed using a variation of the procedure previously described by Nuding and colleagues [14]. Agar diffusion assay was performed by placing purified protein in a well constructed in an agar plate containing an inoculated lawn of bacteria.

High-resolution 1H-NMR

Cells were extracted with methanol/chloroform/water (1:1:0.9) as previously described [38]. High-resolution ^{1}H-NMR spectra were acquired using standard pulse sequences at 300 ± 1 K using a Bruker-600 Avance spectrometer (^{1}H frequency of 600.26 MHz). ^{1}H-NMR spectra were acquired with 256 FIDs, 65,536 complex data points, a spectral width of 7.2 kHz, and a relaxation delay of 1 s. Metabolite assignments were made on the basis of previous reported data and in certain cases confirmed by spiking [39].

Supporting Information

Figure S1   Nod2 localisation of endogenous protein in SW480 intestinal epithelial cells in response to bacteria. SW480 cells were inoculated with *E.coli* (ATCC 25922) at an MOI of 1000:1 as indicated and incubated for 2 hours. Cells were examined by immunofluorescence with αNod2 polyclonal antibody (generated and affinity purified as described in Figure 1) or rabbit IgG (processed over *E.coli* affinity column to remove *E.coli* interacting antibodies), FITC-conjugated phalloidin to detect actin and stained with DAPI to detect DNA (nucleii and bacterial DNA). Nod2 is distributed at low levels throughout the cytoplasm of unstimulated cells and colocalizes with intracellular bacteria following incubation with *E.coli*.

Figure S2   Immunofluorescent detection of recombinant Nod2 LRR domains with *E.faecalis*. Bacteria were incubated with either BSA (left panel) or Nod2 LRR domains (35 μg/ml; centre and right panels). Bacteria were processed and analysed using either anti-Nod2 antibody (left and centre panels) or without primary antibody (right panel) as controls. Insets demonstrate the presence of bacteria following staining with fluorescent membrane dye in each of the images. Bar = 50 μm.

Figure S3   Bacterial aggregation following incubation with recombinant Nod2 LRR domains. Bacteria were incubated overnight with 1 mg/ml (a,c,e) or 20 μg/ml (g) of BSA or equal concentrations of purified Nod2 LRR domains (b,d,f,h). a–f, Treated bacteria were incubated with membrane dye to help visualisation. Each sample was mixed by vortexing, a sample placed on a coverslip and observed by fluorescent microscopy. a,b, *Staphylococcus aureus*, c,d, *Streptococcus pneumoniae*, e,f, *Enterococcus faecalis*. g–h, *E.coli* were incubated as described above and visualised by phase microscopy.

Figure S4   TLR2 and Nalp3 LRR domains inhibit *L.monocytogenes* viability as demonstrated by ATP-coupled luminescent assay. *L.monocytogenes* (5×10^5 bacteria/100 μl) were incubated with increasing concentrations of the indicated recombinant LRR domains for 6 hours at 37°C and ATP levels assessed by luminescent assay (BacTiter-glo: Promega). Values shown are relative to controls incubated in the absence of LRR domains (100%). Results are representative of two experiments for TLR2 and Nalp3. Recombinant LRR domains derived from CIITA and NAIP showed no activity in a single assay up to 50 μg/ml.

Table S1   Metabolite levels in treated *E. coli* (μmol/mg dry wt).

Table S2   LRR anti-bacterial activity against aerobic bacteria.

Acknowledgments

The authors acknowledge the Mucosal Biology Group and the Gastrointestinal Disease Area of NIBR, especially the support of Alyson Fox for this project. In addition we thank Jeff Porter, Susanne Szabo, Andreas Katopodis, Helmut Sparrer, Jennifer Leeds and Mark Fishman for stimulating discussions.

Author Contributions

Conceived and designed the experiments: JDF NR SJP. Performed the experiments: LHP MB TC JDF JG SP AR KS. Analyzed the data: LHP MB TC JDF JG SP AR NR KS PS SJP. Contributed reagents/materials/analysis tools: LHP MB JDF JG NR PS. Wrote the paper: SJP.

References

1. Baumgart DC, Sandborn WJ (2007) Inflammatory bowel disease: clinical aspects and established and evolving therapies. Lancet 369: 1641–1657.
2. Cho J (2008) The genetics and immunopathogenesis of inflammatory bowel disease. Nat Rev Immunol 8: 458–66.
3. Darfeuille-Michaud A, Boudeau J, Bulois P, Neut C, Glasser A-L, et al. (2004) High prevalence of adherent-invasive *Escherichia coli* associated with ileal mucosa in Crohn's disease. Gastroenterology 127: 412–421.
4. Baumgart DC, Carding SR (2007) Inflammatory bowel disease: cause and immunobiology. Lancet 369: 1627–1640.
5. Hugot JP, Laurent-Puig P, Gower-Rousseau C, Olson JM, Lee JC, et al. (1996) Mapping of a susceptibility locus for Crohn's disease on chromosome 16. Nature 379: 821–823.
6. Hugot JP, Chamaillard M, Zouali H, Lesage S, Cézard JP, et al. (2001) Association of NOD2 leucine-rich repeat variants with susceptibility to Crohn's disease. Nature 411: 599–603.
7. Pineton de Chambrun G, Colombel JF, Poulain D, Darfeuille-Michaud A (2008) Pathogenic agents in inflammatory bowel diseases. Curr Opin Gastroenterol 24: 440–447.
8. Ferguson GP, Booth IR (1998) Importance of glutathione for growth and survival of *Escherichia coli* cells: Detoxification of methylglyoxal and maintenance of intracellular K$^+$. J Bacteriol 180: 4314–4318.
9. Bearson S, Bearson B, Foster JS (1997) Acid stress responses in enterobacteria. FEMS Microbiol Lett 147: 173–180.
10. Hisamatsu T, Suzuki M, Reinecker HC, Nadeau WJ, McCormick BA, et al. (2003) CARD15/NOD2 functions as an anti-bacterial factor in human intestinal epithelial cells. Gastroenterology 124: 993–1000.
11. Kobayashi KS, Chamaillard M, Ogura Y, Henegariu O, Inohara N, et al. (2005) Nod2-dependent regulation of innate and adaptive immunity in the intestinal tract. Science 307: 731–734.
12. Meinzer U, Esmiol-Welterlin S, Barreau F, Berrebi D, Dussaillant M, et al. (2008) Nod2 mediates susceptibility to *Yersinia pseudotuberculosis* in mice. PLoS One 3: e2769.
13. Divangahi M, Mostowy S, Coulombe F, Kozak R, Guillot L, et al. (2008) Nod2-deficient mice have impaired resistance to *Mycobacterium tuberculosis* infection through defective innate and adaptive immunity. J Immunol 161: 7157–7165.

14. Nuding S, Fellerman K, Wehkamp J, Mueller HA, Stange EF (2005) A flow cytometric assay to monitor anti-microbial activity of defensins and cationic tissue extracts. J Microbiol Methods 65: 335–345.

15. Zasloff M (2002) Anti-microbial peptides of multicellular organisms. Nature 415: 389–395.

16. Gareau MG, Silva MA, Perdue MH (2008) Pathophysiological mechanisms of stress-induced intestinal damage. Current Molecular Medicine 8: 274–281.

17. Cameron HL, Perdue MH (2005) Stress impairs murine intestinal barrier function: improvement by Glucagon-like peptide-2. J Pharmacol Exp Ther 314: 214–220.

18. Miceli-Richard C, Lesage S, Rybojad M, Prieur A-M, Manouvrier-Hanu S, et al. (2001) CARD15 mutations in Blau syndrome. Nature Genet 29: 19–20.

19. Kanazawa N, Okafuji I, Kambe N, Nishikomori R, Nakata-Hizume M, et al. (2005) Early-onset sarcoidosis and CARD15 mutations with constitutive nuclear factor-kappa-B activation: common genetic etiology with Blau syndrome. Blood 105: 1195–1197.

20. Travassos LH, Carneiro LA, Girardin SE, Boneca IG, Lemos R, et al. (2005) Nod1 participates in the innate immune response to *Pseudomonas aeruginosa*. J Biol Chem 280: 36714–36718.

21. Vinzing M, Eitel J, Lippmann J, Hocke AC, Zahlten J, et al. (2008) NAIP and Ipaf control *Legionella pneumophila* replication in human cells. J Immunol 180: 6808–15.

22. Scharf JM, Damron D, Frisella A, Bruno S, Beggs AH, et al. (1996) The mouse region syntenic for human spinal muscular atrophy lies within the Lgn1 critical interval and contains multiple copies of Naip exon 5. Genomics 38: 405–17.

23. Austin CM, Ma X, Graviss EA (2008) Common nonsynonymous polymorphisms in the NOD2 Gene are associated with resistance or susceptibility to Tuberculosis disease in African Americans. J Infect Dis 197: 1713–1716.

24. Zhang FR, Huang W, Chen SM, Sun LD, Liu H, et al. (2009) Genomewide association study of Leprosy. N Engl J Med 361: 2609–2618.

25. Ferwerda G, Kullberg BJ, de Jong DJ, Girardin SE, Langenberg DML, et al. (2007) *Mycobacterium paratuberculosis* is recognized by toll-like receptors and Nod2. J Leuk Bio 82: 1011–1018.

26. Bochud P-Y, Hawn TR, Aderem A (2003) A Toll-like receptor 2 polymorphism that is associated with lepromatous leprosy is unable to mediate mycobacterial signaling. J Immun 170: 3451–3454.

27. Pierce ES (2009) Where are all the *Mycobacterium avium* subspecies *paratuberculosis* in patients with Crohn's disease? PLoS Pathog 5: e1000234.

28. Nasser SA (2005) Mycobacterium in Crohn's disease is hard to digest. Gastroenterology 129: 1359–61.

29. Sechi, LA, Scanu AM, Molicotti P, Cannas S, Mura M, et al. (2005) Detection and isolation of Mycobacterium avium subspecies paratuberculosis from intestinal mucosal biopsies of patients with and without Crohn's disease in Sardinia. Am J Gastroenterol 100: 1537–8.

30. Lees CW, Satsangi J (2009) Genetics of inflammatory bowel disease: implications for disease pathogenesis and natural history. Expert Rev Gastroenterol Hepatol 3: 513–534.

31. Intemann CD, Thye T, Niemann S, Browne EN, Chinbuah M, et al. (2009) Autophagy gene variant IRGM -261T contributes to protection from tuberculosis caused by *Mycobacterium tuberculosis* but not by *M. Africanum* strains. PLoS Pathog 5: e1000577.

32. DeYoung BJ, Innes RW (2006) Plant NBS-LRR proteins in pathogen sensing and host defense. Nature Immunology 7: 1243–1249.

33. Herrin BR, Alder MN, Roux KH, Sina C, Ehrhardt GRA, et al. (2008) Structure and specificity of lamprey monoclonal antibodies. Proc Natl Acad Sci USA 105: 2040–2045.

34. Pancer Z, Amemiya CT, Ehrhardt GRA, Ceitlin J, Gartland GL, et al. (2004) Somatic diversification of variable lymphocyte receptors in the agnathan sea lamprey. Nature 430: 174–180.

35. Alder MN, Rogozin IB, Iyer LM, Glazko GV, Cooper MD, et al. (2005) Diversity and function of adaptive immune receptors in a jawless vertebrate. Science 310: 1970–1973.

36. Nagawa F, Kishishita N, Shimizu K, Hirose S, Miyoshi M, et al. (2007) Antigen-receptor genes of the agnathan lamprey are assembled by a process involving copy choice. Nature Immunology 8: 206–213.

37. National committee for Clinical Laboratory Standards. Methods for dilution anti-microbial susceptibility tests for bacteria that grow aerobically; Approved standard ã sixth edition. NCCLS document M7-A6, NCCLS, Wayne, PA.

38. Lin CY, Wu H, Tjeerdema RS, Viant MR (2007) Evaluation of metabolite extraction strategies from tissue samples using NMR metabolomics. Metabolomics 3: 55–67.

39. Fan TW (1996) Metabolite profiling by one- and two-dimensional NMR analysis of complex mixtures. Progress in Nuclear Magnetic Resonance Spectroscopy 28: 161–219.

15

Prevalence of *Campylobacter* Species in Adult Crohn's Disease and the Preferential Colonization Sites of *Campylobacter* Species in the Human Intestine

Vikneswari Mahendran[1], Stephen M. Riordan[2,3], Michael C. Grimm[4], Thi Anh Tuyet Tran[1], Joelene Major[1], Nadeem O. Kaakoush[1], Hazel Mitchell[1], Li Zhang[1]*

1 School of Biotechnology and Biomolecular Sciences, University of New South Wales, Sydney, Australia, 2 Gastrointestinal and Liver Unit, The Prince of Wales Hospital, Sydney, Australia, 3 Faculty of Medicine, University of New South Wales, Sydney, Australia, 4 St George Clinical School, University of New South Wales, Sydney, Australia

Abstract

Introduction: Crohn's disease (CD) and ulcerative colitis (UC) are the two major forms of inflammatory bowel disease (IBD). A high prevalence of *Campylobacter concisus* was previously detected in paediatric CD and adult UC. Currently, the prevalence of *C. concisus* in adult CD and the preferential colonization sites of *Campylobacter* species in the human intestine are unknown. In this study, we examined the prevalence of *Campylobacter* species in biopsies collected from multiple anatomic sites of adult patients with IBD and controls.

Methods: Three hundred and one biopsies collected from ileum, caecum, descending colon and rectum of 28 patients IBD (15 CD and 13 UC) and 33 controls were studied. Biopsies were used for DNA extraction and detection of *Campylobacter* species by PCR-sequencing and *Campylobacter* cultivation.

Results: A significantly higher prevalence of *C. concisus* in colonic biopsies of patients with CD (53%) was detected as compared with the controls (18%). *Campylobacter* genus-PCR positivity and *C. concisus* positivity in patients with UC were 85% and 77% respectively, being significantly higher than that in the controls (48% and 36%). *C. concisus* was more often detected in descending colonic and rectal biopsies from patients with IBD in comparison to the controls. *C. concisus* was isolated from patients with IBD.

Conclusion: The high intestinal prevalence of *C. concisus* in patients with IBD, particularly in the proximal large intestine, suggests that future studies are needed to investigate the possible involvement of *C. concisus* in a subgroup of human IBD. To our knowledge, this is the first report of the association between adult CD and *C. concisus* as well as the first study of the preferential colonization sites of *C. concisus* in the human intestine.

Editor: Markus M. Heimesaat, Charité, Campus Benjamin Franklin, Germany

Funding: This work was supported by the Broad Medical Research Program of the Broad Foundation (Grant No: IBD0273-R). The funders had no role in study design, data collection and analysis, decision to publish, or preparation of the manuscript.

Competing Interests: The authors have declared that no competing interests exist.

* E-mail: L.Zhang@unsw.edu.au

Introduction

Campylobacter species have been associated with various diseases in both animals and humans [1]. *Campylobacter jejuni* and *Campylobacter coli* are well established human pathogens, having been associated with a number of clinical conditions such as diarrhoea, abortion, septicaemia and Guillain-Barre syndrome [1]. Some other *Campylobacter* species including *Campylobacter concisus* have been considered as emerging human pathogens [2].

C. concisus is a curved Gram negative bacterium; with a single polar flagellum [3]. *C. concisus* was first isolated by Tanner *et al* in 1981 from human dental plague [4]. In a following-up study, Macuch and Tanner reported a higher isolation rate of *C. concisus* in patients at the initial stage of periodontitis in comparison to individuals with healthy gums [5].

Lately, *C. concisus* has been considered as an emerging human enteric pathogen [6]. Evidence that *C. concisus* may be an important human enteric pathogen has come from a number of recent studies reported that *C. jejuni* and *C. concisus* are the most commonly isolated *Campylobacter* species from diarrheal stool specimens [2,7,8,9]. However, when Engberg *et al* compared the prevalence of *C. concisus* in 107 stool samples subjected to tests for enteric pathogens and in 107 age/sex matched healthy controls, they found that the prevalence of *C. concisus* in these two groups was not significantly different [9]. Furthermore, they found that *C. concisus* was more often isolated from children aged 0–9 years and individuals aged over 60 years as compared with other age groups. These results have led Engberg *et al* to conclude that *C. concisus* should be considered as a commensal bacterium and this bacterium may be an important opportunistic pathogen in individuals with compromised or immature immune systems [9].

In addition to periodontal and diarrheal diseases, recently *C. concisus* has been linked to inflammatory bowel disease (IBD). IBD is a chronic inflammatory condition of the gastrointestinal tract, with the two major forms being Crohn's disease (CD) and ulcerative colitis (UC). The inflammation in CD may occur anywhere along the gastrointestinal tract, however in UC the inflammation often occurs in colon and rectum [10]. The aetiology of IBD is currently unknown. It is understood that a complex interaction of a number of factors including host genetics, environment, immune system and intestinal microflora contributes to the development of IBD [10,11,12]. Despite strong evidence that the intestinal microbial flora plays a key role in the development of IBD, the exact causative agent (s) is still under investigation [11].

Previously, we detected a significantly higher prevalence of *C. concisus* by PCR in intestinal biopsies of children with CD (51%) as compared with the controls (2%) and isolated a *C. concisus* strain from intestinal biopsies of a child with CD [13]. In a later study, we detected high prevalence of *C. concisus* in stool samples of children with CD [14]. A recent study by Mukhopadhya *et al* reported a significantly higher prevalence of *C. concisus* detected by PCR in adult patients with UC as compared with the controls [15].

To date, the prevalence of *C. concisus* in adult patients with CD has not been investigated. Furthermore, no information is available regarding whether *Campylobacter* species preferentially colonize specific sites in the human intestine. In this study, we examined the prevalence of *Campylobacter* species in biopsies collected from four anatomic sites of intestines from adult individuals with normal intestinal histology and patients with IBD by PCR-sequencing and *Campylobacter* cultivation.

Materials and Methods

Ethics statement

Intestinal biopsies were obtained from colonoscopy procedures carried out at the Prince of Wales Hospital and the St George Hospital at Sydney, Australia. Ethics approval for this study was granted by the Ethics Committees of the University of New South Wales and the South East Sydney Area Health Service, Australia (HREC 09237/SESIAHS 09/078 and HREC08335/SESIAHS (CHN)07/48). Written informed consent was obtained from all subjects in this study.

Study subjects and biopsy collection

Sixty-one study subjects, including 28 patients with IBD and 33 controls, were recruited from the Prince of Wales Hospital and the St George Hospital at Sydney, Australia. Among the 28 patients with IBD (15 CD and 13 UC), ten patients (six CD and four UC) were relapsed cases and the remaining eighteen patients were newly diagnosed IBD. Disease location and severity were scored according to the Montreal criteria [16]. The controls, either presenting with gastrointestinal symptoms including abdominal pain and constipation or undertaking a screening colonoscopic examination due to previous history of polyps or a family history of colonic cancer, had no macroscopic or microscopic intestinal inflammation.

Five biopsies were collected from each individual. In the case where macroscopic inflammation was present, biopsies were taken from the edge of the inflamed areas. Of the five biopsies collected from each individual, four biopsies collected from each of the four anatomic sites (ileum, caecum, descending colon and rectum respectively) were used for DNA extraction and detection of *Campylobacter* species by PCR. The additional biopsy collected from caecum was used for *Campylobacter* cultivation.

DNA extraction from intestinal biopsies

Freshly collected intestinal biopsies were directly placed into cell lysis solution and DNA was extracted using the Puregene DNA Extraction kit (Gentra, Minneapolis, USA) according to the manufacturer's instructions.

Detection of *Campylobacter* species in intestinal biopsies by *Campylobacter* genus-PCR

To detect all *Campylobacter* species, DNA extracted from intestinal biopsies were subjected to a nested *Campylobacter* genus-PCR. Bacterial 16S rRNA gene was first amplified from 200 ng of DNA extracted from intestinal biopsies using universal primers F27 and R1496 [17]. The thermal cycling conditions were 94°C for 10 minutes, followed by 35 cycles of 94°C for 10 seconds, 53°C for 10 seconds and 72°C for 1 minute. The PCR reaction volume was 25 µl. The PCR product was then purified using QIAquick PCR purification kit (Qiagen, Hilden, Germany). The purified PCR product (2 µl) was subjected to a *Campylobacter* genus-specific PCR using primers C418 and C1228 designed by Linton *et al* [18]. The thermal cycling conditions for the *Campylobacter* genus-specific PCR were 94°C for 5 minutes, followed by 35 cycles of 94°C for 30 seconds, 55°C for 30 seconds and 72°C for 30 seconds.

Campylobacter species identification

All positive PCR products were sequenced using the BigDyeTM terminator chemistry (Applied Biosystems, Foster City, USA) and the sequencing mixture was analysed on DNA sequence analyser ABI3720 (Applied Biosystems, Foster City, USA). The obtained sequences were compared to gene sequences of known bacterial identities available in GenBank through the National Centre for Biotechonology Information (NCBI website (http://www.ncbi.nlm.nih.gov).

C. concisus specific PCR

Three samples which had mixed sequences in the *Campylobacter* genus-PCR were subjected to a previously described *C. concisus* PCR to examine if *C. concisus* was present [14]. For the *C. concisus* PCR, DNA (50 ng) extracted from biopsies was subjected to the *Campylobacter* genus-PCR, then 1 µl of the *Campylobacter* genus-PCR product was subjected to *C. concisus* PCR as previously described [14].

Cultivation of *Campylobacter* species from intestinal biopsies

One caecal biopsy collected from each individual was subjected to *Campylobacter* cultivation. The biopsy was spread on agar plates prepared using blood agar base no 2 supplemented with 6% sterile defibrinated horse blood, trimethoprim (10 µg/ml), and vancomycin (10 µg/ml). The plates were incubated under microaerophilic conditions generated by a *Campylobacter* gas generating system (Oxoid Limited, Hampshire, United Kingdom) for two days. A bacterial suspension was prepared from the culture plates and filtered through a 0.6 µM filter membrane (Millipore, Billerica, USA) onto a fresh agar plate and further incubated for additional two days.

Candidate colonies were subjected to microscopic examination of morphology, Gram staining, PCR targeting the 16S rRNA gene using primers F27 and R1649 and sequencing of the PCR products.

GenBank Sequence Submission

All 16S rRNA gene sequences of the PCR products were submitted to GenBank.

Statistical analysis

Fisher's exact test (two tailed) was used to compare the prevalence of *Campylobacter* species in patients with IBD and controls. Unpaired *t* test was used to compare the age of patients and controls. Statistical analysis was performed using GraphPad Prism 5 software (San Diego, CA).

Results

Clinical information of patients and controls

The average age of the patients with IBD and controls was 39 ± 13 and 45 ± 11 years old respectively. There were 12 male (43%) patients with IBD and 13 male in controls (39%). The age and sex between patients with IBD and controls were not statistically different.

A total of 301 biopsies (165 biopsies from 33 controls and 136 biopsies from 28 patients with IBD) were collected from four intestinal sites (ileum, caecum, descending colon and rectum) of patients with IBD and controls. Ileal biopsies were not available from two patients with CD, a caecal biopsy was not available from one patient with CD and a rectal biopsy was not available from an additional patient with CD. Both patients and controls did not receive antibiotics one month prior to colonoscopy.

All controls had normal intestinal histology. The Montreal classification of patients with IBD is summarized in Table 1.

Prevalence of *Campylobacter* species in biopsies collected from different intestinal sites of individuals with normal intestinal histology

To examine the possible preferential colonization sites of *Campylobacter* species particularly *C. concisus* in the human intestine, DNA samples extracted from biopsies collected from four intestinal anatomic sites of 33 individuals with normal intestinal histology were subjected to *Campylobacter* genus-PCR. Among the 33 individuals examined, 48% (16/33) were positive for *Campylobacter* genus-PCR (an individual with at least one of the four intestinal biopsies collected from ileum, caecum, descending colon and rectum positive by the *Campylobacter* genus-PCR was considered *Campylobacter* genus-PCR positive). Of the 16 individuals who were positive by the *Campylobacter* genus-PCR, four individuals had one biopsy positive and 12 individuals had 2–4 biopsies positive by the PCR. *Campylobacter* genus-PCR positive

rate in biopsies collected from ileum, caecum, colon and rectum were 27% (9/33), 30% (10/33), 27% (9/33), rectum 27% (9/33) respectively, with no statistical differences observed between sites. *Campylobacter* genus-PCR positive rate in male was 42% (5/12); with no statistical difference from that in females (52%, 11/21).

Sequencing of the positive PCR products yielded 503–766 bp sequences. The obtained sequences were used for identification of *Campylobacter* species. The similarities of 16S rRNA gene sequences between the *Campylobacter* genus-PCR products and the known *Campylobacter* species were 97%–100%. Five *Campylobacter* species were identified from biopsies collected from individuals with normal intestinal histology, including *C. concisus*, *Campylobacter showae*, *Campylobacter hominis*, *Campylobacter ureolyticus* and *Campylobacter hyointestinalis*. Among the 12 individuals who had multiple biopsies positive for the *Campylobacter* genus-PCR, single *Campylobacter* species was identified in eight individuals and two *Campylobacter* species were identified in the remaining four individuals.

Among the 33 individuals examined, 36% (12/33) of individuals were positive for *C. concisus*, 6% (2/33) of individuals were positive for *C. showae*, 9% (3/33) of individuals were positive for *C. hominis*, 6% (2/33) of individuals were positive for *C. ureolyticus* and 3% (1/33) of individuals were positive for *C. hyointestinalis*. For an individual to be classified as *C. concisus* positive, *C. concisus* had to be identified in at least one of the four biopsies collected. The same principle applied for the evaluation of the intestinal prevalence of the other *Campylobacter* species in this study.

Campylobacter species detected in biopsies collected from the four intestinal anatomic sites of individuals with normal histology is shown in Table 2. Ileal, caecal and colonic biopsies showed similar *C. concisus* positive rates and the rectum had a lower *C. concisus* positive rate; however the difference was not statistically significant. Given the low positive rate for the remaining four *Campylobacter* species, no statistical analysis was applied to compare the prevalence of these *Campylobacter* species in different sites of the intestines (Table 2).

Comparison of intestinal prevalence of *Campylobacter* species in patients with IBD and controls

The above 33 individuals with normal intestinal histology were used as controls. *Campylobacter* genus-PCR positive rate in patients with IBD was 82% (23/28), which was significantly higher than that of the controls (48%, 16/33) ($P<0.05$). The *Campylobacter* genus-PCR positive rate was 80% (12/15) in patients with CD and

Table 1. Montreal classification of patients with IBD

Montreal classification (CD)	CD (n = 15)
L1	7% (1/15)
L2	60% (9/15)
L3	33% (5/15)
Montreal classification (UC)-Extent	**UC (n = 13)**
Proctitis E1	8% (1/13)
Left sided UC E2	38% (5/13)
Extensive UC E3	54% (7/13)
Montreal classification (UC)-Severity	**UC (n = 13)**
Clinical remission S0	0
Mild UC S1	54% (7/13)
Moderate UC S2	46% (6/13)
Severe UC S3	0

Table 2. Detection of *Campylobacter* species in biopsies collected from four intestinal anatomic sites of individuals (n = 33) with normal intestinal histology by *Campylobacter* genus-PCR and sequencing*.

	Ileum	Caecum	Colon	Rectum
C. concisus	21% (7/33)	18% (6/33)	18% (6/33)	9% (3/33)
C. showae	3% (1/33)	3% (1/33)	3% (1/33)	6% (2/33)
C. hominis	3% (1/33)	6% (2/33)	3% (1/33)	9% (3/33)
C. ureolyticus	0	0	3% (1/33)	3% (1/33)
C. hyointestinalis	0	3% (1/33)	0	0

*Four biopsies, one each from ileum, caecum, descending colon and rectum of each individual, were examined. Identification of *Campylobacter* species was based on 97–100% similarity of the sequences of PCR products (503–766 bp) to the sequences of known *Campylobacter* species.

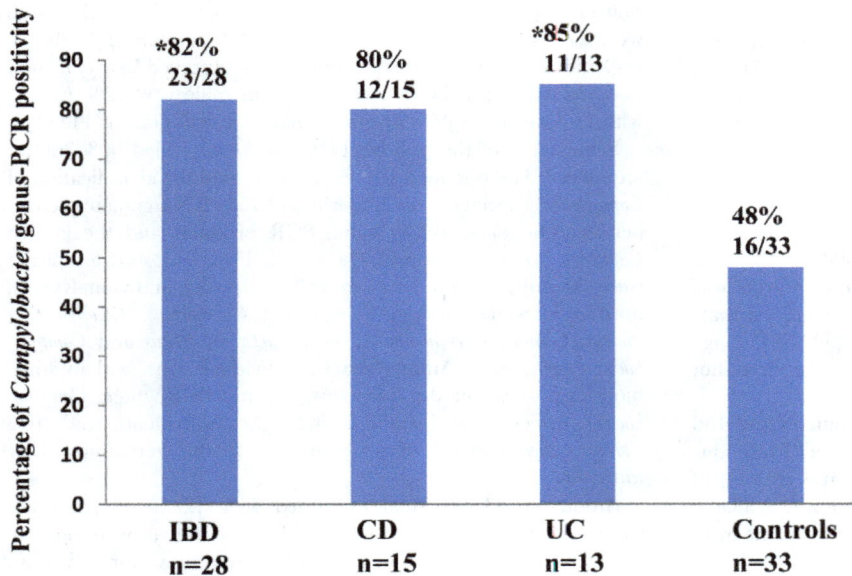

Figure 1. *Campylobacter* **genus-PCR positivity in patients with IBD (CD and UC) and controls.** Four biopsies collected from each individual were examined. A *Campylobacter* genus-PCR positive individual is an individual who had at least one intestinal biopsy positive for *Campylobacter* genus-PCR. *Significantly different as compared with the controls (*P*<0.05).

85% (11/13) in patients with UC; with the difference between UC group and the controls being statistically significant (*P*<0.05) and the difference between CD and controls being not statistically significant (Figure 1).

The prevalence of different *Campylobacter* species in patients with IBD and controls is shown in Table 3. Eight *Campylobacter* species were identified in intestinal biopsies collected from patients with IBD. *C. concisus* was detected in 68% (19/28) patients with IBD, which was significantly higher as compared with the controls 36% (12/33) (*P*<0.05). The *C. concisus* positive rates in patients with CD and UC were 67% (10/15) and 69% (9/13) respectively; the *C. concisus* positive rate between UC and controls was statistically different (*P*<0.05) and the difference between CD and the controls was not significantly different. The prevalence of the remaining seven *Campylobacter* species in patients with IBD and controls was not statistically different (Table 3).

The *C. concisus* positive rate in relapsed CD was 67% (4/6), which was not significantly different as compared with the newly diagnosed CD cases (67%, 6/9). The *C. concisus* positive rate in relapsed UC was 75% (3/4), which was not significantly different from that of the new cases (67%, 6/9).

Of the three biopsies which showed mixed sequences by *Campylobacter* genus-PCR; two samples were positive and one was negative by *C. concisus* PCR.

Comparison of prevalence of *C. concisus* in biopsies collected from different anatomic intestinal sites of patients with IBD and controls

Given that *C. concisus* was the only *Campylobacter* species showing statistical difference between patients with IBD and the controls in this study (Table 3), the prevalence of *C. concisus* in biopsies collected from ileum, caecum, colon and rectum of patients with IBD and controls was further compared and the results are shown in Table 4. Ileal biopsies collected from patients with IBD and controls showed similar *C. concisus* positivity. Caecal biopsies of patients with UC had a low *C. concisus* positive rate; however it was

not statistically different from the other groups. *C. concisus* positive rate of colonic biopsies of patients with IBD was 43% (12/27), which was significantly higher compared to the controls (*P*<0.05). The *C. concisus* positivity in colonic biopsies of patients with CD and UC was 53% (8/15) and 31% (4/13) respectively; with patients with CD showing a statistically significant difference when compared to the controls (*P*<0.05). The *C. concisus* positivity in rectal biopsies of patients with IBD was higher than that of the controls; however it was not statistically different (Table 4).

Prevalence of *C. concisus* in relation to Montreal classification of IBD

No significant differences were noted between the prevalence of *C. concisus* in patients with different Montreal classifications.

Table 3. Percentage of *Campylobacter* species positivity in patients with IBD (CD and UC) and controls [@].

	IBD (n=28)	CD (n=15)	UC (n=13)	Controls (n=33)
C. concisus	68% (19/28)*	67% (10/15)	69% (9/13)*	36% (12/33)
C. showae	11% (3/28)	7% (1/15)	15% (2/13)	6% (2/33)
C. hominis	7% (2/28)	7% (1/15)	8% (1/13)	9% (3/33)
C. ureolyticus	10% (3/28)	13% (2/15)	8% (1/13)	6% (2/33)
C. hyointestinalis	4% (1/28)	7% (1/15)	0	3% (1/33)
C. rectus	4% (1/28)	0	8% (1/13)	0
C. jejuni	4% (1/28)	7% (1/15)	0	0
C. gracilis	7% (2/28)	7% (1/15)	8% (1/13)	0

@A specific Campylobacter species positive individual is an individual who has at least one biopsy positive for the Campylobacter species listed in Table 3, detected by Campylobacter genus-PCR and sequencing. *Significantly higher as compared with the controls (P<0.05).

Table 4. Detection of *C. concisus* in biopsies collected from four intestinal anatomic sites of patients with IBD (CD and UC) and controls [@].

	IBD n = 28	CD n = 15	UC n = 13	Control n = 33
Ileum	23% (6/26)	23% (3/13)	23% (3/13)	21% (7/33)
Caecum	15% (4/27)	21% (3/14)	9% (1/13)	18% (6/33)
Colon	43% (12/28)*	53% (8/15)*	31% (4/13)	18% (6/33)
Rectum	26% (7/27)	21% (3/14)	31% (4/13)	9% (3/33)

[@] Identification of C. concisus was based on Campylobacter genus-PCR and sequencing of the positive PCR products, except for three biopsy samples. The three biopsy samples showed mixed sequences by Campylobacter genus-PCR, therefore were further subjected to C. concisus PCR to examine the presence of C. concisus.
Biopsies collected from four intestinal anatomic sites were examined; ileal biopsies were not available from two patients with CD, caecal biopsy was not available from one patient with CD and rectal biopsy was not available from one patient with CD.
*Significantly higher in patients with IBD as compared with the controls (*P*<0.05).

Isolation of *C. concisus* from intestinal biopsies of patients with IBD and controls

C. concisus was isolated from intestinal biopsies of two patients with IBD, one patient with CD and one patient with UC. The identity of the *C. concisus* isolates was confirmed by bacterial morphology (small curved and spiral rods), Gram stain (Gram negative) and sequence of 1200 bp 16S rRNA gene (100% similarity to the known *C. concisus* in GenBank).

Sequences accession numbers

The accession numbers of the sequences of the PCR products submitted to GenBank were JN544934-JN545008.

Discussion

This study aimed to investigate the prevalence of *C. concisus* in adult patients with CD and the possible preferential colonization sites of *Campylobacter* species in the human intestine; by examining the presence of *Campylobacter* species in 301 intestinal biopsies collected from 28 patients with IBD and 33 controls using PCR-sequencing and *Campylobacter* cultivation.

The high positive rate of *Campylobacter* genus-PCR and intestinal prevalence of *C. concisus* in adult patients with CD and UC observed in this study are consistent with our previous findings in paediatric CD and the findings by Mukhopadhya *et al* in adult UC [13,14,15]. A further finding of this study is the increased prevalence of *C. concisus* in the proximal large intestines (descending colon and rectum) of patients with IBD as compared with the controls (Table 4). In adult patients with CD, only biopsies collected from the descending colon showed a significantly higher prevalence of *C. concisus* as compared with the controls (Table 4).

Different *Campylobacter* species may have preferable intestinal colonization sites in their hosts. For example, a study from Inglis *et al* examining the colonization of *C. jejuni* and *Campylobacter lanienae* in asymptomatic beef cattle, *C. jejuni* was found to colonize the proximal small intestine whereas *C. lanienae* was detected primarily in the caecum, descending colon and rectum [19].

In individuals without intestinal inflammation, biopsies collected from ileum, caecum, descending colon had a similar *C. concisus* positive rate and the rectal biopsies had a lower *C. concisus* positive

rate (Table 2). However, in patients with IBD, a higher prevalence of *C. concisus* in the proximal large intestine (descending colon and rectum) was detected (Table 4). It is not entirely clear why *C. concisus* was more prevalent in the proximal large intestine of patients with IBD, particularly in descending colon of patients with CD (Table 4). It is possible that this may relate to the fact that *C. concisus* requires hydrogen enriched microaerophilic atmosphere for growth [2]. In the human intestine, hydrogen is produced by bacterial flora through fermentation of unabsorbed carbohydrates; previous studies showing that 99% of hydrogen in the intestine is produced in the colon [20]. The amount of hydrogen produced in the intestine is affected by food type and intestinal bacterial composition [20,21]. It may be that the microenvironment of proximal large intestine in some individuals is more suitable for *C. concisus* growth. Whether the high prevalence of *C. concisus* in the proximal large intestine of patients with IBD is a primary event or secondary to the disease is not known. The finding in this study that the prevalence of *C. concisus* in newly diagnosed patients is similar to that of the relapsed cases suggests that the high prevalence of *C. concisus* in patients with IBD is likely a primary event.

The finding that *C. concisus* has a preferable intestinal colonization site (the proximal large intestine) in patients with IBD suggests that different bacterial species may be associated with IBD occurring at different parts of the gastrointestinal tract. Other evidence from both human and animal studies supports this view. For example, in human studies adherent and invasive *Escherichia coli* has been found to be associated with ileal CD only [22]. Furthermore, antibiotics used to treat patients with IBD were effective only in a subgroup of patients [23]. In animal studies, IL-10 −/− mice developed caecal inflammation when monoassociated with *E. coli* but distal colitis when colonized with *Enterococcus faecalis* [24].

Whether *C. concisus* detected in patients with IBD has contributed to the pathogenesis of the disease requires further investigation. *C. concisus* is a bacterium with great diversity; which has been demonstrated by various research groups using different methodologies [25,26,27,28,29]. Intestinal *C. concisus* strains have been shown to be able to induce production of IL-8 in HT-29 cells and some *C. concisus* strains were invasive to Caco2 cells [30,31]. In addition, the presence of bacterial virulence factors such as phospholipase A2 and a cytolethal distending toxin (CDT)-like toxin in some *C. concisus* strains suggest that some *C. concisus* strains may have the enteric pathogenic potential [32,33].

Examination of prevalence of *C. concisus* in patients with gum disease by Macuch and Tanner has revealed an interesting relationship between *C. concisus* and oral mucosal inflammation [5]. In their study, Macuch and Tanner found that the isolation of *C. concisus* from subgingival plaque samples of patients with initial periodontitis was greatly higher than the controls. However the isolation rate of *C. concisus* in patients with established periodontitis was greatly reduced in comparison with the healthy controls [5]. These results suggest that *C. concisus* may be only associated with mild oral mucosal inflammation. A more severe inflammatory microenvironment such as the established periodontitis is certainly no longer a favourable environment for *C. concisus*. We have observed a similar phenomenon in patients with CD. In our previous study in a paediatric population, we found that biopsies taken from macroscopic normal area near the inflamed area had higher *C. concisus* detection than biopsies taken from the centre of the severely inflamed area [13]. Patients with UC included in this study had mild to moderate disease severities (Table 1); we therefore were unable to examine the prevalence of *C. concisus* in patients with severe UC.

These data suggest that the role of *C. concisus* in the pathogenesis of IBD, if there is any, would be most likely to facilitate the establishment of the inflammation in the early stage of the disease or to promote inflammation from a mild form to a more severe form. Recently, we found that *C. concisus* has the ability to modulate the gut mucosal immune system through upregulation of the intestinal epithelial expression of Toll-like receptor (TLR)-4 (unpublished data). The low level intestinal epithelial expression of TLR-4 is one of the mechanisms allowing gut mucosal system to maintain its tolerance to commensal intestinal bacteria flora [34]. Accumulated evidence suggests that some intestinal commensal bacterial species are involved in the pathogenesis of IBD [11]. Perhaps the increased intestinal expression of TLR-4 induced by *C. concisus* has upregulated responses of the gut mucosal immune system to some intestinal commensal bacterial species otherwise it would tolerate. This hypothesis requires further investigation.

Despite the high prevalence of *C. concisus* detected in patients with IBD, the amount of *C. concisus* DNA in the intestinal biopsies was generally low. An initial examination of 20 biopsies collected from 5 patients with CD using direct *Campylobacter* genus-PCR revealed low positivity. Given this, we decided to use a nested PCR method to amplify the 16S rRNA gene of universal bacteria and then use *Campylobacter* genus-PCR. The nested PCR has greatly increased the detection rate of *Campylobacter* species in biopsy samples. It is likely that the preparation procedure for colonoscopy, which involves induction of severe diarrhoea, may have contributed to the low number of *C. concisus* in the biopsies.

In addition to detection of *C. concisus* from intestinal biopsies by PCR, we have isolated *C. concisus* from intestinal biopsies of one patient with CD and one patient with UC.

Some other *Campylobacter* species detected in this study have been shown to be clinically important. However, the prevalence of these *Campylobacter* species in patients with IBD was low and not significantly different from that in the controls (Table 3).

In summary, in this study we detected a significantly higher prevalence of *C. concisus* in colonic biopsies of adult patients with CD as compared with the controls and isolated *C. concisus* from intestinal biopsies of adult patients with IBD. Furthermore, we found that *C. concisus* preferentially colonizes the proximal large intestine of patients with IBD. These results suggest that future studies are needed to investigate the possible involvement of *C. concisus* in a subgroup of human IBD. To our knowledge, this is the first report of the association between adult CD and *C. concisus*; the first study of the preferential colonization sites of *C. concisus* in the human intestine; and the first isolation of *C. concisus* from intestinal biopsies of adult patients with IBD.

Author Contributions

Conceived and designed the experiments: LZ HM SMR MG. Performed the experiments: VM TATT JM NOK. Analyzed the data: VM LZ. Wrote the paper: LZ VM HM MG SMR NOK. Obtained biopsies and clinical data: SMR MG.

References

1. Moore JE, Corcoran D, Dooley JSG, Fanning S, Lucey B, et al. (2005) *Campylobacter.* Vet Res 36: 351–382.
2. Lastovica AJ (2006) Emerging *Campylobacter* spp.: the Tip of the Iceberg. Clin Microbiol Newsl 28: 7.
3. Vandamme P, Dewhirst FE, Paster BJ, On SLW (2005) Genus I. *Campylobacter.* In: Garrity GM, Brenner DJ, Krieg NR, Staley JT, eds. Bergey's Manual of Systematic Bacteriology. 2 ed.. New York: Springer. pp 1147–1160.
4. Tanner ACR, Badger S, Lai CH, Listgarten MA, Visconti RA, et al. (1981) *Wolinella* gen-nov, *Wolinella-succinogenes* (vibrio-succinogenes-wolinet-al) Comb-nov, and description of *Bacteruides-gracilis* sp-nov, *Wolinella-recta* sp-nov, *Campylobacter-concisus* sp-nov and *Eikenella-corrodens* from humans with periodontal-disease. Int J Syst Bacteriol 31: 432–445.
5. Macuch PJ, Tanner ACR (2000) *Campylobacter* species in health, gingivitis, and periodontitis. J Dent Res 79: 785–792.
6. Newell DG (2005) *Campylobacter concisus*: an emerging pathogen? Eur J Gastroen Hepat 17: 1013–1014.
7. Aabenhus R, On SLW, Siemer BL, Permin H, Andersen LP (2005) Delineation of *Campylobacter concisus* genomospecies by amplified fragment length polymorphism analysis and correlation of results with clinical data. J Clin Microbiol 43: 5091–5096.
8. Snijders F, Kuijper EJ, deWever B, vanderHoek L, Danner SA, et al. (1997) Prevalence of *Campylobacter*-associated diarrhea among patients infected with human immunodeficiency virus. Clin Infect Dis 24: 1107–1113.
9. Engberg J, On SLW, Harrington CS, Gerner-Smidt P (2000) Prevalence of *Campylobacter, Arcobacter, Helicobacter,* and *Sutterella* spp. in human fecal samples as estimated by a reevaluation of isolation methods for campylobacters. J Clin Microbiol 38: 286–291.
10. Podolsky DK (2002) Inflammatory bowel disease. New Engl J Med 347: 417–429.
11. Sartor RB (2008) Microbial influences in inflammatory bowel diseases. Gastroenterology 134: 577–594.
12. Fiocchi C (1998) Inflammatory bowel disease: etiology and pathogenesis. Gastroenterology 115: 182–205.
13. Zhang L, Man SM, Day AS, Leach ST, Lemberg DA, et al. (2009) Detection and isolation of *Campylobacter* species other than *C. jejuni* from children with Crohn's disease. J Clin Microbiol 47: 453–455.
14. Man SM, Zhang L, Day AS, Leach ST, Lemberg DA, et al. (2010) *Campylobacter concisus* and Other *Campylobacter* Species in Children with Newly Diagnosed Crohn's Disease. Inflamm Bowel Dis 16: 1008–1016.
15. Mukhopadhya I, Thomson JM, Hansen R, Berry SH, El-Omar EM et al. (2011) Detection of *Campylobacter concisus* and Other *Campylobacter* Species in Colonic Biopsies from Adults with Ulcerative Colitis. Plos One 6: e21490.
16. Silverberg MS, Satsangi J, Ahmad T, Arnott IDR, Bernstein CN, et al. (2005) Toward an integrated clinical, molecular and serological classification of inflammatory bowel disease: Report of a Working Party of the 2005 Montreal World Congress of Gastroenterology. Can J Gastroenterol 19: 5A–36A.
17. Lane DJ (1991) 16S/23S rRNA sequencing. In: Stackebrandt E, Goodfellow M, editors. Nucleic acid techniques in bacterial systematics. Chichester Wiley J & Sons Ltd. 115: 175.
18. Linton D, Owen RJ, Stanley J (1996) Rapid identification by PCR of the genus *Campylobacter* and of five *Campylobacter* species enteropathogenic for man and animals. Res Microbiol 147: 707–718.
19. Inglis GD, Kalischuk LD, Busz HW, Kastelic JP (2005) Colonization of cattle intestines by *Campylobacter jejuni* and *Campylobacter lanienae*. Appl Environ Microbiol 71: 5145–5153.
20. Levitt MD (1969) Production and excretion of hydrogen gas in man. New Engl J Med 281: 122–127.
21. Cummings JH (1983) Fermentation in the human large-intestine-evidence and implications for healthy. Lancet 1: 1206–1209.
22. Darfeuille-Michaud A, Neut C, Barnich N, Lederman E, Di Martino P, et al. (1998) Presence of adherent *Escherichia coli* strains in ileal mucosa of patients with Crohn's disease. Gastroenterology 115: 1405–1413.
23. Guslandi M (2005) Antibiotics for inflammatory bowel disease: do they work? Eur J Gastroenterol Hepat 17: 145–147.
24. Kim SC, Tonkonogy SL, Albright CA, Tsang J, Balish EJ, et al. (2005) Variablephenotypes of enterocolitis in interleukin 10-deficient mice monoassociated with two different commensal bacteria. Gastroenterology 128: 891–906.
25. Vandamme P, Falsen E, Pot B, Hoste B, Kersters K, et al. (1989) Identification of EF group-22 Campylobacters from gastroenteritis cases as *Campylobacter-concisus*. J Clin Microbiol 27: 1775–1781.
26. Matsheka MI, Lastovica AJ, Elisha BG (2001) Molecular identification of *Campylobacter concisus*. J Clin Microbiol 39: 3684–3689.
27. Bastyns K, Chapelle S, Vandamme P, Goossens H, Dewachter R (1995) Specific detection of *Campylobacter concisus* by PCR amplification of 23S rDNA areas. Mol Cell Probe 9: 247–250.
28. Aabenhus R, Permin H, On SLW, Andersen LP (2002) Prevalence of *Campylobacter concisus* in diarrhoea of immunocompromised patients. Scand J Infect Dis 34: 248–252.
29. Zhang L, Budiman V, Day AS, Mitchell H, Lemberg DA, et al. (2010) Isolation and Detection of *Campylobacter concisus* from Saliva of Healthy Individuals and Patients with Inflammatory Bowel Disease. J Clin Microbiol 48: 2965–2967.
30. Man SM, Kaakoush NO, Leach ST, Nahidi L, Lu HK, et al. (2010) Host Attachment, Invasion, and Stimulation of Proinflammatory Cytokines by *Campylobacter concisus* and Other Non-*Campylobacter jejuni Campylobacter* Species. J Infect Dis 202: 1855–1865.
31. Kalischuk LD, Inglis GD (2011) Comparative genotypic and pathogenic examination of *Campylobacter concisus* isolates from diarrheic and non-diarrheic humans. Bmc Microbiology 11: 53–66.

16

Differential Expression of MicroRNAs in Tumors from Chronically Inflamed or Genetic (APC$^{Min/+}$) Models of Colon Cancer

Brian M. Necela[1], Jennifer M. Carr[1], Yan W. Asmann[2], E. Aubrey Thompson[1]*

1 Department of Cancer Biology, Mayo Clinic Comprehensive Cancer Center, Jacksonville, Florida, United States of America, **2** Department of Biomedical Statistics and Informatics, Mayo Clinic College of Medicine, Rochester, Minnesota, United States of America

Abstract

Background: Chronic inflammation associated with ulcerative colitis predisposes individuals to increased colon cancer risk. The aim of these studies was to identify microRNAs that are aberrantly regulated during inflammation and may participate in transformation of colonic epithelial cells in the inflammatory setting.

Methodology/Principal Findings: We have use quantitative PCR arrays to compare microRNA (miRNA) expression in tumors and control colonic epithelial cells isolated from distal colons of chronically inflamed mice and APC$^{Min/+}$ mice. Rank order statistics was utilized to identify differentially regulated miRNAs in tumors that arose due to chronic inflammation and/or to germline APC mutation. Eight high priority miRNAs were identified: miR-215, miR-137, miR-708, miR-31, and miR-135b were differentially expressed in APC tumors and miR-215, miR-133a, miR-467d, miR-218, miR-708, miR-31, and miR-135b in colitis-associated tumors. Four of these (miR-215, miR-708, miR-31, and miR-135b) were common to both tumors types, and dysregulation of these miRNAs was confirmed in an independent sample set. Target prediction and pathway analysis suggests that these microRNAs, in the aggregate, regulate signaling pathways related to MAPK, PI3K, WNT, and TGF-β, all of which are known to be involved in transformation.

Conclusions/Significance: We conclude that these four miRNAs are dysregulated at some very early stage in transformation of colonic epithelial cells. This response is not dependent on the mechanism of initiation of transformation (inflammation versus germline mutation), suggesting that the miRNAs that we have identified are likely to regulate critical signaling pathways that are central to early events in transformation of colonic epithelial cells.

Editor: Eliana Saul Furquim Werneck Abdelhay, Instituto Nacional de Câncer, Brazil

Funding: This work was funded in part by a CCFA Career Development Award to BMN. The funders had no role in study design, data collection and analysis, decision to publish, or preparation of the manuscript.

Competing Interests: The authors have declared that no competing interests exist.

* E-mail: thompson.aubrey@mayo.edu

Introduction

MicroRNAs (miRNAs) are a class of small noncoding RNAs of 19 to 22 nucleotides implicated in a number of important cellular processes such as development, differentiation, proliferation, cell cycle progression, apoptosis, inflammation, and stress responses [1–8]. MicroRNAs are generally believed to function by binding the 3′UTR of target mRNAs and either inhibiting translation or in some cases inducing mRNA degradation [3,9]. Bioinformatic studies suggest that miRNAs may regulate one-third of the transcriptome [10,11]. Given their propensity to regulate numerous processes and target genes, it is no surprise that aberrant expression of miRNAs has been linked to numerous pathological conditions such as asthma, diabetes, kidney, neurodegenerative, and cardiovascular disease. In particular, differential miRNA expression has been implicated in many cancers including breast, thyroid, lung, pancreatic, and colon cancer.

To date, over a dozen studies have reported an association of aberrant miRNA expression in colon cancer [12–31]. Expression of miRNAs in colon tumors can be influenced by numerous clinicopathologic variables such as tumor grade and location, mutation status (p53, APC, MSI) [32–36], and cellular content (*i.e.* inflammatory cells) as well as pre-analytical and analytical variables such extraction method, fixation, and choice of analytical platform (sequence, qPCR, or microarray). As a result of these variables, there is no consensus concerning which miRNAs are differentially expressed in colon tumors. Nevertheless, a few microRNAs have consistently emerged as being dysregulated in colon cancer. Among these, miR-31 is consistently upregulated [12–17,20,22,23,25] and microRNA clusters miR-143/-145 [18,21–23,37–40] and miR-194/-215 [18,21–23,37,38,41] downregulated in colon cancer. MicroRNA −31 has been linked to cell migration and invasion in colon cancer cells [42,43]. MicroRNAs −192 and −215 inhibit cell proliferation and induce cell cycle arrest in a p53-dependent manner [37,44,45]. Likewise, miR-143 and miR-145 inhibit cell growth, with this action, in part, attributed to through inhibition of target genes such as DNMT3A, IRS-1, YES1, STAT1, and FLI1 [21,46–50].

One clinical variable that has not been adequately addressed is the inflammatory status of the colon tumor. A direct link between inflammation and cancer has been firmly established, with NFκB emerging as a key player [51,52]. Inflammation is believed not only to alter and promote the tumor microenvironment, but itself, can lead directly to tumorigenesis. Patients with ulcerative colitis, a chronic, relapsing inflammation of the colon, have increased risk of developing colon cancer. A recent meta-analysis revealed probabilities of colon cancer in ulcerative colitis of 2% after 10 years, 8% after 20 years, and 18% after 30 years of disease [53]. One possible mechanism by which inflammatory pathways may influence transformation is through deregulation of miRNAs. Increasing evidence suggest that miRNAs are capable of regulating inflammatory processes and are dysregulated in various inflammatory diseases [54]. Recently, dysregulation of micro-RNAs has been observed in patients with ulcerative colitis [55,56]. However, little is known about the functional consequence of dysregulation of miRNAs during chronic colitis in epithelial cells, and even less on tumorigenesis. Although limited, these studies do provide the precident that deregulation of a subset of microRNAs during chronic colitis may be associated with neoplastic and metaplastic metaplastic transformation. To this end, microRNAs may be useful biomarkers to help predict risk for malignancy in patients with long standing active disease.

The studies described below were undertaken to begin to test the hypothesis that a subset of microRNAs is dysregulated in the intestinal epithelium during colitis and contribute to carcinogenesis. We measured miRNAs by quantitative PCR low density TaqMan arrays using RNA extracted from colonic epithelial cells of mice induced with acute dextran sulfate colitis (AC), chronic colitis (CC), colitis-associated colon tumors (CAC), and colon tumors in APC$^{Min/+}$ mice. We identified differential expression of miRNAs common and unique to each disease condition. In particular, we demonstrate that a subset of miRNAs is dysregulated in both tumors of both inflammatory and genetic origin. These miRNAs have the potential to control both anti-oncogenic and pro-oncogenic transcriptional networks, thereby influencing tumorigenic outcome.

Results

Comparison of analytical models using acute colitis (AC) samples

Quantification of miRNA expression in tissue samples is complicated by the fact that one has no obvious direct means to identify appropriate endogenous controls that may be used to normalize expression data and correct for differences in the amount of RNA analyzed or the efficiency of miRNA extraction or cDNA conversion in samples from different tissues. This potential problem is particularly acute in the studies such as those that will be described below in which we undertake to compare miRNA abundance in tissues derived from mice of different ages, diets, inflammatory status, and tumor burden. We therefore carried out a pilot experiment to compare different analytical tools and statistical models to identify differentially regulated miRNAs in colonic epithelial cells. To this end we extracted miRNAs from epithelial cell preparations from distal colons of control C57BL/6J mice and mice that had been exposed to 3.5% DSS in drinking water for four days. Histologically, the colons from control and DSS-treated mice were indistinguishable, with no evidence of barrier breakdown, crypt loss, or invasion by immune cells. Although these tissues formally represent a pre-inflamed state, the samples will be designated AC (acute colitis) in the follow discussion, whereas the controls will be identified as Con.

We used AB TaqMan arrays to measure the abundance of 384 miRNAs in AC and Con samples, expressed as critical thresholds (Ct) for each miRNA detector. Three analytical approaches were compared. The simplest of these was rank order statistics. Each miRNA within a given sample was force ranked on analog readout of miRNA abundance (Ct value). Detectors that were scored as 'undetectable' were assigned Ct values of 40, and all miRNAs with Ct = 40 were assigned the same rank within a sample. A t-test (assuming unequal variance) was then carried out to compare the rank order assignments of miRNAs in the two different sample groups so as to identify miRNAs whose mean rank order of expression changed significantly as a result of treatment. The second analytical approach involved a simple median normalization of the samples, followed by a t-test (assuming unequal variance) to compare Ct values between Con and AC samples. Differential expression is expressed as ΔCt (abbreviated DCt), which represents (meanCtMed_Norm_AC) - (meanCtMed_Norm_Con). The third method employed the Integromics Statminer package, which uses a Limma-based empirical Bayesian implementation to calculate a hyperparamter which is in turn used to modulate the variance and increase the degrees of freedom across the samples. The Statminer package also calculates variance among user-defined endogenous controls and identifies those with the least variance across all samples. The Statminer package allows multiple endogenous controls to be used to normalize the dataset. In our case the least variant endogenous controls were sno135 and miR-25, and these were used to normalize the data. Differential expression is expressed as ΔΔCt (abbreviated DDCt), which represents (meanΔCtLimma_SM_Tumor)-(meanΔCtLimma_SM_Con) Thus we compared a relatively simple model in which no attempt was made to normalize the data (rank order statistics, abbreviated Rnk_Diff), a simple median normalization model (Med_Norm), and a more complicated empirical Bayesian model that used multiple endogenous controls to normalize the data (Limma_SM).

A comparison of the changes in rank order of individual miRNAs (Rank Difference AC-Con) and the log2 fold change from median normalized data [Median Normalized DCt (AC-Con)] is shown in Figure 1A, whereas a similar comparison of log2 fold change after Limma normalization to sno135 and miR-25 [DDCt(AC-Con)] is shown in Figure 1B. The distributions are obviously nearly identical, as indicated by Spearman rank correlation coefficients of 0.8324 and 0.8328 for Figures 1A and B, respectively. This similarity results from near identity of the expression data calculated from median normalized and Limma-normalized data (Figure 1C, Spearman rank correlation coefficient = 0.9996). The observation that two very different normalization protocols yielded essentially identical results probably indicates that there is very little variance, either analytical or biological, among our samples.

Using these three approaches we identified 193 miRNAs that were scored as significantly different (P≤0.01) in one or more of the analyses (listed in Table S1). We imposed additional filters of rank difference ≥(±10) and P≤0.01 to identify 73 differentially expressed miRNAs by rank order statistics. When we filtered on log2 fold change≥(±1.0) and P≤0.01 we identified 130 miRNAs that were differentially expressed in the median normalized analysis and 134 miRNAs that were differentially expressed by Limma analysis. A VENN diagram of overlap between these miRNAs is shown in Figure 1D. Somewhat to our surprise, there were only 51 miRNAs that satisfied all conditions for all models. A three dimensional correlation comparing rank difference, DCt (median normalization), and DDCt (Limma normalization) revealed a 3-dimensional correlation coefficient of 1.00 for these 51 samples (data not shown). These miRNAs represent high

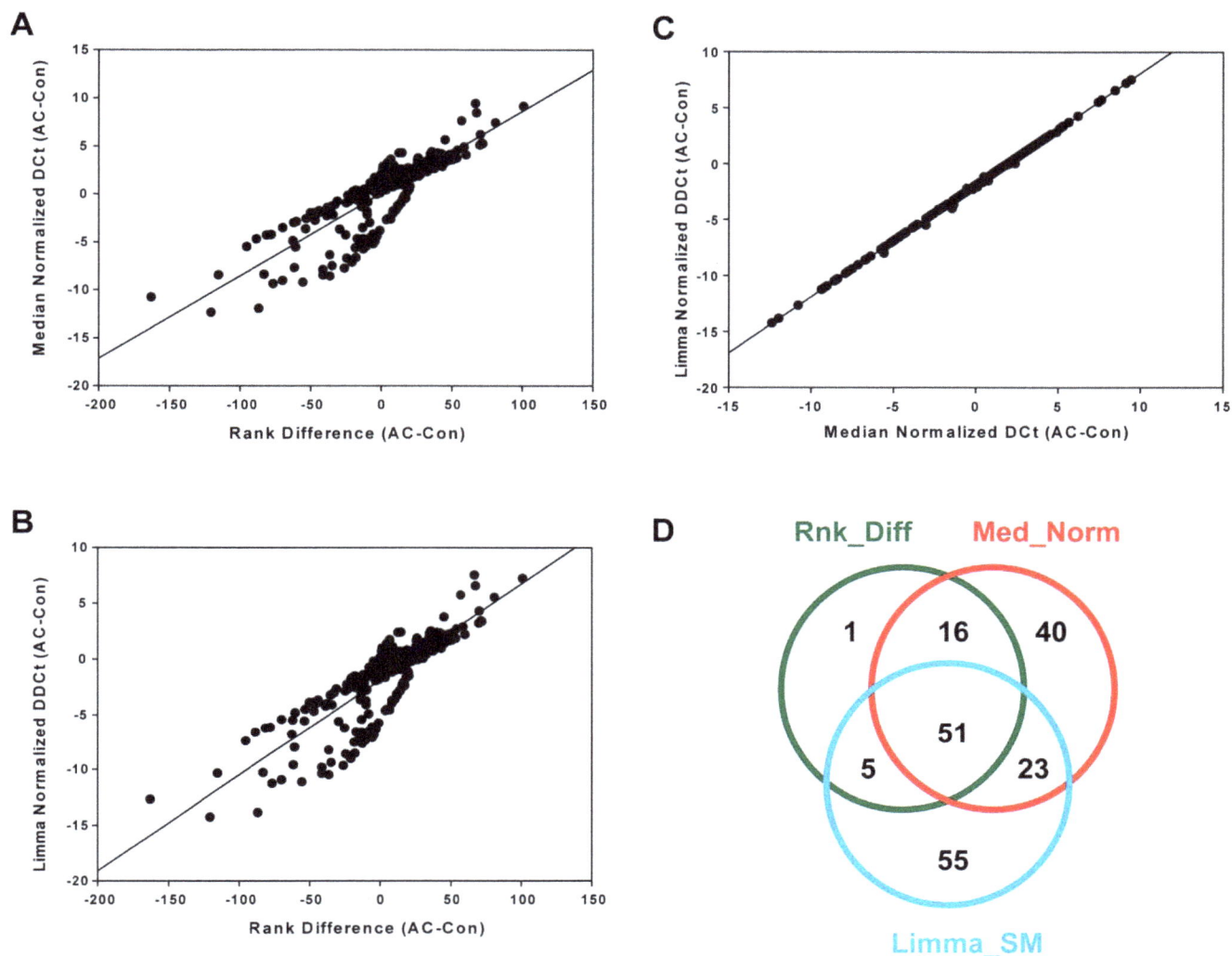

Figure 1. Comparison of three different normalization methods to identify differentially expressed miRNAs in DSS-induced acute colitis. Changes in rank order, defined as mean rank in AC samples minus mean rank in Con samples, are plotted against DCt values (mean Ct_AC minus mean Ct_Con) in **Panel A** or DDCt (mean DCt_AC minus mean DCt_Con) in **Panel B**. Limma normalized DDCt values for individual miRNAs are plotted against median normalized DCt values in **Panel C**. Differentially expressed miRNAs were filtered on P<0.01 and rank order change ≥10 or log2 fold change ≥1.0. Overlap between differentially expressed miRNAs identified by rank order statistics (Rnk_Diff), t-test using median normalized data (Med_Norm), or the Statminer implementation of Limma (Limma_SM) is shown in **Panel D**.

probability targets that are likely to play some role in the very earliest stages of inflammation. (These miRNAs are identified in bold in Table S1.) Both median normalization and Limma yielded significant numbers of outliers, whereas rank order statistical analysis exhibited almost complete overlap with at least one of the other models (Fig. 1D).

Our conclusion from this initial comparison of three different normalization methods is that they all give very similar results, in terms of relative miRNA abundance, in a dataset with little analytical or biological variance within the control and experimental groups. The different statistical models give significantly different p-values, which is probably due in large part to the small number of samples that were included in this analysis as well as the use of moderated variance (Limma) versus unmoderated variance (t-test). Overall the rank order statistics works at least as well as either of the normalized models, tends to be more conservative in terms of number of differentially

regulated miRNAs, and has the additional advantages that it requires no knowledge of appropriate endogenous controls and makes no assumptions about equal amounts of RNA or equal efficiency of miRNA extraction or cDNA conversion from sample to sample. We therefore elected to proceed with our analyses using rank order statistics to identify differentially expressed miRNAs. However, changes in rank order are not informative in terms of absolute (or more precisely analog) miRNA abundance, so we relied on Limma to calculate normalized abundance, expressed as DDCt, which corresponds to −log2 fold change normalized to sno135b/miR-25.

Identification of differentially expressed miRNAs in experimental models of colitis-associated colon cancer and familial adenomatous polyposis coli

We used AB TaqMan miRNA arrays to measure the abundance of 384 miRNAs in tumors isolated from distal colons of APC$^{Min/+}$ mice (APC tumors) and tumors that formed in the distal colons of chronically inflamed mice (CAC tumors). The APC$^{Min/+}$ mice were retired breeders, 120d of age, and maintained on high fat breeder's chow. CAC tumors were isolated from mice that had been subjected to 12 rounds of low level inflammation, induced by DSS as described in Materials and Methods. As control samples, we isolated epithelial cells from adjacent, uninvolved epithelium from APC$^{Min/+}$ (APC control) or chronically inflamed (CC control) mice. Rank order statistics was used to identify candidate differentially expressed miRNAs in APC and CAC tumors. (Raw Ct values for these samples are given in Table S2.)

The Ct values of all miRNAs in individual tumors and control samples were determined and force ranked as described above and the t-test was used to identify miRNAs whose mean rank was significantly different in controls and tumors. The average rank orders for individual miRNAs from APC control and APC tumors are displayed in Figure 2A. There was, in general, a good correspondence between rank order of miRNA abundance in APC control and APC tumor samples (Spearman Rank Order correlation coefficient = 0.973, p = 2.0E^{-07}), however 10 miRNAs (shown as red symbols) fell outside the 95% prediction intervals (shown as parallel lines in Fig. 2A).

Figure 2B compares rank orders of the abundance of miRNAs measured in CCcontrol and CACtumors samples. As with the APC samples, there was a generally high correspondence between rank order abundance of miRNAs in these samples (Spearman Rank Order correlation coefficient = 0.970, p<2.0E^{-07}). However, 10 miRNAs (red symbols) fell outside the 95% prediction intervals (Fig. 2B), indicating that the ranks of these miRNAs were different in controls and tumors, consistent with a high probability that these miRNAs were differentially expressed. It is our experience that very large changes in miRNA abundance (as evidenced in this case by large rank order differences) are occasionally associated with atypical kinetics of amplification of very low abundance miRNAs. We therefore visually inspected the qPCR amplification curves for each of the miRNAs in every sample and eliminated those for which log-linear amplification kinetics (1Ct/cycle) did not obtain. This curation step reduced the number of high probability differentially expressed miRNAs in APC tumors to 5 and the number of such miRNAs in CAC tumors to 7. As shown in Table 1, two miRNAs were repressed in APC tumors (miR-215 and miR-137), compared to adjacent control epithelium, whereas 3 miRNAs were induced (miR-708, miR-31, miR-135b). Only 1 miRNA was repressed in CAC tumors compared to control chronically inflamed epithelium (miR-215), whereas 6 miRNAs were induced in CAC tumors (miR-133a, miR-467d, miR-218, miR-31, miR-135b). Three miRNAs were induced in both APC and CAC samples (miR-31, miR-135b, and miR-708) and 1 miRNA was repressed in both APC and CAC samples (miR-215). In addition, 1 miRNA was uniquely repressed in APC tumors (miR-137), and 3 miRNAs were uniquely induced in CAC tumors (miR-133a, miR-467d, and miR-218). The 8 differentially expressed miRNAs in Table 1 were therefore selected for validation.

Although rank order statistics is a useful tool for nominating miRNAs that are differentially expressed, a more quantitative approach is required to determine the magnitude of the response in any given comparison. To this end we used the Statminer implementation of Limma to carry out normalization and summarization of the TaqMan array expression data. The data are presented in Figure 3 as the log 2 transformation of fold change for each of the 8 focus miRNAs, where Fold Change = −[mean (DCtTumor−DCtControl)]. P-values were calculat-

ed for each comparison using the Limma empirical Bayesian implementation of the t-test to compare normalized (DCt) values for tumors and controls. As shown in Figure 3, all candidate miRNAs exhibited large, statistically significant differences in expression in APC tumors (Fig. 3A) and CAC (Fig. 3B), relative to control samples.

We used conventional TaqMan cDNA conversion primers and qPCR reagents to confirm differential expression of the four miRNAs that exhibited common regulatory responses in the CAC and APC tumor samples used in the initial multiplex qPCR analysis. As shown in Figure 4, repression of miR-215 was confirmed in both CAC and APC tumor samples, whereas induction of miR-708, miR-31, and miR-135b was likewise confirmed in tumors of both origins. We prepared an additional set of controls and tumors from both chronic colitis and APC mice and measured the abundance of miR-215, miR-708, miR-31, and miR-135b. Figure 5 shows that within experimental error the results predicted from the rank order statistical analyses were validated in an independent sample cohort.

Focus miRNA expression in primary human colon cancers

The pattern of expression of the 8 focus miRNAs listed in Table 1 implies that some or all of these miRNAs may play a potential role in the etiology of the early stage adenomas that form in APC$^{Min/+}$ mice and/or mice that have undergone experimental chronic colitis. A literature survey indicates that some of these focus miRNAs have been previously reported to be differentially expressed in primary human colon cancers, as shown in Table 2. MicroRNAs miR-31 and miR-135b have been reported to be induced in colon cancer, similar to the response that we have observed in early stage tumors in chronically inflamed or APC$^{Min/+}$ mice. Likewise, we observed downregulation of miR-215 in tumors of both types, and downregulation of miR-133a in CAC but not APC tumors. Both of these miRNAs are reported to be downregulated in human colon cancers [18,21–23,37]. Our analyses indicate that these miRNA species are induced very early in transformation and probably affect signaling pathways that are central to processes that are independent of the mechanism of initiation.

Analysis of potential miRNA targets and functions in early stage tumors

Several different algorithms have been developed to predict miRNA targets, based upon different parameters to assess complementarily of miRNA seed sequences to sequences within the 3′ untranslated regions of mRNAs [10,57–59]. Although these analyses are far from perfect in terms of predictive ability, they remain the only tools available for predicting miRNA targets, and the output of these analyses is useful for predicting hypothetical connections between miRNAs, targeted pathways, and biological functions. Since different algorithms often yield different results, we used PicTar, MicroCosm, TargetScan, and DianaT to generate lists of potential targets for each of the differentially expressed miRNAs. We included in these lists only targets that were conserved in mouse and human transcripts, and the individual predictions were pooled to form a master list of putative targets for all four miRNAs. This list was then collated with microarray data from isolated mouse distal colonic epithelial cells [60], and targets that were not scored as 'Present' in these cells were eliminated. The curated lists were then used for pathway prediction.

We focused on the 4 miRNAs that were differentially expressed in early stage lesions of both genetic and inflammatory origin (miR-215, miR-31, miR-708, miR-135b). Using the filters

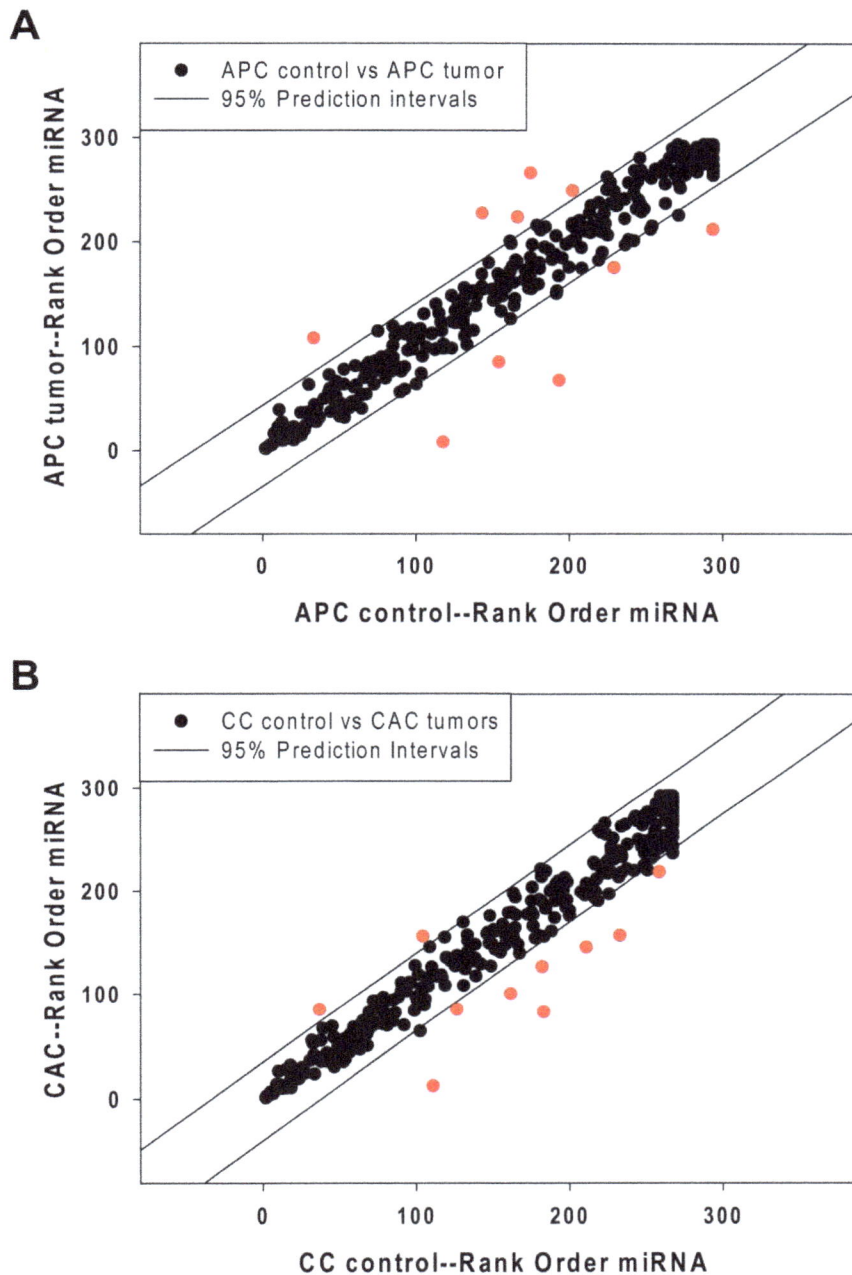

Figure 2. Rank order statistical analysis of differentially expressed miRNAs in tumors from APC$^{Min/+}$ or chronically inflamed mice.
Mean rank orders of miRNA abundance (based on Ct values) were determined for tumors from the distal colons or uninvolved adjacent distal colonic epithelial cells (**Panel A**). SigmaStat was used to calculate 95% confidence intervals for these data (parallel solid lines) and miRNA detectors that fell outside of these intervals are filled in red. Similarly, we compared rank order of expression of miRNAs from tumors that formed in the distal colons of chronically inflamed mice (CAC) and in uninvolved, chronically inflamed distal colonic epithelial cell preparations (CC controls), as shown in **Panel B**. MicroRNA detectors that fell outside of the 95% confidence intervals are filled in red.

described above, we identified 527 potential target mRNAs that were expressed in mouse distal colonic epithelial cells. Gene ontology analysis (Table 3) identified Cancer as the top biological function associated with this gene set, with 130 of the 527 targets linked to Cancer through GO terms (p-value range $5.86E^{-05}$ to $2.87E^{-02}$). GO terms associated with Gene Expression emerged as the top Molecular and Cellular Function, with 131 targets linked to this category (p-value range $5.78E^{-11}$ to $2.87E^{-02}$). The top Tox function was TGF-β Signaling (p = $5.2E^{-04}$, with 9/77

signaling components identified as potential targets). The remaining statistically significant Tox functions were related to nuclear receptors that have been studied extensively within the context of colonic epithelial cell physiology and pathology, including TR/RXR, VDR/RXR, and FXR/RXR.

These hypothetical GO functions predict a strong linkage between the four differentially expressed miRNAs and transformation of colonic epithelial cells. This hypothetical linkage is emphasized by the data shown in Figure 6, in which putative

Table 1. Differentially expressed microRNAs in APC and CAC tumors.

| miRNA | APC control vs APC tumor | | miRNA | CC control vs CAC tumor | |
	Ave rank order diff.	p-value		Ave rank order diff.	p-value
miR-215	−75	0.0014	miR-215	−48	0.0042
miR-137	−57	0.0206	miR-133a	38	0.0014
miR-708	69	0.0022	miR-467d	40	0.0147
miR-31	110	0.0021	miR-218	42	0.0018
miR-135b	126	<0.0001	miR-708	62	0.0014
			miR-31	98	<0.0001
			miR-135b	101	0.0014

Rank order differences were determined by subtracting the average rank order of individual microRNAs in each group of tumor samples from the rank order in the corresponding control (e.g. APC control rank – APC tumor rank = rank order diff.). Signficance (p-value) was assessed using the t-test (assuming unequal variance) to compare rank orders of individual microRNAs in tumors and controls.

miRNA targets (shown in green) are overlaid onto the knowledge-based (Ingenuity) Molecular Mechanisms of Cancer canonical pathway (p = $1.14E^{-06}$, 28 predicted targets/372 pathway components). Critical membrane signaling functions related to Ras/MAPK, PI3K, and WNT/β-catenin represent potential mechanistic links between these miRNAs and transformation, whereas nuclear functions linked to RB/E2F control emerge as potential mediators of cell cycle control. Finally, as indicated by the GO analysis of Tox function, TGF-β/BMP/SMAD signaling is nominated as a very significant potential link between these four miRNAs and transformation of colonic epithelial cells.

Discussion

Our central objective was to compare miRNA expression in colon tumors that arise due to chronic inflammation and germ line mutations in model systems. It was clear early on that normalization of the data would be an issue, since we were comparing very different tissue states (e.g., chronically inflamed mice on standard lab chow versus aged breeders on high fat diets); and there are no well-established objective criteria for identifying appropriate endogenous controls for normalization of miRNA expression under such conditions (For a review of this issue, see [61]). Our first objective was therefore to use an independent sample set to compare different models for normalization. To this end we prepared and analyzed distal colonic epithelial cells from control and acutely inflamed tissues, using a conventional DSS acute colitis model. We examined an early, pre-inflamed, state, prior to detectable loss of histological integrity of the distal colonic epithelium, thinking to minimize changes in miRNA expression that might be associated with massive infiltration of immune cells. Using three different analytical approaches we identified 51 high priority miRNA targets that are likely to play a significant role in controlling gene expression in epithelial cells in the very earliest stages of DSS-induced inflammation. Although these findings represent, to our knowledge, the first detailed report of differential miRNA expression in this colitis model, we have not further analyzed these data. Rather we used these data to validate our choice of rank order statistics to identify differentially expressed miRNAs. This analytical approach does not require identification of appropriate internal controls and is particularly appropriate for analysis of relatively small groups of samples, since no assumptions are required about equal RNA loading or efficiency of extraction of miRNAs or cDNA conversion from very different kinds of tissues [62]. In general, the rank order differences that we

observed correlate well with analog miRNA abundance, expressed as DCt in the median normalized data or DDCt in the sno135/miR-25 normalized (Statminer) analyses. However, the p-values assigned by the different statistical models varied considerably, due at least in part to the small sample size and the use of moderated (Limma empirical Bayesian) versus unmoderated (t-test) approaches to estimating variance. Given that any statistical model is likely to break down with small sample sets, we elected to use the simplest, most conservative approach: rank order statistics. We used Statminer normalization (against sno135 and miR-25) to extract relative miRNA abundance.

Rank order statistics was used to identify 8 differentially expressed miRNAs in tumors that formed in the distal colons of $APC^{Min/+}$ mice and chronically inflamed mice. It should be noted that these tumors are primarily adenomas and thus represent a very early stage in transformation. We should also emphasize that these 8 miRNAs represent only the most prominent, and therefore likely the most reproducible, changes in miRNA expression in these samples. Many other miRNAs exhibited statistically significant changes in rank order (as well as normalized Ct values) in one or another of these sample sets, but our confidence in these targets is limited by the small sample size. We have not undertaken to expand our sample size, given the cost of the TaqMan arrays and the fact that it takes over 40 weeks to generate CAC tumors. Nevertheless, we were able to validate our four most prominent miRNAs (miR-215, miR-708, miR-135b, miR-31) in an independent set of APC and CAC tumors. These four miRNAs are therefore firmly established as differentially expressed in early stage tumors of both genetic and inflammatory origin.

Target identification remains the greatest challenge to determining the functional significance of differential miRNA expression. We have attempted to be as conservative as possible in target prediction, using an approach that combines predicted targets from four of the most popular target prediction programs and curating these predicted targets to include only those that are conserved in mouse and human and are expressed in distal colonic epithelial cells. Our analysis suggests that these four miRNAs, in the aggregate, may affect signaling through a number of important pathways that have been linked to colon carcinogenesis. Notable among these are MAPK, PI3K, WNT, and TGF-β signaling, all of which are well-known to be intimately involved in transformation of colonic epithelial cells. The precise links between any or all of these pathways and individual miRNAs remains to be established. Nevertheless, the observation that these miRNAs are coordinately

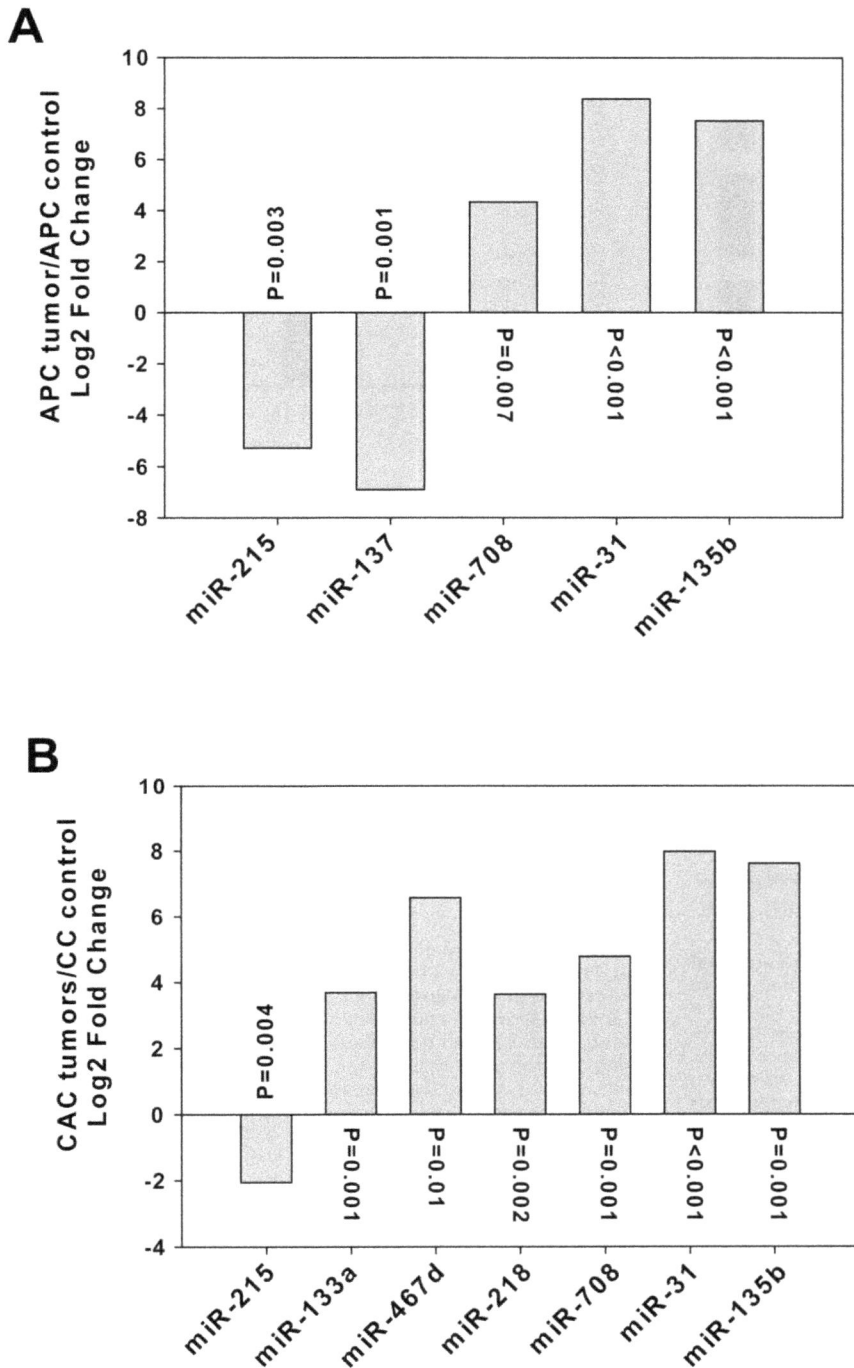

Figure 3. Differential expression of 8 miRNAs in tumors from APC^Min/+ or chronically inflamed mice. MicroRNA abundance in the four different sample cohorts was normalized using Statminer and sno135/miR-25 as endogenous controls. APC controls were normalized to APC tumors (Panel A) and CC controls to CAC tumors (Panel B). The abundance of each of the 8 candidate miRNAs is represented as log2 fold change (mean Ct tumor − mean Ct control) and p-values were calculated using the Limma empirical Bayesian implementation of the moderated t-test.

dysregulated in tumors of very different origins in combination with the hypothetical connections between these miRNAs and known oncogenic signaling pathways strongly suggests that this group of miRNAs plays some critical role or roles in the very earliest stages of transformation of colonic epithelial cells.

One obvious question relates to the link between these focus miRNAs and inflammation. The observation that these miRNAs

are differentially expressed in APC tumors indicates that their identification in the CAC tumors is not simply a reflection of some residual inflammatory state that persists in the colonic epithelium of CC mice. Moreover, most of these miRNAs are only modestly dysregulated in the AC samples, on the order of 2- to 4-fold which may not be significant in these samples. MiR-31 is not induced in AC samples and is clearly not related to inflammation by that

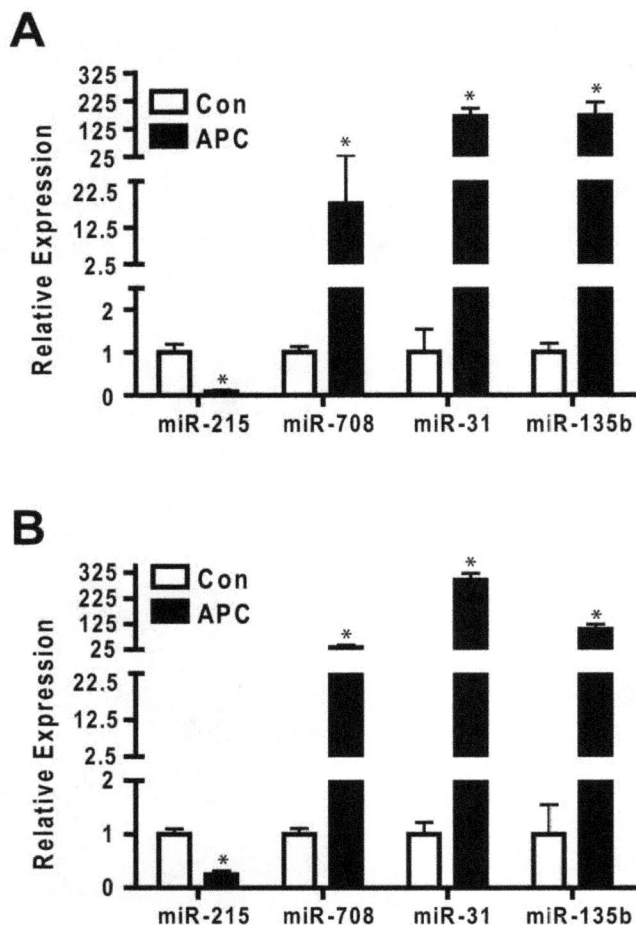

Figure 4. Confirmation of focus miRNAs using conventional qPCR. The RNA samples analyzed in Figures 2 and 3 were converted to cDNA using individual Taqman hairpin RT primers, as opposed to the universal primer mix used for the TaqMan arrays. Thus different cDNA preparations were prepared and assayed for miRNA abundance in APC samples (**Panel A**) and CAC samples (**Panel B**). MicroRNA abundance was normalized with sno135 and p-values calculated with the Statminer Limma protocol. Data for each miRNA were calibrated to expression (2e-DCt) in the relevant control sample. Bars represent the mean and standard deviation for each miRNA, n = 4. * indicates p-value<0.05.

Figure 5. Validation of focus miRNA in an independent sample set. RNA was prepared from an independent set of APC tumors (n = 9) and controls (n = 9) (**Panel A**) or CAC tumors (n = 4) and controls (n = 8) (**Panel B**). MicroRNA abundance was measured by Taqman microRNA specific stem PCR and normalized with sno135. Data were normalized using Statminer and calibrated to expression of individual miRNAs in the control samples. Bars represent mean and standard deviation. * indicates p-value<0.05.

criterion. There have been a limited number of studies on miRNA expression in human inflammatory bowel disease [55,56], and none of our four focus miRNAs was linked to human colitis. MicroRNA expression in human colon tumors has been investigated in some detail. Interpretation of these data is confounded by the fact that there is generally little overlap between the data reported by different groups, using different analytical platforms, different sample cohorts, and different analytical pipelines. Nevertheless, there is evidence that miR-31 [12–17,20,22,23], miR-135b [13–15,20,21,33], and miR-215 [18,21–23,37] are differentially expressed in fully transformed colonic epithelial cells. In addition, a recent publication by Olaru indicates that miR-31 and miR-21 are also upregulated in human colitis-associated neoplasia [25], supporting our data that suggests a role of these miRNAs in transformation of non-IBD and IBD-associated cancer. Of note, our data also indicates that miR-215 is downregulated in APC and CAC tumors and in human colon tumors [18,21–23,37]. In contrast, Olaru et al. observed an

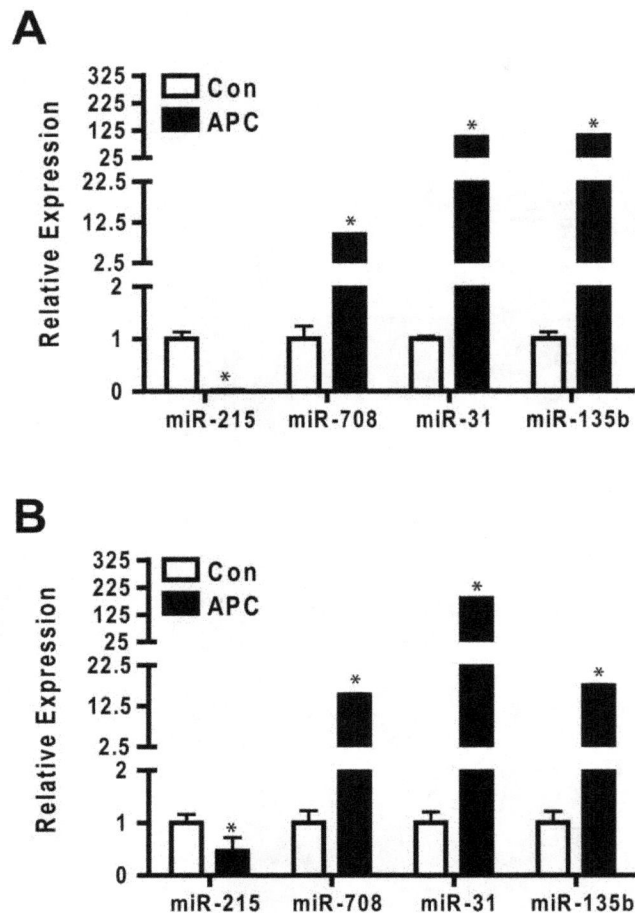

upregulation of miR-215 in colitis-associated neoplasia [25]. The cause of this discrepancy is unclear, but is tempting to speculate the differential expression of miR-215 is reflected by the stage of transformation, dysplasia versus carcinoma. We also note that currently there is no report of miR-708 in human colon cancers, in contrast to our data which indicates that this miRNA is dramatically induced in mouse colonic tumors. Likewise, miR-218 is induced in colitis-associated tumors but is not induced in APC tumors and has not been reported to be induced in human tumors. It is tempting to speculate that miR-218 may play some role that is specific to progression from inflammation to transformation in the colon, but this hypothesis remains to be evaluated. Overall, our analyses indicate that these four focus miRNAs are dysregulated very early in transformation and the observation that these changes appear to be independent of the mechanism of tumorigenesis (genetic versus inflammatory) suggests that these species have some fundamental function(s) that is required for initiation of transformation. The challenge now is to elucidate those functions so as to identify early events that can be manipulated for therapeutic or preventive intervention.

Table 2. Tumor expression levels and validated target genes/functions of the eight focus miRNAs.

miRNA	Tumor Level	References	Validated Targets	Validated Biological Functions	References
miR-31	up	[12–17,22,23,25,39]	TIAM1	migration, invasion	[42]
miR-135b	up	[13–15,20,27,33]	APC		[26]
miR-137	down	[13,15,21,28]	CDC42	cell cycle, invasion	[29]
miR-133a	down	[12,15,21]			
miR-215	down	[18,21–23,37]	TYMS, DTL, DHFR	cell cycle, adhesion, proliferation, chemoresistance	[30,31,35,44,45]
miR-708	not reported				
miR-467d	n.a.*				
miR-218	not reported				

Expression of microRNAs in human colon tumors compared to normal controls as indicated in corresponding references.
*For miR-467d, no human homolog is known. Differential expression of miR-708 and miR-218 was not reported in the literature. Validated gene targets and biological functions of individual miRNAs are indicated with corresponding references. TIAM, t-cell lymphoma invasion and metastasis 1. APC, adenomatosis polyposis coli. TYMS, thymidylate synthetase. DTL, denticleless protein homolog. DHFR, dihydrofolatereductase. CDC42, cell division cycle 42.

Materials and Methods

Ethics Statement

All mice were maintained as part of an American Association for Accreditation of Laboratory Animal Care facility. Animal experimentation was conducted in accordance with accepted standards of humane animal care according to the protocol #A17008 approved by the Mayo Clinic College of Medicine Institutional Animal Care and Use Committee Animal.

Animal studies

Acute and chronic dextran sodium sulfate (DSS) treatment protocols were initiated on six week old female C57BL/6J mice (Jackson Labs) maintained on standard AIN-76A rodent diet. Acute DSS colitis (abbreviated AC) was induced by administering 3.5% dextran sodium sulfate (M.W. 36,000–50,000, MP Biomedicals) *ad libitum* in filter-purified drinking water for four days according to the well-established procedure of Okayasu et al. [63]. To induce chronic colitis (CC) and colitis-associated tumors

Table 3. Summary of top GO functions identified for miR-215, miR-31, miR-135b, and miR-708 by Ingenuity Pathway Analysis.

GO Functions	p-value	# of Genes
Top Biological Function-Disease		
Cancer	5.86E^{-05}-2.87E^{-02}	130
Top Biological Function-Molecular and Cellular Function		
Gene Expression	5.78E^{-11}-2.87E^{-02}	131
Canonical Pathways		
Molecular Mechanisms of Cancer	1.14E^{-06}	28/372
Tox Lists		
TGF-β Signaling	5.3E^{-04}	9/77
TR/RXR Activation	3.63E^{-03}	8/83
VDR/RXR Activation	8.73E^{-03}	7/77
FXR/RXR Activation	1.29E^{-02}	7/83
G1/S Transition of the Cell Cycle	1.60E^{-02}	5/49

(CAC), mice were subjected to 12 cycles of inflammation followed by recovery, to mimic recurrent bouts of colitis in human patients [63,64]. Each cycle consisted of 1% DSS in drinking water for seven days followed by a 10 day recovery (normal water). APC$^{Min/+}$ mice were retired breeders, approximately 120 days of age and maintained on a high fat diet (Breeders Chow).

Mice were sacrificed and colons were dissected and flushed with cold phosphate-buffered saline. Each colon was opened longitudinally to expose the luminal surface and fixed flat in 10% formalin for 12 hr. Tissues were washed three times with colon 1× PBS and stored in 70% ethanol at 4°C. All analyses were performed using tissue from the distal colon since this is the site of tumor formation in both CAC and APC models. A 1 cm section of epithelium was scraped 1 cm from the distal end of colons from mice on the acute colitis, chronic colitis, and control protocols. Some animals that underwent the chronic colitis protocol developed tumors in the distal colon, whereas almost all APC$^{Min/+}$ mice had 1–2 distal colon tumors. Tumors were dissected for RNA extraction. For APC$^{Min/+}$ mice, epithelial scrapings adjacent to isolated distal tumors served as controls. Total number of samples analyzed for each condition were: 4 normal epithelium, 4 acute colitis, 4 chronic colitis, 4 colitis-associated tumors, 4 APC$^{Min/+}$ control epithelium, and 7 APC$^{Min/+}$ tumors. An additional validation set of APC tumors (n = 9) and controls (n = 9) or CAC tumors (n = 4) and controls (n = 8) was also prepared.

RNA isolation and qRT-PCR

Total RNA was extracted with the Recover All™ Total Nucleic Acid isolation kit as described by the manufacturer (Ambion). The abundance of individual miRNAs was determined using conventional two-step quantitative reverse transcriptase-mediated real-time PCR (qPCR). 10 ng of total RNA was converted to cDNA with Taqman mirRNA RT transcription kit and primer specific probes. MicroRNA qPCR reactions were performed in triplicate with 10 ng cDNA and the TaqMan Universal no UMG PCR master mix. All primers and probes were purchased from Applied Biosystems. All amplification data were collected with an Applied Biosystems Prism 7900 FAST sequence detector and analyzed with Sequence Detection System software (SDS ver. 2.3, Applied Biosystems).

TaqMan miRNA low density array

The Taqman© Rodent MicroRNA Array A v2.0 was used to assess miRNA expression in RNA samples from epithelium of

Molecular Mechanisms of Cancer

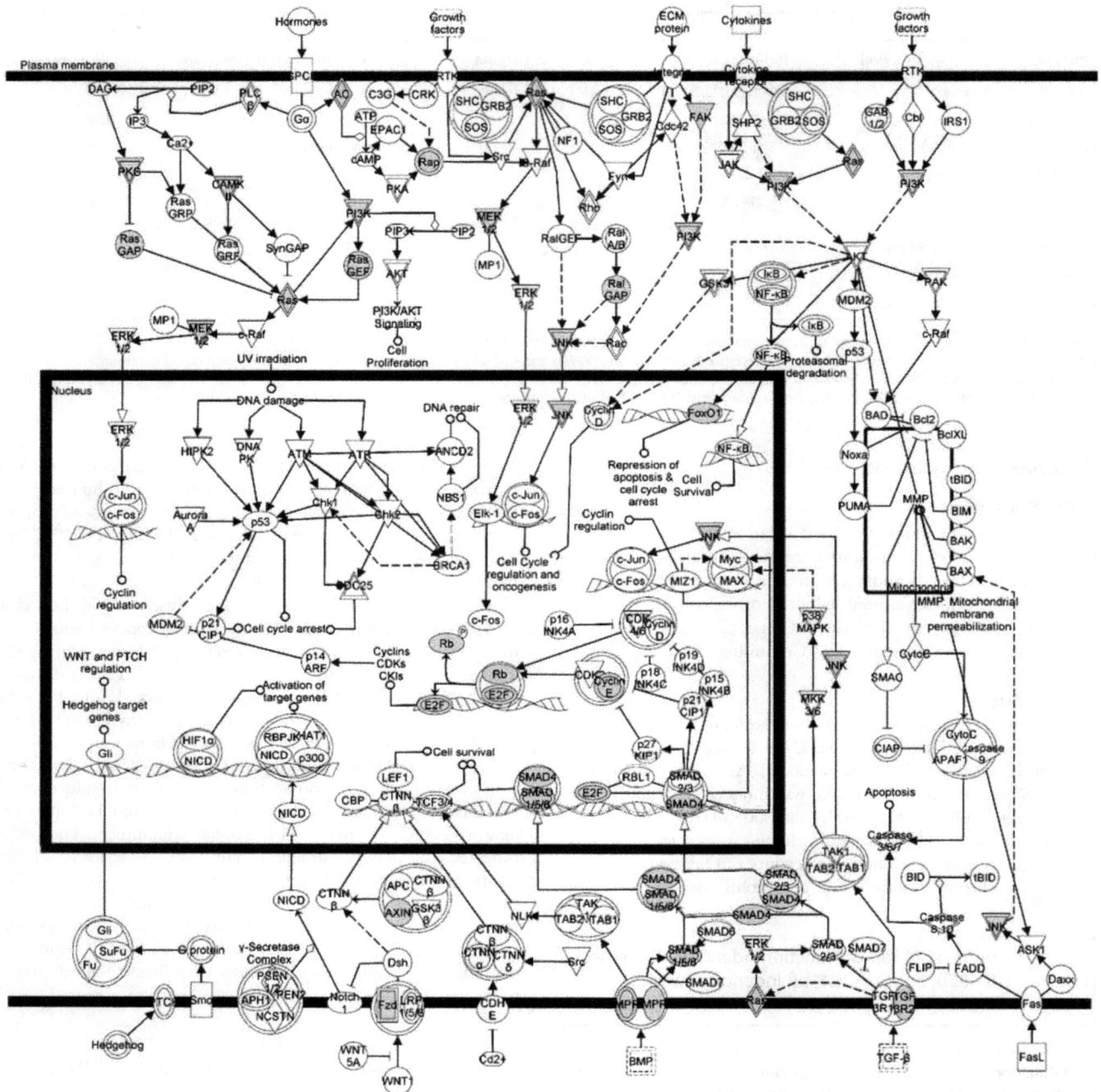

Figure 6. Focus miRNAs are predicted to regulate several key nodal signaling events that are known to be involved in transformation. Putative mRNA targets for the 4 focus miRNAs were compiled using PicTar, MicroCosm, TargetScan, and DianaT databases. Predicted targets were overlaid in gray on the Ingenuity Molecular Mechanisms of Cancer canonical pathway.

normal mouse colon, acute DSS colitis, chronic DSS colitis, chronic colitis tumors, and of APC$^{Min/+}$ tumors and adjacent tissue (see animal studies). Briefly, 500 ng of total RNA was reverse transcribed with Megaplex RT primers and Taqman MicroRNA RT kit. Samples were then amplified with Megaplex Preamp primers and Taqman Preamp master mix. cDNAs were diluted 1:4.33 and loaded with Taqman universal PCR master mix on each low density array according to manufacturer's instructions.

Amplification kinetics were measured on an Applied Biosystems Prism 7900 FAST sequence detector and analyzed with Sequence Detection System software (Applied Biosystems).

Statistical analysis

Stats Direct (ver. 2.6.1) was called from Excel 2007 to carry out t-test and regression analyses. Limma was run in an R environment (ver. 2.4.1) and called from Statminer ver. 4.2

(Integromics, Inc.) to calculate hyperparameters that were then used to moderate variance estimates in a variation of the t-test. Statminer uses this empirical Bayesian approach to estimate variance (defined as M function using the Genorm default) among user-defined endogenous controls. We selected sno135 and miR-25 as normalizers since both had M functions <0.15 individually and a combined M function of <0.1.

miRNA target prediction

Potential miR targets were determined by combining the results from TargetScanv.5.1 (http://www.targetscan.org), MicroCosm v5 (http://www.ebi.ac.uk/enright-srv/microcosm/tdocs/targets/v5/), DIANA-microTv3.0 (http://diana.cslab.ece.ntua.gr/microT/) and Pictar (http://pictar.mdc-berlin.de/). Potential target sequences were pooled for both mouse and human mRNAs and only those targets that were conserved between the two species were retained. Finally, we aligned these predicted targets against our published Affymetrix gene expression profiles from mouse distal colonic epithelial cells [60]. Predicted targets that were not scored as 'Present' in this dataset were eliminated from further analysis. Networks were generated through the use of Ingenuity Pathway Analysis (Ingenuity Systems®, www.ingenuity.com). Functional analysis was used to identify the biological functions and/or diseases that were most significant to the molecules in the network. The network molecules associated with biological functions and/or diseases in Ingenuity's Knowledge Base were considered for the analysis. Right-tailed Fisher's exact test was used to calculate p-value determining the probability that each biological function and/or disease assigned to that network is due to chance alone.

Supporting Information

Table S1 Expression values of differentially expressed miRNAs in DSS-induced acute colitis as determined by three different normalization method. Shown are differentially expressed miRNAs scored as significantly different (P≤0.01) in one or more of the analyses: rank order statistics (Rnk_Diff), t-test using median normalized data (Med_Norm), or the Statminer implementation of Limma (Limma_SM). Using additional filters of ≥(±10),P≤0.01 for rank difference and ≥(±1.0) P≤0.01 for Med_Norm and Limma_SM approaches, 51 miRNAs (shown in bold) overlapped among the three normalization methods. (XLSX)

Table S2 Expression values of miRNAs in CAC and APC tumor samples. Raw Ct values for miRNAs are shown for CAC (n = 4) and APC (n = 5) tumor samples. Detectors that were scored as 'undetectable' were assigned Ct values of 40. Additionally, rank order statistics (Rnk_Diff) was used to compare miRNA profiles in CAC versus APC tumors. Each miRNA within a given sample was force ranked on analog readout of miRNA abundance (Ct value). All miRNAs with Ct = 40 were assigned the same rank within a sample. A t-test (assuming unequal variance) was then carried out to compare the rank order assignments of miRNAs in the two different groups so as to identify miRNAs whose mean rank order of expression changed significantly. (XLSX)

Author Contributions

Conceived and designed the experiments: BMN EAT. Performed the experiments: JMC YWC. Analyzed the data: BMN JMC YWA EAT. Wrote the paper: BMN EAT.

References

1. Ambros V (2004) The functions of animal microRNAs. Nature 431: 350–355.
2. Asli NS, Pitulescu ME, Kessel M (2008) MicroRNAs in organogenesis and disease. Curr Mol Med 8: 698–710.
3. Bartel DP (2004) MicroRNAs: genomics, biogenesis, mechanism, and function. Cell 116: 281–297.
4. Bueno MJ, de Castro IP, Malumbres M (2008) Control of cell proliferation pathways by microRNAs. Cell Cycle 7: 3143–3148.
5. Lee YS, Dutta A (2009) MicroRNAs in cancer. Annu Rev Pathol 4: 199–227.
6. Lu LF, Liston A (2009) MicroRNA in the immune system, microRNA as an immune system. Immunology 127: 291–298.
7. Maatouk D, Harfe B (2006) MicroRNAs in development. Scientific World Journal 6: 1828–1840.
8. Wang Y, Lee CG (2009) MicroRNA and cancer–focus on apoptosis. J Cell Mol Med 13: 12–23.
9. Zeng Y, Yi R, Cullen BR (2003) MicroRNAs and small interfering RNAs can inhibit mRNA expression by similar mechanisms. Proc Natl Acad Sci U S A 100: 9779–9784.
10. John B, Enright AJ, Aravin A, Tuschl T, Sander C, et al. (2004) Human MicroRNA targets. PLoS Biol 2: e363.
11. Lewis BP, Burge CB, Bartel DP (2005) Conserved seed pairing, often flanked by adenosines, indicates that thousands of human genes are microRNA targets. Cell 120: 15–20.
12. Arndt GM, Dossey L, Cullen LM, Lai A, Druker R, et al. (2009) Characterization of global microRNA expression reveals oncogenic potential of miR-145 in metastatic colorectal cancer. BMC Cancer 9: 374.
13. Bandres E, Cubedo E, Agirre X, Malumbres R, Zarate R, et al. (2006) Identification by Real-time PCR of 13 mature microRNAs differentially expressed in colorectal cancer and non-tumoral tissues. Mol Cancer 5: 29.
14. Monzo M, Navarro A, Bandres E, Artells R, Moreno I, et al. (2008) Overlapping expression of microRNAs in human embryonic colon and colorectal cancer. Cell Res 18: 823–833.
15. Sarver AL, French AJ, Borralho PM, Thayanithy V, Oberg AL, et al. (2009) Human colon cancer profiles show differential microRNA expression depending on mismatch repair status and are characteristic of undifferentiated proliferative states. BMC Cancer 9: 401.
16. Slaby O, Svoboda M, Fabian P, Smerdova T, Knoflickova D, et al. (2007) Altered expression of miR-21, miR-31, miR-143 and miR-145 is related to clinicopathologic features of colorectal cancer. Oncology 72: 397–402.
17. Motoyama K, Inoue H, Takatsuno Y, Tanaka F, Mimori K, et al. (2009) Over- and under-expressed microRNAs in human colorectal cancer. Int J Oncol 34: 1069–1075.
18. Schepeler T, Reinert JT, Ostenfeld MS, Christensen LL, Silahtaroglu AN, et al. (2008) Diagnostic and prognostic microRNAs in stage II colon cancer. Cancer Res 68: 6416–6424.
19. Yantiss RK, Goodarzi M, Zhou XK, Rennert H, Pirog EC, et al. (2009) Clinical, pathologic, and molecular features of early-onset colorectal carcinoma. Am J Surg Pathol 33: 572–582.
20. Wang YX, Zhang XY, Zhang BF, Yang CQ, Chen XM, et al. (2010) Initial study of microRNA expression profiles of colonic cancer without lymph node metastasis. J Dig Dis 11: 50–54.
21. Ng EK, Tsang WP, Ng SS, Jin HC, Yu J, et al. (2009) MicroRNA-143 targets DNA methyltransferases 3A in colorectal cancer. Br J Cancer 101: 699–706.
22. Earle JS, Luthra R, Romans A, Abraham R, Ensor J, et al. (2010) Association of microRNA expression with microsatellite instability status in colorectal adenocarcinoma. J Mol Diagn 12: 433–440.
23. Chen X, Guo X, Zhang H, Xiang Y, Chen J, et al. (2009) Role of miR-143 targeting KRAS in colorectal tumorigenesis. Oncogene 28: 1385–1392.
24. Volinia S, Calin GA, Liu CG, Ambs S, Cimmino A, et al. (2006) A microRNA expression signature of human solid tumors defines cancer gene targets. Proc Natl Acad Sci U S A 103: 2257–2261.
25. Olaru AV, Selaru FM, Mori Y, Vazquez C, David S, et al. (2011) Dynamic changes in the expression of MicroRNA-31 during inflammatory bowel disease-associated neoplastic transformation. Inflamm Bowel Dis 17: 221–231.
26. Slattery ML, Wolff E, Hoffman MD, Pellatt DF, Milash B, et al. (2011) MicroRNAs and colon and rectal cancer: differential expression by tumor location and subtype. Genes Chromosomes Cancer 50: 196–206.
27. Ng EK, Chong WW, Jin H, Lam EK, Shin VY, et al. (2009) Differential expression of microRNAs in plasma of patients with colorectal cancer: a potential marker for colorectal cancer screening. Gut 58: 1375–1381.
28. Balaguer F, Link A, Lozano JJ, Cuatrecasas M, Nagasaka T, et al. (2010) Epigenetic silencing of miR-137 is an early event in colorectal carcinogenesis. Cancer Res 70: 6609–6618.
29. Liu M, Lang N, Qiu M, Xu F, Li Q, et al. (2010) miR-137 targets Cdc42 expression, induces cell cycle G1 arrest and inhibits invasion in colorectal cancer cells. Int J Cancer.
30. Boni V, Bitarte N, Cristobal I, Zarate R, Rodriguez J, et al. (2010) miR-192/miR-215 Influence 5-Fluorouracil Resistance through Cell Cycle-Mediated

Mechanisms Complementary to its Posttranscriptional Thymidilate Synthase Regulation. Mol Cancer Ther.

31. Song B, Wang Y, Titmus MA, Botchkina G, Formentini A, et al. (2010) Molecular mechanism of chemoresistance by miR-215 in osteosarcoma and colon cancer cells. Mol Cancer 9: 96.

32. Lanza G, Ferracin M, Gafa R, Veronese A, Spizzo R, et al. (2007) mRNA/microRNA gene expression profile in microsatellite unstable colorectal cancer. Mol Cancer 6: 54.

33. Nagel R, le Sage C, Diosdado B, van der Waal M, Oude Vrielink JA, et al. (2008) Regulation of the adenomatous polyposis coli gene by the miR-135 family in colorectal cancer. Cancer Res 68: 5795–5802.

34. Nakajima G, Hayashi K, Xi Y, Kudo K, Uchida K, et al. (2006) Non-coding MicroRNAs hsa-let-7g and hsa-miR-181b are Associated with Chemoresponse to S-1 in Colon Cancer. Cancer Genomics Proteomics 3: 317–324.

35. Xi Y, Shalgi R, Fodstad O, Pilpel Y, Ju J (2006) Differentially regulated micro-RNAs and actively translated messenger RNA transcripts by tumor suppressor p53 in colon cancer. Clin Cancer Res 12: 2014–2024.

36. Yang L, Belaguli N, Berger DH (2009) MicroRNA and colorectal cancer. World J Surg 33: 638–646.

37. Braun CJ, Zhang X, Savelyeva I, Wolff S, Moll UM, et al. (2008) p53-Responsive micrornas 192 and 215 are capable of inducing cell cycle arrest. Cancer Res 68: 10094–10104.

38. Schetter AJ, Leung SY, Sohn JJ, Zanetti KA, Bowman ED, et al. (2008) MicroRNA expression profiles associated with prognosis and therapeutic outcome in colon adenocarcinoma. Jama 299: 425–436.

39. Wang CJ, Zhou ZG, Wang L, Yang L, Zhou B, et al. (2009) Clinicopathological significance of microRNA-31, −143 and −145 expression in colorectal cancer. Dis Markers 26: 27–34.

40. Michael MZ, SM OC, van Holst Pellekaan NG, Young GP, James RJ (2003) Reduced accumulation of specific microRNAs in colorectal neoplasia. Mol Cancer Res 1: 882–891.

41. Davidson LA, Wang N, Shah MS, Lupton JR, Ivanov I, et al (2009) n-3 Polyunsaturated fatty acids modulate carcinogen-directed non-coding micro-RNA signatures in rat colon. Carcinogenesis 30: 2077–2084.

42. Cottonham CL, Kaneko S, Xu L (2010) miR-21 and miR-31 converge on TIAM1 to regulate migration and invasion of colon carcinoma cells. J Biol Chem 285: 35293–35302.

43. Wang CJ, Stratmann J, Zhou ZG, Sun XF (2010) Suppression of microRNA-31 increases sensitivity to 5-FU at an early stage, and affects cell migration and invasion in HCT-116 colon cancer cells. BMC Cancer 10: 616.

44. Georges SA, Biery MC, Kim SY, Schelter JM, Guo J, et al. (2008) Coordinated regulation of cell cycle transcripts by p53-Inducible microRNAs, miR-192 and miR-215. Cancer Res 68: 10105–10112.

45. Song B, Wang Y, Kudo K, Gavin EJ, Xi Y, et al. (2008) miR-192 Regulates dihydrofolate reductase and cellular proliferation through the p53-microRNA circuit. Clin Cancer Res 14: 8080–8086.

46. La Rocca G, Badin M, Shi B, Xu SQ, Deangelis T, et al. (2009) Mechanism of growth inhibition by MicroRNA 145: the role of the IGF-I receptor signaling pathway. J Cell Physiol 220: 485–491.

47. La Rocca G, Shi B, Badin M, De Angelis T, Sepp-Lorenzino L, et al. (2009) Growth inhibition by microRNAs that target the insulin receptor substrate-1. Cell Cycle 8: 2255–2259.

48. Shi B, Sepp-Lorenzino L, Prisco M, Linsley P, deAngelis T, et al. (2007) Micro RNA 145 targets the insulin receptor substrate-1 and inhibits the growth of colon cancer cells. J Biol Chem 282: 32582–32590.

49. Zhang J, Guo H, Zhang H, Wang H, Qian G, et al. (2011) Putative tumor suppressor miR-145 inhibits colon cancer cell growth by targeting oncogene friend leukemia virus integration 1 gene. Cancer 117: 86–95.

50. Gregersen LH, Jacobsen AB, Frankel LB, Wen J, Krogh A, et al. (2010) MicroRNA-145 targets YES and STAT1 in colon cancer cells. PLoS One 5: e8836.

51. Fantini MC, Pallone F (2008) Cytokines: from gut inflammation to colorectal cancer. Curr Drug Targets 9: 375–380.

52. Karin M, Greten FR (2005) NF-kappaB: linking inflammation and immunity to cancer development and progression. Nat Rev Immunol 5: 749–759.

53. Eaden JA, Abrams KR, Mayberry JF (2001) The risk of colorectal cancer in ulcerative colitis: a meta-analysis. Gut 48: 526–535.

54. Sonkoly E, Stahle M, Pivarcsi A (2008) MicroRNAs: novel regulators in skin inflammation. Clin Exp Dermatol 33: 312–315.

55. Ahmed FE, Jeffries CD, Vos PW, Flake G, Nuovo GJ, et al. (2009) Diagnostic microRNA markers for screening sporadic human colon cancer and active ulcerative colitis in stool and tissue. Cancer Genomics Proteomics 6: 281–295.

56. Wu F, Zikusoka M, Trindade A, Dassopoulos T, Harris ML, et al. (2008) MicroRNAs are differentially expressed in ulcerative colitis and alter expression of macrophage inflammatory peptide-2 alpha. Gastroenterology 135: 1624–1635 e1624.

57. Krek A, Grun D, Poy MN, Wolf R, Rosenberg L, et al. (2005) Combinatorial microRNA target predictions. Nat Genet 37: 495–500.

58. Kiriakidou M, Nelson PT, Kouranov A, Fitziev P, Bouyioukos C, et al. (2004) A combined computational-experimental approach predicts human microRNA targets. Genes Dev 18: 1165–1178.

59. Friedman RC, Farh KK, Burge CB, Bartel DP (2009) Most mammalian mRNAs are conserved targets of microRNAs. Genome Res 19: 92–105.

60. Su W, Bush CR, Necela BM, Calcagno SR, Murray NR, et al. (2007) Differential expression, distribution, and function of PPAR-gamma in the proximal and distal colon. Physiol Genomics 30: 342–353.

61. Gusev Y, ed. MicroRNA Profiling in Cancer: A Bioinformatics Perspective. , Singapore: Pan Stanford Publishing Pte. Ltd.. pp 257.

62. Navon R, Wang H, Steinfeld I, Tsalenko A, Ben-Dor A, et al. (2009) Novel rank-based statistical methods reveal microRNAs with differential expression in multiple cancer types. PLoS One 4: e8003.

63. Okayasu I, Hatakeyama S, Yamada M, Ohkusa T, Inagaki Y, et al. (1990) A novel method in the induction of reliable experimental acute and chronic ulcerative colitis in mice. Gastroenterology 98: 694–702.

64. Seril DN, Liao J, Ho KL, Yang CS, Yang GY (2002) Inhibition of chronic ulcerative colitis-associated colorectal adenocarcinoma development in a murine model by N-acetylcysteine. Carcinogenesis 23: 993–1001.

CD47^{Low} Status on CD4 Effectors is Necessary for the Contraction/Resolution of the Immune Response in Humans and Mice

Vu Quang Van[1], Nobuyasu Baba[1], Manuel Rubio[1], Keiko Wakahara[1], Benoit Panzini[2], Carole Richard[3], Genevieve Soucy[4], Denis Franchimont[5], Genevieve Fortin[6], Ana Carolina Martinez Torres[7,8,9], Lauriane Cabon[7,8,9], Santos Susin[7,8,9], Marika Sarfati[1]*

1 Immunoregulation Laboratory, Centre Hospitalier de l'Université de Montréal, Research Center (CRCHUM), Notre-Dame Hospital, Montreal, Quebec, Canada, 2 Department of Gastroenterology, Centre Hospitalier de l'Université de Montréal (CHUM), Notre-Dame Hospital, Montreal, Quebec, Canada, 3 Department of Digestive Tract Surgery, Centre Hospitalier de l'Université de Montréal (CHUM), Notre-Dame Hospital, Montreal, Quebec, Canada, 4 Department of Pathology, Centre Hospitalier de l'Université de Montréal (CHUM), Notre-Dame Hospital, Montreal, Quebec, Canada, 5 Department de Gastroenterology, Erasme Hospital, Université Libre de Bruxelles (ULB), Bruxelles, Belgique, 6 Research Institute of McGill University Health Centre, McGill University, Montreal, Quebec, Canada, 7 INSERM U872, Mort Cellulaire Programmée et Physiopathologie des Cellules Tumorales, Equipe 19, Centre de Recherche des Cordeliers, Paris, France, 8 Université Pierre et Marie Curie-Sorbonne Universités, UMRS 872, Paris, France, 9 Université Paris Descartes, Paris, France

Abstract

How do effector CD4 T cells escape cell death during the contraction of the immune response (IR) remain largely unknown. CD47, through interactions with thrombospondin-1 (TSP-1) and SIRP-α, is implicated in cell death and phagocytosis of malignant cells. Here, we reported a reduction in SIRP-α-Fc binding to effector memory T cells (T$_{EM}$) and in vitro TCR-activated human CD4 T cells that was linked to TSP-1/CD47-induced cell death. The reduced SIRP-α-Fc binding (CD47^{low} status) was not detected when CD4 T cells were stained with two anti-CD47 mAbs, which recognize distinct epitopes. In contrast, increased SIRP-α-Fc binding (CD47^{high} status) marked central memory T cells (T$_{CM}$) as well as activated CD4 T cells exposed to IL-2, and correlated with resistance to TSP-1/CD47-mediated killing. Auto-aggressive CD4 effectors, which accumulated in lymph nodes and at mucosal sites of patients with Crohn's disease, displayed a CD47^{high} status despite a high level of TSP-1 release in colonic tissues. In mice, CD47 (CD47^{low} status) was required on antigen (Ag)-specific CD4 effectors for the contraction of the IR in vivo, as significantly lower numbers of Ag-specific CD47$^{+/+}$CD4 T cells were recovered when compared to Ag-specific CD47$^{-/-}$ CD4 T cells. In conclusion, we demonstrate that a transient change in the status of CD47, i.e. from CD47^{high} to CD47^{low}, on CD4 effectors regulates the decision-making process that leads to CD47-mediated cell death and contraction of the IR while maintenance of a CD47^{high} status on tissue-destructive CD4 effectors prevents the resolution of the inflammatory response.

Editor: Yoshihiko Hoshino, National Institute of Infectious Diseases, Japan

Funding: This work was supported by Canadian Institutes of Health Research – CIHR (no MOP-102562) and Crohn's and Colitis Foundation of Canada. The funders had no role in study design, data collection and analysis, decision to publish, or preparation of the manuscript.

Competing Interests: The authors have declared that no competing interests exist.

* E-mail: m.sarfati@umontreal.ca

Introduction

During an adaptive immune response (IR), naive T cells responding to Ag proliferate vigorously. While the majority of activated T cells will be killed and eliminated (the contraction phase), effector T cells that have passed this checkpoint will survive and execute their memory T cell differentiation program to generate long-lived memory T cells. Central questions are to determine which cells among proliferating effector T cells will live or die, which cells will be cleared or not, and which factors will dictate these crucial decisions [1]. Although re-expression of IL-7R is a determinant for the survival of effectors that will generate memory T cells [2,3], no surface molecule has been implicated in the control of cell death and elimination during the contraction phase of the IR. Neither differential Fas expression, nor Fas-induced cell death susceptibility can explain why some effectors die during an acute immune response [4,5].

CD47, known as integrin-associated protein (IAP), contains a single IgV-like extracellular domain, a multiple membrane-spanning domain (MMS) and a short intracytoplasmic tail, which is devoid of signaling motifs [6]. CD47, considered as a marker of self, is expressed on hematopoietic and non-hematopoietic cells and regulates two key functions implicated in the IR: cell death and cell elimination [7]. CD47 interacts in cis with integrins and in trans with two ligands, thrombospondin-1 (TSP-1) and signal regulatory protein alpha (SIRP-α). TSP-1 binds two distinct regions on the CD47 IgV loop while it competes with SIRP-α (D1 distal domain) for one of the two CD47 binding sites [8,9]. SIRP-α/CD47 interaction controls immune cell elimination. CD47 delivers a negative signal through SIRP-α expressed on resident macrophages or dendritic cells (DCs) to inhibit the clearance of intact hematopoietic cells [10]. In this regard, CD47 expression must be transiently up-regulated on circulating wild type hematopoietic stem cells to spare them from clearance during bone marrow exit [11]. TSP-1/CD47 interaction induces the caspase-independent cell death of malignant B and T lymphocytes [7,12,13]. TSP-1 is mainly secreted by antigen presenting cells (APCs) and facilitates the clearance of damaged apoptotic cells by APCs [14]. In addition, increased TSP-1 binding facilitates the elimination of aged erythrocytes by SIRP-α^+ macrophages [15]. We recently reported that CD47 status (SIRP-α Fc binding) is transiently regulated on murine CD4 T cells following in vivo immunization. More precisely, CD47^{high} status marked central memory T (T$_{CM}$) CD4 precursors at an early time point of the IR, while CD47^{low} status identified activated CD4 T cells [16].

In the present study, we demonstrated that CD47 expression and more particularly CD47^{low} status on murine activated CD4 T cells, is key for the contraction phase of the IR in vivo. In addition, we showed that TCR activation induced a transient change in the CD47 status on human CD4 T cells, i.e. from CD47^{high} to CD47^{low} to CD47^{high}, which was linked to TSP-1/CD47-mediated cell death in vitro. Importantly, CD47^{low} status was maintained on CD4 effectors cells in inflamed lymphoid and mucosal tissues of patients with Crohn's disease (CD). We thus propose that CD47/SIRP-α/TSP-1 axis is involved in the resolution of the inflammatory response.

Results

1. CD47 Status is Differentially Regulated on TCR-Activated Human CD4 T Cell Subsets

We first investigated the modulation of CD47 expression on in vitro activated human CD4 T cell subsets. To this end, we thought to use a SIRP-α-Fc fusion protein and two anti-CD47 monoclonal antibodies (mAbs) that identify different CD47 conformations [15,17,18,19,20] and/or distinct CD47 epitopes [21]. Hence, B6H12 mAb and SIRP-α-Fc compete for a similar CD47 binding site since B6H12 but not 2D3 inhibits SIRP-α-Fc binding to CD47 [22]. We showed that CD47 expression, as detected by SIRP-α-Fc binding, decreased on a majority of divided naïve CD4 T cells (T$_N$; CD45RA$^+$CCR7$^+$) following stimulation with anti-CD3 and anti-CD28 mAbs (Fig. 1A). The reduced CD47 expression was not observed when activated CD4 T cells were stained with B6H12 anti-CD47 mAb. Thus, decreased SIRP-α-Fc binding to CD47 on activated T$_N$ cells was hereafter referred to as CD47^{low} status when compared to SIRP-α-Fc binding to CD47 on undivided T$_N$ cells as well as on 50% of activated central memory (T$_{CM}$; CD45RA$^-$CCR7$^+$CD27$^+$) T cells hereafter referred to as CD47^{high} status (Fig. 1A). Divided CD47^{low} CD4 T cells displayed an effector phenotype (CCR7^{low}) when compared to undivided CD47^{high} CD4 T cells (Fig. 1B).

Further studies demonstrated that CD47 status was differentially modulated in ex vivo isolated circulating human CD4 T cell subsets (Fig. 1C). Effector memory (T$_{EM}$; CD45RA$^-$CCR7$^-$CD27$^-$) T cells, which represent chronically activated T cells by repeated exposure to Ag in the peripheral blood of healthy individuals, displayed a CD47^{low} status when compared to CD47^{high} T$_N$ and T$_{CM}$ T cells (Fig. 1D). Transitional memory (T$_{TM}$, CD45RA$^-$CCR7$^-$CD27$^+$) and terminally differentiated (T$_{TD}$, CD45RA$^+$CCR7$^-$CD27$^-$) cells were detected as CD47^{low} cells. Alike in vitro TCR-activated CD4 T cells, T$_N$, T$_{EM}$ and T$_{CM}$ expressed similar levels of CD47 expression when they were stained with B6H12 and 2D3 anti-CD47 mAbs, suggesting a change in the conformation rather than in the amount of CD47 protein. Indeed, western blot analysis showed that the three

circulating CD4 T cells subsets possessed similar CD47 protein content (Fig. 1E). We next investigated whether differences seen in SIRP-α- Fc binding to CD47 may reflect a differential distribution of CD47 on the cell surface of T$_N$, T$_{EM}$ and T$_{CM}$. As depicted by confocal microscopy, SIRP-α- Fc staining revealed a homogenous distribution of CD47 molecules on the cell surface of T$_N$ and T$_{CM}$ while a distinct and patchy redistribution was observed on T$_{EM}$ (Fig. 1F). In contrast, no characteristic CD47 distribution was found between T$_N$, T$_{EM}$ and T$_{CM}$ using B6H12 mAb. Additionally, SIRP-α-Fc failed to bind CD47 with a truncated transmembrane domain in a modified human T cell line (Fig. S1). We propose that TCR activation elicits a post transcriptional/translational modification of the CD47 molecule that dictates its ability to bind SIRP-α-Fc but not B6H12 or 2D3 mAbs. These data strongly suggested that CD47 status on T$_{EM}$ and T$_{CM}$ subsets reflect different CD47 protein conformations, as these T cells possessed similar protein content.

2. IL-2 Induces a CD47^{high} Status on Human TCR-activated CD47^{low} CD4 T Cells

Several cytokines that signal through receptors sharing the common γ chain (γc) are critical for peripheral homeostasis and the generation of memory T cells [23,24]. We found that a large proportion of TCR-activated naive CD4 T cells regained a CD47^{high} status when these cells were cultured in the presence of IL-2, with or without CD3 restimulation and co-stimulation (Fig. 2A). This suggested that CFSE^{low}CD47^{high} activated T$_{CM}$ cells arose from CD47^{low} T cells. To rule out the possibility that CD47^{high} T cells originated from a few CD47^{high} T cells, which had proliferated and never modified their CD47 status, CD47^{low} CD4 T cells were purified at the end of T cell primary cultures (day 6) and then were re-stimulated. We demonstrated that, indeed, IL-2 induced the re-establishment of a CD47^{high} and central memory (CCR7^{high}) phenotype in FACS sorted purified TCR-activated CD47^{low} CD4 T cells (Fig. 2B). The appearance of CD47^{high} effectors preceded that of CD127 positive cells (Fig. 2C). Thus, human CD4 T cells transiently modulate their CD47 status in response to polyclonal activation, and T$_{CM}$ phenotype is associated with the reacquisition of a CD47^{high} status.

3. CD47^{low} Status is Linked to TSP-1-induced Cell Death Susceptibility

We next explored whether the transient modulation of CD47 status seen on CD4 T cells might be linked to functional consequences such as T cell death, which occurs during the resolution of the IR. Ligation of CD47 by 4N1K, a peptide that corresponds to the CD47-binding C-terminal domain of TSP-1, kills malignant B cells and T cell lines through a caspase and Fas-independent pathway [13,25,26,27]. We therefore assessed the TSP-1/CD47-mediated cell death of human CD4 T cells in relation to their CD47^{low} or CD47^{high} status. TCR-activated CD47^{low} T cells were susceptible to 4N1K-induced cell death (Fig. 3A). However, they became resistant when they were cultured in the presence of IL-2 and reacquired a CD47^{high} status, linking a change in the CD47 status to susceptibility to TSP-induced cell death. Specific CD47-mediated killing was demonstrated in T$_{EM}$, while T$_N$ and a large fraction of T$_{CM}$ were largely protected from 4N1K-induced cell death (Fig. 3B), corroborating our in vitro findings with TCR-activated T cells. We next asked whether differential CD47 status on CD4 T cell subsets correlated with the switching on of one common "eat me" signal, i.e. calreticulin, which favors cell elimination when CD47/SIRP-α interactions are interrupted [28]. Expression

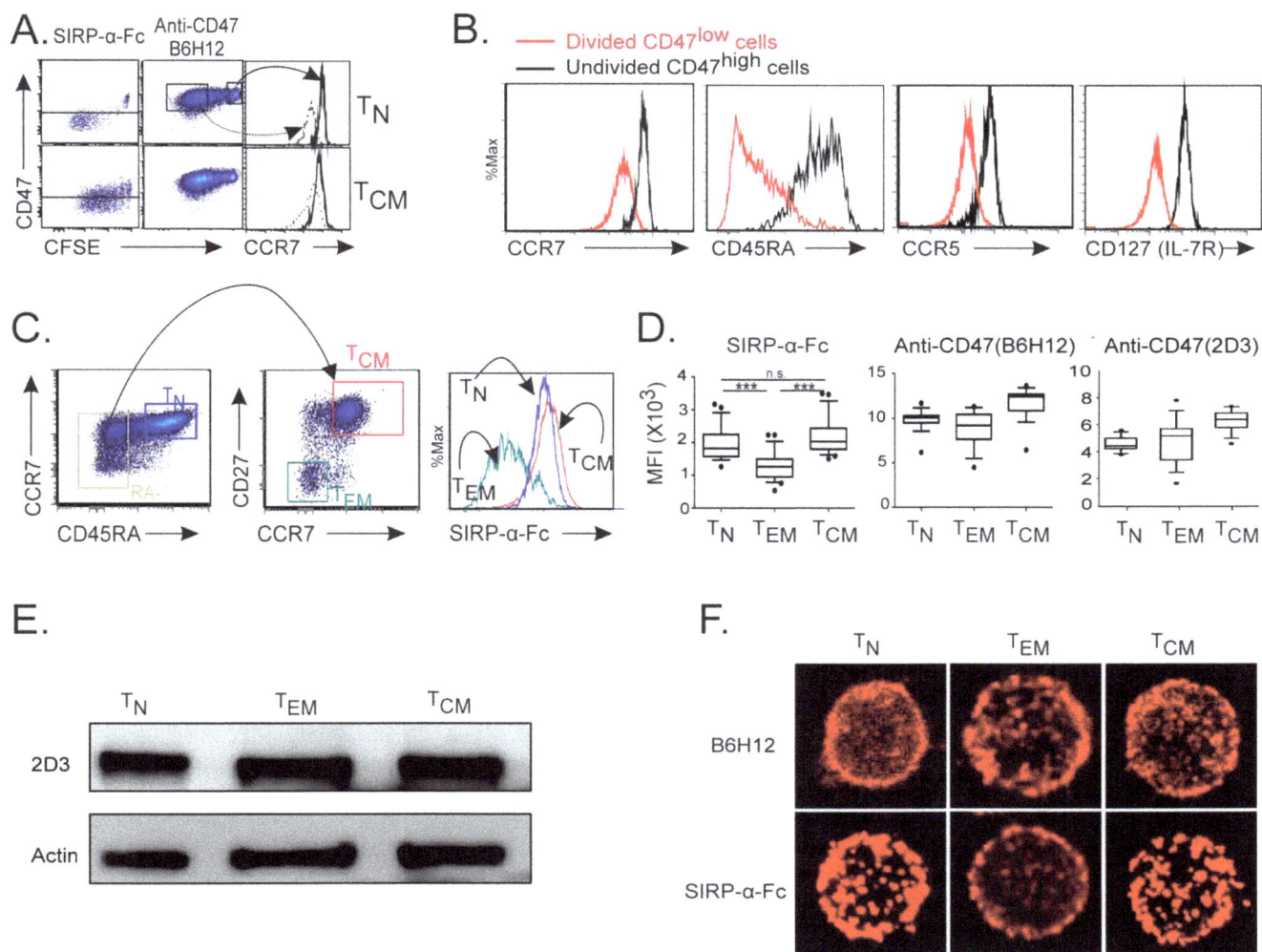

Figure 1. CD47 status is differentially regulated on TCR- activated human CD4 T cell subsets. (**A–B**) CFSE-labeled T_N and T_{CM} cells were stimulated with immobilized anti-CD3 and soluble anti-CD28 mAbs for 6 days. (A) CD47 (using human SIRP-α-Fc protein or anti-CD47 mAb, clone B6H12) and CCR7 expression was analyzed by flow cytometry. (B) Phenotype of divided CD47^{low} and undivided CD47^{high} cells at day 6 of T_N cultures. (**C**) Strategies to examine CD47 expression on *ex vivo* isolated human T cells gated on CD4$^+$ T cells. (**D**) CD47 expression on CD4 T cell subsets using SIRP-α-Fc and anti-CD47 antibodies (B6H12 and 2D3). The mean ± standard deviation (SD) for 16 donors is shown (Anova test: ***p<0.0001). (**E**) Western blot analysis for CD47 protein on whole-cell lysates using 2D3 mAb. (**F**) Confocal immunofluorescence of CD47 using SIRP-α-Fc or anti-CD47 (B6H12) antibodies. (**A–C; E and F**) Data are representative of 3 to 6 independent experiments.

of calreticulin was not detected on viable T_N, T_{EM}, or T_{CM}, although it was significantly induced on T_{EM} killed by 4N1K (Fig. 3C). We propose that killing of CD47^{low} T cells occurs upstream of cell clearance, with the latter being mediated by up-regulation of "eat me" signals combined with the interruption of SIRP-α/CD47 interactions.

4. Chronically Activated T Cells Display a CD47^{high} Status in Lymphoid and Intestinal Tissues of Patients with Crohn's Disease

Survival of auto-aggressive T cells in tissues prevents the resolution of the inflammatory response and perpetuates disease in patients with inflammatory bowel disease (IBD) [29]. More specifically, lamina propria T cells appear resistant to cell death in Crohn's disease (CD). We therefore asked whether escape to cell death of mucosal CD4 T cells correlated with their CD47 status in CD patients. To this end, we examined binding of SIRP-α-Fc to

CD47 on CD4 T cells in blood, mesenteric lymph nodes (mLNs) and intestinal lamina propria mononuclear cells (LPMC) of CD patients. As expected, the frequency of CD4 effectors (CD45RA$^-$CD27$^{+/-}$CCR7$^-$) was increased in mLNs and LPMC when compared to PBMC, whereas that of T_{CM} (CD45RA$^-$CD27$^+$CCR7$^+$) was reduced accordingly (Fig. 4A). Despite abundant TSP-1 release in inflamed colonic CD tissues (Fig. 4B), both CCR7$^+$ and CCR7$^-$ CD4 T cell subsets that infiltrated mLNs and inflamed gut tissues expressed a CD47^{high} status (Fig. 4C) that could explain the maintenance of auto-aggressive T cells. However, as in healthy donors (Fig. 1), circulating T_{EM} and T_{CM} displayed a CD47^{low} and CD47^{high} status, respectively in patients with CD or an unrelated intestinal disorder (non IBD)(Fig. 4). To verify that absence of differential CD47 status on CCR7$^+$ and CCR7$^-$ memory T cells was not a property of T cells that were recruited to peripheral tissues, we also examined mLNs and LPMC of patients with non IBD. As depicted in the same figure, CCR7$^-$ effectors displayed a CD47^{low}

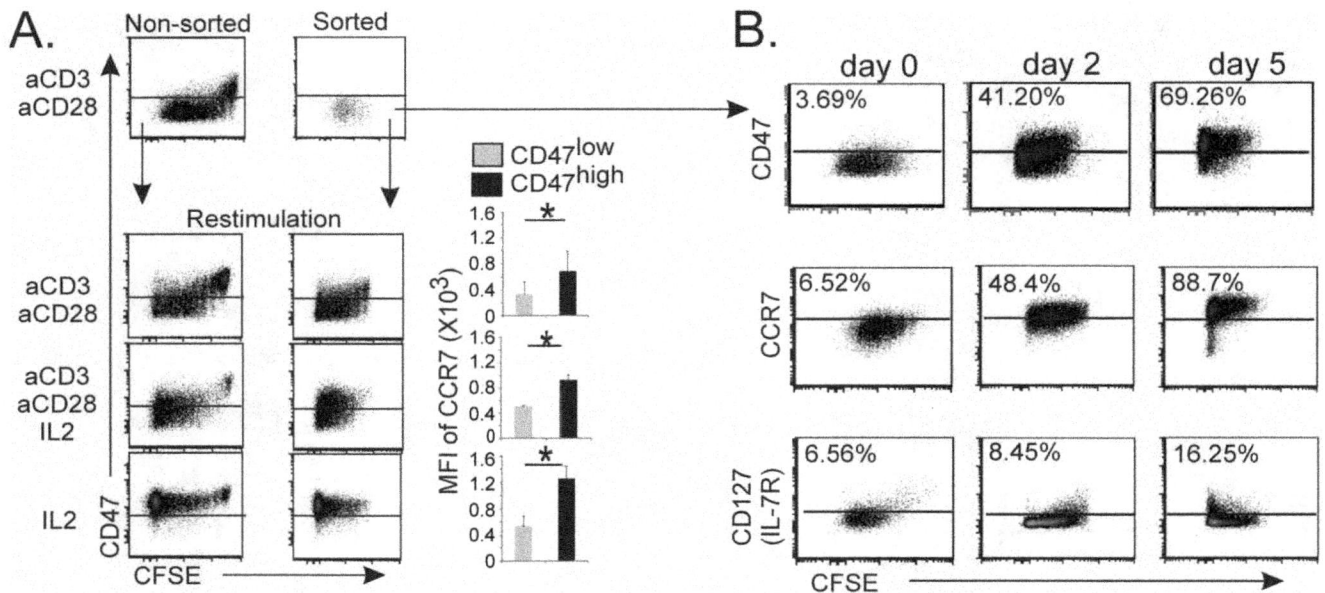

Figure 2. IL-2 induces CD47^{high} status on TCR-activated human CD47^{low} CD4 T cells. (A) CFSE-labeled T$_N$ cells (left panels) were activated with immobilized anti-CD3 and soluble anti-CD28 mAbs for 6 days. Unfractionated activated T cells or FACS sorted CD47^{low} T cells (middle panels) were restimulated for 5 days as indicated. CD47 expression in relation to cell division (CFSE cell dilution) and CCR7 expression in relation to CD47 status. **(B)** T$_N$ were activated as in A and FACS sorted CD47^{low} (day 6) T cells were restimulated in presence of IL-2. Kinetics of CD47 (SIRP-α-Fc protein), CCR7 and CD127 expression is shown. **(A–B)** Data are representative of at least 4 to 6 independent experiments. Right panel A shows the mean ± standard deviation (SD) for 5 independent experiments. Student t test: *p<0.05.

status in mLNs and colons of non IBD donors as reflected by the ratio of CD47 mean fluorescence intensity (MFI) between CCR7$^-$ and CCR7$^+$ T cells. These data suggest that CD4 effectors maintain a CD47^{high} status in inflamed colons, which confers them a resistance to TSP-1-mediated cell death in tissues and favors their accumulation.

6. Expression of CD47 is Required on Murine Ag-specific CD4 T Cells for the Contraction Phase *in vivo*

We recently reported that CD47^{low} status is observed on activated murine CD4 T cells *in vivo*, independently of the route and the methods of immunization [16]. We hypothesized, here, that CD47^{low} status and CD47-mediated cell death are involved in the crash of the IR, while the reestablishment of a CD47^{high} status might offer an advantage to pre-committed T$_{CM}$ cells to escape cell death and elimination. Indeed, CD47^{high} status marked T$_{CM}$ precursors at an early time point of IR [16]. We therefore determined whether CD47 expression and/or CD47 status on murine CD4 T cells had an impact on the contraction phase of the IR *in vivo*. CD47 is implicated in cell elimination [10]. Hence, viable CD47$^{-/-}$ Tg T cells are readily cleared from wild type hosts, whereas they can be adoptively transferred into CD47-deficient hosts without being cleared [30,31]. Here, CD47$^{-/-}$ hosts were passively transferred with Tg CD47$^{-/-}$ or CD47$^{+/+}$ CD4 T cells and immunized subcutaneously with CFA/OVA. Kinetics revealed that proliferation of Tg CD47$^{+/-}$ T cells occurred at an early time point followed by cell contraction (Fig. 5A). The latter correlated with a change to a CD47^{low} status (Fig. 5B). Tg CD47$^{+/+}$ T cells also proliferated, albeit at a lower rate, in DEC205-OVA when compared to CFA/OVA immunized mice before their elimination from hosts (Fig. 5C). Although the recovery of Tg CD47$^{+/+}$ and CD47$^{-/-}$ CD4 T cells was similar until day 9, the absence of CD47 on CD4 T cells significantly

increased the yield of Ag-specific T cells at later time points in both immunogenic (CFA/OVA) and tolerogenic (DEC205-OVA) responses (Fig. 5). Tg CD47$^{-/-}$ T cells were still retraced 70 days after immunization. Therefore, we demonstrate that CD47 expression, and specifically a CD47^{low} status, is required on CD4 T cells for the contraction phase during an acute immune response.

Discussion

The pathway to memory T cell generation can be divided into 3 sequential and critical steps during an acute immune response: 1) resistance to massive cell death, 2) prevention of viable cell elimination, and 3) cell survival. CD47 is implicated in the two first steps [7]. We propose here that a change to a CD47^{low} status is key to determine the cell's decision to die while the commitment to cell clearance occurs as a downstream event. The CD47^{low} status was detected by staining CD4 T cells with a SIRP-α-Fc fusion protein, although it was not observed using two anti-CD47 mAbs that recognize distinct epitopes. Combined with flow cytometry data, the confocal microscopy and Western blot analysis suggest that CD47 status is linked to a post-translational modification and/or cell surface redistribution rather than to differences in the amounts of CD47 protein expression. A change in the CD47 conformation has been reported in several earlier studies. In fact, binding of B6H12, 2D3 mAbs and SIRP-α-Fc to CD47 is regulated by several factors such as temperature, the cell type on which CD47 is expressed and the presence of cholesterol [17,32]. For example, affinity of B6H12 and 2D3 mAb for CD47 is higher when monocytes but not RBC, are incubated at 37C instead of 0C. In addition, CD47 displays a different conformation on sickle RBC when compared to normal RBC [18]. 2D3 binds with greater affinity than B6H12 mAb to CD47 on sickle [18] and aged erythrocytes [15], which results in adhesion to TSP-1 under ow

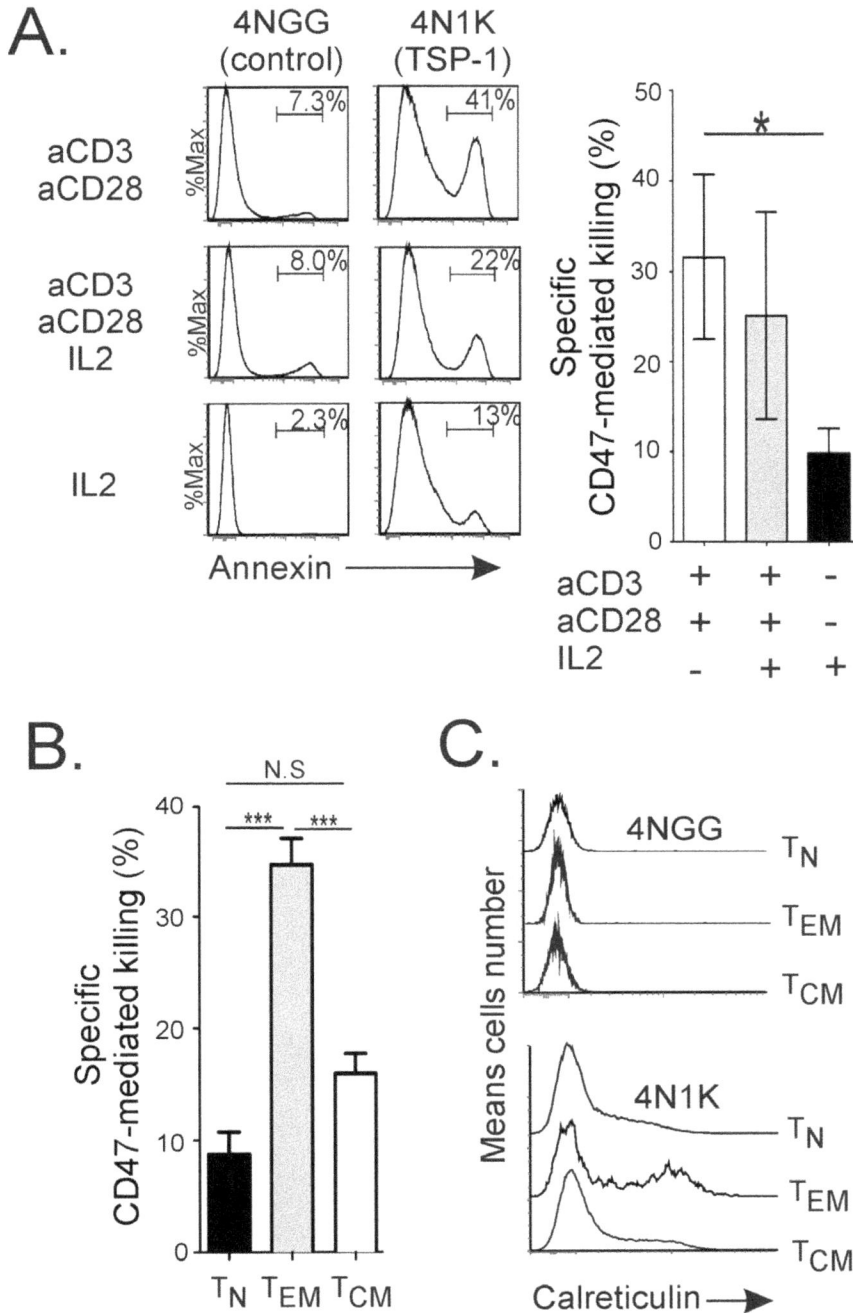

Figure 3. A CD47^low status is linked to TSP-1-induced cell death susceptibility. (A–B) Specific CD47-mediated killing was performed using 4N1K (TSP-1) or 4NGG (control) peptide on *in vitro* restimulated FACS sorted activated CD47^low T cells as in Figure 2 (A) and *ex vivo* isolated CD4 T cell subsets (B). (A–B) The mean ± standard deviation (SD) for 5 independent experiments. Student *t* test: *p<0.05, ***p<0.0001. (C) Calreticulin expression is shown after specific CD47-mediated killing as in B. Data are representative of 4 independent experiments.

and static conditions. A loss of SIRP-α-Fc but not B6H12 and 2D3 binding, thus acquisition of CD47^low status, can be artificially induced either by replacing the transmembrane region of CD47 by CD7, by cholesterol removal, or by a double cysteine mutation that disrupts the S-S disulfide bridge between the transmembrane and extracellular CD47 domains [19,20]. Nonetheless, the precise molecular mechanism behind the physiologic conformational modification of CD47 remains to be elucidated. Reduced or

enhanced binding to SIRP-α-Fc might result from either CD47 association with other surface molecules, since CD47 was originally identified as an integrin-associated molecule [33], CD47 redistribution at the membrane [28], and/or a modified glycosylation pattern [22].

In the present study, we investigated the functional consequences provoked by the change in CD47 status on CD4 T cells. Upon activation, human CD4 T cells transiently displayed

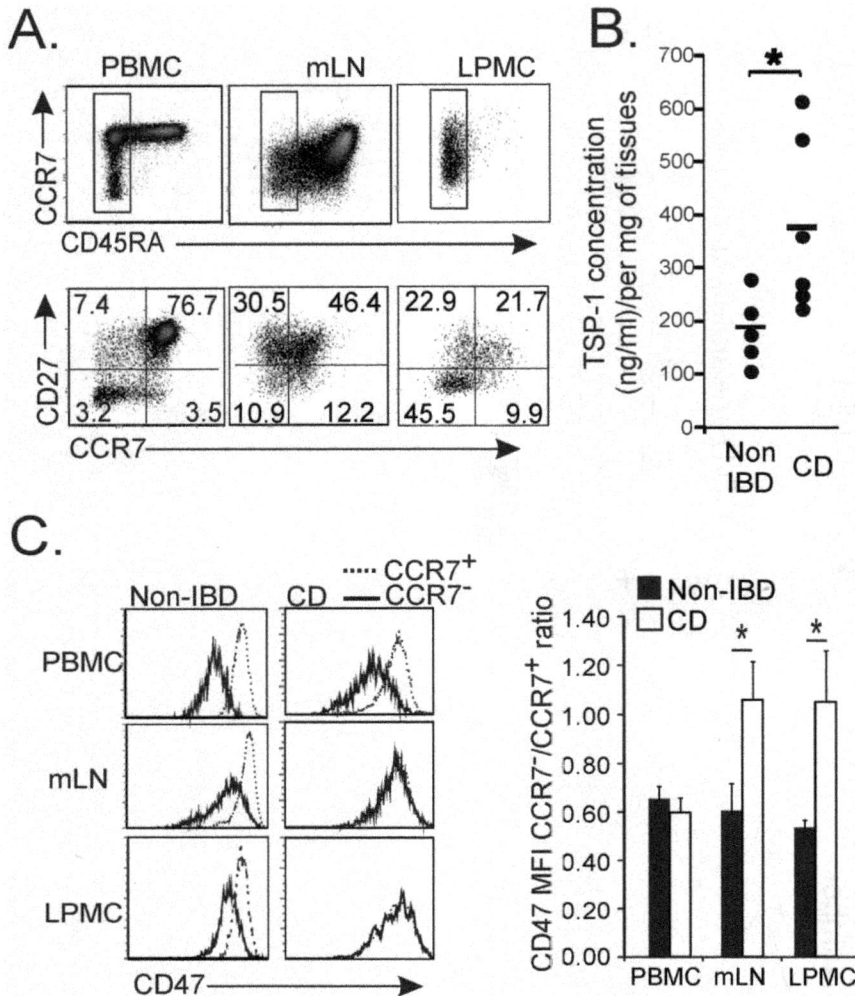

Figure 4. CD4 effectors display a CD47^{high} status in lymph nodes and lamina propria of patients with Crohn's disease. (**A**) CD4 T cell subsets were examined in PBMC, mLNs and LPMC of patients with Crohn's disease. (**B**) TSP-1 concentration in human colon biopsies. (**C**) CD47 expression (SIRP-α-Fc protein) after gating on memory (CCR7$^+$) and effector (CCR7$^-$) CD45RA$^-$CD4$^+$ T cells in PBMC, mLNs and LPMC. Data are representative of 4 to 6 independent experiments. The CD47 Mean Fluorescence Intensity (MFI) CCR7$^-$T/CCR7$^+$ T cell ratio was calculated for patients with CD and unrelated IBD patients. (**A and C**) The mean ± standard deviation (SD) for 5 to 6 independent experiments. Student t test was performed: *$p < 0.05$.

a CD47^{low} status and become sensitive to CD47-mediated cell death by TSP-1. This may represent one mechanism involved in the contraction of the IR, as well as in the resolution of the inflammatory response. We here showed that the absence of CD47 on murine Ag-specific T cells significantly impaired the contraction of the IR *in vivo*, demonstrating that the presence of CD47, and more particularly a CD47^{low} status, was necessary for this process to occur. Furthermore, a transient change of CD47^{low} status on CD4 T cells is required to mediate TSP-1-induced cell death *in vitro* in humans. IL-2 induced a re-expression of CD47^{high} status on human TCR-activated CD4 T cells. T cells themselves represent a source of IL-2 and TSP-1 and CD3 stimulation leads to an increase in the availability of TSP-1 on the cell surface of recently activated T cells [34]. CD47 ligation inhibits early T cell activation, IL-2 production, and CD25 expression [35]. The latter is transiently expressed on activated CD4 T cells *in vivo*, and CD4$^+$CD25$^{-/-}$ or IL-2$^{-/-}$ effector T cells survive very poorly and generate low numbers of memory T cells in non lymphopenic

naive mice [36]. TSP-1 and SIRP-α bind CD47 IgV loop [37] and TSP-1 can inhibit SIRP-α-Fc binding to CD47 expressing Jurkat cells [38]. We therefore postulate that the reestablishment of a CD47^{high} phenotype on T$_{CM}$ and re-encounter with SIRP-α$^+$ myeloid cells (macrophages or DCs) might offer an advantage to avoid TSP-1-induced cell death whereas CD47^{low} status promotes TSP-1 binding that favors cell death and elimination. A direct interaction between CD47^{low} effectors and SIRP-α$^+$ DCs may also induce IL-2 secretion by T cells. Rebres et al. have demonstrated that SIRP-α-Fc ligation synergizes with CD3 for T cell activation and induces PKC θ translocation, resulting in IL-2 production by T cells [19]. DCs, through autocrine secretion of IL-2, trans-present IL-2 to T cells for optimal clonal expansion and effector function [39]. Thus, in addition to T cell-derived IL-2, DCs also could reverse a CD47^{low} to a CD47^{high} status. We showed here that a CD47^{high} status was maintained on CD4 effectors in inflamed CD tissues. This suggests that auto-aggressive T cells that contribute to tissue destruction, might possess a deregulation in the

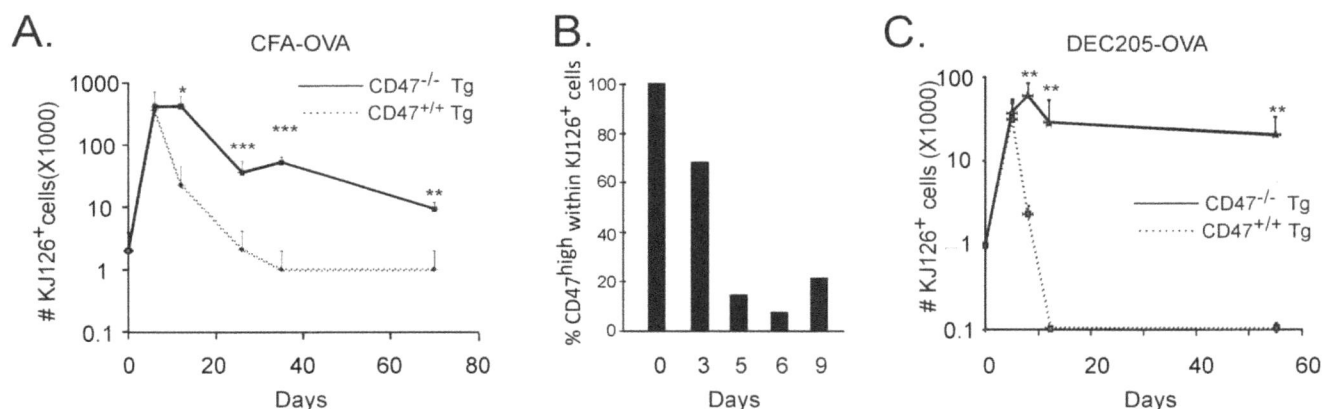

Figure 5. CD47 on CD4 T cells regulates the contraction of the immune response *in vivo*. One day after adoptive transfer of CD47$^{+/+}$ or CD47$^{-/-}$ Tg T cells isolated from DO11.10 mice into CD47$^{-/-}$ BALB/c hosts, mice were immunized s.c. with CFA-OVA or DEC205-OVA. (**A and C**) Kinetic of the recovery of viable Tg T cells is shown. (**B**) CD47 status (SIRP-α-Fc protein) gated on CD4 KJ126$^+$(Tg) T cells post immunization. Data are representative of 4 to 6 independent experiments, student *t* test was performed on 8 to 12 mice. *p<0.05, ***p<0.001.

conformational change process of CD47 which is revealed by an increase in SIRP-α-Fc binding. CD47^{high} status confers resistance to TSP-1-induced killing to CD4 tissue effectors that accumulate in tissues, as we observed abundant TSP-1 release in CD tissues. In that regard, we recently reported that CD47^{high} status on CD4 effectors identifies functional long-lived memory T cell progenitors [16]. Therefore, maintenance of a CD47^{high} status in pathology may be deleterious to the host and perpetuate chronic inflammatory response.

How effector T cell death is regulated during the contraction phase is not fully understood. For many years, the Fas death receptor was considered to be the only T cell surface molecule implicated in the contraction phase of the IR. Fas-mediated signaling leads to activation-induced caspase-dependent apoptosis of TCR-expanded T cells [40,41]. Mice lacking functional genes for Fas or its ligand (FasL), show uncontrolled lympho-proliferation and developed autoimmunity [42,43]. CD47 has been linked to Fas [44]. Yet, CD47$^{-/-}$ mice do not display lympho-proliferative disorders as seen in Fas-deficient mice [45]. Fas signaling, like CD47, kills T_{EM} cells and spares T_{CM} as well as T_N cells. However, unlike differential CD47 status, Fas expression is similar on T_{EM} and T_{CM} cell subsets [46]. CD47 augments Fas-mediated apoptosis, but CD47-initiated signaling is not required to enable Fas killing. This process is unidirectional since Fas is not necessary for CD47-mediated killing [44]. We thus propose that CD47, rather than Fas-mediated cell death, plays a key role in the dampening of an acute response. We showed here an increased yield of Ag-specific CD47$^{-/-}$ T cells in CD47$^{-/-}$ hosts while Ag-specific CD47$^{+/+}$ T cell were barely detectable 70 days after primary immunization. In fact, the role of Fas in contraction phase has been challenged by Alexander *et al*, who showed that the elimination of effector T cells is completely independent of caspase activation. Administration of 11 different regimens of a pan-caspase inhibitor benzyloxycarbonyl-Val-Ala-Asp (OMe)-uoromethylketone (zVAD) *in vivo* showed no significant impact on effector or memory CD8 or CD4 T cell development [4]. Neither the activation of caspases nor that of pro-apoptotic members of the Bcl-2 family, such as Bax, Bak or Bim, or the release of apoptogenic proteins AIF (apoptosis-inducing factor), cytochrome c, endonuclease G (EndoG), Omi/HtrA2 and Smac/DIABLO from mitochondria tocytosol is observed in CD47-mediated cell death [12,25]. Instead, the molecular pathway of CD47-caspase-

independent cell death involves Drp1 translocation from the cytosol to the mitochondria, a process controlled by chymotrypsin-like serine proteases [25]. Once inside the mitochondria, Drp1 provokes an impairment of the mitochondrial electron transport chain, resulting in dissipation of mitochondrial transmembrane potential, reactive oxygen species generation, and a drop in ATP levels. However, a physical interaction between CD47 and the proapoptotic Bcl-2/adenovirus E1B 19-kDa interacting protein 3 (BNIP3), which is expressed upon T cell activation, inhibits BNIP3 degradation by the proteasome, thereby sensitizing T cells to apoptosis [26,47].

At the end of the contraction phase, macrophages and neutrophils must eliminate unwanted (apoptotic or damaged) and "unfit" cells via phagocytosis [48]. CD47 serves as a "don't eat me" signal, which inhibits cell clearance when delivered to SIRP-α$^+$ cells [49]. Viable CD47$^{-/-}$ T cells are quickly eliminated from a CD47$^{+/+}$, but not CD47$^{-/-}$ host, by SIRP-α$^+$ cells [30,31]. Notably, since CD47$^{-/-}$ mice are viable, clearance of CD47$^{-/-}$ cells does not occur in CD47$^{-/-}$ mice because these SIRP-α$^+$ macrophages must be educated by CD47$^{+/+}$ stromal cells to acquire functional phagocytosis via interruption of the CD47/SIRP-α pathway [50]. Nonetheless, the contraction of CD4$^+$CD44^{hi}CD47^{low} T cells occurred in the immunized CD47$^{-/-}$ host. In fact, a CD47^{low} status does not equate to absence of CD47. Of note, only 10% to 20% of normal CD47 expression on RBC is sufficient to prevent cell clearance [51]. Furthermore, Weissman and others demonstrated that concealing CD47 with antibodies on live cells is necessary but insufficient to trigger phagocytosis *in vivo*, since phagocytosis required the expression of calreticulin, which is upregulated on malignant cells [52]. In fact, the "turning off" of non-phagocytic signals must be coupled to the "switching on" of phagocytic signals to provoke cell elimination [48]. Among others, calreticulin serves as a pro-phagocytic signal, which, through binding to its macrophage counter-receptor low-density lipoprotein–related protein (LRP), leads to engulfment of the target cell [28]. In the present study, calreticulin expression was not detected on viable human memory CD4 T cell subsets. In contrast, killing by 4N1K peptide induced calreticulin expression on T_{EM} dying cells, indicating that CD47-mediated cell death represents an upstream event to the elimination of unwanted cells. CD47 expression/

redistribution on apoptotic cells also appear to augment phagocytosis [28,53].

Taken all, we present a key role for CD47 on CD4 T cells in the resolution of an inflammatory response and propose that the following sequence of events accounts for the elimination of a large number of effector T cells. Ag encounter induces a CD47^{low} status on TCR-activated CD4 T cells. Unless rescued by IL-2, which reverses their phenotype to CD47^{high} status, the majority of CD47^{low} T cells will become susceptible to killing by TSP-1 and then augment their expression of pro-phagocytic signals to promote their clearance by SIRP-α^+ cells. Further studies that permit to modulate CD47's status and T cell death may provide novel strategies for improved vaccination and/or the elimination of unwanted, auto-aggressive T cells in inflamed tissues such as in CD.

Materials and Methods

Ethics Statement

All mouse experimental protocols were approved by "Comité institutionnel de protection des animaux (CIPA) du Centre de recherche du Centre hospitalier de l'Université de Montréal (CRCHUM)" that follows the guidelines of the Canadian Council on Animal Care (CCAC). All the experiments were approved by "Comité d'éthique de la recherche du Centre hospitalier de l'Université de Montréal (CHUM)" and written informed consent was obtained from all donors. Human samples were obtained from healthy volunteers, umbilical cord blood and the patients recruited from the Gastroenterology and Surgery Division at CHUM.

Clinical Samples

Peripheral blood samples were collected from all donors, and tissue samples were obtained from endoscopic biopsies or surgically resected specimens. Intestinal tissue samples were taken from unaffected areas of donors with non inflammatory bowel diseases (non IBD) or inflamed regions of Crohn's disease (CD) patients. Mesenteric lymph nodes (mLNs) were collected after surgery by the pathologists.

Animals

CD47$^{-/-}$ 129sv/eg mice were backcrossed onto CD47$^{+/+}$ BALB/c mice for 16 to 18 generations. Mice expressing the DO11.10 TCR transgene, which is specific for the peptide residues 323–339 of chicken OVA, were purchased from Charles River Laboratories and backcrossed into CD47$^{-/-}$ mice. Female mice 6 to 10 weeks old were used in all experimental protocols and were maintained under specific pathogen-free conditions.

Isolation of Cells

Peripheral blood mononuclear cells (PBMC) or umbilical cord blood mononuclear cells (CBMC) were prepared by density gradient centrifugation of heparinized peripheral blood. Lamina propria mononuclear cells (LPMC) were prepared from intestinal specimens using a modified protocol described by Bull and Bookman (1977). Briefly, the dissected mucosal tissue was cut into small pieces, incubated in HBSS (Sigma) with 1 mM DTT (Sigma) and 1 mM EDTA (Sigma) for 45 min at 37°C, followed by enzymatic digestion with 0.25 mg/ml of collagenase D (Roche) and 0.01 mg/ml of DNase I (Roche) for 45–60 min at 37°C, combined with mechanical dissociation by Dissociator (Miltenyi Biotech). Mesenteric LNs were harvested and squeezed on a 70 mm pore mesh to obtain a cellular suspension.

Antibodies and Reagents

All the antibodies were purchased from Biolegend (USA) unless otherwise indicated. 2D3 cell line was obtained from Dr. E. Brown (Genentech, USA). Monoclonal antibodies against the following human antigens were used for labeling and sorting: CD45 (HI30) CD4 (RPA-T4), CD45RA (HI100), CD62L (DREG-56), CCR7 (TG8/CCR7), CD47 (B6H12 and 2D3), CD27 (MT271, BD) CCR5 (2D7/CCR5), CD127 (HIL-7R-M21) and Calreticulin (FMC 75, Assay designs). Antibodies against mouse antigens: CD4 (RM4–5), TCR (DO11.10) (KJ126). Human and mouse CD47 expression was also revealed using huSIRP-α-Fc and muSIRP-α-Fc fusion proteins that contain SIRP-αD1D2D3 domains fused to mutated human Fc IgG (Novartis, Basel, Switzerland), respectively [54]. For in vitro human T cell stimulation, anti-CD3 (OKT3, Janssen-Ortho) and anti-CD28 (CD28.2) mAbs were used.

Flow Cytometry for Phenotypic Analysis

CD47 expression was examined with huSIRP-α-Fc or with anti-CD47 mAbs after gating on naive (T$_N$: CD4$^+$CD45RA$^+$CCR7$^+$), effector memory (T$_{EM}$: CD4$^+$CD45RA$^-$CCR7$^-$CD27$^-$), and central memory (T$_{CM}$: CD4$^+$CD45RA$^-$CCR7$^+$CD27$^+$) T cells. Staining was performed in FACS buffer (PBS supplemented with 2% FCS, 2 mM EDTA, and 0.01% sodium azide at 4°C for 30 min).

Cell Culture

T$_N$ and T$_{CM}$ cells were isolated from PBMC or CBMC using a FACS Aria II sorter (BD). Purity was more than 99%. 1×10^6 CFSE-labeled T$_N$ or T$_{CM}$ cells were stimulated in RPMI (Wisent Inc.) supplemented with 10% fetal calf serum (Wisent Inc), 500 U/ml penicillin, and 500 ug/ml streptomycin with immobilized anti-CD3 (10 ug/ml) and soluble anti-CD28 (2 ug/ml) mAbs for 6 days in 24-well plates (Costar). For secondary cultures, 0.5×10^6 activated T$_N$ cells were restimulated with coated anti-CD3 (10 ug/ml) and soluble anti-CD28 (2 ug/ml) with/without IL-2 (100 U, R&D system) or expanded only in IL-2 for 5 days in 48-well plates (Costar). For some experiments, CFSE-labeled activated CD4 T cells were stained with huSIRP-α-Fc protein and FACS-sorted according to CD47 status before restimulation.

Protein Extractions and Immunoblot

Whole-cell extracts were prepared in 20 mM Tris-HCl pH 7.4, 150 mM NaCl, 1% Triton X-100, 10% glycerol, 2 mM EDTA, and antiprotease mixture (Roche). Protein content was determined with the Bio-Rad DC kit and 10 dodecyl sulfate polyacrylamide gel electrophoresis (SDS-PAGE). After blotting, Nitrocellulose filters were probed with 2D3 mAb and anti β-actin. Both were detected according to standard procedures.

TSP-1 Production by Human Colonic Specimens

TSP-1 concentration (ng/ml) was measured with ELISA kit (Chemicon International) in human colon tissue lysates after homogenization and normalized per milligram of tissue.

Confocal Microscopy

T$_N$, T$_{EM}$ and T$_{CM}$ were FACs sorted from PBMC (purity >99.9%), stained with SIRP-α-Fc or anti-CD47 (B6H12) biotinylated and followed by streptavidin Dylight 649 (Biolegend). Samples were mounted in ProLong Gold (Invitrogen) and analyzed with a confocal microscope (Leica).

CD47-mediated Killing Assays

Purified T cells (4×10^5) isolated from PBMC were labeled with antibodies for CD4 T cell subsets before incubating with 200 uM of TSP-1-specific (4N1K, KRFYVVMWKK) or control (4NGG, KRFYGGMWKK) peptides (McGill University/Sheldon Biotechnology, Montreal) for 30 min at 37°C. Apoptotic cells were revealed with Annexin V binding (BD Bioscience) after gating on T_N, T_{EM}, and T_{CM} T cells. For some experiments, CFSE-labeled T_N were activated for 6 days and then FACS-sorted according to $CFSE^{low}$ before in vitro secondary stimulation. After 5 days, CD47-mediated killing assays were performed under the same conditions as in ex vivo studies. Specific CD47-mediated killing was calculated as follows: percentage of Annexin$^+$ cells in 4N1K-stimulated T cells, minus the percentage of Annexin$^+$ cells in 4NGG-stimulated T cells.

Adoptive Transfer Experiments

BALB/c CD47$^{+/+}$ or CD47$^{-/-}$ mice were passively transferred (intravenously, i.v.) with 2×10^6 CFSE-labeled CD4 T cells isolated from CD47$^{+/+}$ or CD47$^{-/-}$ DO11.10 (Tg) mice. After 1 day, mice were immunized either subcutaneously (s.c.) with OVA protein (100ug/ml, Sigma) emulsified in complete Freund'sFreud adjuvant (MP Biomedicals, LLC) or anti-DEC205 coupled with OVA peptide (gift from R. Steinman, Rockefeller University). The phenotype of Tg T cells was analyzed by flow cytometry at different time points in draining LNs.

Statistical Analysis

Statistical analyses were performed using the unpaired Student t test. One-way Anova test was used to compare the variation of CD47 expression between human CD4 T cell subpopulations. Data represent mean $\pm$ standard deviation (SD). ($***P<.001$; $**P<.01$; $*P<.05$).

Acknowledgments

We would like to thank J-P Wu and G.Delespesse for critical readings and comments, H. Mehta for editing of the manuscript and K. Yurchenko And Janet Crosby Laganière for technical contributions.

Author Contributions

Conceived and designed the experiments: VQV MS. Performed the experiments: VQV NB MR KW. Analyzed the data: VQV NB MR KW ACMT LC GF. Contributed reagents/materials/analysis tools: BP CR GS DF. Wrote the paper: VQV MS SS.

References

1. Gerlach C, van Heijst JW, Schumacher TN (2011) The descent of memory T cells. Ann N Y Acad Sci 1217: 139–153.
2. Li J, Huston G, Swain SL (2003) IL-7 promotes the transition of CD4 effectors to persistent memory cells. The Journal of experimental medicine 198: 1807–1815.
3. Sprent J, Surh CD (2011) Normal T cell homeostasis: the conversion of naive cells into memory-phenotype cells. Nature immunology 131: 478–484.
4. Nussbaum AK, Whitton JL (2004) The contraction phase of virus-specific CD8+ T cells is unaffected by a pan-caspase inhibitor. Journal of immunology 173: 6611–6618.
5. Hughes PD, Belz GT, Fortner KA, Budd RC, Strasser A, et al. (2008) Apoptosis regulators Fas and Bim cooperate in shutdown of chronic immune responses and prevention of autoimmunity. Immunity 28: 197–205.
6. Brown EJ, Frazier WA (2001) Integrin-associated protein (CD47) and its ligands. Trends Cell Biol 11: 130–135.
7. Sarfati M, Fortin G, Raymond M, Susin S (2008) CD47 in the immune response: role of thrombospondin and SIRP-alpha reverse signaling. Curr Drug Targets 9: 842–850.
8. Floquet N, Dedieu S, Martiny L, Dauchez M, Perahia D (2008) Human thrombospondin's (TSP-1) C-terminal domain opens to interact with the CD-47 receptor: a molecular modeling study. Archives of biochemistry and biophysics 478: 103–109.
9. Hatherley D, Graham SC, Turner J, Harlos K, Stuart DI, et al. (2008) Paired receptor specificity explained by structures of signal regulatory proteins alone and complexed with CD47. Molecular cell 31: 266–277.
10. Gardai SJ, Xiao YQ, Dickinson M, Nick JA, Voelker DR, et al. (2003) By binding SIRPalpha or calreticulin/CD91, lung collectins act as dual function surveillance molecules to suppress or enhance inflammation. Cell 115: 13–23.
11. Jaiswal S, Jamieson CH, Pang WW, Park CY, Chao MP, et al. (2009) CD47 is upregulated on circulating hematopoietic stem cells and leukemia cells to avoid phagocytosis. Cell 138: 271–285.
12. Mateo V, Brown EJ, Biron G, Rubio M, Fischer A, et al. (2002) Mechanisms of CD47-induced caspase-independent cell death in normal and leukemic cells: link between phosphatidylserine exposure and cytoskeleton organization. Blood 100: 2882–2890.
13. Pettersen RD, Hestdal K, Olafsen MK, Lie SO, Lindberg FP (1999) CD47 signals T cell death. J Immunol 162: 7031–7040.
14. Ren Y, Savill J (1995) Proinflammatory cytokines potentiate thrombospondin-mediated phagocytosis of neutrophils undergoing apoptosis. J Immunol 154: 2366–2374.
15. Burger P, Hilarius-Stokman P, de Korte D, van den Berg TK, van Bruggen R (2012) CD47 functions as a molecular switch for erythrocyte phagocytosis. Blood.
16. Van VQ, Raymond M, Baba N, Rubio M, Wakahara K, et al. (2012) CD47high Expression on CD4 Effectors Identifies Functional Long-Lived Memory T Cell Progenitors. Journal of immunology.
17. Green JM, Zhelesnyak A, Chung J, Lindberg FP, Sarfati M, et al. (1999) Role of cholesterol in formation and function of a signaling complex involving alphavbeta3, integrin-associated protein (CD47), and heterotrimeric G proteins. J Cell Biol 146: 673–682.
18. Brittain JE, Mlinar KJ, Anderson CS, Orringer EP, Parise LV (2001) Integrin-associated protein is an adhesion receptor on sickle red blood cells for immobilized thrombospondin. Blood 97: 2159–2164.
19. Rebres RA, Green JM, Reinhold MI, Ticchioni M, Brown EJ (2001) Membrane raft association of CD47 is necessary for actin polymerization and protein kinase C theta translocation in its synergistic activation of T cells. J Biol Chem 276: 7672–7680.
20. Rebres RA, Vaz LE, Green JM, Brown EJ (2001) Normal ligand binding and signaling by CD47 (integrin-associated protein) requires a long range disulfide bond between the extracellular and membrane-spanning domains. J Biol Chem 276: 34607–34616.
21. Brown E, Hooper L, Ho T, Gresham H (1990) Integrin-associated protein: a 50-kD plasma membrane antigen physically and functionally associated with integrins. The Journal of cell biology 111: 2785–2794.
22. Subramanian S, Boder ET, Discher DE (2007) Phylogenetic divergence of CD47 interactions with human signal regulatory protein alpha reveals locus of species specificity. Implications for the binding site. J Biol Chem 282: 1805–1818.
23. Osborne LC, Abraham N (2010) Regulation of memory T cells by gammac cytokines. Cytokine 50: 105–113.
24. Kameraa K, Nemoto Y, Kanai T, Shinohara T, Okamoto R, et al. (2010) IL-2 is positively involved in the development of colitogenic CD4(+) IL-7Ralpha(high) memory T cells in chronic colitis. Eur J Immunol.
25. Bras M, Yuste VJ, Roue G, Barbier S, Sancho P, et al. (2007) Drp1 mediates caspase-independent type III cell death in normal and leukemic cells. Mol Cell Biol 27: 7073–7088.
26. Lamy L, Ticchioni M, Rouquette-Jazdanian AK, Samson M, Deckert M, et al. (2003) CD47 and the 19 kDa interacting protein-3 (BNIP3) in T cell apoptosis. J Biol Chem 278: 23915–23921.
27. Mateo V, Lagneaux L, Bron D, Biron G, Armant M, et al. (1999) CD47 ligation induces caspase-independent cell death in chronic lymphocytic leukemia. Nat Med 5: 1277–1284.
28. Gardai SJ, McPhillips KA, Frasch SC, Janssen WJ, Starefeldt A, et al. (2005) Cell-surface calreticulin initiates clearance of viable or apoptotic cells through trans-activation of LRP on the phagocyte. Cell 123: 321–334.
29. Kaser A, Zeissig S, Blumberg RS (2010) Inflammatory bowel disease. Annual Review of Immunology 28: 573–621.
30. Bouguermouh S, Van VQ, Martel J, Gautier P, Rubio M, et al. (2008) CD47 expression on T cell is a self-control negative regulator of type 1 immune response. J Immunol 180: 8073–8082.

31. Oldenborg PA, Zheleznyak A, Fang YF, Lagenaur CF, Gresham HD, et al. (2000) Role of CD47 as a marker of self on red blood cells. Science 288: 2051–2054.

32. Rosales C, Gresham HD, Brown EJ (1992) Expression of the 50-kDa integrin-associated protein on myeloid cells and erythrocytes. Journal of immunology 149: 2759–2764.

33. Lindberg FP, Gresham HD, Schwarz E, Brown EJ (1993) Molecular cloning of integrin-associated protein: an immunoglobulin family member with multiple membrane-spanning domains implicated in alpha v beta 3-dependent ligand binding. J Cell Biol 123: 485–496.

34. Li SS, Liu Z, Uzunel M, Sundqvist KG (2006) Endogenous thrombospondin-1 is a cell-surface ligand for regulation of integrin-dependent T-lymphocyte adhesion. Blood 108: 3112–3120.

35. Avice MN, Rubio M, Sergerie M, Delespesse G, Sarfati M (2001) Role of CD47 in the induction of human naive T cell anergy. J Immunol 167: 2459–2468.

36. Dooms H, Wolslegel K, Lin P, Abbas AK (2007) Interleukin-2 enhances CD4+ T cell memory by promoting the generation of IL-7R alpha-expressing cells. The Journal of experimental medicine 204: 547–557.

37. Floquet N, Dedieu S, Martiny L, Dauchez M, Perahia D (2008) Human thrombospondin's (TSP-1) C-terminal domain opens to interact with the CD-47 receptor: a molecular modeling study. Arch Biochem Biophys 478: 103–109.

38. Isenberg JS, Annis DS, Pendrak ML, Ptaszynska M, Frazier WA, et al. (2009) Differential interactions of thrombospondin-1, -2, and -4 with CD47 and effects on cGMP signaling and ischemic injury responses. The Journal of biological chemistry 284: 1116–1125.

39. Wuest SC, Edwan JH, Martin JF, Han S, Perry JS, et al. (2011) A role for interleukin-2 trans-presentation in dendritic cell-mediated T cell activation in humans, as revealed by daclizumab therapy. Nature medicine 17: 604–609.

40. Krammer PH (2000) CD95's deadly mission in the immune system. Nature 407: 789–795.

41. Ashkenazi A, Dixit VM (1998) Death receptors: signaling and modulation. Science 281: 1305–1308.

42. Nagata S (1998) Human autoimmune lymphoproliferative syndrome, a defect in the apoptosis-inducing Fas receptor: a lesson from the mouse model. Journal of human genetics 43: 2–8.

43. Choi Y, Ramnath VR, Eaton AS, Chen A, Simon-Stoos KL, et al. (1999) Expression in transgenic mice of dominant interfering Fas mutations: a model for human autoimmune lymphoproliferative syndrome. Clinical immunology 93: 34–45.

44. Manna PP, Dimitry J, Oldenborg PA, Frazier WA (2005) CD47 augments Fas/CD95-mediated apoptosis. J Biol Chem 280: 29637–29644.

45. Van VQ, Darwiche J, Raymond M, Lesage S, Bouguermouh S, et al. (2008) Cutting edge: CD47 controls the in vivo proliferation and homeostasis of peripheral CD4+ CD25+ Foxp3+ regulatory T cells that express CD103. J Immunol 181: 5204–5208.

46. Ramaswamy M, Cruz AC, Cleland SY, Deng M, Price S, et al. (2010) Specific elimination of effector memory CD4(+) T cells due to enhanced Fas signaling complex formation and association with lipid raft microdomains. Cell Death Differ.

47. Lamy L, Foussat A, Brown EJ, Bornstein P, Ticchioni M, et al. (2007) Interactions between CD47 and thrombospondin reduce inflammation. J Immunol 178: 5930–5939.

48. Krysko DV, D'Herde K, Vandenabeele P (2006) Clearance of apoptotic and necrotic cells and its immunological consequences. Apoptosis : an international journal on programmed cell death 11: 1709–1726.

49. Blazar BR, Lindberg FP, Ingulli E, Panoskaltsis-Mortari A, Oldenborg PA, et al. (2001) CD47 (integrin-associated protein) engagement of dendritic cell and macrophage counterreceptors is required to prevent the clearance of donor lymphohematopoietic cells. J Exp Med 194: 541–549.

50. Wang H, Madariaga ML, Wang S, Van Rooijen N, Oldenborg PA, et al. (2007) Lack of CD47 on nonhematopoietic cells induces split macrophage tolerance to CD47null cells. Proc Natl Acad Sci U S A 104: 13744–13749.

51. Tsai RK, Discher DE (2008) Inhibition of "self" engulfment through deactivation of myosin-II at the phagocytic synapse between human cells. The Journal of cell biology 180: 989–1003.

52. Chao MP, Jaiswal S, Weissman-Tsukamoto R, Alizadeh AA, Gentles AJ, et al. (2010) Calreticulin Is the Dominant Pro-Phagocytic Signal on Multiple Human Cancers and Is Counterbalanced by CD47. Sci Transl Med 2: 63ra94.

53. Tada K, Tanaka M, Hanayama R, Miwa K, Shinohara A, et al. (2003) Tethering of apoptotic cells to phagocytes through binding of CD47 to Src homology 2 domain-bearing protein tyrosine phosphatase substrate-1. Journal of immunology 171: 5718–5726.

54. Raymond M, Rubio M, Fortin G, Shalaby KH, Hammad H, et al. (2009) Selective control of SIRP-alpha-positive airway dendritic cell trafficking through CD47 is critical for the development of T(H)2-mediated allergic inflammation. The Journal of allergy and clinical immunology 124: 1333–1342 e1331.

18

Relationship between Vagal Tone, Cortisol, TNF-Alpha, Epinephrine and Negative Affects in Crohn's Disease and Irritable Bowel Syndrome

Sonia Pellissier[1,2]*, Cécile Dantzer[3], Laurie Mondillon[4], Candice Trocme[5], Anne-Sophie Gauchez[5], Véronique Ducros[5], Nicolas Mathieu[6], Bertrand Toussaint[5,7], Alicia Fournier[4], Frédéric Canini[8,9], Bruno Bonaz[1,6]

1 Grenoble Institut des Neurosciences (GIN), Centre de Recherche INSERM 836 Equipe : Stress et Interactions Neuro-Digestives (EA3744), Université Joseph Fourier, Grenoble, France, 2 Département de Psychologie, Université de Savoie, Chambéry, France, 3 Laboratoire Interuniversitaire de Psychologie: Personnalité, Cognition, Changement social (LIP/PC2S), Université de Savoie, Chambéry, France, 4 Laboratoire de Psychologie Sociale et Cognitive (LAPSCO, CNRS UMR6024), Université Blaise Pascal, Clermont-Ferrand, France, 5 Institut de Biologie, Centre Hospitalo-Universitaire de Grenoble, Grenoble, France, 6 Clinique Universitaire d'Hépato-Gastroentérologie, Centre Hospitalo-Universitaire de Grenoble, Grenoble, France, 7 Laboratoire TIMC/TheREx UMR 5525, Université Joseph Fourier, Grenoble, France, 8 Unité de Neurophysiologie du Stress, Institut de Recherche Biomédicale des Armées (IRBA), Brétigny-sur-Orge, France, 9 Ecole du Val de Grâce, Paris, France

Abstract

Crohn's disease (CD) and irritable bowel syndrome (IBS) involve brain-gut dysfunctions where vagus nerve is an important component. The aim of this work was to study the association between vagal tone and markers of stress and inflammation in patients with CD or IBS compared to healthy subjects (controls). The study was performed in 73 subjects (26 controls, 21 CD in remission and 26 IBS patients). The day prior to the experiment, salivary cortisol was measured at 8:00 AM and 10:00 PM. The day of the experiment, subjects completed questionnaires for anxiety (STAI) and depressive symptoms (CES-D). After 30 min of rest, ECG was recorded for heart rate variability (HRV) analysis. Plasma cortisol, epinephrine, norepinephrine, TNF-alpha and IL-6 were measured in blood samples taken at the end of ECG recording. Compared with controls, CD and IBS patients had higher scores of state-anxiety and depressive symptomatology. A subgroup classification based on HRV-normalized high frequency band (HFnu) as a marker of vagal tone, showed that control subjects with high vagal tone had significantly lower evening salivary cortisol levels than subjects with low vagal tone. Such an effect was not observed in CD and IBS patients. Moreover, an inverse association (r = −0.48; p<0.05) was observed between the vagal tone and TNF-alpha level in CD patients exclusively. In contrast, in IBS patients, vagal tone was inversely correlated with plasma epinephrine (r = −0.39; p<0.05). No relationship was observed between vagal tone and IL-6, norepinephrine or negative affects (anxiety and depressive symptomatology) in any group. In conclusion, these data argue for an imbalance between the hypothalamus-pituitary-adrenal axis and the vagal tone in CD and IBS patients. Furthermore, they highlight the specific homeostatic link between vagal tone and TNF-alpha in CD and epinephrine in IBS and argue for the relevance of vagus nerve reinforcement interventions in those diseases.

Editor: David L. Boone, University of Chicago, United States of America

Funding: This work was supported by the Association François Aupetit (AFA), the Société Nationale Française de Gastroentérologie (SNFGE) and the Direction Hospitalière de Recherche Clinique (DHRC) of the Grenoble hospital. The funders had no role in study design, data collection and analysis, decision to publish or preparation of the manuscript.

Competing Interests: The authors have declared that no competing interests exist.

* Email: sonia.pellissier@univ-savoie.fr

Introduction

Crohn's disease (CD) is an inflammatory bowel disease (IBD) characterized by a chronic abnormal mucosal immune response with periods of remission of unpredictable duration alternating with acute episodes of flare [1,2]. Irritable bowel syndrome (IBS) is a highly prevalent functional gastrointestinal disorder characterized by abdominal pain and discomfort associated with altered bowel habits [3]. Both pathologies involve brain-gut interaction perturbations and are strongly influenced by narrow interactions between biological and psychosocial factors, and thus considered as bio-psychosocial diseases [4–8]. High perceived stress, negative affects such as anxiety, depression and an imbalanced autonomic nervous system (ANS) are common features in CD and IBS [7,9,10]. The neuroendocrine communication between the brain and the gut is mediated by the parasympathetic and sympathetic branches of the ANS, and by the hypothalamus-pituitary-adrenal (HPA) axis (Bonaz and Bernstein, 2013 for review). These regulatory systems, as a part of the allostatic network, are interrelated and functionally coupled to adapt physiological responses to external and/or internal challenges ensuring homeo-stasis and promoting health [11–13]. Specifically, the parasympa-thetic nervous system plays a major role in gastrointestinal homeostasis [14] and is involved in physiological and psycholog-ical flexibility in reaction to stress [15,16], emotional regulation, and stress recovery [17,18]. Furthermore, the parasympathetic nervous system, through the vagus nerve, modulates the produc-tion of pro-inflammatory cytokines such as TNF-alpha [19] through both vagal afferents and efferents activating respectively the HPA axis and the cholinergic anti-inflammatory pathway [9,20,21]. TNF-alpha is a key pro-inflammatory cytokine involved in CD and anti-TNF therapy is currently the gold standard in the treatment of IBD patients [22]. The vagus nerve is also combined with the HPA axis and under physiological conditions a balance is observed between the parasympathetic nervous system and the HPA axis [23]. This reflects an adapted homeostatic regulation by coupling high vagal tone to low cortisol level. However, in chronic diseases such as alcoholism, where the parasympathetic tone is dramatically blunted, this coupling is altered [24] reflecting an impaired inhibitory control of the HPA axis and an allostatic load as defined by McEwen [25]. An autonomic imbalance with a sympathetic dominance has been described in IBD and IBS [10,26] and should logically have an impact on the HPA axis regulation and thus on catecholamines and pro-inflammatory cytokines levels such as TNF-alpha or IL-6. However, little is known about the nature of the relationship between the vagal tone and the HPA axis in these pathologies and even less with catecholamines and pro-inflammatory cytokines. This raises the question of the correlation, in CD or IBS patients, between the resting vagal tone, which could be considered as a functional parasympathetic fingerprint, on the one hand, and cortisol, catecholamines and pro-inflammatory cytokines levels on the other hand.

Consequently, the principal aim of this study was to examine this functional coupling. If the ANS and the HPA axis are functionally uncoupled in CD and IBS, then we should find no relation between vagal tone and cortisol levels in patients while a high vagal tone will be associated to a low cortisol level (and conversely) in controls. Furthermore, we hypothesized that negative affects (anxiety and depressive symptomatology), cate-cholamines and cytokines levels were dependent on vagal tone in CD and IBS patients but not in controls. For this purpose, heart rate variability (HRV), an index of the parasympathetic nervous system activity, was measured at rest in control healthy subjects, CD patients in remission and IBS patients. Then, a cluster analysis was performed in order to compare, between the low and high vagal tone subgroups, the levels of cortisol, TNF-alpha, IL-6, epinephrine, norepinephrine and negative affects.

Materials and Methods

Subjects and Ethics Statement

The study was performed in agreement with the Declaration of Helsinki and the guidelines of Good Clinical Practice and was approved by the Ethic Committee of the Grenoble Faculty of Medicine and Hospital (ref: 08-CHUG-23, ClinicalTrials.gov Identifier: NCT01095042). Written informed consent was ob-tained from each participant. White subjects, aged 18–60 years, were prospectively recruited between September 2009 and October 2011. CD and IBS patients were recruited in our Department of Gastroenterology while age and sex-matched healthy subjects were recruited by the Grenoble INSERM Clinical Investigation Centre (CIC).

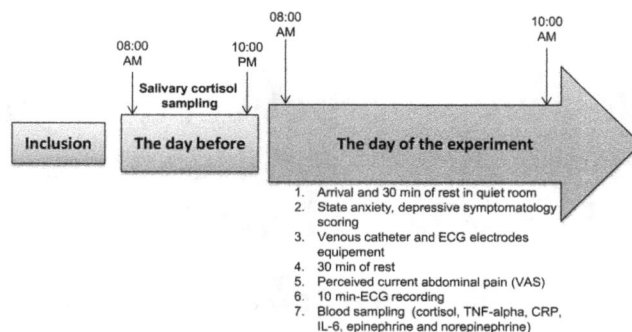

Figure 1. The experimental design.

Criteria for Inclusion

Crohn's Disease (CD) patients. CD patients were selected according to their phenotype as defined by the Montreal classification [27]. CD patients with isolated ano-perineal or upper digestive tract lesions were not eligible. CD activity was evaluated by the Harvey–Bradshaw index (HBI) [28] and patients with an HBI<4 on inclusion were considered in clinical remission. The endoscopic, contrast-enhanced ultrasound and biologic explorations (CRP<5 mg/l) showed that all patients were under mucosal healing and/or parietal healing under their current treatment. Patients were included only if they had a stable dose of *i) 5-aminosalicylates* for at least 2 weeks, *ii) immunosuppressives* for at least 12 weeks, and *iii) biological therapy* (e.g., anti-TNF-alpha) for at least 8 weeks.

Irritable Bowel Syndrome (IBS) patients. Patients were selected according to Rome II criteria [29]: at least 12 weeks, not necessarily consecutive, in the preceding 12 months of abdominal discomfort or pain with two out of the three following features: 1) relieved with defecation; and/or 2) onset associated with a change in frequency of stool; and/or 3) onset associated with a change in form (appearance) of stool. The lack of organicity for patient's symptoms was assumed through: *i)* a negative physical examina-tion; *ii)* a normal colonoscopy performed within the last five years with normal biopsies (i.e., absence of microscopic colitis); *iii)* normal limited laboratory evaluations with a lack of inflammation (i.e., erythrocyte sedimentation rate, C-reactive protein), anaemia, infection (complete blood cell count) and endocrine or metabolic disturbances (i.e., thyroid stimulating hormone, chemical analysis) as well as the absence of IgA anti-transglutaminase (without IgA deficiency).

Criteria for Exclusion

Patients were excluded from the study if: *(i)* they had past or present medical conditions complicated by autonomic dysfunction (e.g., peripheral neuropathy, diabetes, vagotomy, dysthyroidism, amyloidosis, asthma, heart failure, renal insufficiency, alcoholism), *(ii)* they were under medication susceptible to modify the ANS (e.g., anticholinergics, antiarrhytmics, alpha or beta blocking agents, antibiotics). Patients with previous abdominal surgery, except appendectomy and/or cholecystectomy, were excluded from the study.

Experimental Design

All patients underwent an interview concerning their history (disease duration, extent, extra-intestinal manifestations, course, current and past therapies, medications) and a physical examina-tion to determine their inclusion in the study according to the

Table 1. Socio-demographic and psycho-immunologic data of the healthy control subjects, Crohn's disease (CD) and irritable bowel syndrome (IBS) patients who participated to the study.

	Controls	Crohn's Disease (CD)	Irritable Bowel Syndrome (IBS)	p value
Total number of subjects	26	21	26	
Mean age, year ± SD	36±10	40±11	38±11	NS CD or IBS vs controls
Sex, M/F	8/18	9/12	7/19	
BMI (Kg/m²)	23±3.5	22±4.3	22±5.2	NS CD or IBS vs controls
Mean duration of disease, year (range)	-	13.4 (1–28)	10.3 (1–31)	
Localization of Crohn's disease according to Montreal classification		*Ileal:*		
		L1B1: n=3		
		L1B2: n=3		
		B1pB3: n=1		
		Colonic:		
		L2B1: n=6		
		L2B1pB3: n=2		
		Ileocolonic:		
		L3B1: n=2		
		L3B2: n=2		
		L3B2pB3: n=2		
Inflammatory markers (circulating levels)				
CRP level (mg/l)	<4	<5	<5	NS CD or IBS vs controls
Perceived abdominal visceral pain				
VAS	0.30±0.34	1.28±0.38	2.19±0.34	IBS vs controls p<0.001
Mood variables				
State-Anxiety	31±1.90	39±2.15	41±1.91	CD vs controls p<0.05; IBS vs controls p<0.001
Depressive symptomatology	8.94±1.39	13.68±1.58	19.51±1.40	CD vs controls p=0.07; IBS vs controls p<0.001; IBS vs CD p<0.05

inclusion-exclusion criteria. After information and consent, subjects were enrolled and an appointment was fixed. As shown in figure 1, the day before the experiment, salivary cortisol was measured at 08:00 AM and 10:00 PM at home. Participants were asked to have a light breakfast on the morning of their running session. On their arrival in our department (8:00 AM), each participant was oriented to a quiet room to sit and relax during 30 min in a comfortable chair. After explanations on the running of the session, participants completed questionnaires for state-anxiety (State-Trait Anxiety Inventory; STAI) [30] and depressive symptomatology (Center for Epidemiologic Studies-Depression Scale; CES-D) [31,32]. They were then equipped with electrodes for electrocardiogram (ECG) recording and a venous catheter for blood sampling. After a resting period of 30 min, participants were asked to evaluate their current visceral perception through a visual analogic scale (VAS) measuring the intensity of perceived abdominal pain (0: no perceived pain; 10: the maximum perceived pain), then the electrocardiogram (ECG) was recorded for 10 minutes. During this recording period, a technician carefully observed the optimal conditions to ensure that the recording was free of body movements, conversations and any subjective discomfort. Experimental sessions were always performed between 08.00 AM and 10.00 AM to avoid any influence of circadian variations. Catecholamines (epinephrine, norepinephrine), pro-

inflammatory cytokines (TNF-alpha, IL-6), cortisol and C-reactive protein (CRP) were measured in blood samples collected at the end of the resting ECG.

Parasympathetic Assessment: Power spectral analysis of Heart Rate Variability (HRV)

ANS activity was explored using HRV as a reliable and non-invasive method [33]. Initially described by Akselrod [34] to explore cardiovascular control, this tool is now commonly used in gastrointestinal physiology to assess autonomic imbalance related to digestive autonomic regulation [10,35]. ECG signal was acquired through electrodes placed on each wrist. HRV analysis was performed using specific software (Heart Rhythm Scanner, Biocom Technologies, USA). First, QRS complexes were automatically classified. Ectopic or abnormal QRS complexes were visually detected in the software and removed. The signal was then carefully checked and remaining abnormalities were manually removed. Then, a standard spectral analysis was applied on inter-beat intervals using a Fast Fourier Transformation (FFT) according to the standards of measurement of the Task Force on HRV [36]. The following parameters were calculated: (i) Total Power (TP) corresponds to the spectral power density in the range of 0 to 0.40 Hz. It was considered as the net effect of all physiological mechanisms contributing to HRV; (ii) High

Frequency power spectrum (HF, from 0.15 to 0.40 Hz, msec^2) reflected for 90% parasympathetic tone fluctuations caused by respiratory sinus arrhythmia; [37,38] *(iii)* Low Frequency power spectrum (LF, from 0.04 to 0.15 Hz, msec^2) at rest in sitting position, is explained by parasympathetic tone for at least 50% and sympathetic tone for 25%. This HRV component is related to baroreflex modulation [38] *(iv)* Very Low Frequency power spectrum (VLF, from 0.0033 to 0.04 Hz, msec^2) represented various negative emotions or worries in short time recording [39] and various long term endocrine regulations such as renin-angiotensin system and thermoregulation [36,40]. LF and HF variables were also expressed in normalized units: normalized HF [HFnu = HF/(TP–VLF)] and normalized LF [LFnu = LF/(TP–VLF)], respectively. This calculation minimized the effect of changes in Very Low Frequency power on LF and HF power and emphasized the changes in sympathetic or parasympathetic regulation. *(v)* Lastly, LF/HF ratio was calculated as a global marker of the autonomic balance.

Cytokines Measurement

Interleukin-6 and TNF-alpha were evaluated by the Randox Biochip Array technology (Randox Laboratories, Roissy-en-France). This miniaturized ELISA-based technic allows simultaneous quantitative detection of multiple cytokines from a patient low volume single sample. The array used in this study is the Cytokine Array I, which is coated with antibodies against 12 cytokines. Briefly 100 µl of EDTA plasma or standards were added in each well of the biochip and were incubated for 1 hour at 37°C at 370 rpm. Biochip was quickly washed twice with 350 µl of wash buffer, and 4 more washings with a 2-minute soaking step were performed. Then 300 µl of HRP-conjugate antibodies were added and incubated for 1 hour at 37°C at 370 rpm. Washings were realized as previously described and the biochip was briefly air dried. The two components of the signal reagent, luminol and peroxide, were mixed in a ratio of 1:1 and 250 µl were added per well. Signal reading was performed on the Randox Evidence Investigator device, after incubation of the biochip for 2 minutes in the dark. Captured RLU were converted into concentration of cytokines using the 9-point calibration curves run in parallel for each cytokine.

Salivary Cortisol Measurements

Saliva was collected on Salivette (Sarstedt, Marnay, France) the day before the experiment at 8:00 AM and 10:00 PM and stored at −20°C until analysis. Cortisol was evaluated by a commercial radioimmunoassay kit (Cisbio International; Gif-sur-Yvette, France). The principle of the assay is based on the competition between the labelled cortisol and cortisol contained in calibrators or samples to be assayed for a fixed and limited number of antibody binding sites bound to the solid phase (coated tubes). Briefly 150 µl of calibrators, controls or samples were dispensed into the labelled coated tubes and 500 µl of ^{125}I-cortisol was added to each tube. After incubation for 30 minutes at 37°C, unbound tracer was removed by a washing step with 1 ml of distilled water. The remaining radioactivity bound to the tubes was measured with a gamma scintillation counter calibrated for 125 Iodine. The amount of labelled cortisol bound to the antibody was inversely related to the amount of unlabelled cortisol initially present in the sample. Concentration of cortisol in saliva was determined by referring to the radioactivity of the 8-point calibration curve. The range of reference values for the morning and evening salivary cortisol concentrations at the CHU of Grenoble are 6.2–38 nmol/l at 06:00–08:00 AM, 0.8–4.9 nmol/l at 06:00–08:00 PM and < 3 nmol/l at 10:00–00:00 PM.

Catecholamines Measurement

Analysis of catecholamines (epinephrine and norepinephrine) was performed with a commercial kit according to the manufacturer's specifications (Chromsystems, Munich, Germany). Briefly, according to Hue [41], catecholamines were purified from plasma through solid phase extraction by aluminium oxide and secondly measured by reversed phase HPLC on isocratic mode with electrochemical detection (ESA-CoulArray, Eurosep Instruments, Saint Chamond, France).

Psychological Assessments

Anxiety was assessed using the State-Trait Anxiety Inventory (STAI; [30], validated in French by Bruchon-Schweitzer and Paulhan [42] consisting of a scale with 20 items with a score varying from 20 to 80. A high score indicates high anxiety. In the present sample, the internal consistency was high (alpha = 0.91).

Depressive symptomatology was assessed by the Center for Epidemiologic Studies-Depression Scale (CES-D) [31,32]. This brief scale of 20 items assesses symptoms or behaviours often

Table 2. Data representing the sub-group categorization based on HFnu-HRV K-mean classification.

Resting parasympathetic level	Controls		Crohn's Disease (CD)		Irritable Bowel Syndrome (IBS)	
	High (n = 15)	Low (n = 11)	High (n = 8)	Low (n = 13)	High(n = 12)	Low (n = 14)
HR (bpm)	68±2	65±3	71±4	65±3	64±2	66±2
RRI (ms)	894±35	928±41	879±58	938±45	940±30	912±28
Total Power (ms²)	982±134	718±157	492±184	973±134*	885±150	693±140
VLF (ms²)	323±65	275±76	202±89	493±70**	387±73	311±67
LFnu	39±3	68±3***	36±6	63±4**	34±3	66±3***
HFnu	57±2	27±3***	56±3	20±3***	57±2	28±2***
LF/HF	0.74±0.2	2.75±0.2***	0.71±0.8	3.89±0.6***	0.62±0.3	2.79±0.3***

Data are expressed as mean ± sem. Comparisons are made between low and high parasympathetic level using permutations test.
*p<0.05;
**p<0.01;
***p<0.001.

Evening salivary cortisol

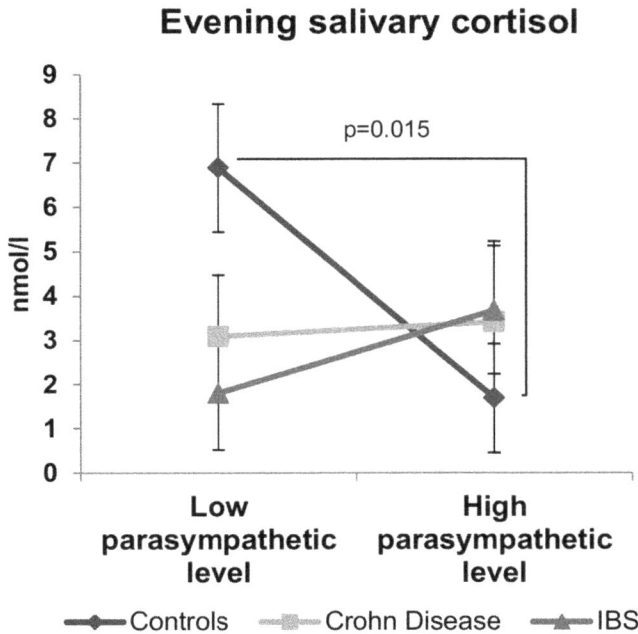

Figure 2. Relationship between the resting parasympathetic vagal tone and the evening salivary cortisol in controls, Crohn's disease (CD) and Irritable bowel syndrome (IBS) patients. A balance was observed between the parasympathetic tone and the evening salivary cortisol in healthy subjects (control group) but not in CD and IBS patients. Data are expressed as mean ± sem. Comparisons are made between the high and low parasympathetic level subgroups using permutations test.

TNF alpha

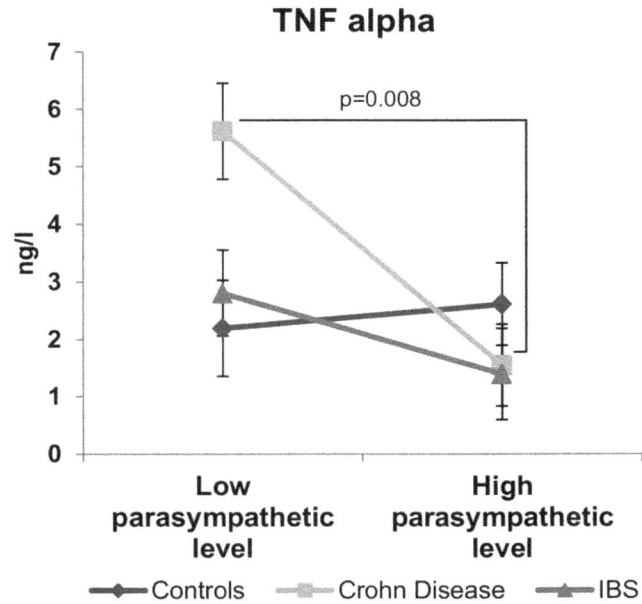

Figure 3. Specific inverse relationship between the resting parasympathetic vagal tone and TNF-alpha plasma level in CD patients. CD patients with low parasympathetic vagal tone exhibit a higher level of TNF-alpha than those with high parasympathetic vagal tone. This inverse relationship was not observed in controls or IBS patients. Data are expressed as mean ± sem. Comparisons are made between the high and low parasympathetic level subgroups using permutations test.

associated with depression. The total score varies from 0 to 60, a high score signifying a high level of depressive symptomatology. An alpha coefficient for internal consistency of 0.85 has been reported in general population samples and 0.90 in psychiatric samples [43]. In the present sample, the alpha coefficient was 0.87.

Statistical Analyses

Statistical analysis was carried out with Statistica 7.1 (Statsoft, Maisons-Alfort, France) and StatExact 9 (Cytel, Paris, France). ANOVA was used to evaluate main effects of group on age, disease duration, visceral pain, state anxiety and depressive symptomatology. When a significant effect was observed, a

Bonferroni *post-hoc* test was applied to determine the differences between each group. Since the high frequency component of HRV is explained for 90% by the parasympathetic activity as described above, the normalized unit of HF (HFnu) has been considered to be the most appropriate, among HRV components, to represent the resting parasympathetic tone. Thus, HFnu was used to categorize subjects in high or low parasympathetic tone using K-means clustering method based on observations. Two clusters of subjects were therefore identified. Non-parametric permutation tests for small samples were performed to make comparisons between the low and high vagal tone subgroups within each group. Spearman correlation coefficients were used to evaluate relationships among vagal tone and cytokines or

Table 3. Influence of the vagal tone on the plasma levels of the morning salivary and plasma cortisol, IL-6, norepinephrine concentrations, state-anxiety and depressive symptomatology scores in Controls, Crohn's disease (CD) and Irritable Bowel syndrome (IBS) patients.

Resting parasympathetic level	Controls		Crohn's Disease (CD)		Irritable Bowel Syndrome (IBS)	
	High (n = 15)	Low (n = 11)	High (n = 8)	Low (n = 13)	High (n = 12)	Low (n = 14)
Morning salivary cortisol (nmol/l)	14.35±2.27	9.75±2.56	9.37±3.21	15.80±2.45	14.30±2.56	16.69±2.36
Morning plasma cortisol (nmol/l)	389.5±61.4	343±69.2	484.9±81.2	419.33±66.3	344.5±66.3	319.1±61.4
IL-6 (ng/l)	0.83±0.28	0.22±0.32	0.50±0.38	0.75±0.31	0.61±0.31	0.65±0.29
Norepinephrine (pmol/l)	1.8±0.18	1.6±0.22	2.3±0.24	2.05±0.2	2.01±0.20	2.38±0.19
State-anxiety score	33.06±2	29.1±3	37.7±4	40.2±2	41.1±3	41.3±2
Depressive symptomatology score	8.5±2	9.3±2	13.7±2	13.6±2	20.3±2	18.7±2

Data are expressed as mean ± sem. Comparisons are made between low and high parasympathetic level using permutations test.

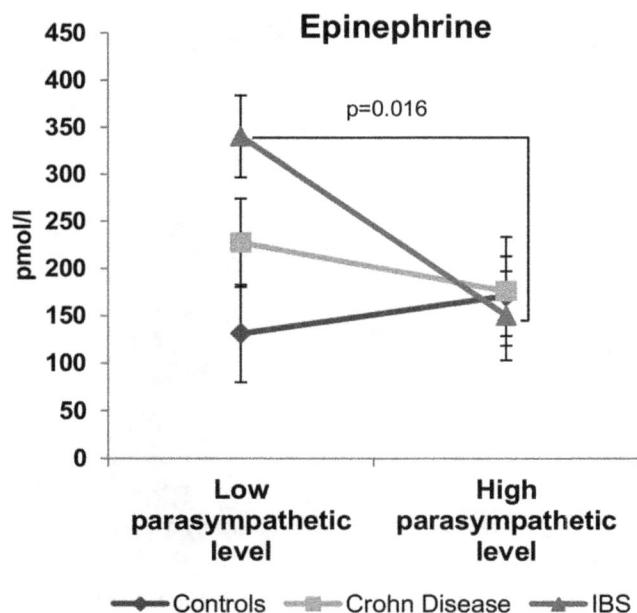

Figure 4. Specific inverse relationship between the resting parasympathetic vagal tone and epinephrine plasma level in IBS patients. IBS patients with low parasympathetic vagal tone exhibit a higher level of plasma epinephrine at rest than those with high parasympathetic vagal tone. This inverse relationship was not observed in controls or CD patients. Data are expressed as mean ± sem. Comparisons are made between the high and low parasympathetic level subgroups using permutations test.

catecholamines within each group (controls, IBS and CD). Data are expressed as means (± standard error of the mean, SEM). The alpha value for statistical significance was set at p<0.05.

Results

Participants

Patients and healthy controls demographics and psycho-immunological data are detailed in table 1. Seventy-three subjects were distributed as healthy volunteers (controls), IBS and CD patients in remission. The mean age of all the participants was 38 ± 10 years old. There was no significant difference in the age ($F_{(2,70)} = 0.85$, p = 0.43) between groups. Among the 26 IBS patients, 7 patients (6 women and 1 man) were diarrhea predominant, 1 patient (woman) constipation predominant and the other 18 patients with alternative diarrhea/constipation. The mean duration of the disease was not significantly different between patients groups ($F_{(1,45)} = 1.46$, p = 0.23). CRP plasmatic level was normal (<5 mg/l) in all groups. There was a significant effect of the disease on the level of perceived visceral pain as evaluated on the day of the experiment ($F_{(2,70)} = 7.48$, p = 0.001). IBS patients had the highest score of perceived visceral pain compared to controls (p<0.001). There was also a significant effect of the disease on the scores of state-anxiety ($F_{(2,66)} = 7.63$, p = 0.001) and depressive symptomatology ($F_{(2.66)} = 14.28$, p< 0.001) with CD and IBS patients exhibiting the highest scores of state-anxiety (p<0.05 and p = 0.001 respectively) and depressive symptomatology (p = 0.07 and p<0.001 respectively) compared to controls. Moreover, the scores of depressive symptomatology were significantly (p<0.02) higher in IBS than CD patients.

Balance between resting vagal tone and cortisol, TNF-alpha, epinephrine and negative affects in CD and IBS patients

The parasympathetic fingerprint. The HRV variable HFnu was used to categorize subjects into low and high parasympathetic tone as a hallmark of the level of their vagal tone. Two clusters of subjects were therefore identified as high or low parasympathetic level within control, CD, and IBS groups. This subgroup classification revealed that about half of the subjects had a high resting parasympathetic tone (HFnu = 56 ± 1.5, n = 35) and the other one a low resting parasympathetic tone (HFnu = 25 ± 1.5; n = 38). Data reporting mean values of HRV variables in low and high subgroups in controls, CD and IBS patients are detailed in table 2.

Interestingly, CD patients with low parasympathetic tone showed significantly higher levels in Total Power (p<0.02) and VLF (p<0.01) HRV variables compared to CD patients with high parasympathetic tone. VLF seemed to be related to visceral sensitivity since (i) CD patients with low parasympathetic tone reported higher scores of perceived abdominal pain than CD patients with high parasympathetic tone (1.76 ± 0.4 and 0.50 ± 0.5 respectively; p<0.05) and (ii) VLF was positively correlated with the score of perceived abdominal pain (r = 0.65; p<0.001). It is interesting to note that this correlation observed in CD was not found in controls (r = −0.29; p = 0.14) or IBS patients (r = 0.30; p = 0.13).

Vagal tone and evening salivary cortisol level (figure 2). Controls with high parasympathetic level (HFnu = 57 ± 2) exhibited significantly (p<0.05) lower evening salivary cortisol (1.69 ± 1.30 nmol/l) than controls with low parasympathetic level (HFnu = 27 ± 3; evening salivary cortisol = 6.89 ± 1.30 nmol/l). Interestingly, this inverse balance between morning vagal tone and evening salivary cortisol level was observed neither in CD (3.41 ± 1.81 nmol/l for high parasympathetic tone and 3.09 ± 1.38 nmol/l for low parasympathetic tone subgroup; p = 0.16) nor in IBS patients (3.68 ± 1.44 nmol/l for high parasympathetic tone and 1.80 ± 1.28 nmol/l for low parasympathetic tone subgroups; p = 0.42). In another way, it is interesting to note that no significant difference was observed between the high and low parasympathetic vagal tone subgroups for the morning plasma and salivary cortisol levels in any group (table 3).

Vagal tone and pro-inflammatory cytokines (figure 3). In CD patients, a significant inverse relationship (r = −0.48; p<0.05) was observed between the parasympathetic tone and TNF-alpha plasma concentration. Thus, CD patients exhibiting a high parasympathetic tone (HFnu = 56 ± 3) had significantly (p<0.01) lower levels of TNF-alpha plasma concentration (1.55 ± 0.98 ng/l) than those with low parasympathetic tone (HFnu = 20 ± 3; TNF-alpha = 5.62 ± 0.80 ng/l). Such a negative correlation was neither observed in IBS patients (r = −0.34; p = 0.09) nor in controls (r = 0.19; p = 0.33) where the TNF-alpha plasma levels did not differ according to the parasympathetic vagal tone. As presented in table 3, IL-6 plasma levels measured in controls, CD and IBS patients were not different between the low and high parasympathetic vagal tone subgroups.

Vagal tone and catecholamines (figure 4). In IBS patients, a significant inverse relationship (r = −0.39; p<0.05) was observed between the parasympathetic tone and the epinephrine plasma concentration. IBS patients exhibiting a high parasympathetic tone (HFnu = 57 ± 2) had significantly (p<0.05) lower levels of epinephrine plasma concentrations (150 ± 47 pmol/l) than those with a low parasympathetic tone (HFnu = 28 ± 2; epinephrine = 340 ± 43 pmol/l). Such a negative correlation was neither observed in CD patients (r = −0.07; p = 0.75) nor in controls (r = −0.05; p = 0.82). Norepinephrine plasma levels did not present any significant difference between high and low parasympathetic tone subgroups in control, CD and IBS patients (table 3).

Vagal tone and negative affects. No significant difference was observed between low and high parasympathetic tone subgroups for state-anxiety and depressive symptomatology scores within any group (table 3). However, in CD group, there was a significant correlation between evening salivary cortisol level and state-anxiety score (r = 0.49; p<0.05) on the one hand, and depressive symptomatology (r = 0.69; p<0.001) on the other hand. Such an association was not observed in IBS group.

Discussion

The present study shows three important results highlighting the strong relationship between the vagal tone and markers of stress regulation and inflammation in CD and IBS patients. *First*, we observed that a high morning vagal tone is associated with a low evening cortisol level in healthy subjects but not in CD and IBS patients suggesting an uncoupling between vagal tone and cortisol level in those patients. *Second*, we found that TNF-alpha plasma level is negatively correlated to vagal tone in CD patients suggesting that the cholinergic anti-inflammatory pathway may be blunted in CD patients with low vagal tone. *Third*, we show that IBS patients with low vagal tone exhibit high plasma level of epinephrine as a mark of an unadapted high sympathetic activity. Finally, even if one limitation of our study may concern the possible impact of gender on the main effects that we observed, data reported here highlight the interest of measuring the resting vagal tone in IBS and CD patients as a marker of homeostatic imbalance that could predict a state of vulnerability to relapse.

The resting vagal tone as a marker of the central homeostatic balance

In the present study, we have categorized individuals according to their resting vagal tone based on the HRV high frequency component (HFnu). The resting vagal tone is strongly involved in the regulation of physiological systems that are important in health and disease and notably those concerning the HPA axis and inflammation [23]. HRV has been previously proposed as an endophenotype marker particularly as a mediator between physiology and behavior [44]. In the present study, we used vagal tone rather like a fingerprint reflecting the balance of the autonomic network. Indeed, Thayer and Lane [44] described a model of neurovisceral integration in which a set of neural structures involved in cognitive, affective, and autonomic regulation referred as the central autonomic network or CAN [45] are related to HRV; thus they proposed HRV as an indicator of CAN-ANS integration. In this integrative interplay, the functional coupling between low cortisol levels and high vagal tone at rest would reflect, at the peripheral level, the central top-down inhibition of the medial prefrontal cortex on subcortical sympatho-excitatory circuits such as the amygdala [23,46]. The hypoactivity of the medial prefrontal cortex enhances amygdala activity and then induce a parasympathetic withdrawal and a sympathetic activation. Thus, according to this model, the lower the vagal tone, the less active the prefrontal cortex will be, reflecting a shift from a homeostatic state to a stress state. This must be associated with emotional and physiological outputs such as an increase in pro-inflammatory cytokines, epinephrine and anxiety. In the present study, we have observed a negative coupling between the vagal tone and cortisol level in healthy subjects. Individuals exhibiting high resting vagal tone in the

morning will have the greater decrease in salivary cortisol levels in the evening. In contrast, this balance between cortisol and HRV (vagal tone) was no more observed in CD and IBS patients. This argues for an uncoupling between the HPA axis and the ANS in both diseases and suggests a breakdown of the functional connectivity between the prefrontal cortex and the amygdala as recently shown in depression and anxiety [47,48]. These results are independent of the circadian cycle since the salivary level of cortisol is high in the morning and low in the evening in the three groups as normally observed [49,50]. According to the McEwen model of stress [11], this uncoupling would be the sign of a costly allostatic regulation with reduced flexibility in the regulatory systems. Such a situation would make CD and IBS patients more reactive to stressful life events or other challenging situations and thus more probable to trigger symptoms. Indeed, a reduced vagal tone could not be in favor of a positive effect of the cholinergic anti-inflammatory pathway (CAP) and thus inflammation and/or pain could be enhanced.

Inverse relationship between vagal tone and TNF-alpha and perceived visceral pain in CD

The second important result reported in this study concerns the inverse relationship between HRV variables representative of the vagal tone and TNF-alpha in CD patients. TNF-alpha is a key pro-inflammatory cytokine in the pathogenesis of CD [51]. TNF-alpha is abundantly expressed in the gastrointestinal tracts of CD patients and contributes to intestinal mucosal inflammation [52]. Currently, the gold standard therapy aims at reducing the activity of TNF-alpha in IBD patients using anti-TNF therapies [53]. The vagus nerve is known to play a dual inhibitory control on inflammation. Its afferent fibers reach the brainstem and activate the HPA axis and cortisol release as an endpoint [4]. Further, more recently, vagal efferent fibers have been shown to exert an anti-inflammatory effect (i.e., the CAP) by inhibiting TNF-alpha production from macrophages [54]. Today, the CAP is a therapeutic target in chronic inflammatory diseases such as CD in which low frequency vagus nerve stimulation is used [55,56]. Recent data, supporting our findings, have described an inverse relationship between HRV indices and TNF-alpha levels in heart failure [57] but also in healthy subjects under stressful situations [18]. In a recent review, Huston and Tracey supported the idea that HRV would be a relevant marker of excessive inflammation [58] in line with our findings. However, in our study, we did not found a significant relationship between HRV and TNF-alpha in healthy volunteers; a similar observation has also been recently reported in patients with chronic heart failure [59]. This is explained by the facts that healthy subjects (i) were under resting and not stressful conditions and (ii) were not under an inflammatory state.

The other interesting result of our study concerns the correlation between the spontaneous visceral abdominal pain perception and the VLF band of HRV. CD patients with low parasympathetic tone had higher levels of VLF than CD patients with high parasympathetic tone, and also reported higher scores of visceral perception. Such an observation has never been reported before. Although the physiological meaning of VLF oscillations has not been completely understood yet, the increase of this HRV variable is related to an important parasympathetic impairment with a loss of coherence between RR intervals and systolic blood pressure variability [60]. Furthermore, VLF power level is influenced by the renin-angiotensin system since the blockade of the angiotensin converting enzyme has been shown to decrease VLF [61]. In another way, VLF oscillations have been related to an increase in peripheral chemosensitivity in patients with congestive heart failure [62]. Angiotensin also acts as a modulator in the spinal transmission of nociceptive information [63]. Interestingly, a recent pilot study revealed an up-regulation of the renin-angiotensin system in inflammatory bowel disease patients [64]. Consequently, one can hypothesize that the increase of VLF oscillations observed in the low vagal tone CD patients, could be related to an impairment of the angiotensin system leading to the increase in visceral pain perception. This could enhance a shift toward hypersensitivity and IBS-like symptoms. If so, VLF oscillations would be a relevant marker of autonomic visceral sensitivity impairment that could be used in the patients' follow-up. Further experiments are currently underway to deepen this question.

Inverse relationship between vagal tone and epinephrine in IBS

Another important finding of our study is the inverse specific relationship between HRV and plasma levels of epinephrine in IBS. Patients with IBS exhibit visceral hypersensitivity (VHS) [65]. In our study, IBS patients reported higher scores of perceived abdominal pain than CD patients or healthy subjects. Besides pain, IBS patients reported more depressive symptoms and anxiety than healthy subjects. Psychosocial factors are often found in IBS patients and IBS is considered as a biopsychosocial model disorder [5]. Indeed, about 20 to 50% of IBS patients have psychiatric disorders, such as major depression, anxiety and somatoform disorders [66]. High perceived stress, negative mood and autonomic imbalance also characterized IBS as reported in previous studies [10,67]. In the present work, we found that IBS patients exhibit higher circulating levels of norepinephrine at rest than healthy subjects. These findings are corroborated by several studies revealing abnormal catecholamines levels in IBS [68,69]. In addition, our study reveals, for the first time, that IBS patients with low vagal tone have higher plasma levels of epinephrine than those with high vagal tone. This inverse relationship in addition to the uncoupling between the vagal tone and cortisol argues for a hyperactivity of the amygdala and a hypo-activation of the prefrontal cortex underlying vulnerability to stress in this disease [46]. This is strengthened by the elevated scores of state-anxiety and depressive symptomatology observed in those patients even if we did not find a linear relationship between the parasympathetic vagal tone at rest and these psychological scores. These affects would be rather associated to the HPA axis and thus to the level of cortisol as previously shown [70] and more probably to the

decrease in the evening cortisol as suggested by the results of our study in CD patients.

Conclusion

The fact that HRV is inversely related to TNF-alpha in CD patients and to norepinephrine in IBS, suggests that HRV would be a reliable marker of the allostatic load in such chronic diseases. This idea supports the fact that HRV that indexes vagal tone is a real marker of homeostasis and autonomic flexibility. In CD patients, the homeostasis of inflammation is imbalanced and a low vagal tone favors an overexpression of TNF-alpha. In IBS, a low vagal tone will be representative of a homeostatic imbalance of the sympatho-adrenergic axis. This is in agreement with the findings that in atherosclerosis, an inflammatory disease characterized by elevated levels of CRP and IL-6, a low vagal tone is inversely correlated with these inflammatory markers [71]. As we could see herein, among patients, only a part of them would require a vagal reinforcement that could be achieved by targeting the vagus nerve through electrical stimulation, pharmacology and/or complementary medicines such as hypnotherapy [9] or Mindfulness Based Stress Reduction a program which increases vagal tone [72]. These therapies would also improve visceral pain perception; reduce epinephrine and TNF-alpha levels allowing remission maintenance.

Acknowledgments

We aknowledge Patricia Raiewski, Nathalie Drivas, David Tartry and Françoise Bardin and Virginie Debard from the Clinique Universitaire d'Hépato-Gastroentérologie of the CHU de Grenoble, for their helpful technical support during the patients enrollment.

This work has been presented at the Digestive Disease Week, Orlando (May 21, 2013), in top ten of the poster presentation (Pellissier S. *et al.* Gastroenterology 2013; 144(5): S-930), and at the meeting of the International Society for Autonomic Neuroscience (ISAN; August 1st, 2013), Giessen, Germany (Pellissier S. et al. Autonomic Neuroscience 2013; 177(2): 315–316).

Author Contributions

Conceived and designed the experiments: SP CD LM BB. Performed the experiments: SP CD. Analyzed the data: SP CD LM FC. Contributed reagents/materials/analysis tools: NM AF CT ASG VD BT. Contributed to the writing of the manuscript: SP BB CD LM. Patients inclusions: NM BB.

References

1. Strober W, Fuss I, Mannon P (2007) The fundamental basis of inflammatory bowel disease. J Clin Invest 117: 514–521.
2. Xie J, Itzkowitz SH (2008) Cancer in inflammatory bowel disease. World J Gastroenterol 14: 378–389.
3. Drossman DA, Dumitrascu DL (2006) Rome III: New standard for functional gastrointestinal disorders. J Gastrointestin Liver Dis 15: 237–241.
4. Bonaz B (2013) Inflammatory bowel diseases: a dysfunction of brain-gut interactions? Minerva Gastroenterol Dietol 59: 241–259.
5. Long MD, Drossman DA (2010) Inflammatory bowel disease, irritable bowel syndrome, or what?: A challenge to the functional-organic dichotomy. Am J Gastroenterol 105: 1796–1798.
6. Grover M, Herfarth H, Drossman DA (2009) The functional-organic dichotomy: postinfectious irritable bowel syndrome and inflammatory bowel disease-irritable bowel syndrome. Clin Gastroenterol Hepatol 7: 48–53.
7. Kovacs Z, Kovacs F (2007) Depressive and anxiety symptoms, dysfunctional attitudes and social aspects in irritable bowel syndrome and inflammatory bowel disease. Int J Psychiatry Med 37: 245–255.
8. Bitton A, Dobkin PL, Edwardes MD, Sewitch MJ, Meddings JB, et al. (2008) Predicting relapse in Crohn's disease: a biopsychosocial model. Gut 57: 1386–1392.
9. Bonaz BL, Bernstein CN (2013) Brain-gut interactions in inflammatory bowel disease. Gastroenterology 144: 36–49.
10. Pellissier S, Dantzer C, Canini F, Mathieu N, Bonaz B (2010) Psychological adjustment and autonomic disturbances in inflammatory bowel diseases and irritable bowel syndrome. Psychoneuroendocrinology 35: 653–662.
11. Peters A, McEwen BS (2012) Introduction for the allostatic load special issue. Physiol Behav 106: 1–4.
12. McEwen BS, Wingfield JC (2010) What is in a name? Integrating homeostasis, allostasis and stress. Horm Behav 57: 105–111.
13. McEwen BS, Wingfield JC (2003) The concept of allostasis in biology and biomedicine. Horm Behav 43: 2–15.
14. Holzer P, Schicho R, Holzer-Petsche U, Lippe IT (2001) The gut as a neurological organ. Wien Klin Wochenschr 113: 647–660.
15. Tran BW, Papoiu AD, Russoniello CV, Wang H, Patel TS, et al. (2010) Effect of itch, scratching and mental stress on autonomic nervous system function in atopic dermatitis. Acta Derm Venereol 90: 354–361.
16. Porges SW (1992) Vagal tone: a physiologic marker of stress vulnerability. Pediatrics 90: 498–504.
17. Goehler LE, Lyte M, Gaykema RP (2007) Infection-induced viscerosensory signals from the gut enhance anxiety: implications for psychoneuroimmunology. Brain Behav Immun 21: 721–726.
18. Weber CS, Thayer JF, Rudat M, Wirtz PH, Zimmermann-Viehoff F, et al. (2010) Low vagal tone is associated with impaired post stress recovery of

cardiovascular, endocrine, and immune markers. Eur J Appl Physiol 109: 201–211.

19. Pavlov VA, Tracey KJ (2006) Controlling inflammation: the cholinergic anti-inflammatory pathway. Biochem Soc Trans 34: 1037–1040.

20. Galvis G, Lips KS, Kummer W (2006) Expression of nicotinic acetylcholine receptors on murine alveolar macrophages. J Mol Neurosci 30: 107–108.

21. Pavlov VA, Wang H, Czura CJ, Friedman SG, Tracey KJ (2003) The cholinergic anti-inflammatory pathway: a missing link in neuroimmunomodulation. Mol Med 9: 125–134.

22. Lichtenstein GR (2013) Comprehensive review: antitumor necrosis factor agents in inflammatory bowel disease and factors implicated in treatment response. Therap Adv Gastroenterol 6: 269–293.

23. Thayer JF, Sternberg E (2006) Beyond heart rate variability: vagal regulation of allostatic systems. Ann N Y Acad Sci 1088: 361–372.

24. Thayer JF, Hall M, Sollers JJ, Fischer JE (2006) Alcohol use, urinary cortisol, and heart rate variability in apparently healthy men: Evidence for impaired inhibitory control of the HPA axis in heavy drinkers. Int J Psychophysiol 59: 244–250.

25. McEwen BS (1998) Stress, Adaptation, and Disease: Allostasis and Allostatic Load. Annals of the New York Academy of Sciences 840: 33–44.

26. Boisse L, Chisholm SP, Lukewich MK, Lomax AE (2009) Clinical and experimental evidence of sympathetic neural dysfunction during inflammatory bowel disease. Clin Exp Pharmacol Physiol 36: 1026–1033.

27. Satsangi J, Silverberg MS, Vermeire S, Colombel JF (2006) The Montreal classification of inflammatory bowel disease: controversies, consensus, and implications. Gut 55: 749–753.

28. Harvey RF, Bradshaw JM (1980) A simple index of Crohn's disease activity. Lancet 1: 514.

29. Thompson WG, Longstreth GF, Drossman DA, Heaton KW, Irvine EJ, et al. (1999) Functional bowel disorders and functional abdominal pain. Gut 45: 43–47.

30. Spielberger CD, Gorsuch RL, Lushene R, Vagg PR, Jacobs GA (1983) Manual for State-Trait Anxiety Inventory (STAI). Alto P, editor: Consulting Psychologists Press Inc.

31. Radloff LS (1977) The CES-D scale: a self-report depression scale for research in the general population. Applied Psychological Measurement 3: 385–401.

32. Fuhrer R, Rouillon F (1989) La version française de l'échelle CES-D (Center for Epidemiologic Studies-Depression Scale). Description et traduction de l'échelle d'autoévaluation Psychiatry and Psychobiology 4: 163–166.

33. Lombardi F, Malliani A, Pagani M, Cerutti S (1996) Heart rate variability and its sympatho-vagal modulation. Cardiovascular Research 32: 208–216.

34. Akselrod S, Gordon D, Ubel FA, Shannon DC, Barger AC, et al. (1981) Power spectrum analysis of heart rate fluctuation: a quantitative probe of beat-to-beat cardiovascular control. Science 213: 220–222.

35. Jarrett ME, Burr RL, Cain KC, Rothermel JD, Landis CA, et al. (2008) Autonomic nervous system function during sleep among women with irritable bowel syndrome. Dig Dis Sci 53: 694–703.

36. (1996) Heart rate variability: standards of measurement, physiological interpretation and clinical use. Task Force of the European Society of Cardiology and the North American Society of Pacing and Electrophysiology. Circulation 93: 1043–1065.

37. Billman GE (2013) The effect of heart rate on the heart rate variability response to autonomic interventions. Front Physiol 4: 222.

38. Billman GE (2013) The LF/HF ratio does not accurately measure cardiac sympatho-vagal balance. Front Physiol 4: 26.

39. Yeragani VK, Sobolewski E, Igel G, Johnson C, Jampala VC, et al. (1998) Decreased heart-period variability in patients with panic disorder: a study of Holter ECG records. Psychiatry Research 78: 89–99.

40. Reyes del Paso GA, Langewitz W, Mulder LJ, van Roon A, Duschek S (2013) The utility of low frequency heart rate variability as an index of sympathetic cardiac tone: a review with emphasis on a reanalysis of previous studies. Psychophysiology 50: 477–487.

41. Hue O, Le Gallais D, Boussana A, Galy O, Chamari K, et al. (2000) Catecholamine, blood lactate and ventilatory responses to multi-cycle-run blocks. Med Sci Sports Exerc 32: 1582–1586.

42. Bruchon-Schweitzer M, Paulhan I (1993) Manuel de l'inventaire d'anxiété état-trait forme Y (STAI-Y). Adapté par Bruchon-Schweitzer et Paulhan; ECPA, editor. Paris.

43. Nunnally JC (1978) Psychometric theory; Hill M, editor. New York.

44. Thayer JF, Lane RD (2009) Claude Bernard and the heart-brain connection: further elaboration of a model of neurovisceral integration. Neurosci Biobehav Rev 33: 81–88.

45. Benarroch EE (1993) The central autonomic network: functional organization, dysfunction, and perspective. Mayo Clin Proc 68: 988–1001.

46. Bonaz B, Pellissier S, Sinniger V, Clarençon D, Peinnequin A, et al. (2012) The irritable bowel syndrome: how stress can affect the amygdala activity and the brain-gut axis. In: Ferry DB, editor. The Amygdala - A Discrete Multitasking Manager: InTech.

47. Kong L, Chen K, Tang Y, Wu F, Driesen N, et al. (2013) Functional connectivity between the amygdala and prefrontal cortex in medication-naive individuals with major depressive disorder. J Psychiatry Neurosci 38: 417–422.

48. Prater KE, Hosanagar A, Klumpp H, Angstadt M, Phan KL (2013) Aberrant amygdala-frontal cortex connectivity during perception of fearful faces and at rest in generalized social anxiety disorder. Depress Anxiety 30: 234–241.

49. Brown GL, McGarvey EL, Shirtcliff EA, Keller A, Granger DA, et al. (2008) Salivary cortisol, dehydroepiandrosterone, and testosterone interrelationships in healthy young males: a pilot study with implications for studies of aggressive behavior. Psychiatry Res 159: 67–76.

50. Shinkai S, Watanabe S, Kurokawa Y, Torii J (1993) Salivary cortisol for monitoring circadian rhythm variation in adrenal activity during shiftwork. Int Arch Occup Environ Health 64: 499–502.

51. Bosani M, Ardizzone S, Porro GB (2009) Biologic targeting in the treatment of inflammatory bowel diseases. Biologics 3: 77–97.

52. Kmiec Z (1998) Cytokines in inflammatory bowel disease. Arch Immunol Ther Exp (Warsz) 46: 143–155.

53. Patil SA, Rustgi A, Langenberg P, Cross RK (2013) Comparative effectiveness of anti-TNF agents for Crohn's disease in a tertiary referral IBD practice. Dig Dis Sci 58: 209–215.

54. Altavilla D, Guarini S, Bitto A, Mioni C, Giuliani D, et al. (2006) Activation of the cholinergic anti-inflammatory pathway reduces NF-kappab activation, blunts TNF-alpha production, and protects againts splanchic artery occlusion shock. Shock 25: 500–506.

55. Bonaz B, Picq C, Sinniger V, Mayol JF, Clarencon D (2013) Vagus nerve stimulation: from epilepsy to the cholinergic anti-inflammatory pathway. Neurogastroenterol Motil 25: 208–221.

56. Meregnani J, Clarencon D, Vivier M, Peinnequin A, Mouret C, et al. (2011) Anti-inflammatory effect of vagus nerve stimulation in a rat model of inflammatory bowel disease. Auton Neurosci 160: 82–89.

57. Nikolic VN, Jevtovic-Stoimenov T, Stokanovic D, Milovanovic M, Velickovic-Radovanovic R, et al. (2013) An inverse correlation between TNF alpha serum levels and heart rate variability in patients with heart failure. J Cardiol 62: 37–43.

58. Huston JM, Tracey KJ (2011) The pulse of inflammation: heart rate variability, the cholinergic anti-inflammatory pathway and implications for therapy. J Intern Med 269: 45–53.

59. Papaioannou V, Pneumatikos I, Maglaveras N (2013) Association of heart rate variability and inflammatory response in patients with cardiovascular diseases: current strengths and limitations. Front Physiol 4: 174.

60. Saul JP, Arai Y, Berger RD, Lilly LS, Colucci WS, et al. (1988) Assessment of autonomic regulation in chronic congestive heart failure by heart rate spectral analysis. Am J Cardiol 61: 1292–1299.

61. Taylor JA, Carr DL, Myers CW, Eckberg DL (1998) Mechanisms underlying very-low-frequency RR-interval oscillations in humans. Circulation 98: 547–555.

62. Ponikowski P, Chua TP, Amadi AA, Piepoli M, Harrington D, et al. (1996) Detection and significance of a discrete very low frequency rhythm in RR interval variability in chronic congestive heart failure. Am J Cardiol 77: 1320–1326.

63. Nemoto W, Nakagawasai O, Yaoita F, Kanno SI, Yomogida S, et al. (2013) Angiotensin II produces nociceptive behavior through spinal AT1 receptor-mediated p38 mitogen-activated protein kinase activation in mice. Mol Pain 9: 38.

64. Garg M, Burrell LM, Velkoska E, Griggs K, Angus PW, et al. (2014) Upregulation of circulating components of the alternative renin-angiotensin system in inflammatory bowel disease: A pilot study. J Renin Angiotensin Aldosterone Syst.

65. Elsenbruch S, Rosenberger C, Enck P, Forsting M, Schedlowski M, et al. (2010) Affective disturbances modulate the neural processing of visceral pain stimuli in irritable bowel syndrome: an fMRI study. Gut 59: 10.1136/gut.2008.175000.

66. Garakani A, Win T, Virk S, Gupta S, Kaplan D, et al. (2003) Comorbidity of irritable bowel syndrome in psychiatric patients: a review. Am J Ther 10: 61–67.

67. Pellissier S, Dantzer C., Fichou C., Bonaz B. (2007) Heart Rate Variability as a marker of stress in inflammatory bowel diseases AGA Institute abstracts. Gastroenterology 132: A-1-A-727.

68. FitzGerald LZ, Kehoe P, Sinha K (2009) Hypothalamic–pituitary– adrenal axis dysregulation in women with irritable bowel syndrome in response to acute physical stress. West J Nurs Res 31: 818–836.

69. Burr RL, Jarrett ME, Cain KC, Jun SE, Heitkemper MM (2009) Catecholamine and cortisol levels during sleep in women with irritable bowel syndrome. Neurogastroenterol Motil 21: 1148–e1197.

70. Vedhara K, Miles J, Bennett P, Plummer S, Tallon D, et al. (2003) An investigation into the relationship between salivary cortisol, stress, anxiety and depression. Biol Psychol 62: 89–96.

71. Richard PS, McCreath H, Tracey KJ, Sidney S, Liu K, et al. (2007) RR interval variability is inversely related to inflammatory markers: The CARDIA Study. Mol Med 13: 178–184.

72. Joo HM, Lee SJ, Chung YG, Shin IY (2010) Effects of mindfulness based stress reduction program on depression, anxiety and stress in patients with aneurysmal subarachnoid hemorrhage. J Korean Neurosurg Soc 47: 345–351.

19

Whole Genome Gene Expression Meta-Analysis of Inflammatory Bowel Disease Colon Mucosa Demonstrates Lack of Major Differences between Crohn's Disease and Ulcerative Colitis

Atle van Beelen Granlund[1,2,9], Arnar Flatberg[1,9], Ann E. Østvik[1,2,4], Ignat Drozdov[7], Bjørn I. Gustafsson[2,4], Mark Kidd[8], Vidar Beisvag[2], Sverre H. Torp[3,5], Helge L. Waldum[2,4], Tom Christian Martinsen[2,4], Jan Kristian Damås[2,6], Terje Espevik[1,2], Arne K. Sandvik[1,2,4]*

1 Centre of Molecular Inflammation Research, Norwegian University of Science and Technology, Trondheim, Norway, 2 Department of Cancer Research and Molecular Medicine, Norwegian University of Science and Technology, Trondheim, Norway, 3 Department of Laboratory Medicine, Norwegian University of Science and Technology, Trondheim, Norway, 4 Department of Gastroenterology and Hepatology, St. Olav's University Hospital, Trondheim, Norway, 5 Department of Pathology, St. Olav's University Hospital, Trondheim, Norway, 6 Department of Infectious Diseases, St. Olav's University Hospital, Trondheim, Norway, 7 Bering Limited, Richmond, United Kingdom, 8 Department of Surgery, Section of Gastroenterology, Yale School of Medicine, New Haven, Connecticut, United States of America

Abstract

Background: In inflammatory bowel disease (IBD), genetic susceptibility together with environmental factors disturbs gut homeostasis producing chronic inflammation. The two main IBD subtypes are Ulcerative colitis (UC) and Crohn's disease (CD). We present the to-date largest microarray gene expression study on IBD encompassing both inflamed and un-inflamed colonic tissue. A meta-analysis including all available, comparable data was used to explore important aspects of IBD inflammation, thereby validating consistent gene expression patterns.

Methods: Colon pinch biopsies from IBD patients were analysed using Illumina whole genome gene expression technology. Differential expression (DE) was identified using LIMMA linear model in the R statistical computing environment. Results were enriched for gene ontology (GO) categories. Sets of genes encoding antimicrobial proteins (AMP) and proteins involved in T helper (Th) cell differentiation were used in the interpretation of the results. All available data sets were analysed using the same methods, and results were compared on a global and focused level as t-scores.

Results: Gene expression in inflamed mucosa from UC and CD are remarkably similar. The meta-analysis confirmed this. The patterns of AMP and Th cell-related gene expression were also very similar, except for *IL23A* which was consistently higher expressed in UC than in CD. Un-inflamed tissue from patients demonstrated minimal differences from healthy controls.

Conclusions: There is no difference in the Th subgroup involvement between UC and CD. Th1/Th17 related expression, with little Th2 differentiation, dominated both diseases. The different *IL23A* expression between UC and CD suggests an IBD subtype specific role. AMPs, previously little studied, are strongly overexpressed in IBD. The presented meta-analysis provides a sound background for further research on IBD pathobiology.

Editor: Mathias Chamaillard, Inserm, France

Funding: Atle van Beelen Granlund is the recipient of a PhD grant from the Norwegian University of Science and Technology (NTNU), Ann Elisabeth Østvik of a PhD grant from The Liaison Committee between the Central Norway Regional Health Authority (RHA) and NTNU. This work was also supported by a research grant from The Liaison Committee between St. Olav's University Hospital and the Faculty of Medicine, NTNU. Mark Kidd is supported by National Institutes of Health (NIH) R01DK080871. BjØrn Munkvold, Kari SlØrdahl and Britt Schulze provided excellent technical assistance. The microarray work was carried out with support from the National Technology Microarray Platform (Norwegian Microarray Consortium) funded by the Functional Genomics Programme (FUGE) of the Norwegian Research Council. The funders had no role in study design, data collection and analysis, decision to publish, or preparation of the manuscript.

Competing Interests: Ignat Drozdov is employed by Bering Limited. There are no patents, products in development or marketed products to declare.

* E-mail: arne.sandvik@ntnu.no

⑨ These authors contributed equally to this work.

Introduction

The term inflammatory bowel disease (IBD) mainly covers ulcerative colitis (UC) and Crohn's disease (CD). IBD is a global health problem, with a reported prevalence as high as 568 and 827 per 100 000 in USA and Europe, respectively[1]. In IBD genetic susceptibility together with environmental factors disturbs intestinal homeostasis, resulting in repeated inflammation-remission cycles. CD can manifest itself anywhere in the gastrointestinal tract, while UC is only seen in the colon with varying length and degree of continuous inflammation extending proximally from the rectum. In UC the inflammation is found in the mucosa, in CD a deeper, often transmural inflammation with fistula formation is seen. Several extraintestinal diseases are associated with IBD, such as skin diseases, seronegative arthritis, uveitis and primary sclerosing cholangitis. Long-standing UC is associated with an increased risk of colorectal cancer. Despite the differences between UC and CD, there are cases where a definite diagnosis cannot be made, resulting in a diagnosis of non-specific colitis.

The coordinated effect of various T helper (Th) subtypes is fundamental to gut homeostasis[2], and UC and CD have been considered different with respect to Th cell activation. In mouse models it was shown that Th1 mechanisms mediated an inflammation similar to CD, and Th2 similar to UC[3]. In later years the concept of Th17 cells has been introduced and it was shown that inflammation previously attributed to Th1 could actually be Th17-driven and that these lymphocytes played an important role in CD[4,5]. Together with a better understanding of the importance of Treg lymphocytes in controlling inflammation, these discoveries have made it necessary to re-evaluate the Th1/Th2 concept of IBD [6].

Since the emergence of whole genome gene expression analysis (WGGE), efforts have been made to identify the transcriptional regulation underlying IBD. Although nearly a hundred susceptibility SNPs for IBD have been found, there has been limited success in translating gene expression results into hypotheses that aid the understanding and treatment of IBD [7]. Previous work in this field differs greatly. Gene expression technology has evolved fromserial analysis of gene expression (SAGE), to the newest WGGE arrays from e.g. Affymetrix and Illumina. Already in 1997 Heller et al. studied CD using spotted cDNA arrays [8]. In 2000 Dieckgraefe et al. examined colonic mucosa samples using Affymetrix Hum 6000 arrays with a coverage of ~6500 genes and expressed sequence tags (ESTs). This study identified 74 differentially expressed genes between inflamed UC and normal mucosa, grouping in functional classes such as immunoregulation and tissue regeneration [9]. Following these initial efforts many studies have been carried out, with great variation in the approach to the subject [10–25].

The WGGE analyses have identified regulation of several genes involved in processes thought to be of importance for IBD. Wu et al. suggested that genes involved in cell adhesion and polarisation processes were down-regulated in un-inflamed UC [11]. Olsen et al. used a set of genes to create a classification model able to discern un-inflamed UC samples from un-inflamed CD/control samples based on expression levels [12]. By comparing samples from IBD patients refractory to corticosteroids and/or immunosuppression before and after infliximab-treatment, Arijs et al. confirmed previous observations that expression of antimicrobial peptide (AMP) genes is changed in IBD [14,26,27]. Other studies have focused on identifying transcriptional regulation that could explain the clinical differences seen between UC and CD. However, the details around the initiation, propagation and maintenance of the chronic inflammation in IBD remain unclear.

When studying gene expression in complex tissues, the choice of sample material is very important. Patient and sample heterogeneity will greatly influence the measured expression levels, often hindering interpretation of the differences between sample groups. In IBD, leukocyte infiltration, Paneth cell metaplasia, crypt hyperplasia and ulceration with loss of epithelial cells are factors that will influence measured gene expression levels. As an example, the increase in α-defensin expression in colonic IBD

has been attributed to colonic Paneth cell metaplasia, while the decrease of α-defensin expression in ileal CD has been linked to loss of epithelial tissue, Paneth cell function and *NOD2* status [14,27–29].

Another effect potentially interfering with IBD microarray analysis is the regional variation in gene expression, with both a dichotomous and a more gradually varying gene expression pattern along the colon [30]. This regional variation has been discussed in several earlier IBD gene expression studies. Wu et al. and Costello et al. identified no such gene expression differences due to regional variation [11,15], In a later study, Noble et al. noted that this was readily identified in healthy controls. It is possible that modest regional variations can be masked when analysing inflamed tissue, but become apparent when un-inflamed biopsies are studied. These observations emphasize the importance of avoiding, or being aware of, confounding effects in the analysis of subtle differences in expression.

In this paper, a microarray-based gene expression analysis of colon pinch biopsies from IBD patients is presented. It is to the best of our knowledge the largest such study undertaken including samples from both inflamed and un-inflamed mucosa from UC and CD patients as well as normal controls. All un-inflamed samples and controls were obtained from the hepatic flexure, minimising any regional effect. The analysis was further supplemented by a meta-analysis of available IBD WGGE data, placing the presented data in the context of previous research on key fields in IBD research; T helper cell activation and antimicrobial peptide expression. The approach used in this work is meant to overcome the challenges of sample size, and heterogeneity in patients and sample material typically seen in gene expression analysis of complex, multifactorial diseases. By exploring the consensus between several data sets for expression related to important aspects of IBD, this analysis serves as a robust validation of suggested hypotheses

Results and Discussion

Gene expression analysis – NTNU data

Clinical material. All biopsies were assessed as either diseased or normal based on endoscopic findings at time of collection. Final diagnosis was done by histopathological evaluation of H–E stained sections. In cases where there was a discrepancy between endoscopic and histological assessment, the sample was excluded from the analysis. Moreover, 6 patients were excluded after a diagnosis of indeterminate colitis. A summary of sample information is provided in Table 1. Full information on the samples used in the analysis is included in Table S1. The final sample population consisted of 20 healthy controls (N), 37 active ulcerative colitis (UC), 7 active Crohn's disease (CD), 44 un-inflamed ulcerative colitis (UCU) and 19 un-inflamed Crohn's disease (CDU) samples. UCU sample group was further divided in two groups based on patient history. Samples originating from patients where sampling area (hepatic flexure) had previously been diagnosed as inflamed (UCUi, 11), and samples where no inflammation of the sample area ever had been observed (UCUu, 23).

Microarray gene expression analysis. Data analyses were performed using Bioconductor for the R software environment (http:www.r-project.org)[31]. Two samples, 226F and 115F, were analysed 8 times on separate chips as technical controls, showing good correlation between technical replicates (226F r2 = 0.989, 115F r2 = 0.992). In the final analysis the replicate closes to median of all replicates was used. Principal component analysis (PCA) analysis identified inflammation status as the dominating

Table 1. Summary of sample information.

	N	CD	UC	CDU	UCU
Number of subjects	20	7	37	19	44
Age, median years (range)	45 (19–71)	31(20–41)	38(19–72)	39(20–61)	45 (21–71)
Female / Male	9/11	2/5	22/15	6/13	24/20
Duration of disease, median years (range)	NA	7 (1–12)	9 (0–40)	6 (0–28)	13 (0–40)
5-ASA/S-ASA (%)	0	2 (29)	23 (62)	6 (32)	27 (61)
Systemic corticosteroids (%)	0	2(29)	9(26)	8 (42)	4(9)

Each column summarizes characteristics for all patients contributing with samples to the corresponding sample groups. 5-ASA – 5-aminosalicylic acid. S-ASA – sulphasalazine. Sample groups are abbreviated N for normal controls, CD for Crohn's disease, UC for ulcerative colitis, CDU for un-inflamed Crohn's disease and UCU for un-inflamed ulcerative colitis.

variation in the dataset, separating CD/UC samples from N/ UCU/CDU as shown in Figure 1A. There was no apparent separation between UC and CD in the PCA analysis. T-testing identified 4187/4189 significantly down/up-regulated genes for inflamed tissue from UC patients (UC), and 2093/2134 for inflamed tissue from CD patients (CD). For un-inflamed tissue (UCU and CDU), a very low number of differentially expressed genes were found (0/3 CDU, 0/0 UCU). Similarly to what was seen for the collected group, no differential expression was detected for the groups UCUi and UCUu when contrasted against normal controls (data not shown). The latter observation stands in contrast to recent finds reported by Planell et al, demonstrating several thousand genes as differentially expressed between UCUi and N[32]. This discrepancy is thought to arise due to differences in sample inclusion criteria. The complete table of results from the analysis is available in Table S2.

A Venn diagram illustrating the relationship between genes differentially expressed in UC and CD is given in Figure 1B. Using normal samples as common reference identified 4063 differentially expressed genes as common for CD and UC, with 4313 unique for UC and 164 unique for CD. This was in contrast to an analysis of CD vs. UC without use of common reference which identifies only 10 differentially expressed genes, of which 7 were included in the two previous analyses. This discrepancy could arise as a result of the imbalance in sample sizes. As the UC sample number is approximately 4 times larger than the CD sample size the variance of UC group is lower, giving higher t-scores in the analysis.

Other gene expression studies of IBD mucosal samples have reported expression differences between UC and CD, and built classifiers based on these results [10,12,24]. All of the classifiers are yet to be confirmed in clinical practice. Based on this observation of similarities between UC and CD gene expression, we chose to focus on defining the consensus set of genes and processes describing IBD, as observed when using whole genome gene expression analysis.

UC and CD samples share similar expression patterns related to T helper cell subtypes. Disease-specific gene co-expression networks were generated by computing Pearson correlation coefficients for the 4227 and 8376 differentially expressed genes in CD and UC respectively. Network analysis for un-inflamed tissue was not undertaken due to low numbers of differentially expressed genes. For each inflamed network, correlations were measured across normal and disease tissue. The CD-specific network (CD.N) and UC-specific network (UC.N) were partitioned into 13 and 9 modules with at least 30

genes. The largest modules in CD.N and UC.N contained 1261 and 4500 genes respectively. Subsequently, an enrichment analysis of each module identified over-represented Gene ontology (GO) terms. The complete lists of enriched GO processes are provided in Table S3 (for CD.N) and Table S4 (for UC.N). To computationally estimate functional similarities between CD.N and UC.N modules, Jaccard coefficient was calculated for all module pairs identified by the WGCNA. The largest overlap was observed between CD.N module 7 and UC.N module 3 (Jaccard = 0.14), enriched for "T cell activation". This similarity between "T cell activation" modules prompted further analysis of gene expression related to T cell differentiation in UC and CD.

The nature of T helper cell development in IBD has been an area of discussion for several years. The predominating theory has been that the adaptive immune response in CD is dominated by Th1 lymphocytes and in UC by Th2 lymphocytes. The identification of Th17 as a unique subset of T helper cells has challenged this view, and today some argue that the adaptive immune response in CD, and to some degree UC, is dominated by Th1/Th17 cells [6]. However, there are still unanswered questions regarding the role of Th2 activation in UC. A set of genes whose expression is known to be related to the four T helper cell lines Th1, Th2, Th17 and Treg were collected. Extracting the differential expression levels given as log2 fold change (log2 FC) and corrected p-values (p) for these genes allows for a characterization of T helper cell function in IBD.

Th1-related transcription factors *STAT1* (log2 FC: 1.62/1.64 for CD/UC, $p<0.001$) and *STAT4* (log2 FC: 0.55/0.76, $p<0.005$), as well as the classical Th1 cytokine *IFNG* (log2 FC:0.76/1.09, $p<0.001$) show increased expression in both CD and UC, a pattern expected during an active Th1 response. This is further supported by the increased expression of *CXCR3* (log2 FC: 0.54/0.42, p 0.001/<0.001), a Th1-associated chemokine receptor[33]. Interestingly there was a small increase in expression of the Th2 transcription factor *GATA3* in UC (log2 FC: 0.11, p: 0.01), but no increase in *IL4* or *STAT6* expression, suggesting an IL4/STAT6-independent activation of the Th2-related transcription factor GATA3. Jenner et al. has suggested an explanation for this unsupported expression of GATA3 by demonstrating that GATA3 may also be expressed in Th1 cells[34]. In this study GATA3 was shown to bind to the promoters of Th1-related genes in a pattern similar to that of the Th1 transcription factor TBX2, suggesting that the absence or presence of TBX2 determines cell lineage [34,35].

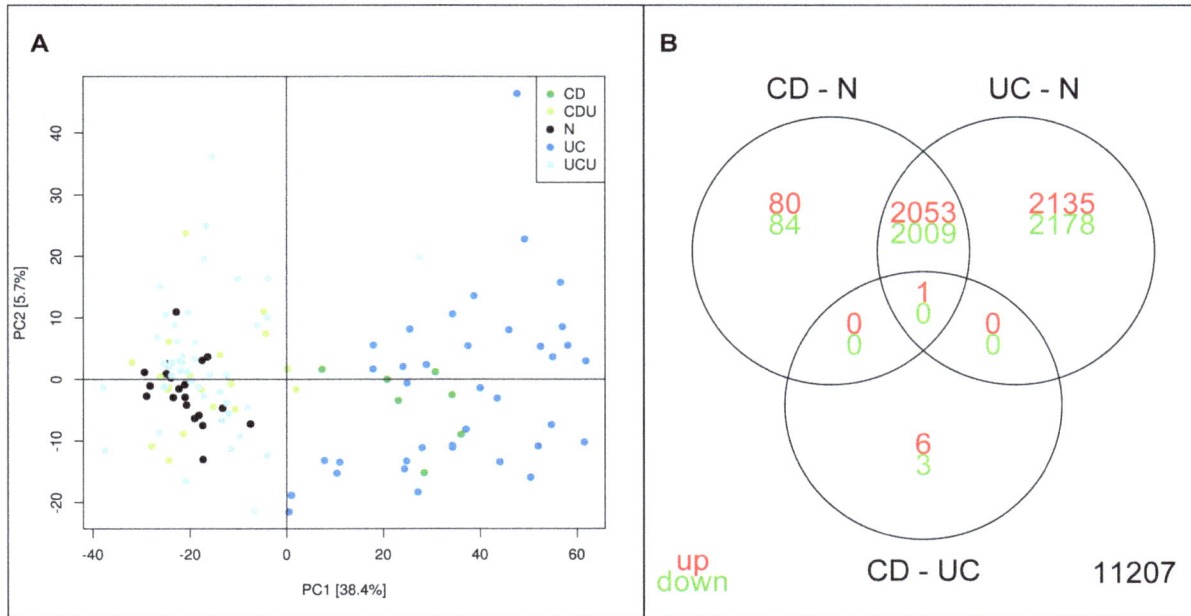

Figure 1. Initial analysis of NTNU data set. A: PCA analysis of NTNU data set. Each point represents one sample, with colour indicating sample groups as described in figure legend. Axis indicate % of total variance explained in each component. B: Venn diagram illustrating the relationship between analyses of sample groups UC and CD directly and using N as common reference. Numbers indicate significant genes (corrected p-val<0.05).

Th17-associated genes are up-regulated in both CD and UC mucosa. The effector cytokines *IL17F* (log2 FC: 0.37/0.24, p<0.002), *IL26* (log2 FC: 0.23/0.24, p: 0.03/<0.001) and *TNF* (log2 FC: 0.49/0.73, p: 0.01/<0.0001) were all up-regulated in CD and UC, suggesting the presence of active Th17-cells in the inflamed mucosa of IBD patients. This is further supported by the overexpression of Th17-associated transcription factors *STAT3* (log2 FC: 0.57/0.58, p<0.001) and *RORA* (log2 FC 0.54/0.48, p: (0.002/<0.001). The cytokines *IL1A* (log2 FC: 1.01/1.45, p<0.001), *IL1B* (log2 FC: 2.38/3.07, p<0.001) and *IL6* (log2 FC: 0.65/1.14, p: 0.01/<0.001), known to stimulate Th17 differentiation, were also up-regulated in IBD tissue[36]. Both Th17-associated chemokine-receptors *CCR4* (log2 FC: 0.26/0.24, p 0.008/<0.001) and *CCR6* (log2 FC: 1.01/0.93, p<0.001), and the Th-17 associated receptor KLRB1/CD161 (log2 FC: 0.83/0.73, p 0.02/<0.01) are differentially expressed in both CD and UC, further substantiating the validity of this observation[37,38].

There is little classical Treg-related expression, with only *STAT5A* exhibiting a marginal up-regulation in CD and UC (log2 FC: 0.35/0.50, p <0.05). However, both subunits of the Treg-cytokine IL35, *IL12A* (log2 FC: 0.17/0.24, p 0.02/0.002) and *EBV3* (log2 FC: 0.95/0.81, p <0.001), were over-expressed, while their other potential co-factors, *IL12B* and *IL27A*, had no significant increase in expression. IL35 is a newly discovered cytokine produced by T regulatory cells [39,40]. A Spearman correlation analysis of the subunits corresponding to IL27 (*IL27A* and *EBI3*), IL35 (*EBI3* and *IL12A*), IL23 (*IL23A* and *IL12B*) and IL12 (IL12A and IL12B) had the following rho values; IL27:0.04, IL23:0.003, IL12: 0.13 and IL35: 0.41. This could suggest an IL35-mediated Treg activity in the inflamed mucosa of IBD patients.

An interesting distinction between UC and CD expression was seen in *IL23A*-expression, with a significant log2 FC of 0.92 in UC but no significant difference in CD. The other subunit of IL23,

IL12B, exhibited no DE in either UC or CD. However, one cannot exclude differential expression of *IL12B*, as expression levels are below the detection limits in the microarray analysis.

Overall, the interpretation of the data in this setting confirms differentiation of activated T cells to Th1 and Th17 cells in both UC and CD, with an apparent absence of Th2-related differential expression. The expression profile of the selected genes in UC and CD are similar in this study, suggesting similar T helper cell population in the mucosa, at least under chronically active conditions.

Antimicrobial peptide genes are overexpressed in both UC and CD. There is increased expression of many AMPs in both inflamed UC and CD mucosa, with only a few interesting exceptions. Defensin 1 beta (*DEFB1*) is significantly down-regulated in both UC (log2 FC -2.19) and CD (log2 FC -1.89), while the gene encoding liver expressed antimicrobial protein 2 (*LEAP2*) showed a similar, but less prominent regulation (UC: log2 FC -0.78, CD: log2 FC -0.68). The loss of DEFB1 expression has previously been reported by Arijs et al., who suggested that alterations may be due to a loss of epithelial tissue in inflamed colon [21]. Our results suggest an alternative explanation. A work by Peyrin-Biroulet et al. describes the role of DEFB1 in maintaining homeostasis, and explores the regulation of colonic DEFB1 expression[41] The study demonstrates that DEFB1 expression is under transcriptional control of PPARG. There was a significant down-regulation of peroxisome-proliferator receptor gamma (*PPARG*) in both UC (log2 FC -1.35) and CD (-1.14), and a strong correlation (rho 0.73) between expression of *PPARG* and *DEFB1* suggesting that *DEFB1* down-regulation could be a result of loss of *PPARG* expression. However, further exploration is needed to conclude with a causal effect of the observed correlation.

Meta-analysis - NTNU data and publicly available datasets

Meta-analysis shows intra-experiment differences in power, but good correlation in regulation. Data from all available datasets fulfilling the search criteria defined in the methods section were included in a meta-analysis to identify gene regulation and processes that were stably correlated with disease status over many analysis settings. The rationale was that regulation consistently identified over a cross-platform, cross-laboratory meta-analysis could be seen as externally verified, thereby increasing the validity of conclusions. Details of the datasets are provided in Table 2. The comparisons were performed both on the gene expression and GO category levels. For the gene level analysis, comparisons were made between both t-score (Figure S1) and by ranking of genes (Figure S2). The rank-based analysis was used to identify an appropriate number of genes to use in the t-score analysis. The number of genes used was chosen based on the top union score of the rankings, as calculated using GeneSelector[42]. The gene comparison demonstrated a wide distribution in the statistical power of the tests performed, with a spread in differentially expressed genes from 7500 to 30 in the comparison UC vs. N. All sets containing both UC and CD samples exhibited a higher number of DE genes for the UC vs. N test than CD vs. N test. However, the cluster analysis does not identify a separation between UC and CD on the basis of mucosal gene expression. For tests of un-inflamed tissue vs. normal there was little consensus, suggesting that each of these tests capture different variation. For comparisons of tests of inflamed tissue vs. normal there was a good agreement between the sets with regard to t-scores, the closest clustering involving inflamed tissue.

There was a high "intra-experiment" similarity, with lists from the same study clustering as neighbours independently of diagnosis. Strong tests of inflamed vs. un-inflamed samples with many DE genes clustered together. The strength of the sets appeared to be the product of two parameters; many samples or well controlled sample groups. Ahrens et al. have relatively few samples (13 patients) in their UC group, but many DE genes in the UC vs. N comparison (>7500) were identified. The samples used in this comparison were uniquely controlled, with a focus on un-medicated paediatric patients. In the dataset collected by Arijs et al. all samples had high degree of inflammation, taken from patients' refractory to corticosteroids/immunosuppressant[21]. In our dataset the number of inflamed UC samples was 37, a number of samples that was sufficient to compensate for the relative heterogeneity in sample set, and resulted in a set of approx. 7500 DE genes.

Some comparisons were divergent. The UCU vs. N test based on samples from Olsen et al. cluster with the affected group, showing high t-scores for genes typically DE in inflamed tissue. This corresponded well with conclusions in the article describing the dataset, suggesting a pre-inflammatory state in un-inflamed tissue from patients diagnosed with UC[12]. The expression pattern seen in this set of sample was however not reproduced in the other sets of unaffected samples.

Gene set analysis of imported data sets identifies consensus processes important in IBD pathology. By using gene set enrichment analysis the results from all the data sets could be compared at a more general level, potentially identifying the fundamental processes underpinning IBD. This reduction into GO categories also helped overcome difficulties in comparing results from many analyses, as similarities in a gene category could be found even when methodological differences limited any gene-for-gene comparison [43]. An initial analysis was undertaken to identify the appropriate number of GO categories to use in the comparison. The result from this analysis is provided in Figure S3.

Figure 2 is a summary of the finds, where categories were chosen on the basis of all data as outlined in the methods section. In this figure all GSEA scores were included, regardless of q value. A supplementary figure with a q value cut-off of 0.25 was included as Figure S4. The analysis showed few gene sets with a significant normalised enrichment score (NES). However, as is seen in figure 2, there is a remarkable consistency in the NES for top ranked categories across studies, suggesting that similar processes are dominating all gene lists based on inflamed samples. As was demonstrated in the t-score based analysis, the cluster analysis readily separated inflamed from un-inflamed comparisons, showing little separation of CD and UC sets. The separation between strong and weak data sets was also repeated.

The list of GO categories was dominated by inflammation-related categories both related to innate and adaptive immunity responses. There were several categories describing cell proliferation, thought to be activated due to the increase in epithelial cell regeneration as a response to tissue damage. Interestingly, several categories related to angiogenesis were broadly activated, supporting the notion that this may be an important process in IBD[44].

Both T helper cell and AMP observations are confirmed by meta-analysis. GSEA analysis based solely on categories related to T helper cell differentiation was performed as described in the methods section. A plot of mean NES scores for UC and CD is given in Figure 3. A Wilcox rank-sum test between UC and CD for each gene category demonstrated no significant difference in NES score for UC and CD. The analysis demonstrated the highest mean NES score for Th1 and Th17-related categories, while the Th2-related categories showed the lowest mean GSEA score for both UC and CD. The GATA3 category showed the largest difference in activity when comparing UC and CD. Of all the categories, this also has the smallest p-value (0.1).

Two lists of gene names were assembled to further investigate T helper cell differentiation and AMP expression in inflamed colonic IBD mucosa. The list of AMPs was based on work by Arijs et al[21]. here was a broad consensus between gene regulation observed in the presented dataset and the meta-analysis both in the subset of T helper cell-associated and AMP genes. Two heat maps were constructed from each gene set, one using only significant t-scores and one with all t-scores irrespective of significance, the rationale being that even non-significant regulation could help interpretation when supported by significant regulation in other analyses. Figures based on scores with corrected p-value <0.05 are included as Figures 4 and 5. The figures based on all scores are given as Figure S5 and S6. Applying p-value cut-off reveals the lack of statistical significance of observed gene regulation for many of the data sets.

The observations made based on our dataset were broadly confirmed by all imported datasets, even when t-scores were not significant. There were few differences in t-scores between UC and CD. *IL23A* expression was only identified as significantly increased in UC vs. N tests. This was an interesting finding when viewed in the light of previous research exploring the IL23-axis in IBD [45,46]. Animal models have suggested an important role for IL23 in Th17 proliferation, and an IBD-susceptibility SNP has been identified in the IL23 receptor [46,47]. The different *IL23A* levels detected in inflamed tissue from UC and CD patients suggest distinct roles for this cytokine in the two diseases. Our dataset is the only analysis showing a DE for *IL6* in CD vs. N, with all other DE shown in UC vs. N tests. Our set together with the data of Noble et al. also identified a DE of *IL17F*, while the other data sets found *IL17A* as DE. A possible explanation for this might be differences in technology, as *IL17F* was found DE on Affymetrix

Table 2. Meta-analysis data source.

Name	Study title	PMID [Ref]	GEO/ArrayExpress accession numbers	N	CD	UC	CDU	UCU	Platform
Ahr	Intestinal macrophage/epithelial cell-derived CCL11/eotaxin-1 mediates eosinophil recruitment and function in pediatric ulcerative colitis.	18981162 [21]	GSE10191	11	0	8	0	0	Affymetrix HG-U133 Plus 2.0
Ari	Mucosal gene expression of antimicrobial peptides in inflammatory bowel disease before and after first infliximab treatment	19956723 [20]	GSE16879	6	19	24	0	0	Affymetrix HG-U133 Plus 2.0
Bje	Genome-wide gene expression analysis of mucosal colonic biopsies and isolated colonocytes suggests a continuous inflammatory state in the lamina propria of patients with quiescent ulcerative colitis	19834973 [22]	GSE13367	10	0	8	0	9	Affymetrix HG-U133 Plus 2.0
Car	Activation of an IL-6:STAT3-dependent transcriptome in pediatric-onset inflammatory bowel disease.	18069684 [17]	GSE9686	8	10	5	0	0	Affymetrix HG-U133 Plus 2.0
Gal	Diagnostic mRNA expression patterns of inflamed, benign, and malignant colorectal biopsy specimen and their correlation with peripheral blood results	18843029 [23]	GSE10714	3	8	3	0	0	Affymetrix HG-U133 Plus 2.0
Gyo	Inflammation, adenoma and cancer: objective classification of colon biopsy specimens with gene expression signature	18776587 [16]	GSE4183	8	6	9	0	0	Affymetrix HG-U133 Plus 2.0
Kug	Loci on 20q13 and 21q22 are associated with pediatric-onset inflammatory bowel disease	18758464 [24]	GSE10616	11	32	10	0	0	Affymetrix HG-U133 Plus 2.0
Nob	Regional variation in gene expression in the healthy colon is dysregulated in ulcerative colitis	18523026 [13]	GSE11223	63	0	62	0	61	Agilent Whole Human Genome microarray
Ols	Diagnosis of ulcerative colitis before onset of inflammation by multivariate modeling of genome-wide gene expression data	19177426 [11]	GSE9452 (UC samples) and GSE11831 (controls), E-TABM-118 (CD samples)	17	0	8	0	9	Affymetrix HG-U133 Plus 2.0
vbG	NTNU study		E-MTAB-184	20	8	37	19	44	Illumina human HT-12 expression BeadChips
Wu	Genome-wide gene expression differences in Crohn's disease and ulcerative colitis from endoscopic pinch biopsies: insights into distinctive pathogenesis.	17262812 [10]	GSE6731	4	7	5	12	4	Affymetrix HG -U95Av2

Information on all data sets used in meta-analysis. Column "Name" refers to abbreviations used in Figure 2- and Figure S1–S5. "Study title" refers to name of original source article, with reference given in column "PMID [Ref]". Column "No. samples" gives number of samples in each group in the relevant data set, with the following group names: N – Normal controls, CD – Crohn's disease, UC – Ulcerative colitis, CDU – Un-inflamed Crohn's disease and UCU – Un-inflamed ulcerative colitis. Column "Platform" refers to microarray technology used in the relevant analysis.

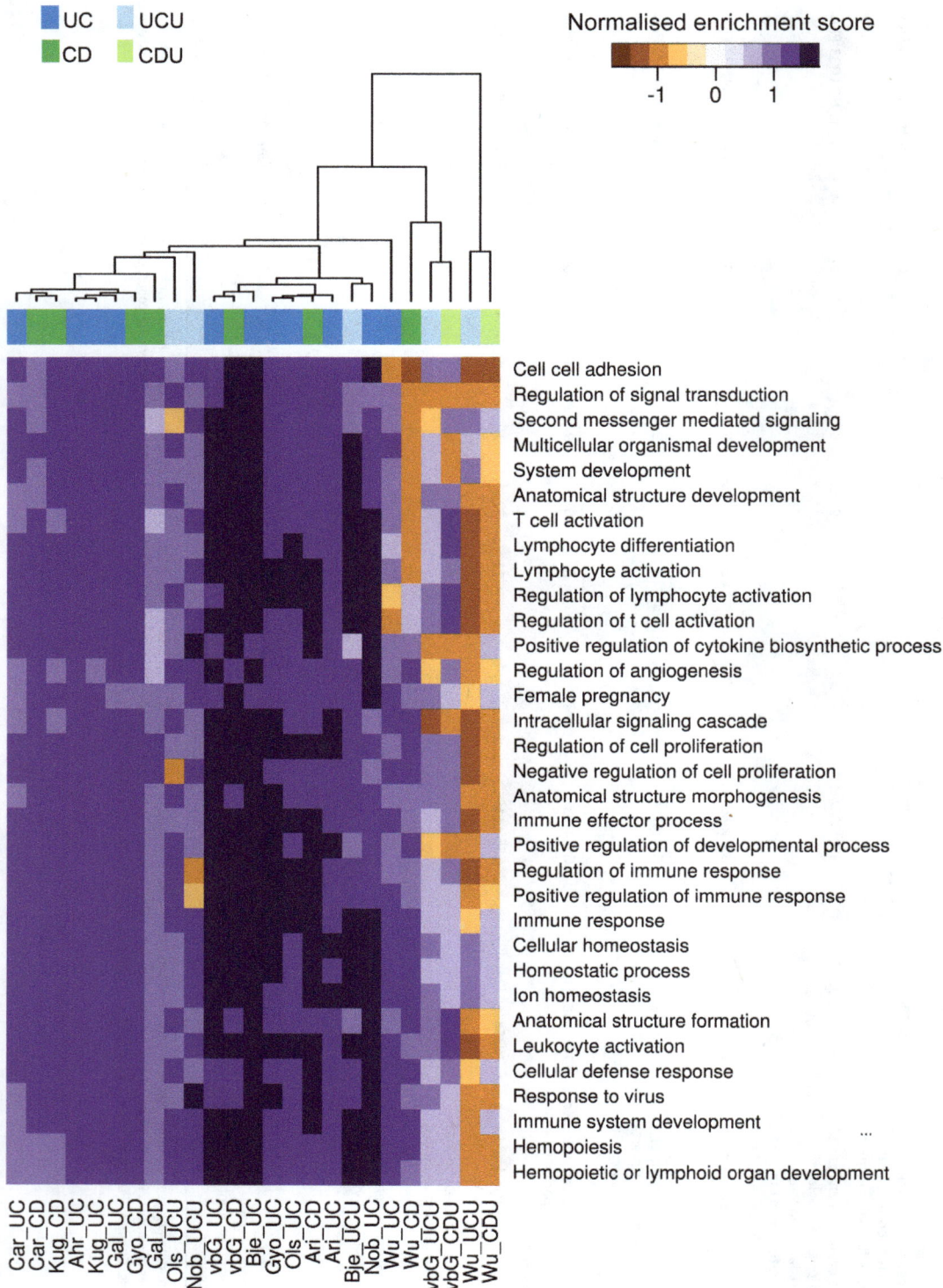

Figure 2. GSEA analysis of all data sets. The figure shows a heat map of GSEA scores for the GO categories selected in the rank-based analysis. Each column in the figure represents the result for one comparison against normal control, with sample source and test group given as column name. The connection between each columns source abbreviation and its related dataset(s) and article(s) are given in table 2.

chips, while *IL17A* was found on Agilent and Illumina microarrays.

An interesting observation was the down-regulation of *RORC*. RORC is seen as a key transcription factor for Th17 cells, that

together with STAT3 and RUNX1 promotes the transcription of the effector cytokines IL17A/F, IL21, IL22, IL26 and CCL20[48]. This down-regulation was unexpected, as both key regulators of *RORC* expression (*TGFB* and *STAT3*), the transcription co-factors

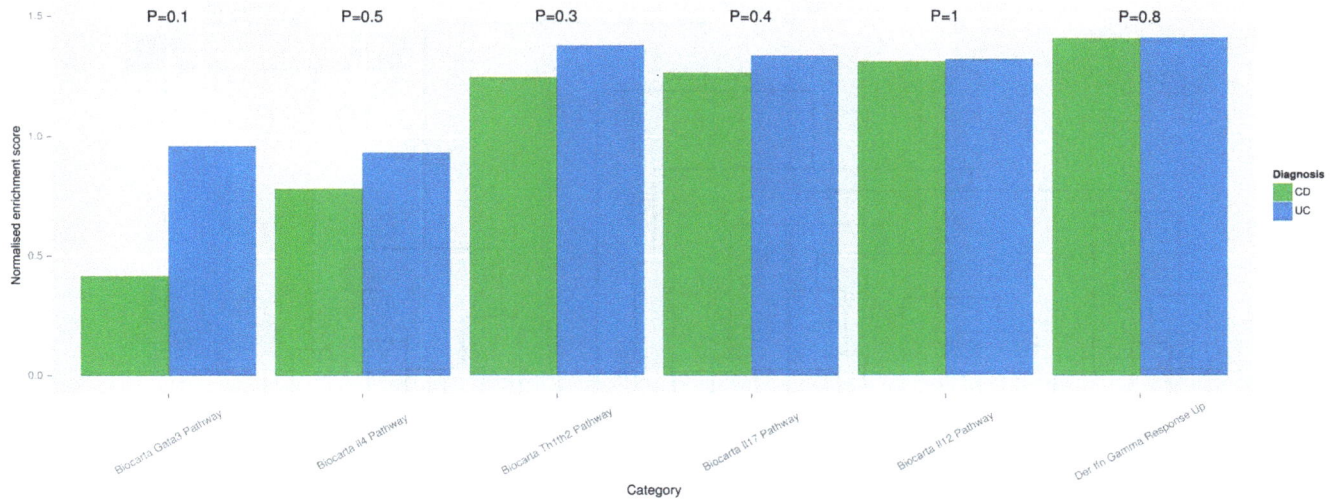

Figure 3. T helper cell associated GSEA analysis. A subset of gene categories thought to represent T helper cell differentiation was selected from MSigDB. The bar plot is a summary of results from GSEA analysis of this subset, where each bar represents the mean GSEA score for a sample group (UC or CD) for the GSEA category in question. A Wilcox rank-sum test was performed between disease groups fails to identify a difference between GSEA scores for the selected categories.

(*RUNX1* and *STAT3*) and the effector cytokines were all over-expressed in many of the datasets included in the analysis. However, the closely related paralog to *RORC*, *RORA*, was over-expressed in several datasets. Studies in mice have demonstrated that RORA expression is sufficient to promote Th17 differentiation, possibly explaining the regulation seen in this meta-analysis[49]. It must also be stressed that even though there was a down-regulation of *RORC* expression, there was no evidence of loss of *RORC* function, possibly suggesting that the relative down-regulation is not enough for RORC to be a limiting factor in the combined transcriptional regulation of RORC, RORA, RUNX1 and STAT3. Interestingly, the sets showing the most distinct regulation of *RORC* was based mainly on un-medicated paediatric patients (Ahrens et al. and Carey et al.), together with data from Kugathasan et al. where no patient age information was given. The same datasets also showed no significant regulation of *STAT3*.

Almost all datasets exhibited over-expression of suppressor of cytokine signalling 3 (*SOCS3*), a gene closely associated with Th2 cell development, while there was a broad down-regulation of other Th2-associated transcription. This apparent paradox has been observed in CD before[50]. It might arise due to another role of SOCS3, namely as an inhibitor of naïve CD4+ cell differentiation to activated T cells. SOCS3 inhibits the production of IL-2, a cytokine crucial for the activation of T cells, effectively inhibiting initial T cell activation. The over-expression of *SOCS3* in this setting might therefore be the result of an effort to limit the activation of T helper cells in the inflamed mucosa, while the increased expression of *STAT3* might be the result of SOCS3-independent activation via IL10[51,52]. It is also possible that the *SOCS3* expression detected stems from cells other than lymphocytes, as both neutrophils, macrophages and epithelial cells have been shown to express *SOCS3* in IBD mucosa[53].

In the AMP set the pattern of expression seen in our dataset was reproduced in the imported sets as shown in Figure 5. The two down-regulated AMPs *DEFB1* and *LEAP2* exhibited similar down-regulation in the other sets, while at the same time confirming the observed up-regulation of AMPs in inflamed mucosa. The down-regulation of *PPARG* was also broadly confirmed in the imported data (data not shown).

Conclusion

The present study is the to-date largest microarray gene expression study examining both inflamed and un-inflamed samples from colonic mucosa of IBD patients. Uniquely, the analysis also includes a gene co-expression network analysis and a meta-analysis of comparable IBD datasets. The analysis shows a similarity between the gene expressions in inflamed mucosa from UC and CD patients, which is confirmed by hierarchical clustering of several independent data sets. This suggests that once established the inflammatory mechanisms at mucosal level are largely the same for the two diseases. Our analysis further demonstrates that the T helper cell-related expression found in the inflamed colonic mucosa of all IBD patients is dominated by Th1/Th17-related expression, with little to no signs of Th2 differentiation. There was no significant difference between GSEA scores for T helper cell related categories between UC and CD. The mean GSEA score was highest for categories related to Th1/Th17, and lowest for Th2-related categories. The only selected gene showing a clear difference in expression between UC and CD was *IL23A*, consistently showing DE in UC vs. N comparisons. This distinction between UC and CD T cell expression seems to be highly reproducible, and is of particular interest given previous research emphasising the importance of the IL23-axis in IBD. Another feature very similar across the diagnoses and the different datasets is the significant change in expression of antimicrobial peptides, the AMPs. The expression of many AMPs in inflamed IBD mucosa is generally increased when compared to un-inflamed mucosa, with the exception of *DEFB1* and *LEAP2*. In the in-house data, the loss of *DEFB1* is highly correlated with loss of *PPARG* expression, a gene known to exert a promoting effect on DEFB1. In addition, mucosal biopsies from un-inflamed colon in patients with IBD had gene expression patterns almost identical to healthy control subjects, with only CDU displaying a few differentially expressed genes in the NTNU dataset.

This IBD WGGE study for the first time integrates external data sets, providing a sound background for further research on IBD pathobiology. The chosen strategy of focusing on consensus

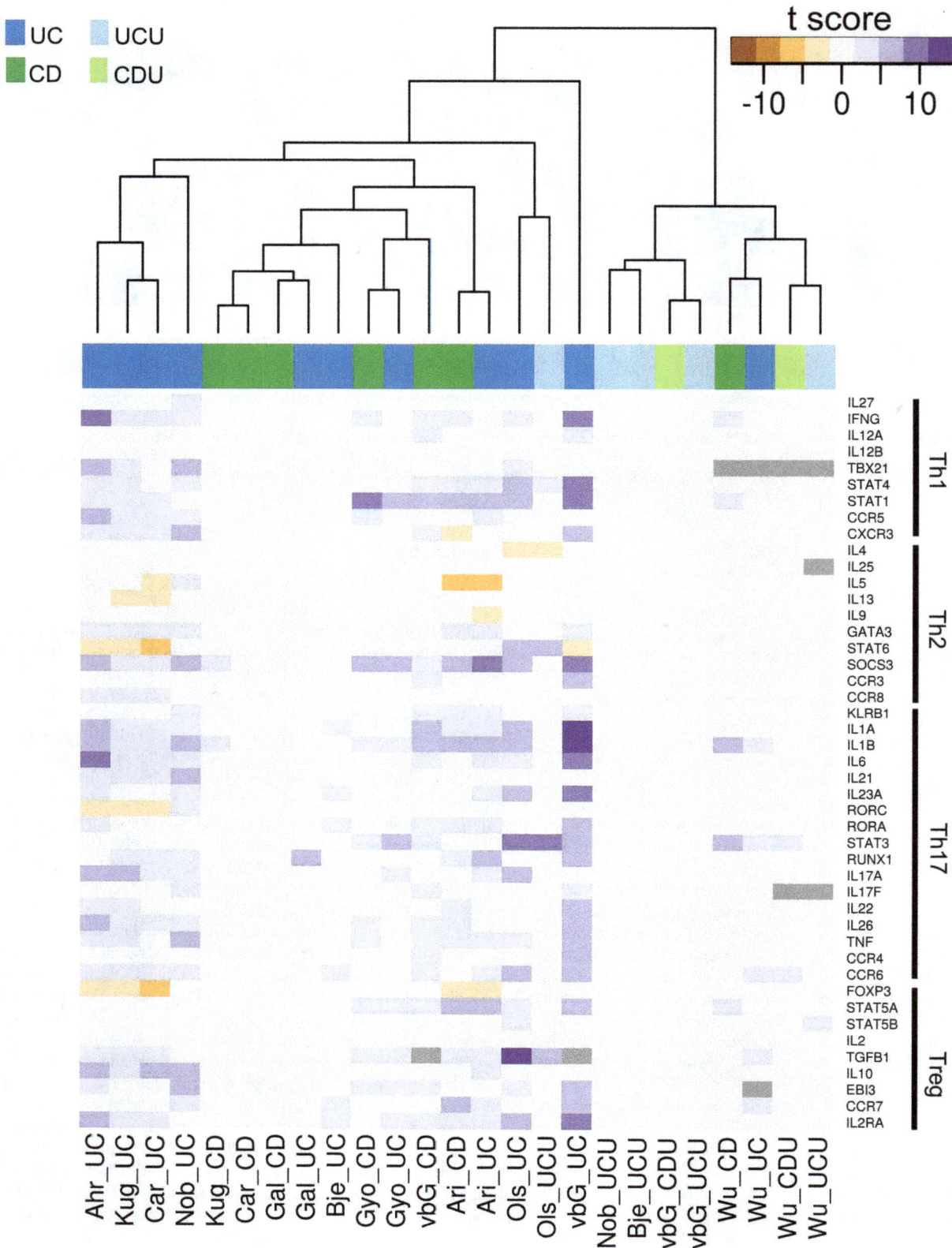

Figure 4. T helper cell-associated genes. The figure shows a heat map of t-scores (corrected p-val <0.05) for genes related to T helper cell differentiation and function. Figure S4 shows the same data with a no p-value cut-off. Genes are grouped in the Th sub-categories Th1, Th2, Th17 and Treg. Each column in the figure represents the result for one comparison against normal control, with sample source and test group given as column name. The connection between each column's source abbreviation and its related dataset(s) and article(s) are given in table 2. Some sets lack measurements for certain genes, in which case a grey marking is used.

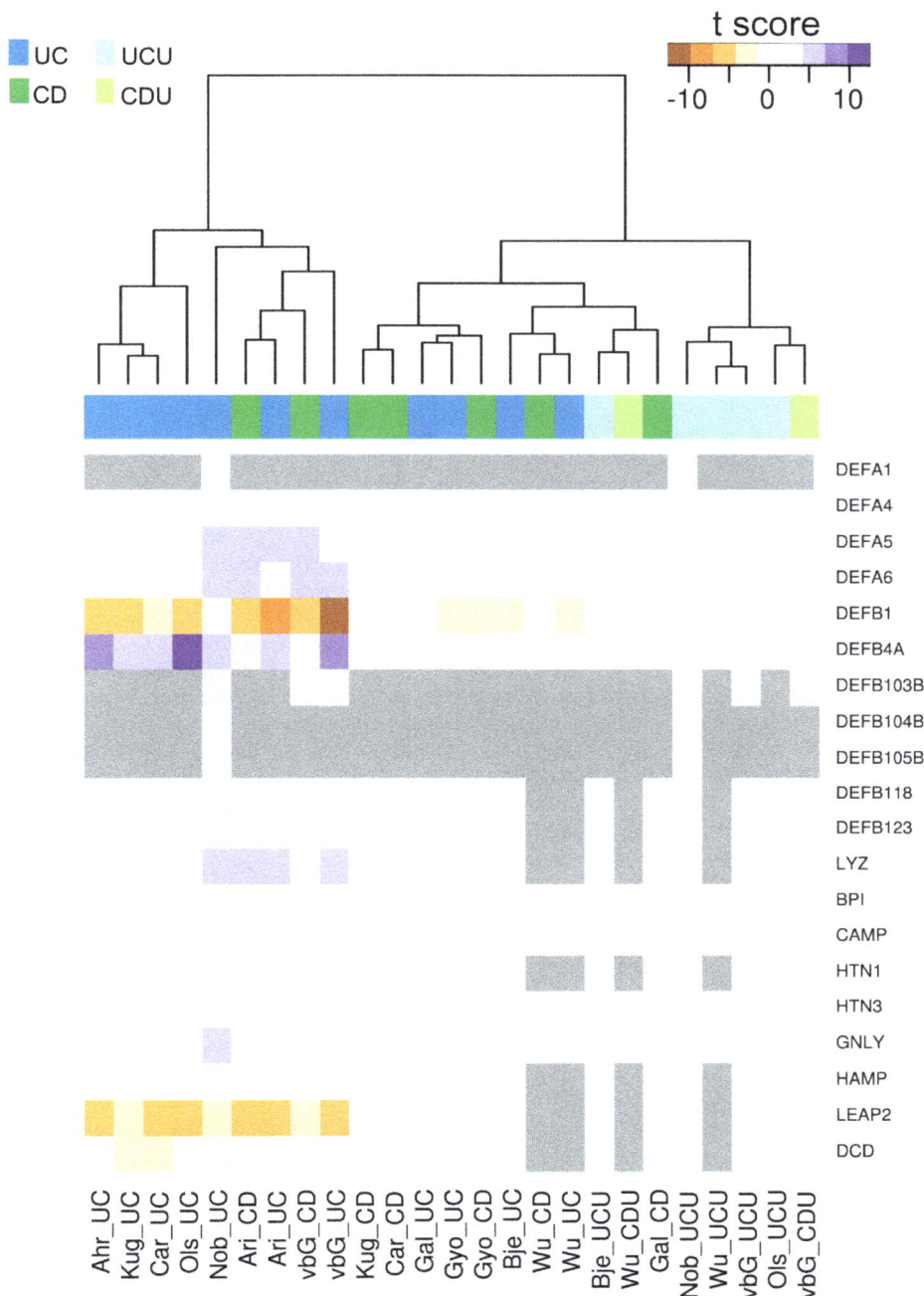

Figure 5. Antimicrobial peptide gene expression. The figure shows a heat map of t-scores (corrected p-val <0.05) for genes coding for known antimicrobial peptides. Figure S5 shows the same data with no p-value cut-off. Each column in the figure represents the result for one comparison against normal control, with the sample source and test group given as column name. The connection between each column's source abbreviation and its related dataset(s) and article(s) are given in table 2. Some sets lack measurements for certain genes, in which case a grey marking is used.

genes and processes over several datasets facilitates result interpretation and validation.

Materials and Methods

Sample material

Samples were collected from an IBD cohort at St. Olav's University Hospital, Trondheim, Norway. Study participants were patients admitted to the Department of Gastroenterology for colonoscopy. Participants were either diagnosed with UC or CD,

or were admitted for diagnostic colonoscopy due to symptoms unrelated to IBD. Patients were only included as normal controls after all clinically indicated examinations had concluded no signs of gastrointestinal disease. In the IBD groups (UC and CD), four endoscopic pinch biopsies were taken from macroscopically maximally inflamed mucosa, as well from the hepatic flexure in cases where this was found to be macroscopically un-inflamed UC unaffected (UCU) and CD unaffected (CDU)). Two UCU samples, 228 F and 118 F were obtained from ascending colon and rectum, respectively. For the normal (N) group, four biopsies were taken from the hepatic flexure. One biopsy from each area was fixed in 4% buffered formaldehyde, while the three remaining biopsies were snap frozen and stored in liquid nitrogen.

Ethics statement

Written informed consent was obtained from all participants, and the study was approved by the Regional Medical Research Ethics Committee (approval no 5.2007.910). The study was registered in the Clinical Trials Protocol Registration System (identifier NCT00516776).

Microarray analysis

RNA extraction and quality control. Frozen biopsies were homogenized in lysis buffer using a rotating knife homogenizer (Zanke & Kunkel IKA-Laboratorie Technik, Staufen, Germany). Total RNA was extracted using the Ambion mirVana miRNA Isolation Kit (Applied Biosystems, CA, USA). Quality control was performed for each extract. Quantity and purity of RNA was assessed using a NanoDrop Spectrophotometer (Thermo Scientific, DE, USA), and the integrity of isolated RNA was determined using Bioanalyzer (Agilent Technologies, CA, USA). Samples were only included in subsequent analysis if the RIN value > 7. Isolated RNA was stored in cryo-tubes in liquid nitrogen.

Hybridization. 250 ng total RNA from each sample was used to generate biotinylated, amplified cRNA using the Illumina TotalPrep RNA Amplification kit (Applied Biosystems/ Ambion, Austin, TX, USA). cRNA was stored at $-80°C$, and the concentration of each cRNA sample was adjusted to 150 ng/ µl prior to hybridization. The samples were all hybridized in parallel on Illumina human HT-12 expression BeadChips (Illumina, San Diego, CA, USA) and scanned on an Illumina BeadStation. Results from the microarray analysis are available at ArrayExpress E-MTAB-184.

Differential expression analysis

Expression data analysis was performed using the R software environment for statistical computing[54]. Methods supplied in the Bioconductor package were used for import, quality assessment, normalization, filtering and statistical analysis of the expression data [31]. Data was log-transformed and quantile normalized. Probes not corresponding to an ENTREZ ID were removed. In cases where several probes corresponded to one ENTREZ ID, the probe showing the highest variance over all samples was chosen for further analysis. Initial interpretation of data was done using the unsupervised method of Principal Component Analysis (PCA). Final differential expression analysis was performed using LIMMA linear models with least squares regression and empirical Bayes moderated t-statistics[55]. P-values were adjusted for multiple comparisons using the Benjamini Hochberg false discovery rate correction (FDR). A corrected p-value of 0.05 was chosen as significance level.

Network analysis

Weighted correlation network formation. From the normalized microarray dataset we followed the protocol for Weighted Correlation Network Analysis (WGCNA) [56,57] to create CD- and UC- specific networks. For each network, only DE genes (Bayes moderated p-values <0.05) in diseased compared to normal samples were analysed and co-expressions were measured across normal and diseased tissue.

Gene module detection, comparison, and enrichment. Genes were hierarchically clustered using 1 − Topological Overlap (TO) [58] as the distance measure and modules were determined by applying a

dynamic tree-cutting algorithm [56]. TO is a biologically meaningful measurement that reflects the similarity of gene co-expression relationships in the network, while the dynamic tree-cutting algorithm allows identification of clusters in a dendrogram depending on their shape. Similarity between CD and UC disease modules was expressed using the Jaccard coefficient - the ratio of the number of genes common to two modules to the number of total genes in both modules. All modules were enriched for over-represented Gene Ontology (GO) functional terms using the Fisher exact test. As background we used all of the supplied genes that were present in at least one term in the GO.

Meta-analysis of available data sets

Choosing data sets for meta-analysis. The microarray data repositories Array Express and NCBI GEO were searched for datasets containing references to "Inflammatory bowel disease", "Ulcerative colitis" or "Crohn's disease" [59,60]. These datasets where then evaluated further by including only analyses done on pinch biopsies from human colon. Data from printed arrays (oligo/cDNA microarrays) were excluded. Only sets where at least one of the groups UC, CD, UCU, CDU in addition to control individuals (N) were included. The total number of external datasets included in the analysis was 10. A full list of included data sets is given in Table 2

Differentially expressed genes meta-analysis. We used the limma software package (ver. 3.12.1) from Bioconductor to assess the effect of DE of IBD subgroups with respect to normal controls. The individual contrast for each dataset was summarised by t-scores and adjusted p-values in the same manner as the original analysis of our data. All analyses following this were based on the resulting "gene x contrast" matrix, where each contrast from each set was represented with two tables containing t-scores and p-values. We determined an aggregated rank score for each gene by a weighted-mean summary across the ranks of inflamed (UC, CD) t-scores. In this method, the weights received are proportional to the logarithm of the number of genes identified as significant in the limma-model, with a minor moderation to accommodate small values. In cases where only a subset of the datasets (due to differences in array types) have a specific gene present we used imputed values for the missing t-scores based on a k-nearest neighbour imputing scheme as implemented in the impute (ver. 1.30.0) Bioconductor package. The imputed values were subsequently removed prior to results visualization.

The (genes x contrasts) table of ranks was visualised as a heat map with genes ordered after aggregated rank score and contrasts ordered by distance to the aggregated rank score. The distance was calculated using linear decay weighting of the Manhattan distance as implemented in the default settings of the GeneSelector package (ver. 2.6.0) and a unionscore was computed from the same package using only the inflamed contrasts. The unionscore measures the similarity between multiple ordered lists by counting the size of the union for each position in the aggregated rank score and normalising with regards to position. A high unionscore indicates high agreement between contrasts. The maximum unionscore was achieved at position 2973 and thus the first 2973 genes were selected for visualising t-scores. The t-scores were visualized in a heat map where both rows and columns were ordered by hierarchical clustering using Euclidean distance and Ward agglomeration. *Gene ontology GSEA meta-analysis*

A GSEA (Gene Set Enrichment Analysis) score was estimated for each of the individual contrasts. The more recent version weighted with correlation to phenotype was used and gene sets were collected from the GO Biological Process part of MSigDB (ver. 3.1) [61]. This relatively reduced set of categories was chosen to improve interpretation, as the goal was not mainly to identify novel categories but rather to provide a well validated representation of the processes at hand in colonic IBD inflammation. A gene set was accepted if it contained between 25 and 1500 genes. Categories were further filtered on q value, including only categories where at least 3 comparisons had q values < 0.25. This resulted in a list of 233 categories. These categories were included in the union score calculation as described for the gene-wise analysis, this time based on ranked q values identifying 33 categories with the top union score. The results were visualised as in the gene meta-analysis. A second GSEA analysis was performed on a subset of the MSigDB categories related to T helper cell differentiation. These categories were "Biocarta GATA3 pathway", Biocarta IL12 pathway", "Biocarta IL17 pathway", "Biocarta IL4 pathway", "Biocarta Th1Th2 pathway", "Biocarta IL4 pathway" and "Der INF gamma response up". A GSEA score was calculated for each of the contrasts, and mean GSEA score for UC and CD contrast were calculated for each category. A Wilcox rank-sum test was performed between GSEA scores for UC and CD.

Supporting Information

Figure S1 T-score analysis of all data sets. A visualisation of the top scoring genes over all available data sets. Each column represents one comparison, with sample group and source given in the column name. Each vertical line represents a t-score from the corresponding analysis. Grey lines replace missing values, where no measurement of the gene in question was given in the source data. The connection between each columns source abbreviation and its related dataset(s) and article(s) are given in table 2.

Figure S2 Gene rank analysis of all data sets. Figure illustrating the method used to choose the number of genes used in t-score based comparison of all data sets. Optimal number of genes was chosen at the maximum unionscore as described in Methods section.

Figure S3 GO rank heat map. GO rank analysis: Figure illustrating the method used to find the optimal number of GO categories to use in a comparison of all data sets. The optimal number of GO categories (33) was chosen at maximum unionscore as described in methods section.

Figure S4 GSEA analysis of all data sets with q value cut-off. The figure shows a heat map of GSEA scores for the GO categories selected in the rank-based analysis. Each column in the figure represents the result for one comparison against normal control, with sample source and test group given as column name. Scores with q-value > 0.25 are removed. The connection between each columns source abbreviation and its related dataset(s) and article(s) are given in table 2.

Figure S5 T helper cell associated genes. Figure shows a heat map of significant t-scores for genes related to T helper cell differentiation and function. Genes are grouped in the Th subcategories Th1, Th2, Th17 and Treg. Each column in the figure represents the result for one comparison against normal control, with sample source and test group given as the column name. The connection between each column's source abbreviation and its related dataset(s) and article(s) are given in table 2. Some sets lack measurements for certain genes, in which case a grey marking is used.

Figure S6 Antimicrobial peptide gene expression. Figure shows a heat map of significant t-scores for genes coding for known antimicrobial peptides. Each column in the figure represents the result for one comparison against normal control, with sample source and test group given as the column name. The connection between each column's source abbreviation and its related dataset(s) and article(s) are given in table 2. Some sets lack measurements for certain genes, in which case a grey marking is used.

Table S1 A table listing the detailed sample description for all samples included in the microarray analysis.

Table S2 The full results from the limma analysis of the NTNU data. P-values given are benjamini-hochberg corrected for multiple comparisons.

Table S3 csv – Comma separated values. Over-represented Gene Ontology terms in the Crohn's disease-specific gene co-expression network.

Table S4 csv – Comma separated values. Over-represented Gene Ontology terms in the Ulcerative colitis-specific gene co-expression network.

Acknowledgments

Bjørn Munkvold, Kari Slørdahl and Britt Schulze provided excellent technical assistance. The microarray gene expression and bioinformatics analysis was performed in collaboration with the Genomics Core Facility, Norwegian University of Science and Technology, and NMC - a national technology platform supported by the functional genomics program (FUGE) of the Research Council of Norway.

Author Contributions

Contributed substantially in results interpretation: TE JKD MK BG AKS. Conceived and designed the experiments: HW AKS ABG AF BG MK JKD TE. Performed the experiments: VB ABG ST. Analyzed the data: AF ABG ID MK TE JKD AKS. Contributed reagents/materials/analysis tools: AEØ TCM AKS HW BG TE. Wrote the paper: ABG AKS AF ID.

References

1. Molodecky NA, Soon IS, Rabi DM, Ghali WA, Ferris M, et al. (2012) Increasing Incidence and Prevalence of the Inflammatory Bowel Diseases With Time, Based on Systematic Review. Gastroenterology 142: 46–54.e42.
2. Nutsch KM, Hsieh C-S (2012) T cell tolerance and immunity to commensal bacteria. Current Opinion in Immunology 24: 385–391.
3. Neurath MF, Finotto S, Glimcher LH (2002) The role of Th1/Th2 polarization in mucosal immunity. Nat Med 8: 567–573.
4. Shale M, Ghosh S (2008) Beyond TNF, Th1 and Th2 in inflammatory bowel disease. Gut 57: 1349–1351.
5. Brand S (2009) Crohn's disease: Th1, Th17 or both? The change of a paradigm: new immunological and genetic insights implicate Th17 cells in the pathogenesis of Crohn's disease. Gut 58: 1152–1167.
6. Di Sabatino A, Biancheri P, Rovedatti L, MacDonald TT, Corazza GR (2012) New pathogenic paradigms in inflammatory bowel disease. Inflammatory Bowel Diseases 18: 368–371.
7. Khor B, Gardet A, Xavier RJ (2011) Genetics and pathogenesis of inflammatory bowel disease. Nature 474: 307–317.
8. Heller RA, Schena M, Chai A, Shalon D, Bedilion T, et al. (1997) Discovery and analysis of inflammatory disease-related genes using cDNA microarrays. Proceedings of the National Academy of Sciences 94: 2150–2155.

9.   Dieckgraefe BK, Stenson WF, Korzenik JR, Swanson PE, Harrington CA (2000) Analysis of mucosal gene expression in inflammatory bowel disease by parallel oligonucleotide arrays. Physiological Genomics 4: 1–11.

10. Lawrance IC, Fiocchi C, Chakravarti S (2001) Ulcerative colitis and Crohn's disease: distinctive gene expression profiles and novel susceptibility candidate genes. Hum Mol Genet 10: 445–456.

11. Wu F, Dassopoulos T, Cope L, Maitra A, Brant SR, et al. (2007) Genome-wide gene expression differences in Crohn's disease and ulcerative colitis from endoscopic pinch biopsies: Insights into distinctive pathogenesis. Inflammatory Bowel Diseases 13: 807–821.

12. Olsen J, Gerds TA, Seidelin JB, Csillag C, Bjerrum JT, et al. (2009) Diagnosis of ulcerative colitis before onset of inflammation by multivariate modeling of genome-wide gene expression data. Inflammatory Bowel Diseases 15: 1032–1038.

13. Ogawa H, Fukushima K, Naito H, Funayama Y, Unno M, et al. (2003) Increased expression of HIP/PAP and regenerating gene III in human inflammatory bowel disease and a murine bacterial reconstitution model. Inflammatory Bowel Diseases 9: 162–170.

14. Noble CL, Abbas AR, Cornelius J, Lees CW, Ho GT, et al. (2008) Regional variation in gene expression in the healthy colon is dysregulated in ulcerative colitis. Gut 57: 1398–1405.

15. Costello CM, Mah N, Häsler R, Rosenstiel P, Waetzig GH, et al. (2005) Dissection of the Inflammatory Bowel Disease Transcriptome Using Genome-Wide cDNA Microarrays. PLoS Med 2: e199.

16. Heimerl S, Moehle C, Zahn A, Boettcher A, Stremmel W, et al. (2006) Alterations in intestinal fatty acid metabolism in inflammatory bowel disease. Biochimica et Biophysica Acta (BBA) - Molecular Basis of Disease 1762: 341–350.

17. Galamb O, Gyorffy B, Sipos F, Spisak S, Nemeth AM, et al. (2008) Inflammation, adenoma and cancer: objective classification of colon biopsy specimens with gene expression signature. Dis Markers 25: 1–16.

18. Carey R, Jurickova I, Ballard E, Bonkowski E, Han X, et al. (2008) Activation of an IL-6:STAT3-dependent transcriptome in pediatric-onset inflammatory bowel disease. Inflammatory Bowel Diseases 14: 446–457.

19. Burczynski ME, Peterson RL, Twine NC, Zuberek KA, Brodeur BJ, et al. (2006) Molecular Classification of Crohn's Disease and Ulcerative Colitis Patients Using Transcriptional Profiles in Peripheral Blood Mononuclear Cells. J Mol Diagn 8: 51–61.

20. Buisine MP, Desreumaux P, Leteurtre E, Copin MC, Colombel JF, et al. (2001) Mucin gene expression in intestinal epithelial cells in Crohn's disease. Gut 49: 544–551.

21. Arijs I, De Hertogh G, Lemaire K, Quintens R, Van Lommel L, et al. (2009) Mucosal gene expression of antimicrobial peptides in inflammatory bowel disease before and after first infliximab treatment. PLoS One 4: e7984.

22. Ahrens R, Waddell A, Seidu L, Blanchard C, Carey R, et al. (2008) Intestinal Macrophage/Epithelial Cell-Derived CCL11/Eotaxin-1 Mediates Eosinophil Recruitment and Function in Pediatric Ulcerative Colitis. The Journal of Immunology 181: 7390–7399.

23. Bjerrum JT, Hansen M, Olsen J, Nielsen OH (2010) Genome-wide gene expression analysis of mucosal colonic biopsies and isolated colonocytes suggests a continuous inflammatory state in the lamina propria of patients with quiescent ulcerative colitis. Inflammatory Bowel Diseases 16: 999–1007.

24. Galamb O, Sipos F, Solymosi N, Spisak S, Krenacs T, et al. (2008) Diagnostic mRNA Expression Patterns of Inflamed, Benign, and Malignant Colorectal Biopsy Specimen and their Correlation with Peripheral Blood Results. Cancer Epidemiology Biomarkers & Prevention 17: 2835–2845.

25. Kugathasan S, Baldassano RN, Bradfield JP, Sleiman PM, Imielinski M, et al. (2008) Loci on 20q13 and 21q22 are associated with pediatric-onset inflammatory bowel disease. Nature genetics 40: 5.

26. Wehkamp J, Schmid M, Stange EF (2007) Defensins and other antimicrobial peptides in inflammatory bowel disease. Current Opinion in Gastroenterology 23: 370–378.

27. Granlund AVB, Beisvag V, Torp SH, Flatberg A, Kleveland PM, et al. (2012) Activation of REG family proteins in colitis. Scandinavian Journal of Gastroenterology 46: 1316–1323.

28. Wehkamp J, Harder J, Weichenthal M, Schwab M, Schäffeler E, et al. (2004) NOD2 (CARD15) mutations in Crohn's disease are associated with diminished mucosal alpha-defensin expression. Gut 53: 1658–1664.

29. Simms LA, Doecke JD, Walsh MD, Huang N, Fowler EV, et al. (2003) Reduced alpha-defensin expression is associated with inflammation and not NOD2 mutation status in ileal Crohn's disease. Gut 57: 903–910.

30. LaPointe LC, Dunne R, Brown GS, Worthley DL, Molloy PL, et al. (2008) Map of differential transcript expression in the normal human large intestine. Physiological Genomics 33: 50–64.

31. Gentleman RC, Carey VJ, Bates DM, Bolstad B, Dettling M, et al. (2004) Bioconductor: open software development for computational biology and bioinformatics. Genome Biology 5: 16.

32. Planell N, Lozano JJ, Mora-Buch R, Masamunt MC, Jimeno M, et al. (2012) Transcriptional analysis of the intestinal mucosa of patients with ulcerative colitis in remission reveals lasting epithelial cell alterations. Gut.

33. Østvik AE, vB Granlund A, Bugge M, Nilsen NJ, Torp SH, et al. (2012) Enhanced expression of CXCL10 in inflammatory bowel disease: Potential role of mucosal toll-like receptor 3 stimulation. Inflammatory Bowel Diseases.

34. Jenner RG, Townsend MJ, Jackson I, Sun K, Bouwman RD, et al. (2009) The transcription factors T-bet and GATA-3 control alternative pathways of T-cell

35. Usui T, Preiss JC, Kanno Y, Yao ZJ, Bream JH, et al. (2006) T-bet regulates Th1 responses through distinct effects on GATA-3 function rather than on IFNG gene acetylation and transcription. The Journal of Experimental Medicine 203: 755–766.

36. Chung Y, Chang SH, Martinez GJ, Yang XO, Nurieva R, et al. (2009) Critical Regulation of Early Th17 Cell Differentiation by Interleukin-1 Signaling. Immunity 30: 576–587.

37. Maggi L, Santarlasci V, Capone M, Peired A, Frosali F, et al. (2010) CD161 is a marker of all human IL-17-producing T-cell subsets and is induced by RORC. Eur J Immunol 40: 2174–2181.

38. Cosmi L, De Palma R, Santarlasci V, Maggi L, Capone M, et al. (2008) Human interleukin 17–producing cells originate from a CD161+ CD4+ T cell precursor. The Journal of Experimental Medicine 205: 1903–1916.

39. Collison LW, Workman CJ, Kuo TT, Boyd K, Wang Y, et al. (2007) The inhibitory cytokine IL-35 contributes to regulatory T-cell function. Nature 450: 566–569.

40. Collison L, Delgoffe G, Guy C, Vignali K, Chaturvedi V, et al. (2012) The composition and signaling of the IL-35 receptor are unconventional. Nature Immunology 13: 290–299.

41. Peyrin-Biroulet L, Beisner J, Wang G, Nuding S, Oommen ST, et al. (2010) Peroxisome proliferator-activated receptor gamma activation is required for maintenance of innate antimicrobial immunity in the colon. Proceedings of the National Academy of Sciences 107: 8772–8777.

42. Boulesteix A-L, Slawski M (2009) Stability and aggregation of ranked gene lists. Briefings in Bioinformatics 10: 556–568.

43. Ramasamy A, Mondry A, Holmes CC, Altman DG (2008) Key Issues in Conducting a Meta-Analysis of Gene Expression Microarray Datasets. PLoS Med 5: e184.

44. Koutroubakis IE, Tsiolakidou G, Karmiris K, Kouroumalis EA (2006) Role of angiogenesis in inflammatory bowel disease. Inflammatory Bowel Diseases 12: 515–523.

45. Kobayashi T, Okamoto S, Hisamatsu T, Kamada N, Chinen H, et al. (2008) IL23 differentially regulates the Th1/Th17 balance in ulcerative colitis and Crohn's disease. Gut 57: 1682–1689.

46. Duerr RH, Taylor KD, Brant SR, Rioux JD, Silverberg MS, et al. (2006) A Genome-Wide Association Study Identifies IL23R as an Inflammatory Bowel Disease Gene. Science 314: 1461–1463.

47. Abraham C, Cho JH (2009) Inflammatory Bowel Disease. New England Journal of Medicine 361: 2066–2078.

48. Maddur MS, Miossec P, Kaveri SV, Bayry J (2012) Th17 Cells: Biology, Pathogenesis of Autoimmune and Inflammatory Diseases, and Therapeutic Strategies. The American Journal of Pathology 181: 8–18.

49. Yang XO, Pappu BP, Nurieva R, Akimzhanov A, Kang HS, et al. (2008) T Helper 17 Lineage Differentiation Is Programmed by Orphan Nuclear Receptors ROR alpha and ROR gamma. Immunity 28: 29–39.

50. Lovato P, Brender C, Agnholt J, Kelsen J, Kaltoft K, et al. (2003) Constitutive STAT3 Activation in Intestinal T Cells from Patients with Crohn's Disease. Journal of Biological Chemistry 278: 16777–16781.

51. Li Y, de Haar C, Peppelenbosch MP, van der Woude CJ (2012) SOCS3 in immune regulation of inflammatory bowel disease and inflammatory bowel disease-related cancer. Cytokine & Growth Factor Reviews 23: 127–138.

52. Yu C-R, Mahdi R, Ebong S, Vistica B, Gery I, et al. (2003) Suppressor of cytokine signaling 3 regulates proliferation and activation of T-helper cells. The Journal of biological chemistry 278: 29752–29761.

53. White G, Cotterill A, Addley M, Soilleux E, Greaves D (2011) Suppressor of cytokine signalling protein SOCS3 expression is increased at sites of acute and chronic inflammation. Journal of Molecular Histology 42: 137–151.

54. R Development Core Team (2008) R: A Language and Enviroment for Statistical Computing. Vienna, Austria: R Foundation for Statistical Computing.

55. Smyth G (2004) Linear models and empirical bayes methods for assessing differential expression in microarray experiments. Statistical applications in genetics and molecular biology 3.

56. Zhang B, Horvath S (2005) A general framework for weighted gene co-expression network analysis. Statistical applications in genetics and molecular biology 4: Article17.

57. Langfelder P, Horvath S (2008) WGCNA: an R package for weighted correlation network analysis. BMC Bioinformatics 9: 559.

58. Ravasz E, Somera AL, Mongru DA, Oltvai ZN, Barabasi AL (2002) Hierarchical organization of modularity in metabolic networks. Science 297: 1551–1555.

59. Parkinson H, Kapushesky M, Kolesnikov N, Rustici G, Shojatalab M, et al. (2009) ArrayExpress update - from an archive of functional genomics experiments to the atlas of gene expression. Nucleic Acids Research 37: D868–D872.

60. Barrett T, Troup DB, Wilhite SE, Ledoux P, Evangelista C, et al. (2011) NCBI GEO: archive for functional genomics data sets - 10 years on. Nucleic Acids Research 39: D1005–D1010.

61. Subramanian A, Tamayo P, Mootha VK, Mukherjee S, Ebert BL, et al. (2005) Gene set enrichment analysis: A knowledge-based approach for interpreting genome-wide expression profiles. Proceedings of the National Academy of Sciences of the United States of America 102: 15545–15550.

20

Tumor Necrosis Factor Alpha Blocking Agents as Treatment for Ulcerative Colitis Intolerant or Refractory to Conventional Medical Therapy

Ruxi Lv[1,2✈], Weiguang Qiao[3✈], Zhiyong Wu[1], Yinjun Wang[2], Shixue Dai[4], Qiang Liu[2*], Xuebao Zheng[1,2*]

1 School of Traditional Chinese Medicine, Southern Medical University, Guangzhou, People's Republic of China, 2 Research Institute of Traditional Chinese Medicine, Guangdong Medical College, Zhanjiang, Guangdong, People's Republic of China, 3 Department of Gastroenterology, Nanfang Hospital, Southern Medical University, Guangzhou, People's Republic of China, 4 Emergency Department of Nanfang Hospital, Southern Medical University, Guangzhou, People's Republic of China

Abstract

Background: Efficacy of tumor necrosis factor alpha (TNF-α) blockers for treatment of ulcerative colitis that is unresponsive to conventional therapy is unclear due to recent studies yielding conflicting results.

Aim: To assess the efficacy and safety of anti-TNF-α agents for treatment of ulcerative colitis patients who were intolerant or refractory to conventional medical therapy.

Methods: Pubmed, Embase, and the Cochrane database were searched. Analysis was performed on randomized controlled trials that assessed anti-TNF-α therapy on ulcerative colitis patients that had previously failed therapy with corticosteroids and/or immunosuppressants. The primary outcome focused on was the frequency of patients that achieved clinical remission. Further trial outcomes of interest included rates of remission without patient use of corticosteroids during the trial, extent of mucosal healing, and the number of cases that resulted in colectomy and serious side effects.

Results: Eight trials from seven studies (n = 2122) met the inclusion criteria and were thus included during analysis. TNF-α blockers demonstrated clinical benefit as compared to placebo control as evidenced by an increased frequency of clinical remission (p<0.00001), steroid-free remission (p = 0.01), endoscopic remission (p<0.00001) and a decrease in frequency of colectomy (p = 0.03). No difference was found concerning serious side effects (p = 0.05). Three small trials (n = 57) comparing infliximab to corticosteroid treatment, showed no difference in frequency of clinical remission (p = 0.93), mucosal healing (p = 0.80), and requirement for a colectomy (p = 0.49). One trial compared infliximab to cyclosporine (n = 115), wherein no difference was found in terms of mucosal healing (p = 0.85), colectomy frequency (p = 0.60) and serious side effects (p = 0.23).

Conclusion: TNF-α blockers are effective and safe therapies for the induction and maintenance of long-term remission and prevention of treatment by colectomy for patients with refractory ulcerative colitis where conventional treatment was previously ineffective. Furthermore, infliximab and cyclosporine were found to be comparable for treating acute severe steroid-refractory ulcerative colitis.

Editor: Fabio Cominelli, CWRU/UH Digestive Health Institute, United States of America

Funding: This study was funded by National Natural Science Foundation of China, grant number [No. 81173240]. The funders had no role in study design, data collection and analysis, decision to publish, or preparation of the manuscript.

Competing Interests: The authors have declared that no competing interests exist.

* E-mail: lvrucy@126.com (QL); xuebaozheng1964@gmail.com (XBZ)

✈ These authors contributed equally to this work.

Introduction

Ulcerative colitis (UC) is a chronic disease characterized by diffuse mucosal inflammation within the colon, often with alternating periods of exacerbation and remission. This disease has conventionally been treated with 5-aminosalicylic acid, corticosteroids and oral immunosuppressant (e.g. azathioprine, 6-mercaptopurine) with the goals of achieving clinical or mucosal remission, and/or eliminating long-term corticosteroid use [1]. However, these conventional therapies are in many instances ineffective or cannot be tolerated by the patients. This failure to

pervasively treat UC patients is apparent in the frequency of colectomies performed; the cumulative probability of colectomy from the time of diagnosis is 13.1% at 5 years, 18.9% at 10 years, and 25.4% at 20 years [2]. This deficit in widespread, effective treatment of UC patients therefore warrants the development and study of alternative treatments.

One potential alternative therapy is inhibition of tumor necrosis factor alpha (TNF-α) as previous studies have established a correlation between increased production of TNF-α and UC pathophysiology [3–6].

Currently, the anti-TNF-α agents most commonly used for UC treatment are infliximab (IFX) and adalimumab (ADA). Intravenous and subcutaneous administration of IFX and ADA, respectively, has been shown by some studies to be effective for treating moderately to severely active UC [7–10]. However, other studies pertaining to IFX treatment have yielded conflicting results [11]. Another anti-TNF-α agents, golimumab, induces and maintains clinical remission in patients with moderate to severe UC as evidenced by two recent trials [12,13]. The need for alternative UC therapies, as well as the range and conflicting reports found from studies on anti-TNF-α therapeutics, encouraged us to perform a meta-analysis to analyze the efficacy of these agents for UC patients who were intolerant or refractory to conventional medical therapy.

Several systematic reviews and meta-analyses of TNF-α blockers as treatment for UC have been published in recent years [14–17]_ENREF_10. However, these failed to fully take into account heterogeneity between the trials analyzed, including differences in the severity of UC in patients studied, drugs administered within the control group, and the point at which patient follow-up concluded. Moreover, the doses of the anti-TNF-α agent varied between different studies that had been included. As expected, these discrepancies skewed the results of the previous meta-analyses. Because of this need to account for inconsistencies within previous analyses, as well as include recent findings concerning anti-TNF-α treatment, we conducted a meta-analysis of TNF-α blockers as therapy for UC patients intolerant or refractory to conventional medical treatment. It would be very helpful for decision-making for patients with UC who do not respond well to conventional treatments if we could provide currently available evidence for or against anti-TNF-α therapeutics in UC. To reduce heterogeneity and enhance comparability between studies during our meta-analyses, trials wherein only a single infusion of anti-TNF-α was administered or patient follow-up concluded within 12 weeks post first treatment were excluded. Furthermore, sub-analyses were executed within our meta-analyses to account for whether the control group received placebos or active intervention.

Methods

Search strategy

The databases Pubmed, Cochrane Library and Embase were searched for studies published between 1991 and July 20, 2013 containing the terms "(infliximab or adalimumab or certolizumab or golimumab or tumor necrosis factor alpha) and (inflammatory bowel disease or ulcerative colitis) and (trial*)." Furthermore, the reference lists of any studies previously identified as having met the inclusion criteria were manually reviewed to find additional relevant publications.

Study selection

The titles and abstracts of published studies were screened independently by two investigators to determine whether they fulfilled the following inclusion criteria: (i) the studies had to be randomized controlled trials (RCTs) comparing anti-TNF-α therapies (e.g. adalimumab, certolizumab, golimumab, or infliximab) with the administration of a placebo or other intervention, and published in the English language, (ii) the UC patients of any age included had to have UC resistant to conventional therapy of corticosteroids and/or immunosuppressive agents, or refractory to intravenous corticosteroids, and, (iii) the patients had to have been given TNF-α blockers at least twice and monitored for at least 12 weeks after the initial dose of TNF-α blocker or control drug. The primary outcome measured was frequency of clinical remission,

which was defined by each of the primary studies. Secondary outcomes recorded were the frequency of long-term mucosal healing, steroid-free remission, colectomy and severe side effects. Furthermore, reviews, case reports and abstracts that lacked sufficient information to determine if the above parameters were met were excluded.

Outcome assessment

Unless otherwise defined in the primary study, clinical remission was defined either as a total Mayo score≤2 with no individual subscore exceeding 1 points, mucosal healing was defined as an endoscopy subscore of 0 or 1. The decision to perform a colectomy was made on clinical grounds. Serious side effects were defined by each primary study.

Data extraction

All data and inclusion decisions were performed independently by two investigators. When there was disagreement between the reviewers, the cases in question were discussed and a decision to include or exclude a study was made by reviewer consensus. The information collected from each study included the type of study, number of patients enrolled in the study, experimental and control therapies used, side effects observed, duration of patient follow-up, patient baseline demographics, patient medical and UC-related history, concomitant therapy received by the patient and the trial outcomes. For instances where a patient dropped out of the study or where data was missing, an intention-to-treat principle was applied and these cases were considered as treatment failure.

Assessment of risk of bias

This data collection and assessment was performed independently by two investigators, wherein any disagreements were resolved by discussion. Risk of bias was assessed as described in the Cochrane handbook [18]: by recording the method of random sequence generation, the method of allocation concealment, whether blinding was implemented, whether incomplete outcome data was reported, whether an intention-to-treat analysis was conducted, and whether there was evidence of selective reporting of outcomes. The quality of the RCTs was assessed by the Jadad scoring system by two independent investigators [19].

Statistical Analysis

The meta-analyses were performed by using relative risk (RR) for dichotomous outcomes. Pooled estimates were presented with 95% confidence intervals (CIs). Sub-analyses were chosen based on the type of control group within the study (placebo or active interventions). Heterogeneity between studies was quantified by calculating I^2 where p<0.10 was determined significant. Where there was evidence of heterogeneity, a random-effects model was used for pooling. Otherwise, a fixed-effects model was used. Funnel plots were not conducted to investigate publication bias as there were not enough studies included in each comparison to produce a meaningful analysis. All statistical analyses were executed on RevMan 5.2 software. Results were analyzed according to the intention-to-treat principle.

Results

Literature retrieval

The previously described search strategy identified 1911 citations, of which, 1890 were excluded after examination of the title and abstract (Figure 1). 21 articles reporting on the efficacy of anti-TNF-α therapies in UC were then further evaluated [8–13,20–33]. 14 of these 21 articles were excluded: 4 due to use of only a single infusion of anti-TNF-α agents [20–23], 3 because the duration of patient follow-up lasted fewer than 12 weeks[10–12], 4 because the enrolled participants [13,29,30]or outcome(s) assessed[24] failed to meet the inclusion criteria, 1 because there was no placebo used [31], and 2 because the papers were published only as an abstract [32,33].

The remaining 7 studies were used for meta-analysis [8,9,25–28], 1 study reported on 2 separate trials [8], bringing the total number of trials analyzed to 8. Of these trials, 4 compared infliximab or adalimumab treatment to placebo, 3 compared infliximab treatment to corticosteroid, and 1 compared infliximab to cyclosporine. The characteristics and trial design of the included studies were shown in Table 1 and Table 2, respectively.

Methodological quality of included studies

The assessment of the risk of bias was summarized in Figures 2 and Figure 3. Overall, the quality of the studies ranged from moderate to high (Jadad score≥3). Two studies were rated at high risk of bias due to lack of proper blinding controls [25,27]. All data were analyzed in accordance with the intention-to-treat principle. Due to an insufficient number of studies to produce a meaningful analysis, funnel plots were not used to investigate publication bias.

Data synthesis: Clinical remission

The frequency of clinical remission of patients treated with TNF-α blockers was studied in 6 trials that consisted of 1279 patients. Of these 6 trials, 3 trials were controlled by administering a placebo. Patients were treated with infliximab in 2 of the trials and adalimumab in 1. No significant heterogeneity was detected between these trials ($I^2 = 0\%$, p = 0.57). A pooled analysis using fixed-effects models showed that the TNF-α blocker was significantly superior to placebo for maintenance of clinical remission (RR = 2.29; 95% [1.73, 3.03], Z = 5.78, p<0.00001, Figure 4). In 3 of the trials, infliximab treatment was compared with glucocorticoid. The control group within these trials consisted of patients given methylprednisolone in 2 of the trials and prednisolone in the other trial. There was no significant heterogeneity found among the trials ($I^2 = 0\%$, p = 0.61). Based on fixed-effects models, there was no significant difference in clinical remission rates between the anti-TNF-α agents and

glucocorticoid treatment (RR = 1.01; 95% [0.73, 1.42], Z = 0.09, p = 0.93, Figure 4).

Data synthesis: Mucosal healing

Mucosal healing was evaluated in 5 trials, consisting of 1345 patients, to determine TNF-α blocker treatment efficacy. Of these, 3 trials compared anti-TNF-α agents with a placebo control. Patients were given infliximab in 2 trials and adalimumab in the third trial. No heterogeneity was detected when comparing these 3 trials ($I^2 = 37\%$, p = 0.20). A pooled analysis using fixed-effects models showed the TNF-α blocker was significantly superior to placebo for healing of the mucosa (RR = 1.89; 95% [1.55, 2.31], p<0.00001, Figure 5). Only 1 trial included in our analysis compared infliximab with prednisolone. This trial found that infliximab and prednisolone are equally effective for sustaining mucosal healing in UC (RR = 0.88; 95% [0.31, 2.44], p = 0.80, Figure 5), although with the caveat of a small trial population. In another trial, patients within the control group were given cyclosporine, and it was concluded that infliximab is as effective as cyclosporine in sustaining mucosal healing in UC (RR = 1.04; 95% [0.70, 1.55], p = 0.85).

Data synthesis: Steroid-free remission

Of the trials included in our analysis, 3, consisting of 698 patients, reported discontinued corticosteroid use and sustained steroid-free remission during their study. Of these, infliximab treatment efficacy was examined in 2 trials and adalimumab in 1 trial. No heterogeneity was detected when comparing the 3 trials ($I^2 = 4\%$, p = 0.35). A pooled analysis utilizing fixed-effects models was conducted. It was shown that the proportion of patients who achieved steroid-free remission was higher in groups that received the TNF-α blockers than in the placebo treated groups (RR = 2.97; 95% [1.77, 4.96], p<0.0001, Figure 6).

Data synthesis: Colectomy rate

The rate of colectomy was only reported within 3 of the included trials, which evaluated a total of 863 patients. The data demonstrated that more patients in the placebo group (36/244) than in the infliximab group (46/484) had a colectomy, as shown in Figure 7. This difference in colectomy rate is statistically significant (RR = 0.64; 95% [0.43, 0.97], p = 0.03, Figure. 7), indicating the benefit of infliximab treatment. In another trial, methylprednisolone was showed that the colectomy rate was equivalent between those receiving infliximab and those receiving prednisolone (RR = 3.00; 95% [0.14, 65.90], p = 0.49, Figure 7). Finally, 1 trial administered cyclosporine within the control group. This trial found that infliximab is as effective as cyclosporine in preventing patient colectomy (RR = 1.22; 95% [0.57, 2.60], p = 0.60, Figure 7).

Data synthesis: Serious side effects

Serious side effects were reported in 6 of the trials, consisting of 2088 patients. Within these trials, the frequency of serious side effects was 16.9% in the anti-TNF-α group, 20.0% in the placebo group and 24.7% in cyclosporine group. Of these, 4 trials administered a placebo as a control and 1 used cyclosporine. Significant heterogeneity was not detected when comparing these trials ($I^2 = 34\%$, p = 0.19). A pooled analysis using fixed effects models showed the occurrence of serious side effects was equivalent between TNF-α and placebo receiving patients (RR = 0.83; 95%[0.69, 1.00], Z = 1.98, p = 0.05, Figure 8). Also, no significant difference was found between the anti-TNF-α group

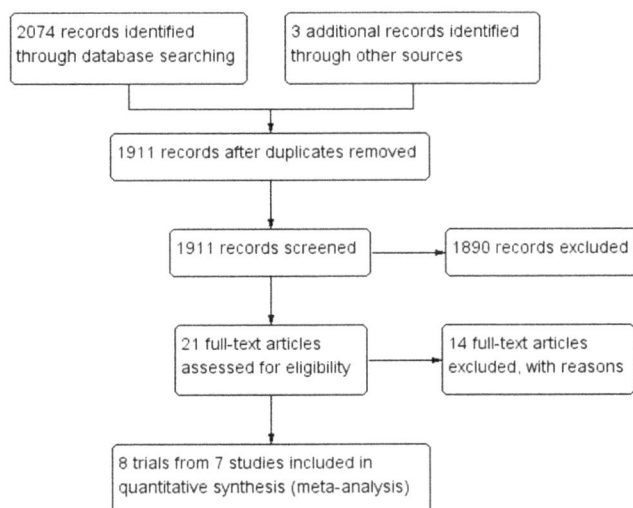

Figure 1. Study flow diagram.

Table 1. Baseline characteristics of included studies.

Study	Case (n)	Mean age (years)	Male (%)	Duration (years)	Co-therapy permitted	Type of study (Jadad score)
Armuzzi 2004	20	36.3	-	5.15	NR	Open-label, RCT(2)
Gavalas 2007	24	47.8	58	4.64	AZA,Steriods,5-ASA	Controlled trial (3)
Laharie 2012	115	37.5	52.2	1.7	AZA, Antibiotics, nutritional; CS tapered.	Open-label, RCT (5)
Ochsenkühn 2004	13	37.4	46.2	5.5	Mesalazine, sulfasalazine, antibiotics, or anti-diarrheal drugs at stable doses	Double-blind, RCT (3)
Rutgeerts 2005 ACT1	364	41.9	74	6.8	CS alone or in combination with AZA or MP	Double-blind, RCT (6)
Rutgeerts 2005 ACT2	364	40.0	71.7	6.6	CS alone or in combination with AZA or MP and 5-ASA	Double-blind, RCT (6)
Sandborn 2009	728	41.0	60.0	6.7	CS and/or AZA or 6-MP and/or 5-ASA	Double-blind, RCT (6)
Sandborn 2012	294	40.4	59.5	8.3	CS and/or AZA or 6-MP; CS tapered	Double-blind, RCT (4)

Note: NR, Not reported; AZA, Azathioprine; 5-ASA, 5-aminosalicylates; CS, corticosteroids; MP, mercaptopurine; RCT, randomized controlled trail.

recipients and the cyclosporine recipients in terms of serious side effects (RR = 0.63; 95% [0.30, 1.34], Z = 1.19, p = 0.23, Figure 8).

Discussion

Refractory UC treatment is one of the most challenging aspects in the clinical practice of luminal gastroenterology. UC patients who have frequent disease relapse, despite receiving the optimal conventional medical treatments, have few remaining non-surgical options. However, TNF-α inhibition offers a possible alternative therapy for UC patients who are treatment refractory or intolerant to corticosteroids and/or immunosuppressants. In the present study, we analyzed RCTs studying the efficacy of TNF-α blockers where the duration of patient follow-up continued for at least 12 weeks post initial treatment. We found that TNF-α blockers are effective and relatively safe therapies for maintaining long-term remission and preventing colectomy in patients with refractory UC. Of the available TNF-α blockers, infliximab and cyclosporine are comparable when used as rescue therapy in acute severe steroid-refractory UC.

UC is a chronic inflammation of the colon with states of disease that can range from dormant to refractory. Conventional therapy against UC includes a wide range of drugs, such as aminosalicylic acids, thiopurines, and corticosteroids. However, these agents fail to adequately control the disease in a large proportion of UC patients and are associated with many adverse side effects [34,35]. It has now been recognized that treatment goals should go beyond just controlling the symptoms of UC. Rather, UC treatment should aim to rapidly induce steroid-free remission, and achieve complete mucosal healing, while minimizing serious complications and side effects [36]. Due to the introduction of newer biological therapies, such as anti-TNF-α, these treatment goals are within the realm of possibility.

Of the developed anti-TNF-α therapies, infliximab, adalimumab and golimumab have been approved by the Food and Drug Administration (FDA) for the treatment of UC. The efficacy of such agents in steroid-refractory UC was first shown in a controlled pilot study [23]. Later, however, a larger placebo controlled trial (n = 43) failed to support the efficacy of infliximab in active glucocorticoid resistant cases [11]. Subsequently,

Table 2. Trial design of included studies.

Study	Participants(UC)	Intervention	Control	Follow-up	Outcome
Armuzzi 2004	Steroid-dependent	Infliximab	Methylprednisolone	9.8±1.1 months	Clinical remission; colectomy rate
Gavalas 2007	Steroid-dependent	Infliximab	Methylprednisolone	21months	Clinical remission
Laharie 2012	Not respond to intravenous steroid	Infliximab	Ciclosporin	98 days	Mucosal healing; colectomy rate; safety; serious adverse events.
Ochsenkühn 2004	Refractory to 5-aminosalicylates.	Infliximab	Prednisolone	13 weeks	Clinical remission; mucosal healing
Rutgeerts 2005 ACT 1	Not respond to conventional therapy	Infliximab	Placebo	54 weeks	Clinical remission; mucosal healing; steroid-free remission; serious adverse events.
Rutgeerts 2005 ACT2	Not respond to conventional therapy	Infliximab	Placebo	30-week	Clinical remission; mucosal healing; steroid-free remission; serious adverse events.
Sandborn 2009	Not respond to conventional therapy	Infliximab	Placebo	54 weeks	Colectomy rate; serious adverse events.
Sandborn 2012	Not respond to conventional therapy	Adalimumab	Placebo	54 weeks	Clinical remission; mucosal healing; steroid-free remission; serious adverse events.

Note: UC, Ulcerative colitis.

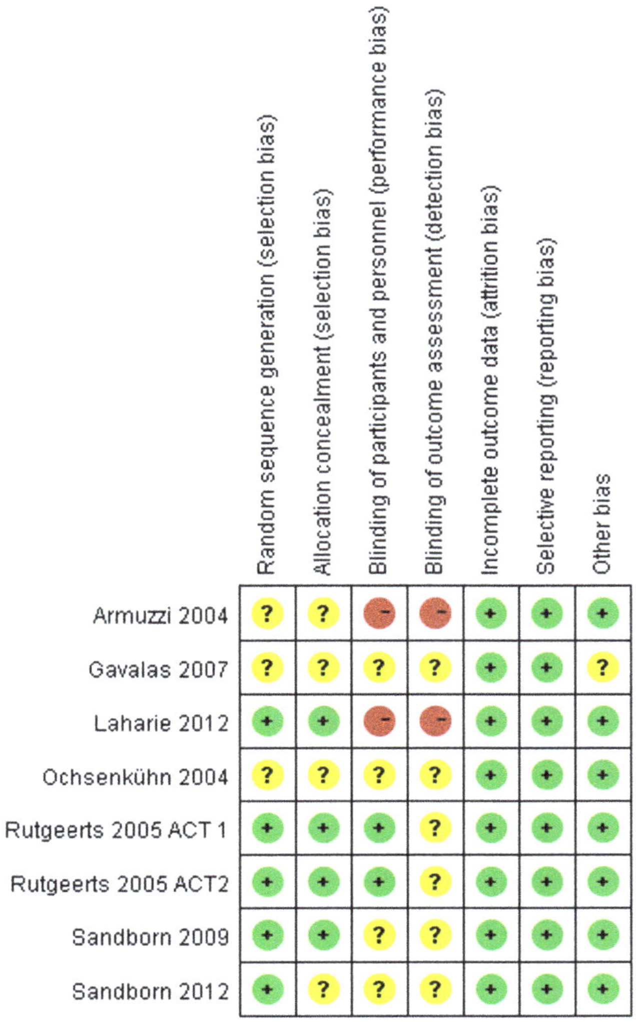

Figure 2. Risk of bias summary: review of authors' judgements about each risk of bias item for included studies.

increasingly controlled trials were designed to assess the effect of infliximab and adalimumab on refractory UC. Two recent well controlled trials showed that golimumab could induce a clinical response, as evidenced by clinical remission and mucosal healing in patients with active UC [12,13]. Unfortunately, both trials were excluded in our analyses due to a failure to follow-up with patients for at least 12 weeks after the initial treatment [12] and the enrolled patients are these who were response to golimumab therapy [13], respectively. Therefore, only infliximab and adalimumab were pooled for analysis within this study.

The rigorous inclusion criteria employed during our literature search returned 8 trials described in 7 published studies (n = 1922) that were hence pooled for meta-analysis. Among these studies, infliximab and adalimumab were compared to a placebo controlled group in 3[8,28] and 1 trial(s) [9], respectively. The patients in the first 3 trials were randomized to receive infliximab at doses of 5 or 10 mg/kg via intravenous, or the matched placebo at weeks 0, 2, and 6, and then every 8 weeks[8,28]. The patients in the fourth trial(s) were randomly assigned to receive subcutaneous injections of 160 mg adalimumab at week 0, 80 mg at week 2 and then 40 mg EOW beginning at week 4, or the matched placebo[9]. These studies concluded that anti-TNF-α therapy was slightly a little superior than administration of a placebo for treatment of UC patients in terms of clinical remission, mucosal healing, steroid-free remission, and reduction of colectomy rate, without causing serious side effects. Therefore, TNF-α blockers are an effective and relatively safe therapy to maintain long-term remission and avoid colectomy for patients who are not responsive to conventional treatment. Additionally, 3 small trials (n = 57) compared infliximab to steroid treatment. There were no statistically significant difference found in terms of frequency of clinical remission, mucosal healing and colectomies. However, this conclusion is unreliable due to the low number of patients in these trials. Moreover, one RCT trial (n = 115) compared infliximab to cyclosporine for use as rescue therapy for acute severe UC patients who were not responsive to intravenous steroid treatment. It was found that these drugs were comparable for rate of clinical remission, mucosal healing, colectomies rate and serious side effects. This result confirmed the conclusions from a previous meta-analysis, which pooled six retrospective cohort studies but did not include RCTs [37].

Besides the efficacy, the possible side effects of TNF-α blocker treatment were of interest when conducting this study. The main

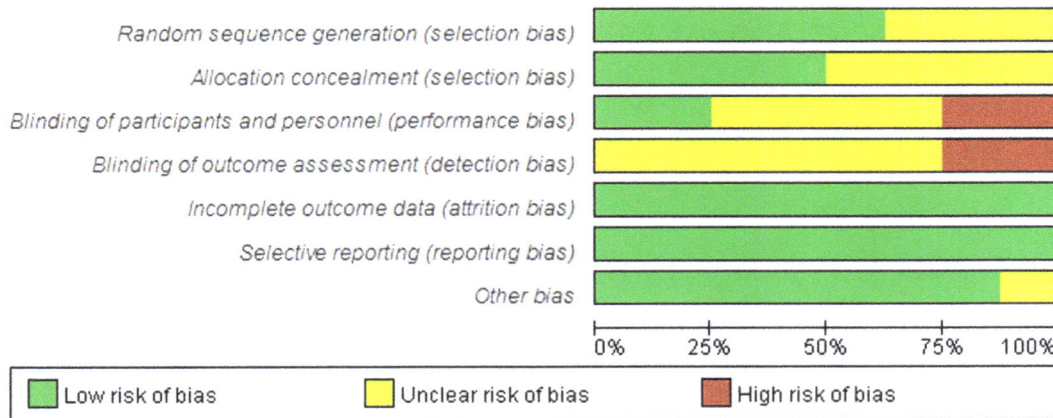

Figure 3. Risk of bias graph: review of authors' judgements about each risk of bias item presented as percentages across all included studies.

Study or Subgroup	TNF-α blocker Events	TNF-α blocker Total	Control Events	Control Total	Weight	Risk Ratio M-H, Fixed, 95% CI
1.1.1 Infliximab/ Adalimumab VS placebo						
Rutgeerts 2005 ACT 1	84	243	20	121	31.7%	2.09 [1.35, 3.23]
Rutgeerts 2005 ACT2	74	241	13	123	20.4%	2.91 [1.68, 5.03]
Sandborn 2012	43	248	21	246	25.0%	2.03 [1.24, 3.32]
Subtotal (95% CI)		732		490	77.1%	2.29 [1.73, 3.03]
Total events	201		54			
Heterogeneity: Chi² = 1.12, df = 2 (P = 0.57); I² = 0%						
Test for overall effect: Z = 5.78 (P < 0.00001)						
1.1.2 Infliximab VS glucocorticoid						
Armuzzi 2004	9	10	8	10	9.5%	1.13 [0.78, 1.63]
Gavalas 2007	11	16	5	8	7.9%	1.10 [0.59, 2.07]
Ochsenkühn 2004	3	6	5	7	5.5%	0.70 [0.28, 1.77]
Subtotal (95% CI)		32		25	22.9%	1.01 [0.73, 1.42]
Total events	23		18			
Heterogeneity: Chi² = 0.97, df = 2 (P = 0.61); I² = 0%						
Test for overall effect: Z = 0.09 (P = 0.93)						
Total (95% CI)		764		515	100.0%	2.00 [1.57, 2.53]
Total events	224		72			
Heterogeneity: Chi² = 19.30, df = 5 (P = 0.002); I² = 74%						
Test for overall effect: Z = 5.70 (P < 0.00001)						
Test for subgroup differences: Chi² = 13.32. df = 1 (P = 0.0003). I² = 92.5%						

0.02   0.1   1   10   50

Favours control   Favours TNF-α blocke

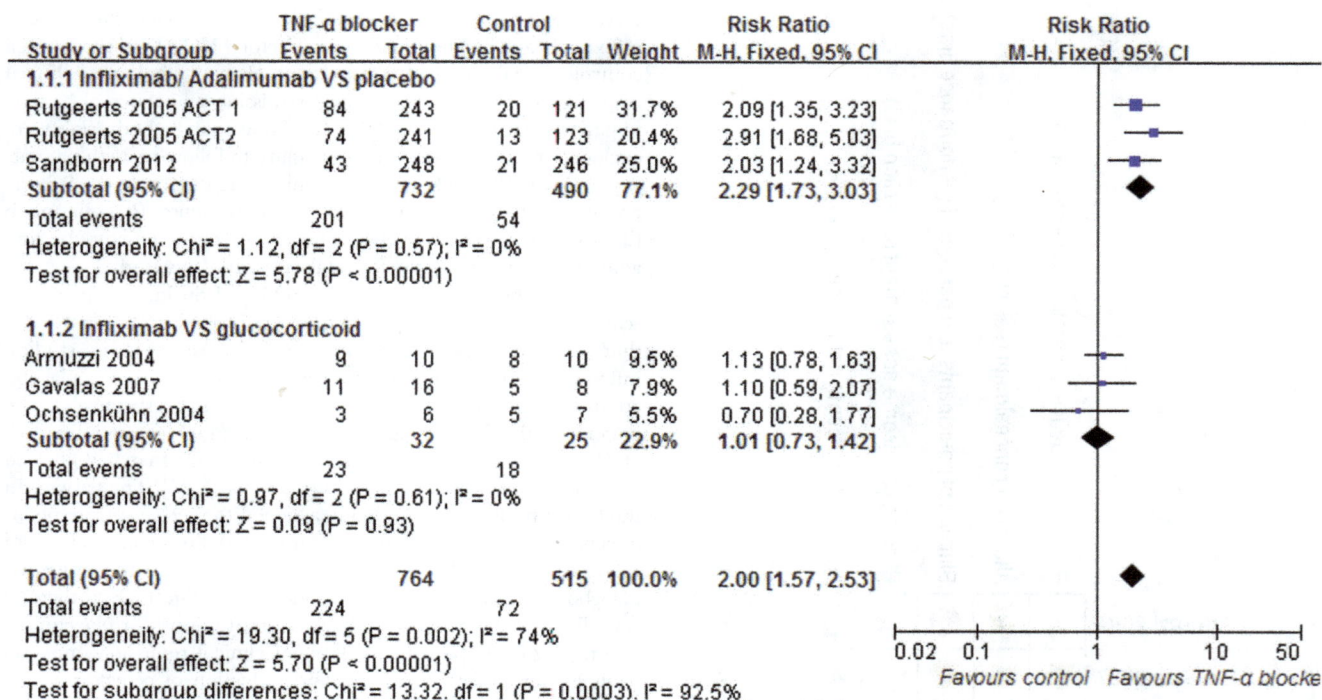

Figure 4. Pooled outcome for clinical remission in patients exposed to TNF-α blocker vs. controls.

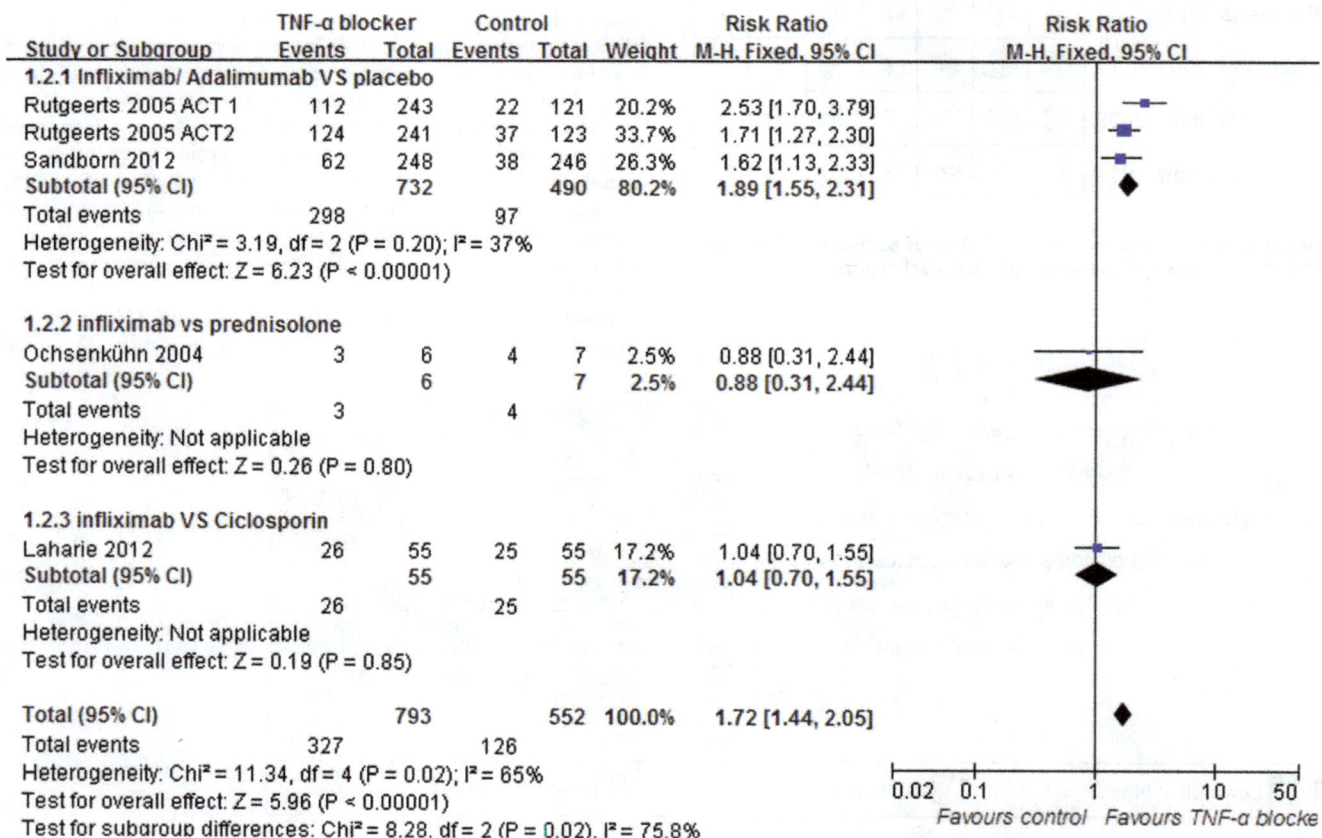

Study or Subgroup	TNF-α blocker Events	TNF-α blocker Total	Control Events	Control Total	Weight	Risk Ratio M-H, Fixed, 95% CI
1.2.1 Infliximab/ Adalimumab VS placebo						
Rutgeerts 2005 ACT 1	112	243	22	121	20.2%	2.53 [1.70, 3.79]
Rutgeerts 2005 ACT2	124	241	37	123	33.7%	1.71 [1.27, 2.30]
Sandborn 2012	62	248	38	246	26.3%	1.62 [1.13, 2.33]
Subtotal (95% CI)		732		490	80.2%	1.89 [1.55, 2.31]
Total events	298		97			
Heterogeneity: Chi² = 3.19, df = 2 (P = 0.20); I² = 37%						
Test for overall effect: Z = 6.23 (P < 0.00001)						
1.2.2 infliximab vs prednisolone						
Ochsenkühn 2004	3	6	4	7	2.5%	0.88 [0.31, 2.44]
Subtotal (95% CI)		6		7	2.5%	0.88 [0.31, 2.44]
Total events	3		4			
Heterogeneity: Not applicable						
Test for overall effect: Z = 0.26 (P = 0.80)						
1.2.3 infliximab VS Ciclosporin						
Laharie 2012	26	55	25	55	17.2%	1.04 [0.70, 1.55]
Subtotal (95% CI)		55		55	17.2%	1.04 [0.70, 1.55]
Total events	26		25			
Heterogeneity: Not applicable						
Test for overall effect: Z = 0.19 (P = 0.85)						
Total (95% CI)		793		552	100.0%	1.72 [1.44, 2.05]
Total events	327		126			
Heterogeneity: Chi² = 11.34, df = 4 (P = 0.02); I² = 65%						
Test for overall effect: Z = 5.96 (P < 0.00001)						
Test for subgroup differences: Chi² = 8.28. df = 2 (P = 0.02). I² = 75.8%						

0.02   0.1   1   10   50

Favours control   Favours TNF-α blocke

Figure 5. Pooled outcome for mucosal healing in patients exposed to TNF-α blocker vs. controls.

Study or Subgroup	TNF-α blocker Events	Total	Control Events	Total	Weight	Risk Ratio M-H, Fixed, 95% CI	Risk Ratio M-H, Fixed, 95% CI
1.3.1 infliximab VS placebo							
Rutgeerts 2005 ACT 1	30	143	7	79	45.1%	2.37 [1.09, 5.14]	
Rutgeerts 2005 ACT2	29	126	2	60	13.5%	6.90 [1.70, 27.99]	
Subtotal (95% CI)		269		139	58.6%	3.42 [1.74, 6.72]	
Total events	59		9				
Heterogeneity: Chi² = 1.83, df = 1 (P = 0.18); I² = 45%							
Test for overall effect: Z = 3.56 (P = 0.0004)							
1.3.2 Adalimumab VS placebo							
Sandborn 2012	20	150	8	140	41.4%	2.33 [1.06, 5.13]	
Subtotal (95% CI)		150		140	41.4%	2.33 [1.06, 5.13]	
Total events	20		8				
Heterogeneity: Not applicable							
Test for overall effect: Z = 2.11 (P = 0.03)							
Total (95% CI)		419		279	100.0%	2.97 [1.77, 4.96]	
Total events	79		17				
Heterogeneity: Chi² = 2.08, df = 2 (P = 0.35); I² = 4%							
Test for overall effect: Z = 4.15 (P < 0.0001)							
Test for subgroup differences: Chi² = 0.52, df = 1 (P = 0.47), I² = 0%							

0.01 0.1 1 10 100
Favours control   Favours TNF-α blocke

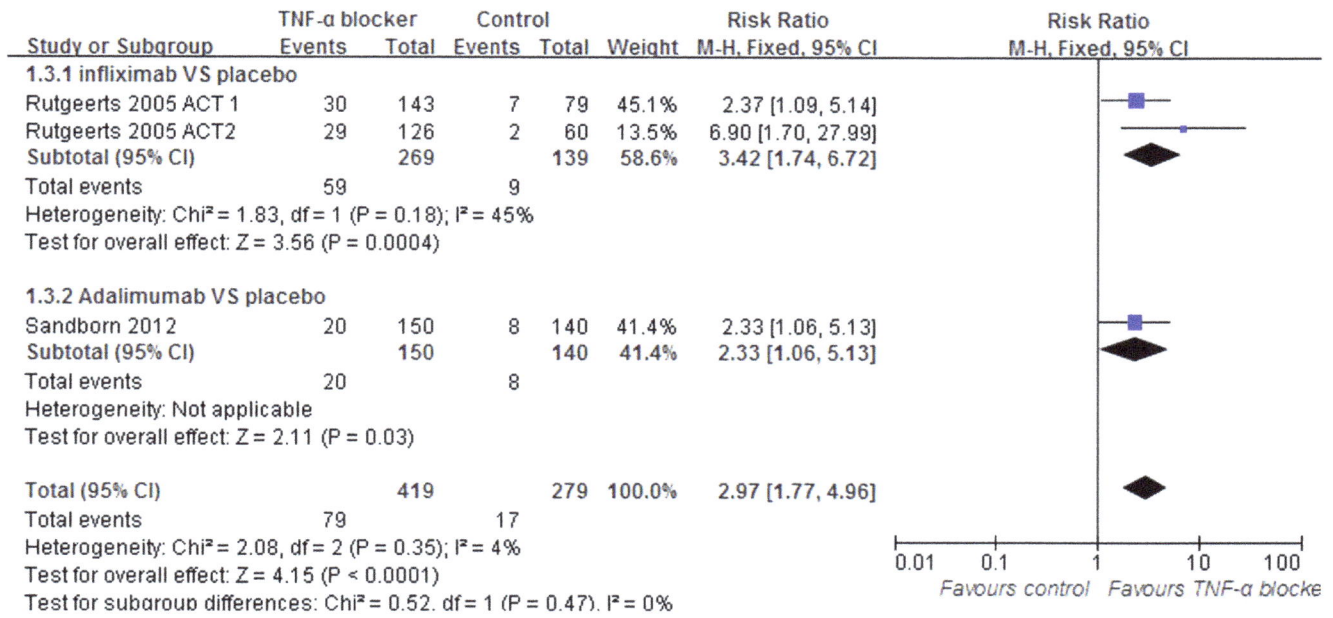

Figure 6. Pooled outcome for steroid-free remission in patients exposed to TNF-α blocker vs. controls.

side effects that have been recorded are an increased risk of infections, occurrence of autoimmune disorders [28], and risk of lymphoma or other malignancy [9]. In the present study, we found the risk of serious side effects were similar between anti-TNF-α and the control (p<0.00001, Figure 8), Overall, serious side effects occurred in 20% of patients within the placebo group and 16.9% of patients within the anti-TNF-α group. However, the rate of adverse events (AE) for AE's for combined immunomodulator/

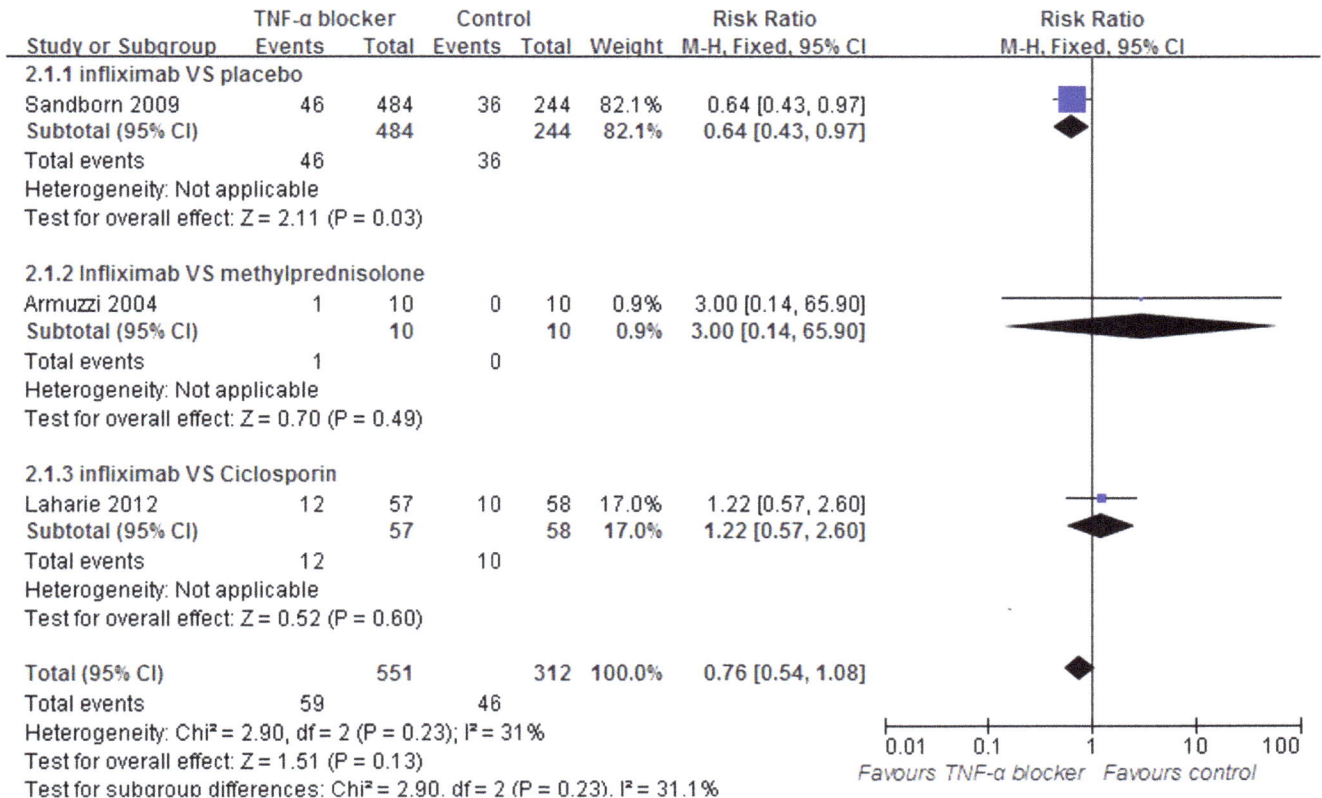

Study or Subgroup	TNF-α blocker Events	Total	Control Events	Total	Weight	Risk Ratio M-H, Fixed, 95% CI	Risk Ratio M-H, Fixed, 95% CI
2.1.1 infliximab VS placebo							
Sandborn 2009	46	484	36	244	82.1%	0.64 [0.43, 0.97]	
Subtotal (95% CI)		484		244	82.1%	0.64 [0.43, 0.97]	
Total events	46		36				
Heterogeneity: Not applicable							
Test for overall effect: Z = 2.11 (P = 0.03)							
2.1.2 Infliximab VS methylprednisolone							
Armuzzi 2004	1	10	0	10	0.9%	3.00 [0.14, 65.90]	
Subtotal (95% CI)		10		10	0.9%	3.00 [0.14, 65.90]	
Total events	1		0				
Heterogeneity: Not applicable							
Test for overall effect: Z = 0.70 (P = 0.49)							
2.1.3 infliximab VS Ciclosporin							
Laharie 2012	12	57	10	58	17.0%	1.22 [0.57, 2.60]	
Subtotal (95% CI)		57		58	17.0%	1.22 [0.57, 2.60]	
Total events	12		10				
Heterogeneity: Not applicable							
Test for overall effect: Z = 0.52 (P = 0.60)							
Total (95% CI)		551		312	100.0%	0.76 [0.54, 1.08]	
Total events	59		46				
Heterogeneity: Chi² = 2.90, df = 2 (P = 0.23); I² = 31%							
Test for overall effect: Z = 1.51 (P = 0.13)							
Test for subgroup differences: Chi² = 2.90, df = 2 (P = 0.23), I² = 31.1%							

0.01 0.1 1 10 100
Favours TNF-α blocker   Favours control

Figure 7. Pooled outcome for colectomy rate in patients exposed to TNF-α blocker vs. controls.

Study or Subgroup	TNF-α blocker Events	TNF-α blocker Total	Control Events	Control Total	Weight	Risk Ratio M-H, Fixed, 95% CI
3.1.1 Infliximab/ Adalimumab VS placebo						
Rutgeerts 2005 ACT 1	55	243	31	121	20.7%	0.88 [0.60, 1.29]
Rutgeerts 2005 ACT2	24	241	24	123	15.9%	0.51 [0.30, 0.86]
Sandborn 2009	89	484	57	244	37.9%	0.79 [0.59, 1.06]
Sandborn 2012	41	257	37	260	18.4%	1.12 [0.74, 1.69]
Subtotal (95% CI)		1225		748	92.9%	0.83 [0.69, 1.00]
Total events	209		149			

Heterogeneity: Chi² = 5.62, df = 3 (P = 0.13); I² = 47%
Test for overall effect: Z = 1.98 (P = 0.05)

Study or Subgroup	TNF-α blocker Events	TNF-α blocker Total	Control Events	Control Total	Weight	Risk Ratio M-H, Fixed, 95% CI
3.1.3 infliximab VS Ciclosporin						
Laharie 2012	9	58	14	57	7.1%	0.63 [0.30, 1.34]
Subtotal (95% CI)		58		57	7.1%	0.63 [0.30, 1.34]
Total events	9		14			

Heterogeneity: Not applicable
Test for overall effect: Z = 1.19 (P = 0.23)

Study or Subgroup	TNF-α blocker Events	TNF-α blocker Total	Control Events	Control Total	Weight	Risk Ratio M-H, Fixed, 95% CI
Total (95% CI)		1283		805	100.0%	0.81 [0.68, 0.98]
Total events	218		163			

Heterogeneity: Chi² = 6.07, df = 4 (P = 0.19); I² = 34%
Test for overall effect: Z = 2.22 (P = 0.03)
Test for subgroup differences: Chi² = 0.46, df = 1 (P = 0.50), I² = 0%

Risk Ratio M-H, Fixed, 95% CI (scale: 0.02 0.1 1 10 50)
Favours TNF-α blocker   Favours control

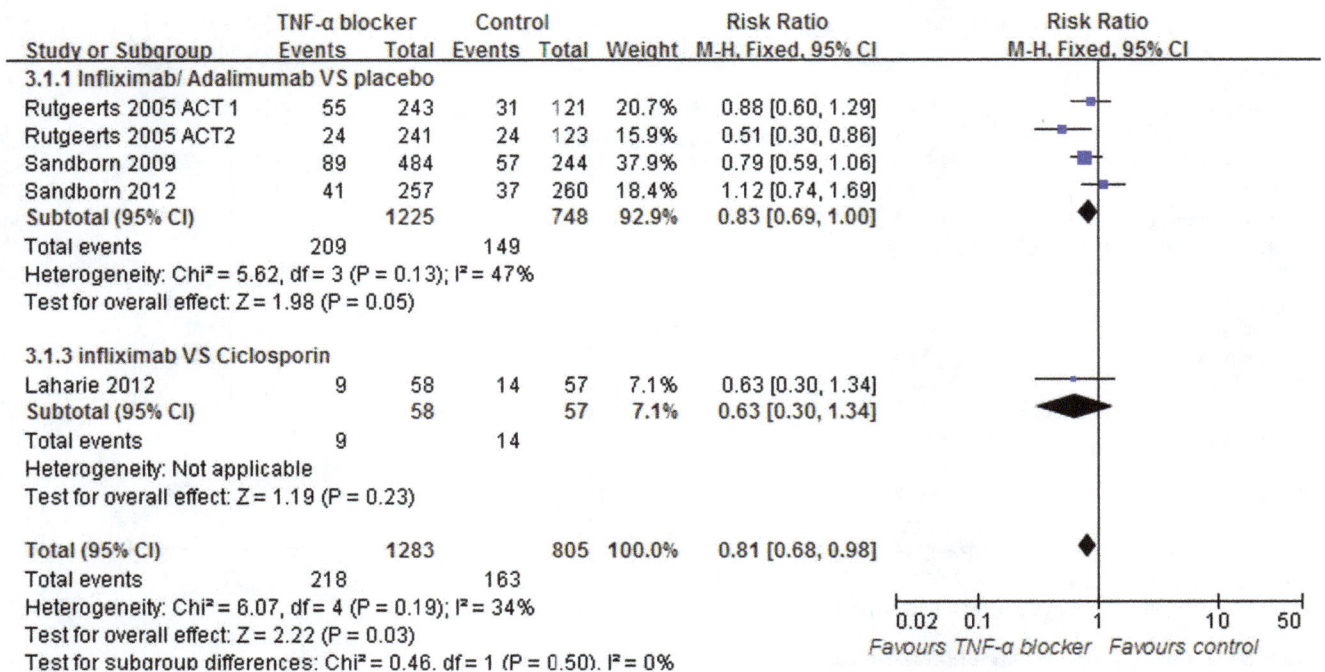

Figure 8. Pooled outcome for serious side effects in patients exposed to TNF-α blocker vs. controls.

anti-TNF therapy compared to each used as monotherapy beyond conventional treatment is a source of controversy. More studies with larger sample size are needed in future trials to further evaluate the rate serious infection due to the limit sample size in the current ones.

When performing a meta-analysis, caution needs to be used when drawing conclusions based on pooled studies of heterogeneous patient populations. To control for this heterogeneity, only the studies that had enrolled patients refractory to conventional treatment (e.g. steroid-dependent, nonresponsive to intravenous steroid or nonresponsive to conventional therapy) were included. Furthermore, trials of only a single infusion of anti-TNF-α and/or and a patient follow up duration of less than 12 weeks were excluded. To statistically control any further heterogeneity in the meta-analysis, we used a random effects model to analyze if there was heterogeneity among the trials. Also, subgroup analyses were performed based on the interventions applied in the control group. It should be noted that the majority of the included studies were judged to be of "moderate to high" quality without publication bias during our analysis.

Despite rigorous inclusion criteria that have been made to reduce the heterogeneity there are still several limitations within this study. First, the duration of patient follow up within the analyzed trials was still variable, ranging from 13 weeks to 54 weeks. Second, UC severity was not uniform upon trial initiation. Some trials enrolled patients that were steroid-dependent/refractory, while others enrolled those nonresponsive to intravenous steroid therapy and/or oral conventional drugs treatment. Third, the co-therapy scheme and dose administered of TNF-α blockers differed between trials. All of these instances of variability could affect the results drawn from our analysis.

In summary, this meta-analysis has updated the UC treatment field and demonstrated that TNF-α blockers were superior for patient treatment as compared to placebo. This conclusion was based on increased achievement of clinical remission and mucosal healing and reduction in the need for colectomy, combined with no significant, severe side effects. Using anti-TNF-α also spares patients the effects of corticosteroid treatment, which is used when the patients have refractory UC nonresponsive to conventional treatment. Additionally, infliximab and cyclosporine are comparable when used as rescue therapy in acute severe steroid-refractory UC, although, more randomized trials are needed to further evaluate the efficacy of these agents. So, in selected patients with moderate to severe active ulcerative colitis who have failed to respond or are poorly responsive to standard pharmacologic forms of treatment with corticosteroids and immunosuppressive agents, therapy with an anti-TNF-α agent may be considered. In addition, it may be necessary to identify biomarkers that indicative of patients who will respond to the TNF-α inhibitor.

Author Contributions

Conceived and designed the experiments: RXL WGQ XBZ. Performed the experiments: RXL ZYW QL. Analyzed the data: WGQ YJW SXD. Contributed reagents/materials/analysis tools: ZYW QL. Wrote the paper: RXL WGQ. Provided clinical advice: XBZ QL.

References

1. Ordas I, Eckmann L, Talamini M, Baumgart DC, Sandborn WJ (2012) Ulcerative colitis. Lancet 380: 1606–1619.

2. Samuel S, Ingle SB, Dhillon S, Yadav S, Harmsen WS, et al. (2013) Cumulative Incidence and Risk Factors for Hospitalization and Surgery in a Population-based Cohort of Ulcerative Colitis. Inflammatory Bowel Diseases 19: 1858–1866.

3. Braegger CP, Nicholls S, Murch SH, Stephens S, MacDonald TT (1992) Tumour necrosis factor alpha in stool as a marker of intestinal inflammation Lancet 339: 89–91.

4. MacDonald TT, Hutchings P, Choy MY, Murch S, Cooke A (1990) Tumour necrosis factor-alpha and interferon-gamma production measured at the single cell level in normal and inflamed human intestine. Clinical and Experimental Immunology 81: 301–305.

5. Murch SH, Lamkin VA, Savage MO, Walker-Smith JA, MacDonald TT (1991) Serum concentrations of tumour necrosis factor alpha in childhood chronic inflammatory bowel disease. Gut 32: 913–917.

6. Breese EJ, Michie CA, Nicholls SW, Murch SH, Williams CB, et al. (1994) Tumor necrosis factor alpha-producing cells in the intestinal mucosa of children with inflammatory bowel disease. Gastroenterology 106: 1455–1466.

7. Mowat C, Cole A, Windsor A, Ahmad T, Arnott I, et al. (2011) Guidelines for the management of inflammatory bowel disease in adults. Gut 60: 571–607.

8. Rutgeerts P, Sandborn WJ, Feagan BG, Reinisch W, Olson A, et al. (2005) Infliximab for induction and maintenance therapy for ulcerative colitis. The New England Journal of Medicine 353: 2462–2476.

9. Sandborn WJ, Assche G, Reinisch W, Colombel JF, D'Haens G, et al. (2012) Adalimumab induces and maintains clinical remission in patients with moderate-to-severe ulcerative colitis. Gastroenterology 142: 257–265.

10. Reinisch W, Sandborn WJ, Hommes DW, D'Haens G, Hanauer S, et al. (2011) Adalimumab for induction of clinical remission in moderately to severely active ulcerative colitis: results of a randomised controlled trial. Gut 60: 780–787.

11. Probert CS, Hearing SD, Schreiber S, Kühbacher T, Ghosh S, et al. (2003) Infliximab in moderately severe glucocorticoid resistant ulcerative colitis: a randomised controlled trial. Gut 52: 998–1002.

12. Sandborn WJ, Feagan BG, Marano C, Zhang H, Strauss R, et al. (2014) Subcutaneous golimumab induces clinical response and remission in patients with moderate to severe ulcerative colitis. Gastroenterology 146: 85–95.

13. Sandborn WJ, Feagan BG, Marano C, Zhang H, Strauss R, et al. (2014) Subcutaneous golimumab maintains clinical response in patients with moderate to severe ulcerative colitis. Gastroenterology 146: 96–109.

14. Rahimi R, Nikfar S, Abdollahi M (2007) Meta-analysis technique confirms the effectiveness of anti-TNF-alpha in the management of active ulcerative colitis when administered in combination with corticosteroids. Medical Science Monitor: International Medical Journal of Experimental and Clinical Research 13: 13–18.

15. Huang X, Lv B, Jin HF, Zhang S (2011) A meta-analysis of the therapeutic effects of tumor necrosis factor-alpha blockers on ulcerative colitis. European Journal of Clinical Pharmacology 67: 759–766.

16. Lawson MM, Thomas AG, Akobeng AK (2006) Tumour necrosis factor alpha blocking agents for induction of remission in ulcerative colitis. Cochrane Database of Systematic Reviews DOI: 10.1002/14651858.

17. Ford AC, Sandborn WJ, Khan KJ, Hanauer SB, Talley NJ, et al. (2011) Efficacy of biological therapies in inflammatory bowel disease: systematic review and meta-analysis. The American Journal of Gastroenterology 106: 644–59.

18. Tarsilla M (2010) Cochrane Handbook for Systematic Reviews of Interventions. Journal of Multidisciplinary Evaluation 6: 142–148.

19. Jadad AR, Moore RA, Carroll D, Jenkinson C, Reynolds DJ, et al. (1996) Assessing the quality of reports of randomized clinical trials: is blinding necessary? Controlled Clinical Trials 17: 1–12.

20. Croft A, Walsh A, Doecke J, Cooley R, Howlett M, et al. (2013) Outcomes of salvage therapy for steroid-refractory acute severe ulcerative colitis: ciclosporin vs. infliximab. Alimentary Pharmacology & Therapeutics 38: 294–302.

21. Gustavsson A, Jarnerot G, Hertervig E, Friis-Liby I, Blomquist L, et al. (2010) Clinical trial: colectomy after rescue therapy in ulcerative colitis - 3-year follow-up of the Swedish-Danish controlled infliximab study. Alimentary Pharmacology & Therapeutics 32: 984–989.

22. Jarnerot G, Hertervig E, Friis-Liby I, Blomquist L, Karlén P, et al. (2005) Infliximab as rescue therapy in severe to moderately severe ulcerative colitis: a randomized, placebo-controlled study. Gastroenterology 128: 1805–1811.

23. Sands BE, Tremaine WJ, Sandborn WJ, Rutgeerts PJ, Hanauer SB, et al. (2001) Infliximab in the treatment of severe, steroid-refractory ulcerative colitis: a pilot study. Inflammatory Bowel Diseases 7: 83–88.

24. Feagan BG, Reinisch W, Rutgeerts P, Sandborn WJ, Yan S, et al. (2007) The effects of infliximab therapy on health-related quality of life in ulcerative colitis patients. The American Journal of Gastroenterology 102: 794–802.

25. Armuzzi A, De Pascalis B, Lupascu A, Fedeli P, Leo D, et al. (2004) Infliximab in the treatment of steroid-dependent ulcerative colitis. European Review for Medical and Pharmacological Sciences 8: 231–233.

26. Gavalas E, Kountouras J, Stergiopoulos C, Zavos C, Gisakis D, et al. (2007) Efficacy and safety of infliximab in steroid-dependent ulcerative colitis patients. Hepatogastroenterology 54: 1074–1079.

27. Laharie D, Bourreille A, Branche J, Allez M, Bouhnik Y, et al. (2012) Ciclosporin versus infliximab in patients with severe ulcerative colitis refractory to intravenous steroids: a parallel, open-label randomised controlled trial. Lancet 380: 1909–1915.

28. Sandborn WJ, Rutgeerts P, Feagan BG, Reinisch W, Olson A, et al. (2009) Colectomy rate comparison after treatment of ulcerative colitis with placebo or infliximab. Gastroenterology 137: 1250–1260.

29. Ochsenkühn T, Sackmann M, Göke B (2004) Infliximab for acute, not steroid-refractory ulcerative colitis: a randomized pilot study. European Journal of Gastroenterology & Hepatology 16: 1167–1171.

30. Sandborn WJ, Colombel JF, D'Haens G, Van Assche G, Wolf D, et al. (2013) One-year maintenance outcomes among patients with moderately-to-severely active ulcerative colitis who responded to induction therapy with adalimumab: Subgroup analyses from ULTRA 2. Alimentary Pharmacology & Therapeutics 37: 204–213.

31. Sjoberg M, Magnuson A, Bjork J, Benoni C, Almer S, et al. (2013) Infliximab as rescue therapy in hospitalised patients with steroid-refractory acute ulcerative colitis: a long-term follow-up of 211 Swedish patients. Alimentary Pharmacology & Therapeutics 38: 377–387.

32. Sands B, Podolsky D, Tremaine W, Sandborn W, Rutgeerts P, et al. (1996) Chimeric monoclonal anti-tumor necrosis factor antibody (cA2) in the treatment of severe, steroid-refractory ulcerative colitis (UC). Gastroenterology 110: A1008–A1008.

33. Probert C, Hearing S, Schreiber S, Kuhbacher T, Ghosh S, et al. (2002) Infliximab in steroid-resistant ulcerative colitis: a randomised controlled trial. Gastroenterology 122: A99–A99.

34. Reinisch W, Van Assche G, Befrits R, Connell W, D'Haens G, et al. (2012) Recommendations for the treatment of ulcerative colitis with infliximab: a gastroenterology expert group consensus. Journal of Crohn's & Colitis 6: 248–258.

35. Lee KM, Jeen YT, Cho JY, Lee CK, Koo JS, et al. (2013) Efficacy, safety, and predictors of response to infliximab therapy for ulcerative colitis: a Korean multicenter retrospective study. Journal of Gastroenterology and Hepatology 28: 1829–1833.

36. Panaccione R, Rutgeerts P, Sandborn WJ, Feagan B, Schreiber S, et al. (2008) Review article: treatment algorithms to maximize remission and minimize corticosteroid dependence in patients with inflammatory bowel disease. Alimentary Pharmacology & Therapeutics 28: 674–688.

37. Chang KH, Burke JP, Coffey JC (2013) Infliximab versus cyclosporine as rescue therapy in acute severe steroid-refractory ulcerative colitis: a systematic review and meta-analysis. International Journal of Colorectal Disease; 28: 287–293.

21

Fecal Microbial Composition of Ulcerative Colitis and Crohn's Disease Patients in Remission and Subsequent Exacerbation

Edgar S. Wills[1,2], Daisy M. A. E. Jonkers[1], Paul H. Savelkoul[2], Ad A. Masclee[1], Marieke J. Pierik[1], John Penders[2,3]*

1 School for Nutrition, Toxicology and Metabolism (NUTRIM), Division Gastroenterology-Hepatology, Maastricht University Medical Center+, Maastricht, The Netherlands,
2 School for Nutrition, Toxicology and Metabolism (NUTRIM), Department of Medical Microbiology, Maastricht University Medical Center+, Maastricht, The Netherlands,
3 School for Public Health and Primary Care (Caphri), Department of Epidemiology, Maastricht University, Maastricht, The Netherlands

Abstract

Background: Limited studies have examined the intestinal microbiota composition in relation to changes in disease course of IBD over time. We aimed to study prospectively the fecal microbiota in IBD patients developing an exacerbation during follow-up.

Design: Fecal samples from 10 Crohn's disease (CD) and 9 ulcerative colitis (UC) patients during remission and subsequent exacerbation were included. Active disease was determined by colonoscopy and/or fecal calprotectine levels. Exclusion criteria were pregnancy, antibiotic use, enema use and/or medication changes between consecutive samples. The microbial composition was assessed by 16S rDNA pyrosequencing.

Results: After quality control, 6,194–11,030 sequences per sample were available for analysis. Patient-specific shifts in bacterial composition and diversity were observed during exacerbation compared to remission, but overarching shifts within UC or CD were not observed. Changes in the bacterial community composition between remission and exacerbation as assessed by Bray-Curtis dissimilarity, were significantly larger in CD versus UC patients (0.59 vs. 0.42, respectively; p = 0.025). Thiopurine use was found to be a significant cause of clustering as shown by Principal Coordinate Analysis and was associated with decreases in bacterial richness (Choa1 501.2 vs. 847.6 in non-users; p<0.001) and diversity (Shannon index: 5.13 vs. 6.78, respectively; p<0.01).

Conclusion: Shifts in microbial composition in IBD patients with changing disease activity over time seem to be patient-specific, and are more pronounced in CD than in UC patients. Furthermore, thiopurine use was found to be associated with the microbial composition and diversity, and should be considered when studying the intestinal microbiota in relation to disease course.

Editor: Jack Anthony Gilbert, Argonne National Laboratory, United States of America

Funding: This study was financially supported by grants form the Academic Foundation of Maastricht University Medical Center+ and by the IBD Research Foundation. The funders had no role in study design, data collection and analysis, decision to publish, or preparation of the manuscript.

Competing Interests: MP has acted as a consultant for MSD and received payments for lectures from MSD, Falk, Pharma, Abvie and Ferring. The other authors have declared that no competing interests exist.

* E-mail: j.penders@mumc.nl

Introduction

Crohn's disease (CD) and ulcerative colitis (UC) are chronic inflammatory diseases of the gastrointestinal tract, collectively referred to as inflammatory bowel disease (IBD). IBD is a heterogenous disease ith respect to disease location, disease course, occurrence of extra-intestinal manifestations and therapeutic response. The disease course is characterized by exacerbations and remissions. IBD is generally considered to arise from the interaction between host genetics, environmental factors, dysregulated immune responses and alterations in the intestinal microbiota composition [1]. IBD, especially active disease, is associated with a decreased quality of life and high health care costs, [2,3] especially due to the use of medication [2,4]. Treatment is mainly based on symptom reduction by nonspecific immune-modulating drugs and can be associated with serious side effects [5]. Further insight in causative factors associated with the development of exacerbations (i.e. active mucosal inflammation) may contribute to new specific treatment options for IBD.

The intestinal microbiota is considered to play a central role in the pathogenesis of IBD and numerous studies have corroborated evidence for intestinal dysbiosis in IBD patients compared to healthy controls [6–9]. The gut microbiota of healthy individuals is dominated by the bacterial phyla Firmicutes and Bacteroidetes, and to a lesser extent by Proteobacteria, Actinobacteria and Verrucomicrobia [10]. In IBD patients, members of the

Firmicutes phylum appear to be reduced, [9,11,12] whereas members of Gammaproteobacteria seem to bloom [13–16]. In CD patients the Clostridia cluster IV group, in particular *Faecalibacterium prausnitzii*, has shown to be decreased [15,17]. Members of Clostridia group XIVa, belonging to the *Roseburia* genus, also seem to be decreased in all IBD patients [17–19]. Data on Bacteroidetes are more ambiguous; inconsistent findings have been reported for their presence in IBD compared to controls [20–25]. In addition to these differences in relative abundances of specific phylotypes, there appears to be a general decrease in biodiversity in IBD patients [25,26].

Altogether, these studies provide compelling evidence for changes in the gut microbial communities in IBD patients as compared to healthy controls. Only a few studies, however, investigated the intestinal microbiota in relation to disease activity. Differences in bacterial species or groups (e.g. *F. prausnitzii*, Clostridia, *E. coli* and *Fusobacterium varium*) were found, when comparing active with inactive UC and CD patients,[7,9,20,27–29] but could not always be confirmed [17]. These studies are prone to confounding effects due to their cross-sectional designs and differences in medication use. Studies monitoring the microbiota composition within patients with changing disease activity over time and controlling for medication use are currently lacking. Therefore, the aim of the present study was to prospectively monitor the microbial composition in UC and CD patients during remission and subsequent exacerbation by means of 16S rDNA pyrosequencing.

Materials and Methods

Population and Design

The current study was conducted within the context of a prospective follow-up cohort of IBD outpatients, in which standardized demographic and clinical data, feces and blood samples were collected at study entry, at every subsequent outpatient visit and during an exacerbation [30].

The diagnosis of IBD was based on clinical and endoscopic or radiological findings. For case definition of CD, the Lennard-Jones criteria were applied [31]. UC was defined as continuous mucosal inflammation with granulomata, affecting the rectum and/or some or all of the colon in continuity with the rectum. Data of concomitant use of medication, body mass index (BMI), disease duration since diagnosis and disease phenotype (Montreal classification) were obtained using the computer-based medical registration databases. Furthermore at each visit, the occurrence of infections was checked by medical history and culture if indicated, and questions on overall changes in dietary habits were completed.

Fecal samples were collected at home on the evening before or the morning of each visit and stored at 4°C. Upon arrival at the hospital, the faecal samples were split directly. Part was sent to the laboratory of Clinical Chemistry for routine analysis of fecal calprotectine and the remaining part was frozen at −80°C within 24 hours after defecation for analyses of the microbiota.

Within the prospective cohort, patients with faecal samples at remission as well as after subsequent development of an exacerbation during a one-year follow-up period were eligible for the present study.

As clinical indices do not correlate very well with endoscopic scores [32,33] and as we aimed to assess the association of the fecal microbiota with the presence of mucosal inflammation, an exacerbation was defined by colonoscopy, a calprotectin value > 150 μg/g feces or >5-fold increase in calprotectin as compared to remission levels. For CD, only patients with colonic involvement were included as fecal samples are not likely to reflect microbial composition in the small intestine. For UC, eligible patients had pancolitis, left-sided colitis or proctosigmoiditis. Exclusion criteria were pregnancy, use of rectal enemas, use of antibiotics in the 3 months prior to inclusion or during follow-up, and/or a change in immunosuppressive medication between sampling at remission and subsequent development of disease exacerbation.

Ethics Statement

The study was approved by the Medical Ethics Committee of the Maastricht University Medical Center+ (NL31636.068.10), and written informed consent was obtained from all subjects.

16S rRNA V1–V3 Amplicon Library Preparation

Approximately 200 milligram feces was used for DNA isolation by the PSP SPIN Stool DNA plus kit (Stratec Molecular GmbH, Berlin, Germany) according to the manufacturer's instructions and eluted in a final volume of 200 μL.

Amplicon libraries for pyrosequencing of the 16S rDNA V1–V3 regions were generated using a barcoded forward primer consisting of the 454 Titanium platform A linker sequence (5′-CCATCCCTGCGTGTCTCCGACTCAG-3′), a key (barcode) that was unique for each sample, and the 16S rRNA 534R primer sequence 5′- ATTACCGCGGCTGCTGG -3′, and a reverse primer consisting of a 9:1 mixture of two oligonucleotides, 5′-*B*-AGAGTTTGATCMTGGCTCAG-3′ and 5′-*B*- AGGGTTCGATTCTGGCTCAG-3′, where *B* represents the B linker (5′-CCTATCCCCTGTGTGCCTTGGCAGTCTCAG-3′) followed by the 16S rRNA 8F and 8F-Bif primers, respectively (Table S1) [34].

PCR amplifications (in a volume of 50 μL) were performed using 1× FastStart High Fidelity Reaction Buffer, 1.8 mM MgCl$_2$, 1 mM dNTP solution, 5 U FastStart High Fidelity Blend Polymerase (from the High Fidelity PCR System (Roche, Indianapolis, USA)), 0.2 μM reverse primer, 0.2 μM of the barcoded forward primer (unique for each sample) and 1 μL of template DNA. PCR was performed using the following cycle conditions: an initial denaturation at 94°C for 3 min, followed by 25 cycles of denaturation at 94°C for 30 s, annealing at 51°C for 45 s and extension at 72°C for 5 min, and a final elongation step at 72°C for 10 min. Amplicons (20 μL) were purified using AMPure XP purification (Agencourt, Massachusetts, USA) according to the manufacturer's instructions and eluted in 25 μl 1× low TE (10 mM Tris-HCl, 0.1 mM EDTA, pH 8.0).

Amplicon concentrations were determined by Quant-iT Pico-Green dsDNA reagent kit (Invitrogen, New York, USA) using a Victor3 Multilabel Counter (Perkin Elmer, Waltham, USA). Amplicons were mixed in equimolar concentrations to ensure equal representation of each sample. A one-region 454 sequencing run was performed on a GS FLX Titanium PicoTiterPlate with a GS FLX pyrosequencing system (Roche, Branford, USA).

Data Analysis

The V1–V3 16S rDNA bacterial sequences analyzed in this paper have been deposited in the MG-RAST database (project ID: 4728).

Raw pyrosequencing reads were initially passed through quality filters to reduce the overall error rate using Mothur version 1.23 [35]. Only those sequences with perfect proximal primer fidelity and a threshold quality score of ≥20, a read length between 200 and 540 nucleotides, a maximum of one ambiguous base call and a maximum homopolymer length of 9 were retained for further analysis.

Subsequent data processing was conducted using Quantitative Insights Into Microbial Ecology (QIIME) version 1.5.1 [36].

Barcodes were used to identify sequences belonging to each patient sample. The UCLUST algorithm was used to cluster sequences into operational taxonomic units (OTUs) or phylotypes based on 97% similarity (species level) against the Greengenes reference set [37]. The following nondefault search parameters for UCLUST were applied: maxrejects = 100 and stepwords = 16. Creation of new clusters for sequences that did not cluster to reference sequences within the given similarity threshold was disabled, to further reduce the influence of pyrosequencing errors.

Species richness and diversity within communities (alpha-diversity) was measured by means of the observed OTUs (observed richness), Chao1 index (estimated richness), and the Shannon diversity index. Beta-diversity or diversity shared across patient communities was determined by UniFrac distance and Bray-Curtis dissimilarity (BC). UniFrac distances are based on the fraction of branch length shared between two communities within a phylogenetic tree constructed from the 16S rRNA gene sequences from all communities being compared. A relatively small UniFrac distance implies that two communities are compositionally similar, harboring lineages sharing a common evolutionary history [38]. Both weighted and unweighted UniFrac were used, respectively taking into account the abundance of each bacterial species for creating branch length or not.

Statistical Analysis

BC and Unweighted UniFrac distances were calculated for each patient (remission versus active sample) and distances were subsequently compared between CD and UC patients using the Mann-Whitney U test. Distances between subsequent samples from the same patient (within subjects) and distances between remission samples of different patients (between subjects) were also compared using the Mann-Whitney U test. The above mentioned statistical analyses were conducted using SPSS version 20.

All subsequent statistical analyses were conducted within QIIME 1.5.1, unless stated otherwise.

Age was dichotomized in two groups with 52 years (median age) as cut-off. Differences in alpha-diversity with respect to IBD type, disease location, age, gender and medication use (thiopurines, TNF-α inhibitors, aminosalicylates, prednisone or methotrexate) were tested using a nonparametric two-sample t-tests (i.e. using Monte Carlo permutations to calculate the p-value) at a rarefaction intensity of >6,190 sequences per sample. To test for differences in alpha-diversity within patients with respect to disease activity, the Wilcoxon Signed-Rank test was applied (conducted within SPSS v. 20).

OTU coverage was estimated using the conditional uncovered probability method [39]. Analysis of similarities (ANOSIM) was used to test for differences in community structure (UniFrac) among the various groups (IBD type, disease location, age, gender and medication use) in remission state. ANOSIM is a permutation-based test of the null hypothesis that within-group distances are not significantly smaller than between-group distances [40].

To test for associations between OTUs (presence) and IBD type, disease location, age, gender and medication use, the G-test statistic was used. To test for differences in the relative abundance of OTUs, the paired-sample T-test was used with respect to disease activity (within group comparisons) and ANOVA was used to test for differences with respect to IBD type, disease location, age, gender and medication use between groups. The false discovery rate (FDR) method was used to correct for multiple testing at a cutoff of 0.25. The relatively high value was used so as not to miss possible associations.

Results

Study Population

Out of the 323 patients from the prospective IBD cohort, with an average of three subsequent samples per subject, ten CD and nine UC patients that fulfilled our criteria could be selected. Patient characteristics are presented in Table 1. All patients, except one, had calprotectin levels above 150 µg/g feces at time of active disease. The single patient with a calprotectin level below 150 µg/g, showed a 9-fold increase (from 14 toward 126 µg/g faeces) during the flare as compared to remission.

454 Sequencing

In total, 230,026,772 bases and 551,607 sequences were recovered following pyrosequencing. After trimming, filtering and binning 324,085 sequences (mean length ±SD: 310±72.7 bases), ranging from 6,194 to 11,030 sequences per sample, remained for downstream analysis. A total of 2,839 OTUs were found with an OTU coverage of 97.1% ±1.1% (mean ± s.d.).

Dominant phyla across all samples included Firmicutes (81.3%), Bacteroidetes (15.9%), Proteobacteria (3.8%), Actinobacteria (3.7%), Verrucomicrobia (2.5%) and Tenericutes (1.1%) (Figure 1).

Patient-specific shifts in bacterial composition were observed in all patients. In a subgroup of patients, major shifts were observed for specific bacteria. Two CD patients (labeled #10 and 11 in Figure 1) showed strong increases in the relative abundances of *Bacteroides fragilis* during active disease, i.e. from 0.1% to 10.1% and from 0.1% to 81.9% respectively, whereas another CD patient (#17) showed a large increase in relative abundance of *Akkermansia muciniphila* (1.6% to 62.9%) during activity. Similarly, one UC patient (#8) showed a strong increase in the relative abundance of *Bacteroides dorei* (2.6% to 18.3%) and another UC patient (#3) showed an increase (1.2% to 13.9%) of an undefined *Lactobacillus* species. Despite these shifts in the individual microbial profiles, no significant difference in presence or relative abundance of any particular species or group was detected based on disease activity on a group level neither in the CD nor in the UC patients. Furthermore, no sequences from pathogenic species such as *Campylobacter spp.*, *Helicobacter spp.*, *Salmonella spp.* or *Mycobacterium spp.* were detected.

Effects on Richness and Diversity

No significant differences in any alpha-diversity metrics were found comparing subgroups based on IBD type, or disease activity (Table 2), nor for disease location, age, gender or use of TNF-α inhibitor, aminosalicylate, prednisone or methotrexate (data not shown). Alpha-diversity seemed to be affected in only one CD patient (#11) during follow up. This patient showed a large relative increase of fecal *B. fragilis* abundance during relapse compared to remission as reported above.

Thiopurine was used by 7 patients both at remission and during exacerbation (median treatment duration 49.5 (2–182) months), and was found to be associated with a lower number of observed OTUs, Chao1 and Shannon index (Table 2). The median daily dose expressed as 6-mercaptopurine (6-MP) equivalences [41] was 57.9 mg per day.

The number of observed OTUs in thiopurine users was significantly decreased among IBD patients in general (p = 2.37 * 10^{-4}), but also when studying CD patients (p = 2.57*10^{-5}) and UC patients (p = 7.93 * 10^{-4}) separately (Figure 2).

Effects on Community Membership and Composition

Unweighted UniFrac-based principal coordinate analysis (PCoA) did not show clustering according to disease activity,

Table 1. Patient characteristics[a.]

	CD (n = 10)	UC (n = 9)
Age (years)	42.5 (22–73)	65.0 (30–79)
Gender	6 ♂, 4 ♀	7 ♂, 2 ♀
Time since diagnosis (years)	7.5 (1–29)	10 (3–28)
Location	3 ileocolonic[c]	2 proctosigmoid
	7 colonic[c]	5 left-sided
		2 pancolitis
Medication use (n) [b]:		
TNF-α inhibitor	7	1
Thiopurine	4	3
Aminosalicylate	1	4
Methotrexate	1	1
Prednisone	1	1
Calprotectin (μg/g feces):		
- Remission	37.0 (17–82)	15.0 (15–115)
- Activity	365.0 (126–4,900)	231.0 (161–1,120)
Time between samples (remission to activity, in months)	1.5 (1–10)	3.0 (1–6)

[a]Age (year), calprotectin level (Calp) and time from remission to activity (months) displayed as median with the range in parentheses.
[b]No change in IBD medication, except doubling of mesalazine in one patient (#5 in subsequent figures and text) and use of lactulose in another patient (#6) during exacerbation.
[c]Disease extent in colon at time of inclusion was left-sided (n = 5), right sided (n = 2), pancolonic (n = 2) and cecal (n = 2).

IBD type, TNF-α inhibitor, aminosalicylate, prednisone or methotrexate use (Figures S2, S3, S4). Age ($R^2 = 0.16$; p = 0.001), thiopurine use ($R^2 = 0.41$; p = 0.001), gender ($R^2 = 0.35$; p = 0.003), disease location of UC ($R^2 = 0.34$; p = 0.008) were related to clustering (Figure 3 and Figure S1), as tested by ANOSIM. For thiopurine use, Fusobacteria and Verrucomicrobia phyla appeared to explain clustering for users, whereas especially Lentisphaerae appeared to determine clustering for non-users (Figure S5).

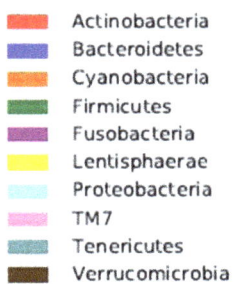

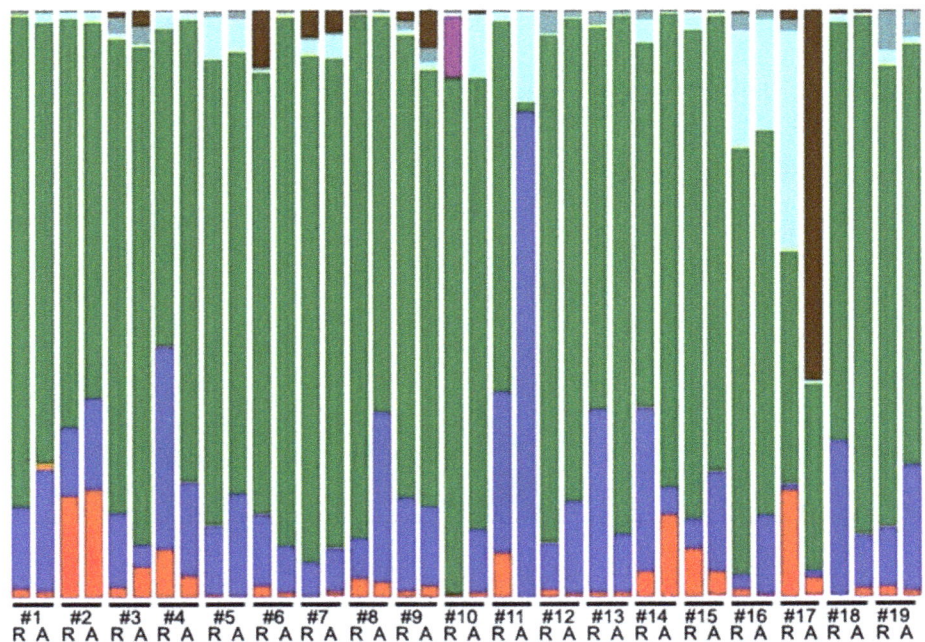

Figure 1. Relative abundance of bacterial phyla in fecal samples of nine UC (#1–9) and ten CD (#10–19) patients during remission and subsequent exacerbation.

Table 2. Alpha-diversity metrics for IBD subtype, disease activity, 6-MP use (Median (range)).

	Reads per sample	Coverage (%)	Observed OTUs	Chao1	Shannon
CD	8,053.5	97,4	477.2	684.0	6.6
	(6,503.0–10,033.0)	(94.8–99.3)	(72.1–652.8)	(99.7–1087.6)	(1.4–7.1)
UC	8,097.0	97.0	499.3	753.4	6.7
	(6,194–11,030)	(95.8–98.6)	(272.7–675.7)	(433.1–1047.3)	(5.5–7.7)
Exacerbation	7,921.0	97.4	493.3	726.3	6.7
	(6,194.0–11,030.0)	(95.8–99.3)	(72.1–664.5)	(99.7–1087.6)	(1.4–7.7)
Remission	8,169.0	97.0	493.9	747.7	6.6
	(6,503.0–10,013.0)	(94.8–99.1)	(160.6–675.7)	(308.9–1067.3)	(2.8–7.4)
Thiopurine use	8,193.0	97.8	338.9	489.3	5.8
	(6,465.0–10,013.0)	(96.2–99.3)	(72.1–517.4)[a]	(99.7–868.4)[a]	(1.4–7.0)[b]
No thiopurine use	7,929.0	96.6	569.4	875.9	6.7
	(6,194.0–11,030.0)	(94.8–98.0)	(406.9–675.7)	(605.9–1087.6)	(5.8–7.7)

[a]significantly lower in thiopurine users, p<0.001.
[b]significantly lower in thiopurine users, p<0.01.

Unweighted UniFrac distances of patients were significantly closer (p<0.001) between their own remission and exacerbation samples than to samples of other patients (Figure 4). Only the remission sample of patient #11 showed more similarity to the other patients' remission samples than to his own exacerbation sample.

Interestingly, the mean distance in community membership between paired Crohn's disease samples (0.51; s.d. 0.12) was significantly larger as compared to UC samples (0.42; s.d. 0.04; p = 0.027). Using Bray-Curtis dissimilarity distances, the same trend was observed with CD at 0.59 (s.d. 0.18) and UC at 0.42 (s.d. 0.09) (figure 5). This difference between the means was also statistically significant as determined by Mann-Whitney U test with p = 0.027.

Several associations were found between specific OTUs and patient characteristics as determined by G-test and ANOVA, but none of these withstood correction for multiple testing by means of FDR (Tables S2, S3, S4, S5).

Discussion

To our knowledge, this is the first prospective study using next-generation sequencing to examine the fecal microbiota composition in UC and CD during a quiescent disease phase and a subsequent exacerbation.

Similar to previous studies on the human fecal microbiota, the divisions of Firmicutes and Bacteroidetes predominated [42–44]. Although no overarching shifts in microbial communities could be

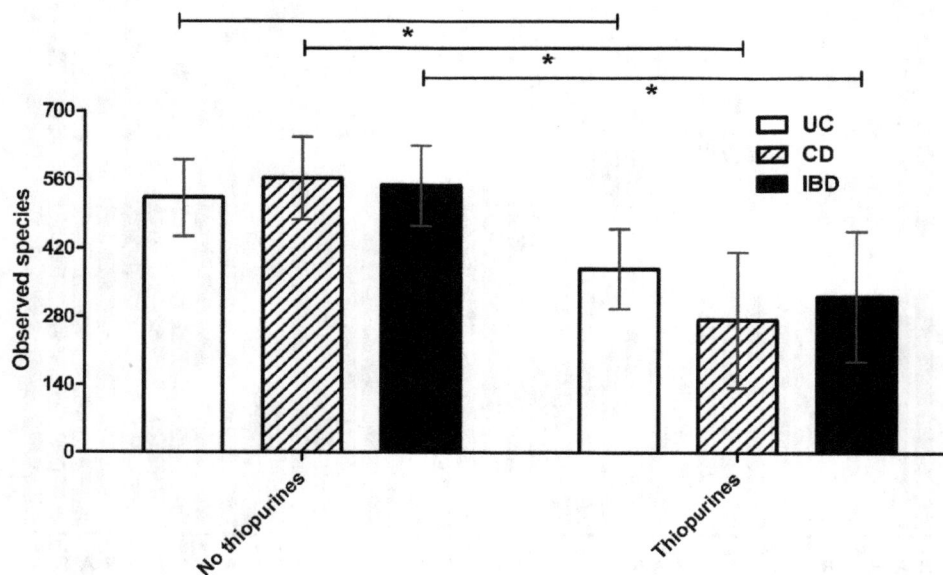

Figure 2. Mean number of observed species (OTUs) according to thiopurine use in Crohn's disease (p = 2.57*10^{-5}), total Inflammatory Bowel Disease (p = 2.37*10^{-4}) and Ulcerative Colitis (p = 7.93*10^{-4}) patients. *: Significantly different (p<0.001).

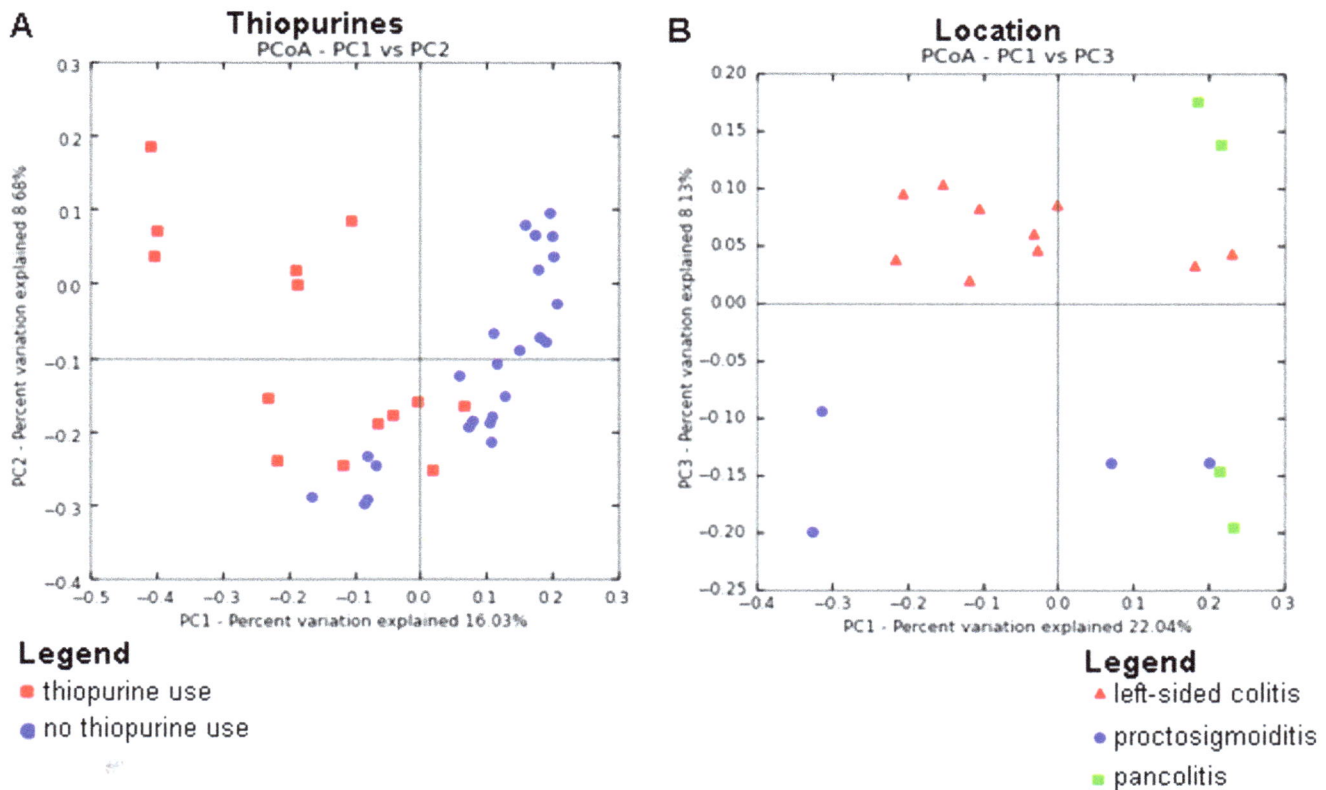

Figure 3. Communities clustered using Principal Coordinates Analysis (PCoA) of the unweighted UniFrac distance matrix. (A) PC1 and PC2 are plotted on x- and y-axes. Each point corresponds to a community colored according to thiopurine use. All samples are shown. The percentage of variation explained by the plotted principal coordinates is indicated on the axes. (B) PC1 and PC3 are plotted on x- and y-axis. Each point corresponds to a community colored according to disease location. Only samples from UC patients are included.

detected in the CD and UC populations, shifts in composition and decreased diversity were observed in individual patients. Moreover, it was demonstrated that the microbiota within CD patients was less stable compared to the microbiota from UC patients. Finally, thiopurines appear to affect the gut microbial composition and diversity.

In the present study, we were not able to identify overall patterns in microbial changes related to the presence of an exacerbation. An exacerbation was defined by endoscopic scores and/or fecal calprotectin levels as indicators for mucosal inflammation, as clinical scores are reported not to correlate very well with endoscopy findings [32,33]. Mucosal inflammation is increasingly recognized as outcome parameter for active disease and is important for optimization of therapeutic strategies and to prevent complications [45].

Previous studies did show microbial differences comparing active with inactive IBD patients. For example, a combination of leucocytes in the fecal-mucosal transition zone and the concentration of *F. prausnitzii* were found to be strong predictors of active CD and UC [7]. Diminished *F. prausnitzii*, as well as a lower Firmicutes/Bacteroidetes ratio was also associated with active disease in another study on 49 IBD patients [9]. Furthermore, a decrease in the Clostridium family was found in active UC and inactive and active CD compared to inactive UC and healthy controls [20]. A decrease of *C. coccoides*, *C. leptum* subgroup, Atophium cluster and *B. ovatus* was reported in feces of active compared to inactive UC, [8] while increased counts of

bifidobacteria, *E. coli* and Clostridia were found in tissue specimens of active compared to inactive UC by others [27].

The above-mentioned studies had a cross-sectional design and are therefore more vulnerable to selection bias and confounding. None of these studies did match patients with quiescent disease to patients with active disease based on characteristics such as disease location, medication, diet and other possible confounders, nor did they adjust for these factors in their statistical analyses. In contrast, two more recent studies that used pyrosequencing did not show clustering based on disease status. A study by Willing et al. used a multivariate statistical approach (partial least-squares discriminant analysis) to distinguish disease phenotypes based on microbial composition in 40 twin pairs [17]. Six patients had active disease based on clinical scores, which could not be distinguished from 34 patients with inactive disease. In the second study, analyzing 231 biopsies and stool samples of IBD patients and healthy subjects, disease activity was not associated with specific shifts in the microbiome composition even after adjusting for other factors such as sample type (i.e. stool or biopsy), IBD type, age, smoking and medication [29].

A potential explanation for the lack of overarching shifts in microbial composition at time of exacerbation in our study may be due to the relatively small study population. Although we included only CD patients with colonic disease and excluded IBD patients with changes in medication over time, some heterogeneity in the study population cannot be excluded. IBD can be considered a set of diseases with overlapping phenotypes rather than a single disease [46,47]. This may contribute to the patient-specific

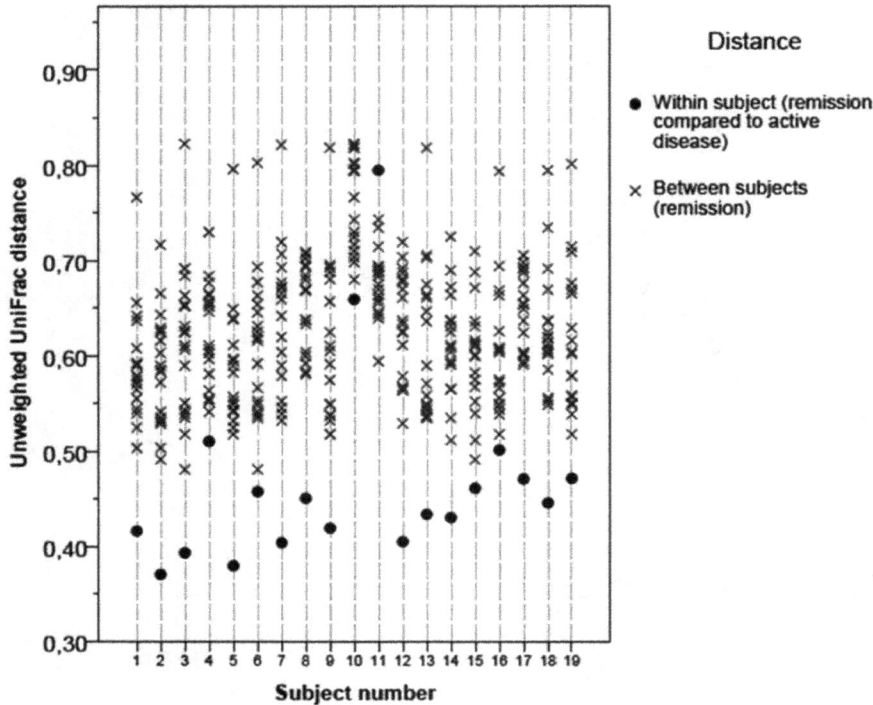

Figure 4. Within and between subjects pair-wise unweighted UniFrac distances for ulcerative colitis (#1–9) and Crohn's disease (#10–19) patients.

microbial composition shifts, and lack thereof at group level. The fact that from a large cohort of 323 subjects, only 19 fulfilled our selection criteria, illustrates that it is very difficult to include a rather large homogenous subpopulation.

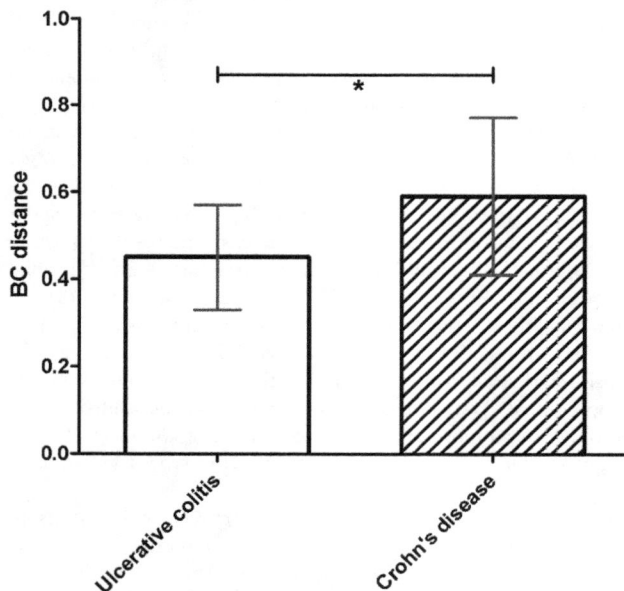

Figure 5. Mean within subjects pair-wise Bray-Curtis distances for ulcerative colitis and Crohn's disease patients (p = 0.027). *: Significantly different (p<0.05).

The main strength of the present study is the prospective design comparing the microbiota in association to disease activity within the same patients followed over time, particularly considering the interindividual differences in microbiota composition. Clear subject-specific changes have been observed. As modifications of medication use over time were not allowed, these changes were most likely associated with the changing disease activity. Major increases (up to 81.9%) in specific bacterial subspecies were observed in five patients, being *Lactobacillus spp.* (in one UC patient), *B. dorei* (in one UC patient), *A. muciniphila* (in one CD patient), and *B. fragilis* (in two CD patients (#10 and #11)). These two latter patients were both non-smoking females (age 35 and 50 years respectively) using a combination of thiopurines and TNF-inhibitors continuously during the period of interest. Apart from developing an exacerbation, no major changes in clinical or environmental factors did occur during the follow-up period in any of these patients that could have contributed to the observed findings. Although larger patient numbers need to be studied before final conclusions can be drawn on the role of the individual commensal in the pathogenesis of IBD, the potential importance of *B. fragilis* is supported by findings from others. *B. fragilis* was found to be significantly more abundant in biopsies from CD patients compared to UC patients and healthy subjects [23]. In another study, the mucosal biofilm mass in IBD patients appeared to be dominated by *B. fragilis* [24]. Some strains of *B. fragilis* are enterotoxigenic by producing a zinc-dependent metalloprotease toxin, and appear to be more prevalent in active IBD patients as compared to inactive patients and control subjects [48]. Animal models have confirmed that enterotoxigenic *B. fragilis* alone is sufficient to induce colitis [49]. Furthermore, a potential role for the eukaryotic-like ubiquitin gene in *B. fragilis* in the pathophysiology of CD has recently been postulated [50].

In the present study, we found a different level of microbial variability contributing to exacerbations in either CD or UC. This may indicate that changes in gut bacterial composition play a more important role in CD than in UC exacerbation development. These findings are in line with findings by others. Willing et al. (2010) found different microbial profiles between CD and controls but not between UC and controls based on 454 sequencing [17]. In addition, Andoh et al. found inactive UC patients to cluster with healthy controls, while inactive and active CD clustered separately together with active UC [20].

Although the numbers were small, we found that thiopurine treatment was associated with the microbial composition and the diversity. Based upon the Principal Coordinate analysis, thiopurine use was found to be the most important factor responsible for clustering and was furthermore associated with a significant decrease in alpha-diversity. It has previously been found that the thiopurines 6-mercaptopurine (6-MP) and azathioprine inhibit growth of *M. avium* subspecies *paratuberculosis in vitro* [51,52]. We could not demonstrate an antimicrobial effect of 6-MP in vitro as tested on *Bacillus subtilis* by disc diffusion test (test range 1–64 µg, data not shown). This does however not exclude the possibility of an (indirect) effect of 6-MP or one of its metabolites on the intestinal microbiota in vivo.

As such, the present findings indicate that thiopurine use, especially changes in administration or dosage over time, should be considered as a potential confounding factor when studying the microbiota composition in IBD. Replication of our findings on the association between thiopurine use and shifts in microbiota composition as well as more mechanistic insight on the potential underlying mechanisms is warranted to prove a causal relationship.

Conclusion

Although we did observe patient-specific shifts in microbial composition, we could not demonstrate general changes in microbial composition or diversity in IBD patients at time of exacerbation as compared to a quiescent disease state. Patient-specific shifts in fecal microbial composition seemed to be associated with larger Bray-Curtis dissimilarity between remission and active disease for CD as compared to UC. Furthermore, thiopurine use was found to have significant impact on the microbial composition and diversity, and should be considered when studying the intestinal microbiota in relation to disease course.

Larger prospective studies that enable controlling for potential confounders such as medication, disease subtype and location, are needed to unravel potential general shifts in the microbiota related to exacerbations in IBD.

Supporting Information

Figure S1 Communities clustered using Principal Coordinates Analysis (PCoA) of the unweighted UniFrac distance matrix. (A) PC1 and PC2 are plotted on x- and y-axes. Each point corresponds to a community colored according to age (red, <52 years; blue ≥52 years). All samples are shown. The percentage of variation explained by the plotted principal coordinates is indicated on the axes. (B) PC1 and PC2 are plotted on x- and y-axis. Each point corresponds to a community colored according to gender (blue, male; red, female).

Figure S2 Communities clustered using Principal Coordinates Analysis (PCoA) of the unweighted UniFrac distance matrix. (A) PC1 and PC2 are plotted on x- and y-axes. Each point corresponds to a community colored according to aminosalicylate use (red, no aminosalicylate use, blue, aminosalicylate use). All samples are shown. The percentage of variation explained by the plotted principal coordinates is indicated on the axes. (B) PC1 and PC2 are plotted on x- and y-axis. Each point corresponds to a community colored according to IBD type (red, CD; blue UC).

Figure S3 Communities clustered using Principal Coordinates Analysis (PCoA) of the unweighted UniFrac distance matrix. (A) PC1 and PC2 are plotted on x- and y-axes. Each point corresponds to a community colored according to TNF-α inhibitor use (red, TNF-α inhibitor use; blue, no TNF-α inhibitor use). All samples are shown. The percentage of variation explained by the plotted principal coordinates is indicated on the axes. (B) PC1 and PC2 are plotted on x- and y-axis. Each point corresponds to a community colored according to disease activity (red, exacerbation; blue, remission).

Figure S4 Communities clustered using Principal Coordinates Analysis (PCoA) of the unweighted UniFrac distance matrix. (A) PC1 and PC2 are plotted on x- and y-axes. Each point corresponds to a community colored according to methotrexate use (red, methotrexate use; blue, no methotrexate use). All samples are shown. The percentage of variation explained by the plotted principal coordinates is indicated on the axes. (B) PC1 and PC2 are plotted on x- and y-axis. Each point corresponds to a community colored according to prednisone use (red, no prednisone use; blue, prednisone use).

Figure S5 Communities plotted together with phyla using Principal Coordinates Analysis (PCoA) of the unweighted UniFrac distance matrix. PC1, PC2 and PC3 are plotted on x-, y- and z-axes. Each point corresponds to a community colored according to thiopurine use (red, thiopurine use; blue, no thiopurine use). Note: Axes were deliberately skewed to most clearly depict relation of clustering to bacterial groups.

Table S1 Primers used in this study.

Table S2 Species associations to thiopurine use in resting disease.

Table S3 Species associations to age (<52 years/>52 years) in remission state.

Table S4 Species associations to gender in remission state; F– indicates decreased presence in female subjects.

Table S5 Species associations to IBD type in remission state.

Author Contributions

Conceived and designed the experiments: DJ MP AM PS JP. Performed the experiments: EW. Analyzed the data: EW JP. Contributed reagents/materials/analysis tools: DJ MP. Wrote the paper: EW DJ AM PS MP JP. Drafting the article or revising it critically for important intellectual content: EW DJ AM PS MP JP. Final approval of the version to be published: EW DJ AM PS MP JP.

References

1. Scharl M, Rogler G (2012) Inflammatory bowel disease pathogenesis: what is new? Curr Opin Gastroenterol 28: 301–309.

2. Blumenstein I, Bock H, Weber C, Rambow A, Tacke W, et al. (2008) Health care and cost of medication for inflammatory bowel disease in the Rhein-Main region, Germany: a multicenter, prospective, internet-based study. Inflamm Bowel Dis 14: 53–60.

3. Buchanan J, Wordsworth S, Ahmad T, Perrin A, Vermeire S, et al. (2011) Managing the long term care of inflammatory bowel disease patients: The cost to European health care providers. J Crohns Colitis 5: 301–316.

4. van der Valk ME, Mangen MJ, Leenders M, Dijkstra G, van Bodegraven AA, et al. (2014) Healthcare costs of inflammatory bowel disease have shifted from hospitalisation and surgery towards anti-TNFalpha therapy: results from the COIN study. Gut.

5. Talley NJ, Abreu MT, Achkar JP, Bernstein CN, Dubinsky MC, et al. (2011) An evidence-based systematic review on medical therapies for inflammatory bowel disease. Am J Gastroenterol 106 Suppl 1: S2–25; quiz S26.

6. Frank DN, St Amand AL, Feldman RA, Boedeker EC, Harpaz N, et al. (2007) Molecular-phylogenetic characterization of microbial community imbalances in human inflammatory bowel diseases. Proc Natl Acad Sci U S A 104: 13780–13785.

7. Swidsinski A, Loening-Baucke V, Vaneechoutte M, Doerffel Y (2008) Active Crohn's disease and ulcerative colitis can be specifically diagnosed and monitored based on the biostructure of the fecal flora. Inflamm Bowel Dis 14: 147–161.

8. Takaishi H, Matsuki T, Nakazawa A, Takada T, Kado S, et al. (2008) Imbalance in intestinal microflora constitution could be involved in the pathogenesis of inflammatory bowel disease. Int J Med Microbiol 293: 463–472.

9. Sokol H, Seksik P, Furet JP, Firmesse O, Nion-Larmurier I, et al. (2009) Low counts of Faecalibacterium prausnitzii in colitis microbiota. Inflamm Bowel Dis 15: 1183–1189.

10. Eckburg PB, Bik EM, Bernstein CN, Purdom E, Dethlefsen L, et al. (2005) Diversity of the human intestinal microbial flora. Science 308: 1635–1638.

11. Sokol H, Seksik P, Rigottier-Gois L, Lay C, Lepage P, et al. (2006) Specificities of the fecal microbiota in inflammatory bowel disease. Inflamm Bowel Dis 12: 106–111.

12. Rehman A, Lepage P, Nolte A, Hellmig S, Schreiber S, et al. (2010) Transcriptional activity of the dominant gut mucosal microbiota in chronic inflammatory bowel disease patients. J Med Microbiol 59: 1114–1122.

13. Seksik P, Rigottier-Gois L, Gramet G, Sutren M, Pochart P, et al. (2003) Alterations of the dominant faecal bacterial groups in patients with Crohn's disease of the colon. Gut 52: 237–242.

14. Sokol H, Lay C, Seksik P, Tannock GW (2008) Analysis of bacterial bowel communities of IBD patients: what has it revealed? Inflamm Bowel Dis 14: 858–867.

15. Martinez-Medina M, Aldeguer X, Gonzalez-Huix F, Acero D, Garcia-Gil LJ (2006) Abnormal microbiota composition in the ileocolonic mucosa of Crohn's disease patients as revealed by polymerase chain reaction-denaturing gradient gel electrophoresis. Inflamm Bowel Dis 12: 1136–1145.

16. Kotlowski R, Bernstein CN, Sepehri S, Krause DO (2007) High prevalence of Escherichia coli belonging to the B2+D phylogenetic group in inflammatory bowel disease. Gut 56: 669–675.

17. Willing BP, Dicksved J, Halfvarson J, Andersson AF, Lucio M, et al. (2010) A pyrosequencing study in twins shows that gastrointestinal microbial profiles vary with inflammatory bowel disease phenotypes. Gastroenterology 139: 1844–1854 e1841.

18. Nagalingam NA, Lynch SV (2011) Role of the microbiota in inflammatory bowel diseases. Inflamm Bowel Dis.

19. Rajilic-Stojanovic M, Shanahan F, Guarner F, de Vos WM (2013) Phylogenetic analysis of dysbiosis in ulcerative colitis during remission. Inflamm Bowel Dis 19: 481–488.

20. Andoh A, Imaeda H, Aomatsu T, Inatomi O, Bamba S, et al. (2011) Comparison of the fecal microbiota profiles between ulcerative colitis and Crohn's disease using terminal restriction fragment length polymorphism analysis. J Gastroenterol 46: 479–486.

21. Sepehri S, Kotlowski R, Bernstein CN, Krause DO (2007) Microbial diversity of inflamed and noninflamed gut biopsy tissues in inflammatory bowel disease. Inflamm Bowel Dis 13: 675–683.

22. Bibiloni R, Mangold M, Madsen KL, Fedorak RN, Tannock GW (2006) The bacteriology of biopsies differs between newly diagnosed, untreated, Crohn's disease and ulcerative colitis patients. J Med Microbiol 55: 1141–1149.

23. Gophna U, Sommerfeld K, Gophna S, Doolittle WF, Veldhuyzen van Zanten SJ (2006) Differences between tissue-associated intestinal microfloras of patients with Crohn's disease and ulcerative colitis. J Clin Microbiol 44: 4136–4141.

24. Swidsinski A, Weber J, Loening-Baucke V, Hale LP, Lochs H (2005) Spatial organization and composition of the mucosal flora in patients with inflammatory bowel disease. J Clin Microbiol 43: 3380–3389.

25. Ott SJ, Musfeldt M, Wenderoth DF, Hampe J, Brant O, et al. (2004) Reduction in diversity of the colonic mucosa associated bacterial microflora in patients with active inflammatory bowel disease. Gut 53: 685–693.

26. Manichanh C, Rigottier-Gois L, Bonnaud E, Gloux K, Pelletier E, et al. (2006) Reduced diversity of faecal microbiota in Crohn's disease revealed by a metagenomic approach. Gut 55: 205–211.

27. Mylonaki M, Rayment NB, Rampton DS, Hudspith BN, Brostoff J (2005) Molecular characterization of rectal mucosa-associated bacterial flora in inflammatory bowel disease. Inflamm Bowel Dis 11: 481–487.

28. Ohkusa T, Sato N, Ogihara T, Morita K, Ogawa M, et al. (2002) Fusobacterium varium localized in the colonic mucosa of patients with ulcerative colitis stimulates species-specific antibody. J Gastroenterol Hepatol 17: 849–853.

29. Morgan XC, Tickle TL, Sokol H, Gevers D, Devaney KL, et al. (2012) Dysfunction of the intestinal microbiome in inflammatory bowel disease and treatment. Genome Biol 13: R79.

30. Masclee GM, Penders J, Pierik M, Wolffs P, Jonkers D (2013) Enteropathogenic Viruses: Triggers for Exacerbation in IBD? A Prospective Cohort Study Using Real-time Quantitative Polymerase Chain Reaction. Inflamm Bowel Dis 19: 124–131.

31. Lennard-Jones JE (1989) Classification of inflammatory bowel disease. Scand J Gastroenterol Suppl 170: 2–6; discussion 16–19.

32. af Bjorkesten CG, Nieminen U, Turunen U, Arkkila P, Sipponen T, et al. (2012) Surrogate markers and clinical indices, alone or combined, as indicators for endoscopic remission in anti-TNF-treated luminal Crohn's disease. Scand J Gastroenterol 47: 528–537.

33. Regueiro M, Kip KE, Schraut W, Baidoo L, Sepulveda AR, et al. (2011) Crohn's disease activity index does not correlate with endoscopic recurrence one year after ileocolonic resection. Inflamm Bowel Dis 17: 118–126.

34. Dethlefsen L, Huse S, Sogin ML, Relman DA (2008) The pervasive effects of an antibiotic on the human gut microbiota, as revealed by deep 16S rRNA sequencing. PLoS Biol 6: e280.

35. Schloss PD, Westcott SL, Ryabin T, Hall JR, Hartmann M, et al. (2009) Introducing mothur: open-source, platform-independent, community-supported software for describing and comparing microbial communities. Appl Environ Microbiol 75: 7537–7541.

36. Caporaso JG, Kuczynski J, Stombaugh J, Bittinger K, Bushman FD, et al. (2010) QIIME allows analysis of high-throughput community sequencing data. Nat Methods 7: 335–336.

37. McDonald D, Price MN, Goodrich J, Nawrocki EP, DeSantis TZ, et al. (2011) An improved Greengenes taxonomy with explicit ranks for ecological and evolutionary analyses of bacteria and archaea. ISME J 6: 610–618.

38. Lozupone C, Knight R (2005) UniFrac: a new phylogenetic method for comparing microbial communities. Appl Environ Microbiol 71: 8228–8235.

39. Lladser ME, Gouet R, Reeder J (2011) Extrapolation of urn models via poissonization: accurate measurements of the microbial unknown. PLoS One 6: e21105.

40. Clarke K (1993) Non-parametric multivariate analyses of changes in community structure. Austral J Ecol 18: 117–143.

41. Sandborn WJ (2001) Rational dosing of azathioprine and 6-mercaptopurine. Gut 48: 591–592.

42. Nam YD, Jung MJ, Roh SW, Kim MS, Bae JW (2011) Comparative analysis of Korean human gut microbiota by barcoded pyrosequencing. PLoS One 6: e22109.

43. Claesson MJ, O'Sullivan O, Wang Q, Nikkila J, Marchesi JR, et al. (2009) Comparative analysis of pyrosequencing and a phylogenetic microarray for exploring microbial community structures in the human distal intestine. PLoS One 4: e6669.

44. van den Bogert B, de Vos WM, Zoetendal EG, Kleerebezem M (2011) Microarray analysis and barcoded pyrosequencing provide consistent microbial profiles depending on the source of human intestinal samples. Appl Environ Microbiol 77: 2071–2080.

45. Vaughn BP, Shah S, Cheifetz AS (2014) The Role of Mucosal Healing in the Treatment of Patients With Inflammatory Bowel Disease. Curr Treat Options Gastroenterol.

46. Kaser A, Zeissig S, Blumberg RS (2010) Genes and environment: how will our concepts on the pathophysiology of IBD develop in the future? Dig Dis 28: 395–405.

47. Young VB, Kahn SA, Schmidt TM, Chang EB (2011) Studying the Enteric Microbiome in Inflammatory Bowel Diseases: Getting through the Growing Pains and Moving Forward. Front Microbiol 2: 144.

48. Prindiville TP, Sheikh RA, Cohen SH, Tang YJ, Cantrell MC, et al. (2000) Bacteroides fragilis enterotoxin gene sequences in patients with inflammatory bowel disease. Emerg Infect Dis 6: 171–174.

49. Rabizadeh S, Rhee KJ, Wu S, Huso D, Gan CM, et al. (2007) Enterotoxigenic bacteroides fragilis: a potential instigator of colitis. Inflamm Bowel Dis 13: 1475–1483.

50. Patrick S, Blakely GW (2012) Crossing the eukaryote-prokaryote divide: A ubiquitin homolog in the human commensal bacterium Bacteroides fragilis. Mob Genet Elements 2: 149–151.

51. Greenstein RJ, Su L, Haroutunian V, Shahidi A, Brown ST (2007) On the action of methotrexate and 6-mercaptopurine on M. avium subspecies paratuberculosis. PLoS One 2: e161.

52. Shin SJ, Collins MT (2008) Thiopurine drugs azathioprine and 6-mercaptopurine inhibit Mycobacterium paratuberculosis growth in vitro. Antimicrob Agents Chemother 52: 418–426.

Permissions

List of Contributors

Tiago Rodrigues-Sousa, Helena Carvalheiro and M. Margarida Souto-Carneiro
ImmunoMetabolic Pharmacology Group, CNC- Centro de Neurociências e Biologia Celular, Universidade de Coimbra, Coimbra, Portugal

Ana Filipa Ladeirinha, Lina Carvalho and Ana Alarcão
Departamento de Anatomia Patológica, Faculdade de Medicina, Universidade de Coimbra, Coimbra, Portugal

Ana Raquel Santiago
Instituto Biomédico de Investigação da Luz e Imagem, Faculdade de Medicina, Universidade de Coimbra, Coimbra, Portugal

Bruno Raposo and Rikard Holmdahl
Medical Inflammation Research, Karolinska Institute, Stockholm, Sweden

António Cabrita
Departamento de Patologia Experimental, Faculdade de Medicina, Universidade de Coimbra, Coimbra, Portugal

Julia Seiderer, Florian Beigel, Cornelia Tillack, Johannes Stallhofer, Christian Steib Burkhard Göke, Thomas Ochsenkühn and Stephan Brand
Department of Medicine II - Grosshadern, Ludwig-Maximilians-University, Munich, Germany

Matthias Friedrich, Johanna Wagner and Julia Diegelmann
Department of Preventive Dentistry and Periodontology, Ludwig- Maximilians-University, Munich, Germany
Department of Medicine II - Grosshadern, Ludwig-Maximilians-University, Munich, Germany

Torsten Olszak
Gastrointestinal Division, Brigham & Women's Hospital, Harvard Medical School, Boston, Massachusetts, United States of America
Department of Medicine II - Grosshadern, Ludwig-Maximilians-University, Munich, Germany

Martin Wetzke
Department of Pediatrics, Hannover Medical School,Germany,
Department of Medicine II - Grosshadern, Ludwig-Maximilians-University, Munich, Germany
Department of Preventive Dentistry and Periodontology, Ludwig- Maximilians-University, Munich, Germany

Jürgen Glas
Department of Medicine II - Grosshadern, Ludwig-Maximilians-University, Munich, Germany
Department of Preventive Dentistry and Periodontology, Ludwig- Maximilians-University, Munich, Germany
Department of Human Genetics, Rheinisch-Westfälische Technische Hochschule (RWTH), Aachen, Germany

Darina Czamara and Nazanin Karbalai
Max-Planck-Institute of Psychiatry, Munich, Germany

Tania O. Crişan, Theo S. Plantinga, Frank L. van de Veerdonk, Marius F. Farcaş, Monique Stoffels, Bart-Jan Kullberg, Jos W. M. van der Meer, Leo A. B. Joosten and Mihai G. Netea
Department of Medicine, Radboud University Nijmegen Medical Center, Nijmegen, The Netherlands
Nijmegen Institute for Infection, Inflammation and Immunity (N4i), Radboud University Nijmegen Medical Center, Nijmegen, The Netherlands

Andrea Mencarelli, Barbara Renga, Claudio D'Amore, Sabrina Cipriani, Giuseppe Palladino and Stefano Fiorucci
Dipartimento di Medicina Clinica e Sperimentale, University of Perugia, Facoltàdi Medicina e Chirurgia, Via Gerardo Dottori nu 1 S. Andrea delle Fratte, Perugia, Italy

Eleonora Distrutti
Azienda Ospedaliera di Perugia, Ospedale Santa Maria della Misericordia, S. Andrea delle Fratte, Perugia, Italy

Annibale Donini and Patrizia Ricci
Dipartimento di Scienze Chirurgiche, Radiologiche e Odontostomatologiche, Nuova Facoltàdi Medicina e Chirurgia Sant' Andrea delle Fratte, Perugia, Italy

Poonam Dharmani, Pearl Leung and Kris Chadee
Department of Microbiology, Immunology and Infectious Diseases, Gastrointestinal Research Group, Health Sciences Centre, University of Calgary, Calgary, Alberta, Canada

Julia Seiderer, Melinda Nagy, Christoph Fries, Florian Beigel, Maria Weidinger, Simone Pfennig, Burkhard Göke, Thomas Ochsenkühn and Stephan Brand
Department of Medicine II - Grosshadern, University of Munich, Munich, Germany

Julia Diegelmann
Department of Medicine II - Grosshadern, University of Munich, Munich, Germany
Department of Preventive Dentistry and Periodontology, University of Munich, Munich, Germany

Jürgen Glas
Department of Medicine II - Grosshadern, University of Munich, Munich, Germany
Department of Preventive Dentistry and Periodontology, University of Munich, Munich, Germany
Institute of Human Genetics, RWTH Aachen, Aachen, Germany

Matthias Folwaczny
Department of Preventive Dentistry and Periodontology, University of Munich, Munich, Germany

Wolfram Klein and Jörg T. Epplen
Department of Human Genetics, Ruhr-University Bochum, Bochum, Germany

Peter Lohse
Institute of Clinical Chemistry - Grosshadern, University of Munich, Munich, Germany

Darina Roeske and Bertram Müller-Myhsok
Max-Planck-Institute of Psychiatry, Munich, Germany

Koichi Yanaba, Yoshihide Asano, Yayoi Tada, Makoto Sugaya, Takafumi Kadono and Shinichi Sato
Department of Dermatology, Faculty of Medicine, University of Tokyo, Tokyo, Japan

Xin Liu
College of Pharmaceutical Sciences, Zhejiang University, Hangzhou, China

Jian Ming Wang
Academy of Traditional Chinese Medicine, Heilongjiang University of Chinese Medicine, Harbin, China

Birte Zurek, Andreas Neerin, Katharina Birkner and Thomas A. Kufer
Institute for Medical Microbiology, Immunology and Hygiene, University of Cologne, Cologne, Germany

Ida Schoultz, Maria Lerm and Johan D. Söderholm
Department of Clinical and Experimental Medicine, Faculty of Health Sciences, Linköping University, Linköping, Sweden, and Department of Surgery, Linköping, Sweden

Germana Meroni
Cluster in Biomedicine (CBM), AREA Science Park, Trieste, Italy

Luisa M. Napolitano
Cluster in Biomedicine (CBM), AREA Science Park, Trieste, Italy
Telethon Institute of Genetics and Medicine, Naples, Italy

Eveline Bennek and Gernot Sellge
Department of Medicine III, University Hospital Aachen, Aachen, Germany

Benjamin Lehne and Thomas Schlitt
Department of Medical and Molecular Genetics, King's College London, London, United Kingdom

Cathryn M. Lewis
Social, Genetic and Developmental Psychiatry Centre, Institute of Psychiatry, King's College London, London, United Kingdom
Department of Medical and Molecular Genetics, King's College London, London, United Kingdom

Martin Storr
Division of Gastroenterology, Department of Medicine, University of Calgary, Calgary, Alberta, Canada

Dominik Emmerdinger, Julia Diegelmann, Simone Pfennig, Thomas Ochsenkühn, Burkhard Göke and Stephan Brand
Department of Medicine II – Grosshadern, Ludwig-Maximilians- University Munich, Munich, Germany

Peter Lohse
Department of Clinical Chemistry – Grosshadern, Ludwig-Maximilians-University Munich, Munich, Germany

Melanie Craven, Belgin Dogan and Kenneth W. Simpson
Department of Clinical Sciences, College of Veterinary Medicine, Cornell University, Ithaca, New York, United States of America

Charlotte E. Egan, Eric Y. Denkers and Dwight Bowman
Department of Microbiology and Immunology, College of Veterinary Medicine, Cornell University, Ithaca, New York, United States of America

Scot E. Dowd
MR DNA (Molecular Research), Shallowater, Texas, United States of America

Sean P. McDonough
Department of Pathology, College of Veterinary Medicine, Cornell University, Ithaca, New York, United States of America

Ellen J. Scherl
Division of Gastroenterology and Hepatology, Jill Roberts Inflammatory Bowel Disease Center, Weill Cornell Medical College, Cornell University, New York, New York, United States of America

Marco Gerling, Rainer Glauben, Martin Zeitz and Britta Siegmund
Medical Clinic I, Charité – Universitätsmedizin Berlin, Campus Benjamin Franklin, Berlin, Germany

Jens K. Habermann
Laboratory for Surgical Research, Department of Surgery, University of Lübeck, Lübeck, Germany

Anja A. Kühl and Christoph Loddenkemper
Institute of Pathology / RCIS, Charité – Universitätsmedizin Berlin, Campus Benjamin Franklin, Berlin, Germany

Hans-Anton Lehr
Centre Hospitalier Universitaire Vaudois (CHUV), Institut Universitaire de Pathologie, Lausanne, Switzerland

Laurent-Herve Perez, Matt Butler, Tammy Creasey, Stephanie Petit, Anna Ropenga, Kathryn Smith, Philip Smith and Scott J. Parkinson
Gastrointestinal Disease Area, Novartis Institutes for Biomedical Research, Horsham, United Kingdom

John Gounarides
Analytical Sciences, Novartis Institutes for Biomedical Research, Cambridge, Massachusetts, United States of America

JoAnn Dzink-Fox and Neil Ryder
Infectious Disease Area, Novartis Institutes for Biomedical Research, Cambridge, Massachusetts, United States of America

Vikneswari Mahendran, Thi Anh Tuyet Tran, Joelene Major, Nadeem O. Kaakoush, Hazel Mitchell and Li Zhang
School of Biotechnology and Biomolecular Sciences, University of New South Wales, Sydney, Australia

Stephen M. Riordan
Gastrointestinal and Liver Unit, The Prince of Wales Hospital, Sydney, Australia
Faculty of Medicine, University of New South Wales, Sydney, Australia

Michael C. Grimm
St George Clinical School, University of New South Wales, Sydney, Australia

Brian M. Necela, Jennifer M. Carr and E. Aubrey Thompson
Department of Cancer Biology, Mayo Clinic Comprehensive Cancer Center, Jacksonville, Florida, United States of America

Yan W. Asmann
Department of Biomedical Statistics and Informatics, Mayo Clinic College of Medicine, Rochester, Minnesota, United States of America

Vu Quang Van, Nobuyasu Baba, Manuel Rubio, Keiko Wakahara and Marika Sarfati
Immunoregulation Laboratory, Centre Hospitalier de l'Universitéde Montréal, Research Center (CRCHUM), Notre-Dame Hospital, Montreal, Quebec, Canada

Benoit Panzini
Department of Gastroenterology, Centre Hospitalier de l'Universitéde Montréal (CHUM), Notre-Dame Hospital, Montreal, Quebec, Canada

Carole Richard
Department of Digestive Tract Surgery, Centre Hospitalier de l'Universitéde Montréal (CHUM), Notre-Dame Hospital, Montreal, Quebec, Canada

Genevieve Soucy
Department of Pathology, Centre Hospitalier de l'Universitéde Montréal (CHUM), Notre-Dame Hospital, Montreal, Quebec, Canada

Denis Franchimont
Department de Gastroenterology, Erasme Hospital, UniversitéLibre de Bruxelles
(ULB), Bruxelles, Belgique

Genevieve Fortin
Research Institute of McGill University Health Centre, McGill University, Montreal, Quebec, Canada

Ana Carolina Martinez Torres, Lauriane Cabon and Santos Susin
INSERM U872, Mort Cellulaire Programmée et Physiopathologie des Cellules Tumorales, Equipe 19, Centre de Recherche des Cordeliers, Paris, France UniversitéPierre et Marie Curie-Sorbonne Universités, UMRS 872, Paris, France, UniversitéParis Descartes, Paris, France

Bruno Bonaz
Grenoble Institut des Neurosciences (GIN), Centre de Recherche INSERM 836 Equipe : Stress et Interactions Neuro-Digestives (EA3744), UniversitéJoseph Fourier, Grenoble, France
Clinique Universitaire d'Hépato-Gastroentérologie, Centre Hospitalo-Universitaire de Grenoble, Grenoble, France

Sonia Pellissier
Département de Psychologie, Universitéde Savoie, Chambéry, France
Grenoble Institut des Neurosciences (GIN), Centre de Recherche INSERM 836 Equipe: Stress et Interactions Neuro-Digestives (EA3744), Université Joseph Fourier, Grenoble, France

Cécile Dantzer
Laboratoire Interuniversitaire de Psychologie: Personnalité, Cognition, Changement social (LIP/PC2S), Universitéde Savoie, Chambéry, France

Laurie Mondillon and Alicia Fournier
Laboratoire de Psychologie Sociale et Cognitive (LAPSCO, CNRS UMR6024), UniversitéBlaise Pascal, Clermont-Ferrand, France

Candice Trocme, Anne-Sophie Gauchez, Bertrand Toussaint and Véronique Ducros
Institut de Biologie, Centre Hospitalo-Universitaire de Grenoble, Grenoble, France

Nicolas Mathieu
Clinique Universitaire d'Hépato-Gastroentérologie, Centre Hospitalo-Universitaire de Grenoble, Grenoble, France

Bertrand Toussaint
Laboratoire TIMC/TheREx UMR 5525, UniversitéJoseph Fourier, Grenoble, France
Institut de Biologie, Centre Hospitalo-Universitaire de Grenoble, Grenoble, France

Frédéric Canini
Unitéde Neurophysiologie du Stress, Institut de Recherche Biomédicale des Armées (IRBA), Brétigny-sur-Orge, France, Ecole du Val de Grâce, Paris, France

Arnar Flatberg
Centre of Molecular Inflammation Research, Norwegian University of Science and Technology, Trondheim, Norway

Atle van Beelen Granlund and Terje Espevik
Centre of Molecular Inflammation Research, Norwegian University of Science and Technology, Trondheim, Norway
Department of Cancer Research and Molecular Medicine, Norwegian University of Science and Technology, Trondheim, Norway

Arne K. Sandvik and Ann E. Østvik
Centre of Molecular Inflammation Research, Norwegian University of Science and Technology, Trondheim, Norway
Department of Cancer Research and Molecular Medicine, Norwegian University of Science and Technology, Trondheim, Norway
Department of Gastroenterology and Hepatology, St. Olav's University Hospital, Trondheim, Norway

Vidar Beisvag
Department of Cancer Research and Molecular Medicine, Norwegian University of Science and Technology, Trondheim, Norway

Tom Christian Martinsen, Bjørn I. Gustafsson and Helge L. Waldum
Department of Cancer Research and Molecular Medicine, Norwegian University of Science and Technology, Trondheim, Norway
Department of Gastroenterology and Hepatology, St. Olav's University Hospital, Trondheim, Norway

Kristian Damås
Department of Cancer Research and Molecular Medicine, Norwegian University of Science and Technology, Trondheim, Norway
Department of Infectious Diseases, St. Olav's University Hospital, Trondheim, Norway

Sverre H. Torp
Department of Laboratory Medicine, Norwegian University of Science and Technology, Trondheim, Norway
Department of Pathology, St. Olav's University Hospital, Trondheim, Norway

Ignat Drozdov
Bering Limited, Richmond, United Kingdom

Mark Kidd
Department of Surgery, Section of Gastroenterology, Yale School of Medicine, New Haven, Connecticut, United States of America

Zhiyong Wu
School of Traditional Chinese Medicine, Southern Medical University, Guangzhou, People's Republic of China

Yinjun Wang and Qiang Liu
Research Institute of Traditional Chinese Medicine, Guangdong Medical College, Zhanjiang, Guangdong, People's Republic of China

Weiguang Qiao
Department of Gastroenterology, Nanfang Hospital, Southern Medical University, Guangzhou, People's Republic of China

Shixue Dai
Emergency Department of Nanfang Hospital, Southern Medical University, Guangzhou, People's Republic of China

Ruxi Lv and Xuebao Zheng
School of Traditional Chinese Medicine, Southern Medical University, Guangzhou, People's Republic of China
Research Institute of Traditional Chinese Medicine, Guangdong Medical College, Zhanjiang, Guangdong, People's Republic of China

Daisy M. A. E. Jonkers, Ad A. Masclee and Marieke J. Pierik
School for Nutrition, Toxicology and Metabolism (NUTRIM), Division Gastroenterology-Hepatology, Maastricht University Medical Center+, Maastricht, The Netherlands

Paul H. Savelkoul
School for Nutrition, Toxicology and Metabolism (NUTRIM), Department of Medical Microbiology, Maastricht University Medical Center+, Maastricht, The Netherlands

John Penders
School for Public Health and Primary Care (Caphri), Department of Epidemiology, Maastricht University, Maastricht, The Netherlands
School for Nutrition, Toxicology and Metabolism (NUTRIM), Department of Medical Microbiology, Maastricht University Medical Center+, Maastricht, The Netherlands

Edgar S. Wills
School for Nutrition, Toxicology and Metabolism (NUTRIM), Division Gastroenterology-Hepatology, Maastricht University Medical Center+, Maastricht, The Netherlands
School for Nutrition, Toxicology and Metabolism (NUTRIM), Department of Medical Microbiology, Maastricht University Medical Center+, Maastricht, The Netherlands

Index

www.ingramcontent.com/pod-product-compliance
Lightning Source LLC
Chambersburg PA
CBHW070154240326

41458CB00126B/4601